Ocular Pathology

Geeta K. Vemuganti
Somasheila Murthy
Dilip K. Mishra
Editors

Ocular Pathology

Basics to Clinico-pathologic Correlation

Springer

Editors
Geeta K. Vemuganti
School of Medical Sciences
University of Hyderabad
Hyderabad, Telangana, India

Dilip K. Mishra
Ophthalmic Pathology Laboratory
L V Prasad Eye Institute
Hyderabad, Telangana, India

Somasheila Murthy, MD, DOMS, FCPS
Medical Director, Specialist in Corneal Diseases, Uveitis, Cataract and Refractive Surgery
Shantilal Shanghvi Eye Institute,
Mumbai, Maharashtra, India

ISBN 978-981-96-8613-1 ISBN 978-981-96-8614-8 (eBook)
https://doi.org/10.1007/978-981-96-8614-8

This Springer imprint is published by the registered company Springer Nature Singapore Pte Ltd.
The registered company address is: 152 Beach Road, #21-01/04 Gateway East, Singapore 189721, Singapore

We dedicate our textbook firstly to two great institutions:

LV Prasad Eye Institute, which has a mission of "providing equitable and quality eye care to all and to prevent blindness and provide visual rehabilitation", and to the University of Hyderabad, a premier university with a mission of "promoting, nurturing and achieving excellence in health sciences by offering novel teaching and research programs".

Secondly, we dedicate this book to our senior pathology technicians at the LV Prasad Pathology Laboratory: Mr Chenchu Naidu and Mr B Sreedhar Rao, who have been part of our team for over 25 years, and with their technical expertise have significantly contributed to the growth of the Ophthalmic Pathology services, thus benefitting our patients.

Our gratitude to our teachers and mentors to whom we dedicate this book: late Professor K S Ratnakar, Professor Narsing A Rao and Dr Gullapalli N Rao, for their teaching, encouragement and constant guidance to achieve higher goals.

And last but not least, we dedicate this book to each member of our families and dear friends, for their unconditional support and encouragement.

Foreword by Gullapalli N. Rao

Ophthalmic Pathology is an invaluable component of every aspect of ophthalmology—clinical care, education and research. The critical role played by this function is often poorly understood. Most education programmes lack any such support, depriving future clinicians of offering better quality of care. Trainees are also deprived of a deeper understanding of pathological processes and their effects. This will also impair their access to research, which is a whole other issue. Instead of addressing this lacuna, we are seeing the opposite: A disturbing trend globally is the closure of an ever-increasing number of ophthalmic pathology laboratories, including some hallowed institutions. As eye hospitals proliferate, especially in low- and middle-income countries, the need for a high-quality introduction to ophthalmic pathology is critical. Against such a background, this volume on "Ophthalmic Pathology" by Prof. Geeta Vemuganti will be a welcome addition to educational resources of both trainees and faculty of ophthalmology.

The book includes a diverse selection of topics, and the contributing authors meticulously fill the gaps in current literature and present a comprehensive picture. The chapter on general pathology at the very beginning is a positive feature. Inclusion of some of the aspects from current scientific knowledge is yet another valuable addition. The numerous illustrations add strength to the book and make learning easier for readers. The wide plethora of various pathologic conditions is covered in a very lucid manner. Today, there is an almost total lack of exposure to pathology in most ophthalmology departments, which makes this a valuable and necessary resource for such places.

Overall, this contribution of Drs Geeta K Vemuganti, Somasheila Murthy and Dilip K. Mishra will be a great asset to all groups in ophthalmology and pathology. I commend the authors for creating such a great resource and recommend it highly to all ophthalmology educational institutions.

Distinguished Chair of Eye Health
LV Prasad Eye Institute
Hyderabad, India

Gullapalli N. Rao

Foreword by Narsing A. Rao

In general, both anatomic pathology and ophthalmology share a common feature of being image-oriented disciplines; the former in vitro and the latter in vivo. Such imaging approaches are a part of the diagnosis and management of ocular diseases. In recent years, there have been several advances in imaging in both of these fields, such as molecular techniques and immunohistochemical methods in pathology and optical coherence tomography (OCT) and OCT angiography of the retina in ophthalmology. Moreover, the validation of such ophthalmic imaging in the diagnosis of several ophthalmic disorders is supported in part by histopathologic and clinicopathologic correlations.

The book entitled *Ocular Pathology: Basics to Clinicopathologic Correlation* focuses on covering recent advances in the clinicopathologic features of ocular diseases, with an emphasis on the case-based nature of the diseases and the inclusion of numerous superb clinical and histopathologic illustrations. These features are displayed throughout the book's chapters, covering ophthalmic disorders that are organized primarily based on an anatomic approach. The editors and chapter contributors are leaders in their respective fields of pathology and/or ophthalmology. Their vast experience in teaching, diagnostic ocular histopathology and/or research is clearly reflected in highlighting the main clinicopathologic correlations succinctly. I had the privilege of mentoring and/or interacting with the editors and several contributing authors over three decades and visiting their outstanding ophthalmic pathology laboratories at LV Prasad Eye Institute, Hyderabad and Sankara Nethralaya, Chennai. These laboratories are treasure troves of well-documented clinical cases supported by histopathologic diagnoses.

The chapters covering general principles of pathology and pathogenesis, ocular tissue processing of surgical specimens, and systematic case-based coverage of ocular diseases offer a valuable resource for teaching and practicing the subspeciality of ophthalmic pathology. The editors and contributors should be congratulated for their superbly illustrated chapters with clinicopathologic correlations. Medical students, post-graduates, residents, and fellows pursuing training in ophthalmology and pathology will find this book a valuable resource in learning evidence-based eye pathology and excelling in clinical ophthalmology through the proper diagnosis of ophthalmic disorders. The illustrations, tables, and pertinent references will aid in pursuing the subject further and in research. Surgical pathologists and ophthalmologists may find this book useful in their practice when faced with submitting surgically removed tissue and fluids for histopathologic diagnosis and processing. I am honored and privileged to review the chapters and provide a foreword. I am confident that students and surgical pathologists interested in the field of ophthalmic pathology will find this book essential in the proper diagnosis, management, and prevention of blindness from various ophthalmic diseases.

Narsing A. Rao

Grace and Emery Beardsley Professor
of Ophthalmology, Co-Director of the
USC Roski Eye Institute
Department of Ophthalmology and
Pathology Keck School of Medicine
University of Southern California
Los Angeles, CA, USA

Preface

Pathology is one of the disciplines of medicine that provides diagnostic information about the disease to clinicians and patients. This science impacts all aspects of patient care, from appropriate diagnosis to treatment and prognosis through appropriate and applicable laboratory testing. While pathology plays a vital role in all subspecialties, its role in ophthalmology is unique. Globally, the field of ophthalmic pathology is taken up as an additional specialization by ophthalmologists and pathologists. While it may appear easy to practice, it depends heavily on the knowledge, skills, training, expertise, and attitude of the pathologists, but also on the clinical information provided to the pathologist at the time of diagnosis. This is more so for the histopathologic diagnosis of the cases wherein accurate diagnosis can be made only if one is familiar with the normal tissues of the eye and their histology and is aware and updated with the abundance of pathologies that can occur in various tissues of the eye.

While one may believe that the knowledge of ocular pathology is mandatory for an ophthalmic pathologist, it is equally important for all clinicians involved in patient care related to eye and vision to be well-versed in pathological findings and diagnosis.

The proposed book covers the basic pathology of eye diseases with an emphasis on clinic-pathologic correlation. Since the understanding of pathology is an integral part of clinical medicine, the book will assist eye care professionals in integrating basic or general and clinical pathology. The book covers various diseases of the eye including infection, inflammation, and tumors of all parts of the eye with appropriate illustrations of pathology microphotographs. On the one hand, it includes the processing and handling of eye tissues, and on the other hand, it covers the use of special tests that aid in making the final diagnosis. As it has components of both subjects, the book will be of use to all eye professionals and students of optometry, ophthalmologists, as well as pathologists. It focuses more on an integrated approach to understanding disease biology. Being an upcoming specialty mostly restricted to the hospitals and institutes with tertiary eye care services, it is also rare for general pathologists to see the diverse spectrum of diseases that affect the eye. Hence, we sincerely believe that it will improve the understanding of ophthalmic pathology as a distinct yet integrated part of the related specialties, i.e., ophthalmology, optometry, as well as pathologists.

Hyderabad, Telangana, India Geeta K. Vemuganti
Hyderabad, Telangana, India Somasheila Murthy
Hyderabad, Telangana, India Dilip K. Mishra

Acknowledgments

We acknowledge the significant contribution of our pathology technicians and pathology team, our institutions for their support, the photography department, LV Prasad Eye Institute, our patients and the EyeSmart electronic medical record system for patient data, and Hyderabad Eye Research Foundation.

Contents

About the Editors and Contributors

Editors

Geeta K. Vemuganti is a renowned ocular pathologist with over 25 years of experience in eye pathology and research. A graduate of J.L.N. Medical College, Ajmer, she completed her pathology residency at Nizam's Institute of Medical Sciences. At the LV Prasad Eye Institute (LVPEI), she established a globally recognized eye pathology lab and served as Head of Ophthalmic Pathology Services. She was the founding Dean of LVPEI's School of Medical Sciences and a fellow of ARVO and the National Academy of Medical Sciences and currently serves as Professor of Eminence and senior mentor at LVPEI, Hyderabad.

She has authored 300+ peer-reviewed publications, with 8,585 citations and an H-index of 53. In her checkered career, she has secured multiple prestigious national and international grants and awards, including ARVO's prestigious Mildred Weisenfeld Award. Some of her contributions include the WHO Classification of Eye Tumors (2018) and several seminal publications.

Somasheila Murthy is a cornea and anterior segment specialist, trained at BYL Nair Hospital and Lokmanya Tilak Municipal Medical College, Mumbai. She completed two fellowships, one at LVPEI in cornea and anterior segment and a research fellowship in uveitis and ocular pathology at the Doheny Eye Institute, USC, under Prof. Narsing A. Rao.

She led the Cornea and Anterior Segment Services at LVPEI for over a decade and served on its faculty for 23 years. Now the founding Medical Director of the Shantilal Shanghvi Eye Institute, Mumbai, her expertise spans corneal disease, ocular inflammation, trauma, refractive surgery, and complex cataract procedures. She has published over 200 articles and 12 book chapters, with 4,473 citations and an H-index of 37. An invited speaker at national and international forums, she has earned awards for research and leadership and serves on the Scientific Committee of the All-India Ophthalmological Society. She has a passion for teaching and mentorship, especially women's empowerment.

Dilip K. Mishra MD in Pathology from the Rajendra Institute of Medical Sciences, is a consultant at the Ophthalmic Pathology Laboratory, LVPEI,

Hyderabad. Formerly with Manipal Medical College and several accredited labs in Hyderabad, he has received specialized training in onco-pathology and cytopathology from Apollo Hospital, University College London, and Moorfields Eye Institute.

His research centers on cancer stem cells, squamous neoplasia, infections, and corneal dystrophies, and he is currently pursuing a PhD. Dr. Mishra has authored over 100 peer-reviewed publications and a chapter in a cell and molecular biology textbook. He has presented at international conferences, including SACH and BAOP at Oxford University. A life member of multiple pathology societies, he was selected to present at the Government of India's Young Scientists Conclave and has trained pathologists in African nations. He serves as Associate Editor of *BMC Ophthalmology* and reviewer for various journals, earning both national and international accolades.

Contributors

Manisha Acharya Department of Cornea and Refractive Services, Dr. Shroff's Charity Eye Hospital, New Delhi, India

Akshay Badakere Department of Pediatric Ophthalmology, Sankara Nethralaya, Chennai, India

Manjushree Bhate Jasti V Ramanamma Children's Eye Care Center, Kallam Anji Reddy Campus, Hyderabad, Telangana, India

Triveni Bandi Government Medical College, Maheshwaram, Hyderabad, Telangana, India

Jyotirmay Biswas Uveitis and Ocular Pathology Department, Medical Research Foundation, Sankara Nethralaya, Chennai, India

Indranil Chakrabarti Department of Pathology and Laboratory Medicine, All India Institute of Medical Sciences, Kalyani, West Bengal, India

Isha Chaudhari Department of Cornea and Refractive Services, Dr. Shroff's Charity Eye Hospital, New Delhi, India

Dipankar Das Department of Ocular Pathology, Uveitis and Neuro-ophthalmology Services, Sri Sankaradeva Nethralaya, Guwahati, Assam, India

Sujata Das Shantilal Shangvi Cornea Institute, L V Prasad Eye Institute, Bhubaneswar, Odisha, India

Tarjani Vivek Dave Ophthalmic Plastic Surgery Service, Kallam Anji Reddy Campus, L V Prasad Eye Institute, Hyderabad, Telangana, India

Arpan Gandhi Chairperson Laboratory Services, Dr Shroff's Charity Eye Hospital, Secondary Centres, New Delhi, India

Neha Ghose Ophthalmic Plastic Surgery Service, Kallam Anji Reddy Campus, L V Prasad Eye Institute, Hyderabad, Telangana, India

Shilpa Goyal Sattvaguna Lab & Healthcare Private Limited, Ambala City, Haryana, India

Anirudh Heroor Academy of Eye Care Education, L V Prasad Eye Institute, Hyderabad, Telangana, India

Neha Jain Cornea Service, Shantilal Shangvi Cornea Institute, L V Prasad Eye Institute, Hyderabad, Telangana, India

Saumya Jakati Ophthalmic Pathology Laboratory, Kallam Anji Reddy Campus, L V Prasad Eye Institute, Hyderabad, Telangana, India

Swathi Kaliki Ophthalmic Plastics, Ocular Oncology, Dacryology, and Aesthetics Services, Kallam Anji Reddy Campus, L V Prasad Eye Institute, Hyderabad, Telangana, India

Operation Eyesight Universal, Kallam Anji Reddy campus, L V Prasad Eye Institute, Hyderabad, Telangana, India

Dilip K. Mishra Ophthalmic Pathology Laboratory, Kallam Anji Reddy Campus, L V Prasad Eye Institute, Hyderabad, Telangana, India

Sanchita Mitra Jhaveri Microbiology Centre, Kallam Anji Reddy Campus, L V Prasad Eye Institute, Hyderabad, Telangana, India

Kaustubh Mulay National Reporting Centre for Ophthalmic Pathology (NRCOP), Centre For Sight, Hyderabad, India

Somasheila Murthy, MD, DOMS, FCPS Medical Director, Specialist in Corneal Diseases, Uveitis, Cataract and Refractive Surgery, Shantilal Shanghvi Eye Institute, Mumbai, Maharashtra, India

Milind Naik Ophthalmic Plastic Surgery Service, LV Prasad Eye Institute, Hyderabad, India

Anamika Patel Department of Vitreo-retina and Uveitis, GMRV Campus, L V Prasad Eye Institute, Visakhapatnam, Andhra Pradesh, India

Avinash Pathengay Department of Vitreo-retina and Uveitis, GMRV Campus, L V Prasad Eye Institute, Visakhapatnam, Andhra Pradesh, India

Arkaprava Pradhan Vitreo Retina Consultant, Medical Research, Foundation, Sankara Nethralaya, Chennai, India

Muralidhar Ramappa Cornea Service, Shantilal Shangvi Cornea Institute, L V Prasad Eye Institute, Hyderabad, Telangana, India

Varsha M. Rathi Allen Foster Community Eye Health Research Centre, Gullapalli Pratibha Rao International Centre for Advancement of Rural Eye care, LV Prasad Eye Institute, Hyderabad, Telangana, India

Aravind Roy Cornea & Anterior Segment Service, L V Prasad Eye Institute, Vijayawada, Andhra Pradesh, India

Seema Sen Ocular Pathology, Dr. R.P Centre for Ophthalmic Sciences, AIIMS, New Delhi, India

Alan Treviño-Herrera Department of Vitreo-retina and Uveitis, GMRV Campus, L V Prasad Eye Institute, Visakhapatnam, Andhra Pradesh, India

Swathi Vallabh Smt. Jadhavbai Nathamal Singhvee Glaucoma Services, Sankara Nethralaya, Chennai, India

Vijitha S. Vempuluru Ophthalmic Plastics, Ocular Oncology, Dacryology, and Aesthetics Services, Kallam Anji Reddy Campus, L V Prasad Eye Institute, Hyderabad, Telangana, India

Operation Eyesight Universal, Kallam Anji Reddy campus, L V Prasad Eye Institute, Hyderabad, Telangana, India

Dr. Geeta K. Vemuganti School of Medical Sciences, University of Hyderabad, Hyderabad, India

Distinguished Pathologist and Scientist, LVPEI, School of Medical Sciences, Hyderabad, Telangana, India

Abbreviations

5 HETE	5-Hydroxyeicosatetraenoic acid
AAION	Arteritic Anterior ION
ABC	Activated B-cell
ABG	Arterial gas analysis
AC	Anterior chamber
ACC	Adenoid cystic carcinoma
ACG	Angle closure glaucoma
aCT	Activated clotting time
ACTH	Adrenocorticotropic hormone
AD	Alzheimer's disease
ADP	Adenosine diphosphate
ADVIRC	Autosomal dominant vitreoretinochoroidopathy
AF	Acid-fast/autofluorescence
AFB	Acid-fast bacillus
AFP	Alpha foetoprotein
AGE	Advanced glycation end
AGV	Ahmed glaucoma valve
AIDS	Acquire immunodeficiency syndrome
AIF	Apoptosis-inducing factor
AIS	Anemia-inducing substance
AJCC	American Joint Committee on Cancer
AMD	Age-related macular degeneration
AML	acute myeloid leukemia
ANA	Antinuclear antibody
ANCA	Antineutrophil cytoplasmic antibody
AP	Arterial pressure
APAF	Apoptotic protease activating factor
APC	Argon plasma coagulation
APP	Amyloid precursor protein
APR	Acute phase reactants
aPTT	Activated partial thromboplastin time
ARMD	Age-related macular degeneration
ARMS	Alveolar rhabdomyosarcoma
ARN	Acute retinal necrosis
ASD	Anterior segment dysgenesis
ATLL	Adult T-cell leukemia/lymphoma
ATP	Adenosine triphosphate

AV	Atrioventricular
AV	Arteriovenous
AVM	Arteriovenous malformations
BAD	Bipolar affective disorder
BAK	Benzalkonium chloride
BAX	Bcl-2-associated X protein
BCC	Basal cell carcinoma
BD	Behçet's disease
BETT	Birmingham Eye Trauma Terminology
BFGF	Basic fibroblastic growth factor
BMA	Bone marrow aspiration
BMB	Bone marrow biopsy
BP	Blood pressure
BRAF	v-raf murine sarcoma viral oncogene homolog B1
BRAO	Branch retinal artery
BRCA	Breast cancer gene
BRVO	Branch retinal vein
BSK	Band-shaped keratopathy
BUN	Blood urine nitrogen
C3F8	perfluoropropane
Ca	Calcium
CAR	Chimeric antigen receptors
CBC	Complete blood count
CC14	Carbon tetrachloride
CCDF	Central cloudy dystrophy of François
CD4+T	Clusters of differentiation 4 and T stands for helper cell
CD62L	L-selectins
CDK	Cyclin-dependent kinase
CEA	Carcinoembryonic antigen
CEME	Clinically significant macular edema
CHARGE	Coloboma, Heart defects, Atresia of the choanae (blocked nasal passages), Retardation of growth and/or development, Genital anomalies, and Ear abnormalities.
CHED	Congenital hereditary endothelial dystrophy
CHED	Congenital hereditary endothelial dystrophy
CHF	Congestive heart failure
CHRPE	Congenital hypertrophy of the retinal pigment epithelium
CHR-RPE	Combined hematoma of the retina and retinal pigment epithelium
CI	Chromosomal instability
CIMP	CpG island methylator phenotype
CK	Creatine kinase
Ck-MB	Creatine Kinase-Myocardial Band
CLL	Chronic lymphocytic leukemia
CLRA	Cilioretinal artery
CLRAO	Cilioretinal artery occlusion
CM	Confocal microscopy
CM	Capillary malformation

CME	Cystoid macular edema
CML	Chronic myeloid leukemia
CMV	Cytomegalovirus
CNS	Central nervous system
CNVM	Choroidal neovascular membranes
CONS	Coagulase-negative staphylococci
CoV	Coronavirus
CPA	Congenital primary aphakia
CPG	5′—C—phosphate—G—3′
CRAI	Cilioretinal arteriolar insufficiency
CRAO	Central retinal artery occlusion
CRION	Chronic relapsing inflammatory optic neuropathy
CRP	C-reactive protein
CRVO	Central retinal vein occlusion
CSCD	Congenital stromal corneal dystrophy
CSF	Cerebrospinal fluid
CSW	Capsular warning syndrome
CT	Computed tomography
CTC	Circulating tumor cells
CTL	Cytotoxic T lymphocytes
CTLA	Cytotoxic T lymphocyte-associated antigen
CTNNB1	Catenin Beta 1
CTX	Cerebrotendinous xanthomatosis
CVC	Chronic venous congestion
CWF	Calcofluor white
CWS	Cotton wool spots
CXL	Corneal collagen cross-linking
DAB	Text
DALK	Deep anterior lamellar keratoplasty
DBS	Dried blood spots
DDR	DNA damage response
DH	Dystrophia Helsinglandica
DIC	Disseminated intravascular coagulation
DICER	Endoribonuclease dicer
DISC	Death-inducing signalling complex
DLBCL	Diffuse large B-cell lymphoma
DLBL	Diffuse B-cell lymphoma
DLE	Discoid lupus erythematosus
DM	Descemet's membrane
DM	Diabetes mellitus
DME	Diabetic macular edema
DMEK	Descemet's membrane endothelial keratoplasty
DNA	Deoxyribonucleic acid
DR	Death receptor
DR	Diabetic retinopathy
DRs	Diabetic retinopathy study
DS	Dystrophia smolandiensis
DSAEK	Descemet's stripping automated endothelial keratoplasty

DSRCT	Desmoplastic small round cell tumors
DVT	Deep vein thrombosis
EBMD	Epithelial basement membrane dystrophy
EBV	Epstein-Barr virus
ECG	Electrocardiogram
ECM	Extracellular matrix
ED	Equatorial diameter
EDTA	Ethylenediaminetetraacetic acid
EGF	Epidermal growth factor
EGPA	Eosinophilic granulomatosis with polyangiitis
EL	Ectopia lentis
EL	Endolaser
ELISA	Enzyme-linked immunosorbent assay
EM	Electron microscopy
EMA	European Medicines Agency
EMT	Epithelial-mesenchymal transition
EMZL	Extranodal marginal zone lymphoma
ENMZL	Extranodal marginal zone lymphoma
ER	Endoplasmic reticulum
ER	Estrogen receptors
ERD	Exudative retinal detachment
ERED	Epithelial recurrent erosion dystrophies
ERMS	Embryonal rhabdomyosarcoma
ESR	Erythrocyte sedimentation rate
ETDR	Early Treatment Diabetic Retinopathy Study
EUGOGO	The European Group on Graves' Ophthalmopathy
EVP	elevated episcleral venous pressure
EVS	Endophthalmitis Vitrectomy Study
FADD	Fas-associated death domain
FAP	Familial adenomatous polyposis
FAS	Fetal alcohol syndrome
FC	Fragment crystallizable
FCD	Fleck corneal dystrophy
FDG	F-fluorodeoxyglucose
Fe	Ferrous
FECD	Fuchs endothelial corneal dystrophy
FFA	Fundus fluorescein angiography
FFPE	Formalin-fixed paraffin embedding
FGF	Fibroblast growth factor
FHI	Text
FISH	Fluorescent in situ hybridization
FL	Follicular lymphoma
FNA	Fine needle aspiration
FNAB	Fine needle aspiration biopsy
FNAC	Fine needle aspiration cytology
FOXE3	Forkhead box protein E3
FPN	ferroprotein
FRCD	Franceschetti corneal dystrophy

GA	Geographic atrophy
GAGs	Glycosaminoglycans
GAIL	Text
GALK	Galactokinase
GALT	Galactose-1-phosphate uridyl transferase
GCA	Giant cell arteritis
GCB	Germinal center B-cell
GCD 1	Granular corneal dystrophy, type 1
GDG	Congenital disorders of glycosylation
GFAP	Glial fibrillary acidic protein
GI	Gastrointestinal
GIT	Gastrointestinal tract
GLC	Gas-liquid chromatography.
GLD	Globoid cell leukodystrophy
GLUT	Glucose transporter
GMS	Gomori methenamine silver
GOLD	Gelatinous drop-like corneal dystrophy
GPA	Granulomatosis with polyangiitis
GPCR	G Protein-coupled receptors
GSD	Glycogen storage diseases
GWCD	Grayson-Wilbrandt corneal dystrophy
H	Hydrogen
H&E	Hematoxylin and eosin
H2O	Water
H2O2	Hydrogen peroxide
HAMP	Hepcidin antimicrobial peptide
HBsAg	Hepatitis B surface antigen
HBV	Hepatitis B virus
HCV	Hepatitis C virus
Hexa	Hexosaminidase
HFE	Human homeostatic iron regulator protein
HHV	Human herpesvirus
HIF	Hypoxia-inducible transcription factor
HIV	Human immunodeficiency virus
HJV	Hemojuvelin
HLA	Human leukocyte antigens
HLAB	Human leukocyte antigen B HMB Human Melanoma Black
HNPCC	Hereditary nonpolyposis colon cancer
HOCL	Hypochlorous acid
HPA	Hypothalamic-pituitary-adrenal axis
HPV	Human papillomavirus
HRC	High risk criteria
HRVO	Hemiretinal vein occlusion
HSIL	High-grade squamous intraepithelial lesion
HSP	Heat shock proteins
HSV	Herpes simplex virus
HTLV	Human T-lymphotropic virus
HTN	Hypertension

HZO	Herpes zoster ophthalmicus
IAP	Inhibitors of apoptosis proteins
ICAM	Intercellular adhesion molecule
ICE	Iridocorneal endothelial
IFN	Intravenous Infusion
IFN	Interferon
IgA	Immunoglobin A
IgE	Immunoglobulin E
IGF	Insulin-like growth factor
IgG	Immunoglobulin G
IHC	Immunohistochemistry
IMD	Inherited metabolic disorders
IMG	Intussusceptive microvascular growth
INR	International Normalized Ratio
IOFB	Intraocular foreign body
IOID	Idiopathic orbital inflammatory disease
IOL	Intraocular lens-related anterior uveitis
ION	Ischemic optic neuropathy
IOP	Intraocular pressure
IPE	Iris pigment epithelial
IRMA	intraretinal microvascular abnormalities
ISSVA	International Society for the Study of Vascular Anomalies
ITP	Immune thrombocytopenic purpura
ITVA	Intravitreal triamcinolone acetonide
IV	Intravenous
JAK	Janus kinase
JIA	Juvenile idiopathic arthritis
JXG	Juvenile xanthogranuloma
K	Potassium
KCS	Keratoconjunctivitis sicca
KF	Kayser-Fleischer
KOH	Potassium hydroxide
KRAS	Kirsten rat sarcoma viral oncogene homolog
LASIK	Laser-assisted in situ keratomileusis
LCAM	Leucocyte adhesion molecules
LCD 1	Lattice corneal dystrophy, type 1
LCED	Lisch epithelial corneal dystrophy
LDH	Lactate dehydrogenase
LECD	Lisch epithelial corneal dystrophy
LEL	Lymphoepithelial lesions
LFA	Lymphocyte function-associated antigen
LH	Lymphoid hyperplasia
LM	Lymphatic Malformation
LMP	Latent membrane protein
LPS	Levator palpebrae superioris muscle
LSD	Lysergic acid diethylamide
LT	Leukotriene
MABS	Monoclonal antibodies

MAC	Mycobacterium avium complex
MALT	Mucosa-associated lymphoid tissue
MBL	Mannose-binding lectin
MBP	Major basic protein
MCD	Macular corneal dystrophy
MCHC	Mean corpuscular hemoglobin concentration
MCL	Medial collateral ligament
MCV	Mean corpuscular volume
MECD	Meesmann corneal dystrophy
MEWDS	Multiple evanescent white dot syndrome
MGDA	Morning Glory disc anomaly
MGG	Molecular Genetics and Genomics
MHC	Major histocompatibility complex
MHC	Text
MI	Myocardial infarction
MiNEN	Mixed neuroendocrine non-neuroendocrine neoplasms
MMMT	Malignant mixed Mullerian tumors
MMP	Matrix metalloproteinases
MMR	Mismatch repair
MNG	Multinucleate giant cells
MOG	Myelin oligodendrocyte glycoprotein
MOG IgG	Myelin oligodendrocyte glycoprotein antibody
MOMP	Mitochondrial outer membrane permeabilization
MPA	Microscopic polyangiitis
MPNST	Malignant peripheral nerve sheath tumor
MPO	Myeloperoxidase
MPS	Mucopolysaccharidoses
MRD	Minimum residual disease
MRI	Magnetic resonance imaging
MRNF	Myelinated retinal nerve fiber layers
MS	Multiple sclerosis
MSA	Multiple system atrophy
MSI	microsatellite instability
MSVI	Moderate to severe visual impairment
MYC	Text
MYCN	v-myc avian myelocytomatosis viral oncogene neuroblastoma derived homolog
Na	Sodium
NAAION	Text
NADP	Nicotinamide adenine dinucleotide phosphate
NADPH	Nicotinamide adenine dinucleotide phosphate
NBS	New born screening
NDC	Nieman Pick disease type C
NDPR	Non-proliferative diabetic retinopathy
NEMOS	Neuromyelitis Optica Study group
NER	Nucleotide excision repair
NF	Neurofibromatosis
NF1	Neurofibromatosis type 1

NFkB	Nuclear factor kappa B
NGS	Next-generation sequencing
NHL	Non-Hodgkin's lymphoma
NICH	Noninvoluting congenital hemangioma
Nk	Natural killer
NMO	Neuromyelitis optica
NMOSD	Neuromyelitis optica spectrum disorders
NO	Nitric oxide
NOS	Not otherwise specified
NSAID	Non-steroidal anti-inflammatory drugs
NSE	Neuron-specific enolase
NSK	Necrotizing stromal keratitis
NSOID	Nonspecific inflammatory orbital disease
NTM	Non-tuberculous mycobacterial
NVA	Neovascularization of the angle
NVD	Neovascularization of the disc
NVE	Neovascularization elsewhere
NVG	Neovascular Glaucoma
NVI	Neovascularization of the iris
NVI	Neurological visual impairment
O2	Oxygen
OA	Ocular albinism
OAG	Open-angle glaucoma
OALD	Ocular adnexal lymphoproliferative disease
OALs	Ocular adnexal lymphomas
OCA	Oculocutaneous albinism
OCT	Optimal cutting temperature
OCT	Optical coherence tomography
OD	Oculus dexter
ODFR	Oxygen-derived free radicals
OH-	Hydroxyl radical
OIF	Oil-immersion field
OMIM	Online Mendelian Inheritance in man
ONH	Optic nerve head
ONOO	Peroxynitrous acid
ONTT	Optic Neuritis Treatment Trial
OTB	Ocular tuberculosis
OTS	Ocular Trauma Score
P450	Cytochrome P450
PACD	Posterior amorphous corneal dystrophy
PAF	Platelet-activating factor
PAH	Pulmonary arterial hypertension
PAP	Positive airway pressure
PAS	Periodic Acid-Schiff
PAX6	Paired box 6
PBS	Peripheral blood smear
PCG	Primary congenital glaucoma
PCNSL	Primary central nervous system lymphomas

PCR	Polymerase chain reaction
PCV	Pack cell volume
PDCD	Pre-Descemet corneal dystrophy
PDGF	Platelet-derived growth factor
PDR	Proliferative diabetic retinopathy
PDS	Pigment dispersion syndrome
PE	Pulmonary embolism
PECAM	Platelet endothelial cell adhesion molecule
PET	Positron emission tomography
PEX	Pseudoexfoliation syndrome
PG	Pigmentary glaucoma
PH	Potential of hydrogen
PHMB	Polyhexamethylene biguanide
PHPV	Persistent hyperplastic primary vitreous
PI	Perfusion index
PI	Peripheral iridotomy
PICH	Partially involuting congenital hemangioma
PIRW	Patchy ischemic retinal whitening
PKP	Penetrating keratoplasty
PKU	Phenylketonuria
PLEX	Plasma exchange
PMD	Pellucid marginal degeneration
PNET	Primitive neuroectodermal tumor
PNS	Paraneoplastic syndromes
P-O	Pupil optic nerve
POAG	Primary open angle glaucoma
PPCD	Posterior polymorphous corneal dystrophy
PPL	Pars plana lensectomy
PPV	Pars plana vitrectomy
PRP	pan retinal photocoagulation
PSS	Primary Sjögren syndrome
PT	Prothrombin time
PTAH	Phosphotungstic acid hematoxylin
PTI	Protein thiolation index
PUFA	Polyunsaturated fatty acids
PUK	Peripheral ulcerative keratitis
PUMA	p53-upregulated modulator of apoptosis
PUMA	Polyurethane methyl acrylate
PVD	Posterior vitreous detachment
PVR	Proliferative vitreoretinopathy
PVRL	Pulmonary vascular resistance
PXG	Pseudoexfoliation glaucoma
PXS	Pseudoxfoliation syndrome
RA	Rheumatoid arthritis
RAPD	Relative afferent pupillary defect
RAS	Reticular activating system
RB	Retinoblastoma
RBC	Red blood cell

RBCD	Reis–Bücklers corneal dystrophy
RBS	Random blood sugar
RDD	Rosai–Dorfman disease
rER	Rough endoplasmic reticulum
RetNet	The Retinal Information Network online
RICH	Rapidly involuting congenital hemangioma
RIP	Receptor-interacting protein
RLH	Reactive lymphoid hyperplasia
RMS	Rhabdomyosarcoma
RNA	Ribonucleic acid
RNFL	Retinal nerve fiber layer
ROS	Reactive Oxygen Species
RPAD	Relative afferent pupillary defect
RPE	Retinal pigment epithelium
RRD	Rhegmatogenous retinal detachments
RT-PCR	Real-time polymerase chain reaction
SARS	Severe Acute Respiratory Syndrome
SB	Scleral buckle
SC	Schlemm canal
SC	Sebaceous carcinoma
SCC	Squamous cell carcinoma
SCD	Schnyder's corneal dystrophy
SCG	Sebaceous gland carcinoma
SF6	Sulfur hexafluoride
SFT	Solitary fibrous tumor
SGOT	Serum glutamic oxaloacetic transaminase
SIADH	Syndrome of inappropriate antidiuretic hormone secretion
SIDS	Surgically induced diffuse scleritis
SINS	Surgically induced necrotizing scleritis
SLC	Secondary lymphoid-tissue chemokine
SLE	Systemic lupus erythematosus
SMA	Spinal muscular atrophy
SMAC	Second mitochondrial activator of caspases
SMAD	Suppressor of Mothers against Decapentaplegic
SMCD	Subepithelial mucinous corneal dystrophy
SO	Sympathetic ophthalmia
SOD	Superoxide dismutase
SOD	Septo-optic dysplasia
SOL	Space-occupying lesions
SPP	Skin perfusion pressure
SRCT	Small round cell tumors
STAT protein	cytokine-induced signal transducer and activator of transcription
SUN	Standard Uveitis Nomenclature
TBCD	Thiel-Behnke corneal dystrophy
TBPCR	polymerase chain reaction for *Mycobacterium tuberculosis*.
TED	Thyroid eye disease
TERT	Telomerase reverse transcriptase

TF	Tissue factor
TFR	Transferrin receptor
TGF-α	Transforming growth factor-α
TGF-β	Transforming growth factor-β
TIGR	Trabecular Meshwork I-inducible glucocorticoid response
TIL	Tumor-infiltrating lymphocytes
TIMP	Tissue inhibitors of metalloproteinases
TLR	Toll-like receptors
TM	Trabecular meshwork
TMD	Terrien's marginal degeneration
TME	Tumor microenvironment
TNF	Tumor necrosis factor
TNFR	Tumor Necrosis Factor Receptor
TNM	T—Tumor, N—lymph node involvement, M—metastasis
TON	Traumatic optic neuropathy
T-PA	Tissue plasminogen activator
TRADD	TNF receptor–associated death domain
TRAILR	Text
TRD	Tractional retinal detachments
TS	Tuberous sclerosis
TT	Thrombin time
UBM	Ultrasound biomicroscopy
UV	Ultraviolet
VCAM	Vascular cell adhesion molecule
VEGF	Vascular endothelial growth factor
VHL	Von Hippel-Lindau Syndrome
VIP	Vasoactive intestinal polypeptide
VKC	Vernal keratoconjunctivitis
VKH	Vogt Koyanagi Harada
VLA 4	Integrin very late antigen-4
VLM	Veno-lymphatic malformations
VM	Vascular mimicry
VM	Venous malformation
VTE	Venous thromboembolism
vWD	Von Willebrand disease
VWF	Von Willebrand factor
VZV	Varicella Zoster virus
WBC	White blood cell
WES	Whole exome sequencing
WGS	Whole-genome sequencing
WHO	World Health Organization
XECD	X-linked endothelial corneal dystrophy
YAG	Yttrium aluminum garnet
α-SMA	Alpha-smooth muscle actin

Part I

General Pathology

Introduction to Ocular Pathology

1

Geeta K. Vemuganti

Contents

1.1 Introduction

As Franklin defined research as a "Systematic investigation" to lead to "communicable knowledge," similarly, pathology investigates the etiology of disease and the mechanisms involved that result in clinical signs and symptoms. While the study of pathology started with a detailed study of the gross appearance of the organ and bodies, the armamentarium of tools is increasing with each passing day. From the time of morphology, routine staining with hematoxylin (violet) and eosin (lilac) of nuclear and cytoplasmic staining, respectively [1–3], we have come a long way adapting to the application of molecular, genetic, immunologic techniques, automated processing at all levels, digital pathology, and Artificial intelligence into routine clinical practice [4–7].

G. K. Vemuganti (✉)
School of Medical Sciences, University of Hyderabad, Gachibowli, Hyderabad, India
e-mail: gkvemuganti@gmail.com

1.2 Sections of the Book

Traditionally, the histopathology section is divided into general pathology and systemic pathology; the first elucidates the pathobiology of all the disease processes that occur in the body at the cellular, tissue, and organ levels, followed by the same in each system of the body.

General Pathology The topics covered under this section include Cellular injury, adaptation and wound healing, Hemostasis, Inflammation, Infections, Neoplasia, Metabolic Diseases, Congenital, and Inherited diseases. In addition, an effort has been made to introduce the readers to the principles and interpretation of some of the routine investigations so that the integration of knowledge from all of these, that is, the pathobiology of the disease, the evaluation of the same through common investigations with the clinical presentation, contributes significantly to a better understanding of the cases and also paves way for evidence-based practice. Arriving at a diagnosis is based on tissue or cytologic diagnosis

G. K. Vemuganti et al. (eds.), *Ocular Pathology*, https://doi.org/10.1007/978-981-96-8614-8_1

(histopathology/cytology) as well as clinical pathology, which deals with the tests done on biological fluid samples like blood, serum, urine, cerebrospinal fluid, etc. While it is not in the scope of the book to cover all investigations, a brief description of some of the routine tests is provided in the chapter on clinical pathology [8].

Ophthalmic Pathology While the second part of Ocular Pathology attempts to build the pathology of each layer of the eye elaborating on the epidemiology, pathogenesis, classifications, morphologic description, and genetic testing as applicable, followed by clinical presentation, differential diagnosis, principles of management, prognosis, and clinical outcome.

Ocular pathology deals with the pathology of different layers of the eye, namely, the anterior segment (cornea, conjunctiva, sclera, lens), middle layer vascular layer of the eye (uvea), neuroretina, optic nerve, and vitreous. It also covers the diseases of the eyelid, orbit, and lacrimal gland. While the general pathology is a reference guide to the pathobiology of the disease, the specific findings of each layer of the ocular tissue are unique and are the basis of clinical findings observed during the examination of the eye, that is, more evidence-based approach. Therefore, knowledge of pathology not only helps in diagnosing the clinical condition, but also aids in assessing the prognosis, and treatment outcomes, and exploring newer treatment modalities.

The second section starts with a chapter on the handling and grossing of ocular tissues for histopathologic examination [1, 9, 10]. The tissues removed during any surgical procedure are a storehouse of information. It is therefore important for the ophthalmologist to communicate with the pathologists before, during, and after surgical procedures so that a good clinicopathological correlation is established and the pathologist can provide the most accurate interpretation of the tissue submitted. This chapter gives a simple description of the routine and special techniques adopted by most ophthalmic pathology laboratories. It covers routine procedures like techniques of fixation, gross examination and cutting, tissue processing, embedding, cutting, and staining of the tissues received from the eye for diagnostic or therapeutic purposes, for example, cornea, conjunctiva, lid, orbit, and intraocular structures. It also describes the handling of specimens obtained from special procedures like vitreous biopsy, scrape cytology, fine need aspiration cytology, impression cytology, etc. Urgent processing of tissues for rapid intraoperative diagnosis of the lesion using frozen sections and imprint and squash cytology is also described [11, 12]. Most importantly, it is the responsibility of the pathologist to ensure that all the information on the disease including the known prognostic features seen in the specimen is well captured in the report by following the appropriate checklist. This is more important in ocular tumors [13]. This chapter aims to reiterate that the primary responsibility is with the referring ophthalmologist to ensure the appropriate handling and transport of tissues along with adequate clinical data.

Another salient feature of this book is that in each chapter, the focus is the clinic-pathologic correlation with case illustrations. Some important take-home messages are highlighted as practical tips for arriving at a correct diagnosis. This innovative approach meets the criteria of applying the knowledge of pathology to clinical practice.

It is interesting to note that there is some evidence that much of pathology is still based on empiricism, which is defined as a method that is predicated on observation and experience [14]. In pathology, it surely is the most efficient way of solving clinical problems. Anatomic pathologists can recognize and diagnose tumors based on the combined knowledge of gross examination, microscopy, and molecular methods. So, if this is combined with adequate training, training, knowledge, and judgment, then it becomes an important tool to overcome the limitations of so-called empiricism in pathology.

1.3 Benefits of This Book

The anticipated outcome of this book is it would help the reader to integrate the knowledge of pathology into clinical practice and will facilitate evidence-based evaluation, diagnosis, and treatment. It will also be a valuable tool to develop and evaluate novel treatment modalities, thus contributing to management strategies. It meets the curricula for bachelor's and master's degrees and for continuous medical education of practicing professionals. Integrating basic and clinical pathology also promotes the behavior and attitude of the scholars to integrate knowledge rather than segregate each subject into structured courses of anatomy, physiology, pathology, and pharmacology.

The vision and mission of health-care professionals in the field of vision and ophthalmology is the application of knowledge and be able to diagnose and treat ocular diseases. Another program learning objective is to prepare for research in the field of ophthalmology, optometry, and vision sciences. Hence, the objective of this book is to shift the focus from the traditional teaching to learner-centric approach. An interesting study by Ahmed et al. [15] showed that there is a similarity in the learning styles of fellows and faculty, revealing predominantly observational learning styles, which is logical as pathology is a visual field. In contrast, residents showed the dominance of "learn by doing" styles ("converging" and "accommodating"). So, we hope the in-depth knowledge acquired from this book would help the reader to examine the patient, apply the knowledge acquired in evaluating the patient for ocular and systemic conditions, derive an appropriate diagnosis, and treat or refer appropriately to the concerned expert. With the understanding of the disease process in the context of clinical application, it also paves the way for new ideas and research in basic and clinical research.

References

1. Rosai J. Gross techniques in surgical pathology. In: Ackerman's surgical pathology. 7th ed. St. Loius: CV Mosby Co; 1989. p. 13–29.
2. Gravanis MB, Rietz CW. The problem-oriented postmortem examination and record: an educational challenge. Am J Clin Pathol. 1973;60:522–35.
3. Vemuganti GK, Murthy SI, Mishra DK. Role of histopathology in the diagnosis of corneal and conjunctival infections. In: Das S, Jhanji V, editors. Infections of the cornea and conjunctiva. Singapore: Springer; 2020.
4. Mullis K, Faloona F, Scharf S, Saiki R, Hom G, Erlich H. Specific enzymatic amplification of DNA *in vitro*: the polymerase chain reaction. Cold Spring Harb Symo Quant Biol. 1986;51:263–73.
5. Krauthammer M, Kong Y, Ha BH, et al. Exome sequencing identifies recurrent somatic RAC1 mutations in melanoma. Nat Genet. 2012;44(9):1006–14.
6. Onken MD, Worley LA, Ehlers JP, Harbour JW. Gene expression profiling in uveal melanoma reveals two molecular classes and predicts metastatic death. Cancer Res. 2004;64(20):7205–9.
7. Cui M, Zhang DY. Artificial intelligence and computational pathology. Lab Investig. 2021;101:412–22.
8. Lilleyman JS. De Gruchy's clinical haematology in medical practice. J Clin Pathol. 1990;43(4):352.
9. Eagle RC Jr. Specimen handling in the ophthalmic pathology laboratory. Ophthalmol Clin North Am. 1995;8:1–15.
10. Vemuganti GK. Ocular pathology for clinicians. In: Choudhary Z, Vanathi M, editors. Post graduation ophthalmology, vol. 1. New Delhi: Pubs Jaypee brothers; 2020. p. 206–2016.
11. Vemuganti GK, Naik MN, Honavar SG, Sekhar GC. Rapid intraoperative diagnosis of tumors of the eye and orbit by squash and imprint cytology. Ophthalmology. 2004;111(5):1009–15.
12. Font RL, Lauciricia R, Ramzy I. Cytological evaluation of tumours of the orbit and ocular adnexa: an analysis of 84 cases studied by the "squash technique". Diagn Cytopathol. 1994;10:135–42.
13. Folberg R, Salomao D, Grossniklaus HE, Proia AD, Rao NA, Cameron JD. Recommendations for the reporting of tissues removed as part of the surgical treatment of common malignancies of the eye and its adnexa. Mod Pathol. 2003;16:725–30.
14. Wick MR, Marchevsky AM. Evidence-based principles in pathology: existing problem areas and the development of "quality" practice patterns. Arch Pathol Lab Med. 2011;135:1398–404.
15. Ahmed A, Wojcik EM, Ananthanarayanan V, Mulder L, Mirza KM. Learning styles in pathology: a comparative analysis and implications for learner-centered education. Acad Pathol. 2019;6:237428951985231.

Cell Injury: Causes, Mechanisms and Response to Injury

2

Kaustubh Mulay, Shilpa Goyal,
and Geeta K. Vemuganti

Contents

K. Mulay
National Reporting Centre for Ophthalmic Pathology (NRCOP), Centre For Sight, Hyderabad, India
e-mail: kaustubh.m@hotmal.com

S. Goyal
Sattvaguna Lab & Healthcare Private Limited, Ambala City, Haryana, India

G. K. Vemuganti (✉)
School of Medical Sciences, University of Hyderabad, Hyderabad, Telangana, India
e-mail: gkvemuganti@gmail.com

G. K. Vemuganti et al. (eds.), *Ocular Pathology*, https://doi.org/10.1007/978-981-96-8614-8_2

2.1 Introduction

To study the pathology of the body, it is important to understand the process at a cellular level; hence, this chapter explains in detail the magnitude of changes that the cell undergoes in health and disease. Cell injury spectrum therefore extends from a physiological process of ageing to the effect of stresses due to etiologic agents a cell encounters resulting in changes in its internal and external environment [1, 2]. The cell thus exposed to various injuries undergoes biochemical changes, structural changes, morphological tissue changes, and functional changes, thus resulting in the disease process [1, 3, 4]. The chapter deals with the following aspects of cell injury

1. Causes of cellular injury
2. Sequence of cellular injury
    2.1. Reversible
    2.2. Irreversible cell death
3. Reperfusion injury
4. Gangrene
5. Calcification
6. Intracellular accumulations
7. Cellular adaptation
8. Cellular ageing

2.2 Causes of Cell Injury

Cell injury may be caused due to *Genetic* or *Acquired* causes.

Acquired causes can be subcategorized as follows [1, 3, 5, 6]:

2.2.1 Hypoxia and Ischemia

Hypoxia or Ischemia (reduction in supply of oxygen) is one of the most common and clinically important causes of cellular injury. Hypoxia results from inadequate oxygenation of blood (cardiopulmonary dysfunction), inadequate oxygen transport to the tissues (e.g.,: anemia or carbon monoxide poisoning), or inhibition of respiratory enzymes (e.g., cyanide toxicosis). Ischemia also hampers with the elimination of wastes, thus perpetuating the damage.

2.2.2 Physical Agents

These include radiation, mechanical trauma, electric shock, changes in atmospheric pressure, and extremes of temperature like heat and cold.

2.2.3 Toxins, Drugs and Chemicals

These include chemical poisons (e.g., arsenic, cyanide etc.), environmental pollutants, insecticides and pesticides, high oxygen, high levels of glucose, electrolyte imbalance, substances of abuse (e.g., alcohol), and therapeutic drugs when used above therapeutic indications and dosage.

2.2.4 Microbial (Infectious) Agents

Microbe-induced cell injury may be triggered by microorganisms like bacteria, rickettsiae, viruses, fungi, and parasites. Unlike other causes of injury, these organisms can multiply within the body, hence perpetuate the diseases unless treated.

2.2.5 Immunologic Agents

Immune system, though protective in nature, may induce cell injury due to inadequate function, that is, immunodeficiency or overactivity to foreign antigens (hypersensitivity) or self-antigens (autoimmunity), both of which can cause cell injury.

2.2.6 Nutritional Imbalance

Nutritional deficiency includes overall nutrition deficiency as seen in starvation or deficiency of a specific nutrient like protein calorie (e.g., marasmus, kwashiorkor), minerals (e.g., goiter, anemia), trace elements (e.g., zinc, selenium, copper, etc. deficiencies). Another emerging burden is that of nutritional excess, which results in obesity and thus many associated diseases like atherosclerosis, heart disease, and hypertension. Obesity is one of the most common risk factors for the noncommunicable diseases.

2.2.7 Ageing

Each cell is believed to be having a biologic clock, and thus, the accumulated changes to the cellular constituents or organelles result in cellular senescence with replicative senescence, inability of cells to respond to stress and eventual cell death.

2.2.8 Psychogenic Diseases

Substance abuses like drug addiction, alcoholism, and smoking contribute to various kinds of diseases such as cirrhosis, chronic bronchitis, cancer, hypertension, ischemic heart disease, peptic ulcers, etc.

2.2.9 Iatrogenic Factors

Iatrogenic (treatment-associated) cell injury could be due to ingestion of drugs, due to medical or surgical interventions, radiation exposure, and other nonmedical events in medical environment.

2.2.10 Idiopathic Diseases

The diseases are labelled as Idiopathic when the exact cause of injury cannot be truly determined based on the existing tools of evaluation.

The Genetic causes of Death include congenital conditions like Down syndrome or genetic mutations like sickle cell anemia or metabolic diseases that are dealt in another chapter.

2.3 Sequence of Cell Injury

The factors that influence the outcome of cell injury include nature of cell injury; type, duration, and severity of injurious agent; type, and adaptability of the affected cells [1, 5]. While skeletal muscle withstands hypoxic injury for long-time, cardiac muscle suffers irreversible cell injury when ischemia persists for over 20 min [7].

2.4 Pathogenesis of Hypoxic Injury

2.4.1 Reversible Cell Injury

The changes of hypoxia are related to the duration and the rapidity of onset as well as restoration of circulation.

The sequence of the biochemical changes includes (a) decreased generation of cellular ATP; (b) intracellular lactic acidosis resulting in nuclear clumping; (c) damage to plasma pumps resulting in hydropic swelling; (d) reduced protein synthesis and dispersed ribosomes [1, 5, 7–9]. The cellular changes thus culminate in the tissue changes, which if massive are grossly visible to the naked eye or identified in the histologic sections of the tissues. Based on the morphology of the tissues, the reversible cell injury is classified as

(i) Hydropic change
(ii) Hyaline change
(iii) Mucoid change
(iv) Fatty change

2.4.1.1 Hydropic Change

Hydropic change results in the accumulation of water within the cytoplasm of the cell leading to cloudy swelling, or vacuolar degeneration [1, 3]. This causes swelling and enlargement of tissues, which with increased turgor appear to bulge when cut. Histologically, they appear as enlarged cells with pale eosinophilic or vacuolated cytoplasm [5, 10]. Ultrastructurally, chromatin is clumped, the cytosol is electron-lucent, ribosomes detach from RER, and the ER becomes vesiculated. Myelin figures result from coiling of damaged membranes. Cytoskeletal damage causes the plasma membrane to lose microvilli or other specialized structures and to undergo blebbing.

2.4.1.2 Hyaline Change

Hyaline change appears as glassy, homogeneous, eosinophilic appearance of proteinaceous material in routine sections (Fig. 2.1) and may be seen both within or outside the cell [5]. While intracellular hyaline is mainly seen in epithelial cells, its extracellular counterpart is seen in connective tissues. Some examples include.

Intracellular hyaline

1. Nuclear inclusions seen in some viral infections, for example, Molluscum contagiosum (Fig. 2.2) [11].
2. Russell's bodies (excessive immunoglobulins) in the RER of the plasma cells [12].

Extracellular hyaline

Hyalinized fibrocollagenous tissues in sclerosing idiopathic orbital inflammation [13].

2.4.1.3 Mucoid Change

The mucoid or myxoid change could be seen in both epithelial tissues and connective tissue and are best demonstrated by the use of mucin stains like periodic acid-Schiff (PAS) for epithelial mucins (respiratory and GIT tract), and colloidal

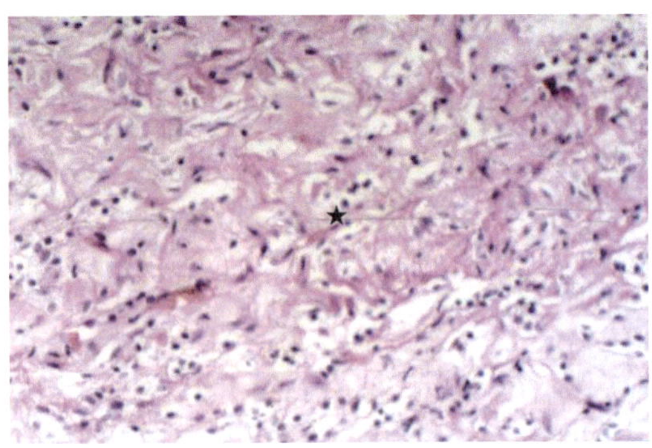

Fig. 2.1 Hyaline degeneration in a glioma. Eosinophilic, glassy, homogenous hyaline material seen in Rosenthal fibers of glioma (asterix)

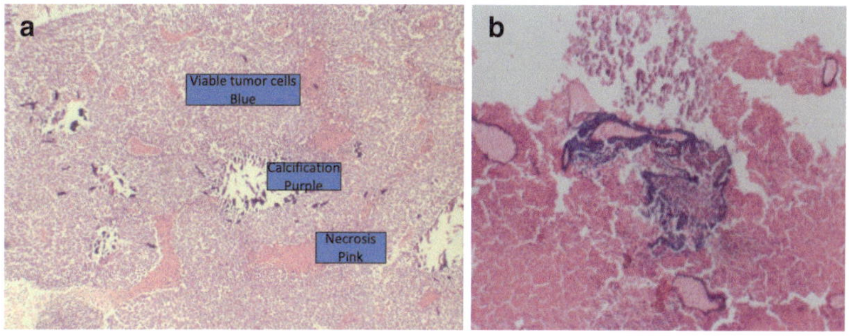

Fig. 2.2 Coagulative necrosis in a tumor. A shows viable blue tumor cells with pink necrotic areas, and purple areas of calcification. Large pink areas of necrotic tumor cells with no nuclear details. A few blood vessels show basophilic appearance due to diffusion of chromatin from the ghost cells (Azzopardi effect)

iron for connective tissue mucins (tumors) [5, 12, 14–19].

2.4.1.4 Fatty Change

Fatty change refers to abnormal accumulation of fats in the cytoplasm of the parenchymal cells, liver being the most commonly affected organ, along with muscles, heart, and kidneys [1]. This may occur because of increased lipid levels due to excessive alcohol intake, diabetes mellitus, impaired lipid metabolism, obesity, etc. Grossly, the affected organ is enlarged and smooth with greasy appearance [3]. Microscopically, the cytoplasm shows fat globule, which appears as a pale vesicle on routine histopathology staining. If large, the fat vesicle may push the nucleus to cell periphery and is called macrovesicular steatosis, and if the fat accumulation is seen only as small globules in cell, then it is called microvesicular steatosis. Oil red O stain may be applied on fresh frozen tissue section to see the fat globules, which stain red highlighting the fat.

2.4.2 Irreversible Cell Injury

Irreversibility is caused by perpetuating injury and is characterized by a) inability to restore mitochondrial function, b) structural and functional loss of plasma membrane and membrane of the cellular organelles, or c) loss of DNA, cytoskeletal damage, and chromatin structural integrity [48]. The nuclear damage results in pyknosis of the nucleus (condensation), karyorrhexis, or karyolysis: The damage to lysosomes results in the release of the enzymes and cell death. The enzymes released into the blood are the basis of blood/serum investigations to assess cell injury: for example, serum glutamic oxaloacetic transaminase, SGOT and creatine kinase isoenzyme, CK-MB in myocardial infarction, amylase in pancreatitis etc.

2.4.3 Morphology of Irreversible Cell Injury

2.4.3.1 Cell Death

Cell death could be of two morphologic forms: necrosis or apoptosis [4–6]. Necrosis derived from Greek word *necros*, that is, death is caused by swelling of the cell (*oncosis*) followed by the rupture of cell membranes. Based on the pattern of necrosis, it could be present as a zonal phenomenon [10]. Widespread necrotic cell death results in local or systemic inflammatory response due to the release of cell contents into the extracellular space (Fig. 2.3).

Apoptosis, on the other hand, occurs when injury is less severe or physiological [4, 6]. It is an orchestrated cell death resulting from cellular signaling cascades and typically affects individual cells. It results in sequential changes of the nuclear chromatin as well as cytoplasmic blebs with eventual fragmentation of the cell. Importantly, apoptotic cell fragments remain membrane bound; hence, they do not evoke any

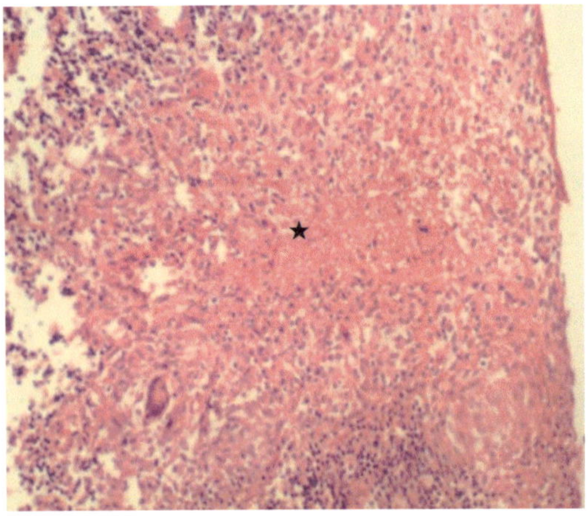

Fig. 2.3 Caseous necrosis. Large areas of acellular cheesy pink necrotic material (asterix) flanked by a Langhans' type giant cell and a granuloma (bottom), suggestive of tuberculosis

inflammatory response in the tissues. Existence of both forms of cell death is referred to as *necroptosis* (Table 2.1) [20].

Table 2.1 Differentiating features of necrosis and apoptosis [1, 9, 22–27]

Features	Necrosis	Apoptosis
Definition	Passive accidental cell death due to ravaging external causes	Active programmed autonomous cellular breakdown
Area of involvement	Large field of cells affected	Individual or a group of cells involved
Key mechanism	Cell membrane damage	DNA breakage due to endonuclease activation
Physiology	Complete dismantling of cytoskeleton structure with enzymatic digestion of cellular components	Controlled removal of cellular components by apoptotic bodies without their destruction
Morphology	Cell swelling, nuclear pyknosis, loss of cellular details with presence of inflammation	Shrinkage of cells with formation of cytoplasmic blebs (apoptotic bodies), nuclear condensation. No inflammation seen
Terminal phase	Disposal and digestion of cell corpses by phagocytic cells	Apoptotic bodies taken up by phagocytic cells and degraded within lysosomes
Pathologic role	Inflammation, ischemia	Normal physiologic process. Dysregulation can lead to cancers

2.4.3.2 Autolysis

Autolysis (self-digestion) refers to the disintegration of the cell by its own hydrolytic enzymes liberated from lysosomes [5]. It is generally seen as postmortem change and lacks the inflammatory response, which is the hallmark of a living tissue. Autolyzed cells show loss of nuclear and cellular details with remains of cell ghosts or cell debris.

Morphology of Necrosis

Macroscopically, the necrotic tissue may appear swollen and pale, followed by loss of structural detail and demarcation from adjacent viable tissue [1, 3, 5]. Zonal necrosis can be indistinguishable in its early stages from reversible degeneration. In contrast, unifocal or multifocal necrosis or segmental zonal necrosis is more easily recognized macroscopically given its difference from adjacent viable tissue.

Microscopically, the cells appear eosinophilic due to denatured cytoplasmic proteins [4, 5, 28]. Loss of lighter-staining glycogen imparts a glassy, homogenous appearance to the cytoplasm. Relative to normal cells, necrotic ones contain more myelin figures. The cells show a vacuolated or moth-eaten appearance due to digestion of cellular organelles. Ultrastructurally, necrotic cells have increased myelin figures, breaks in the plasma/organelle membrane, mitochondrial dilatation with increased density and disruption of lysosomes. Nuclear changes include *pyknosis* (nuclear shrinkage and increase basophilia resulting from condensation of DNA), *karyorrhexis* (nuclear fragmentation), and eventually *karyolysis* occurs with fading of basophilia due to action of DNases resulting in digestion of nuclear DNA. Necrotic may, at times, lack nuclei completely.

2.4.4 Types of Tissue Necrosis

2.4.4.1 Coagulative Necrosis

It is the most common type of necrosis caused by irreversible focal injury and refers to the denaturation of cytoplasmic proteins, which imparts an opaque and intense cytoplasmic eosinophilia. It follows infarction in all solid organs except brain, which shows liquefactive necrosis. In early stages, focus of coagulative necrosis in the is pale, firm, and slightly swollen and is called infarct (Fig. 2.4). With progression, the affected area becomes more yellowish, softer, and shrunken. The tissue architecture is preserved until a few days after cell death. Proteolysis is delayed or absent due to the denaturation of the structural protein and enzymes. The hallmark is the conversion of normal cells into their "tombstones," that is, outlines of the cells are retained but cytoplasmic and nuclear details are lost). With the infiltration of the leukocytes and release of lysosomal enzymes, the degradation of the necrotic cells is initiated, which is cleared by recruited neutrophils and macrophages.

2.4.4.2 Liquefactive (Colliquative) Necrosis

It usually follows ischemic injury, focal bacterial and occasionally fungal infections [5, 29]. Due to the chemotactic nature of the microbes, the inflammatory cells accumulate and cause hydrolytic degeneration of the native tissue. Common site of such necrosis is the brain. The liquefactic necrosis is subsequently removed by the phagocytes leaving behind a cyst-like structure filled with necrotic debris. When superadded with infection, it could lead to bacterial infections. Microscopically, the cystic space contains necrotic cell debris and macrophages filled with phagocytosed material. The cyst wall is formed by proliferating capillaries, inflammatory cells, and proliferating glial cells in the brain and proliferating fibroblasts in abscess cavity elsewhere in the human body.

2.4.4.3 Caseous Necrosis

Caseous refers to the curdled or cheese-like gross appearance of this form of necrosis within the center of an epithelioid granulomatous inflammatory reaction [1, 5]. This type of necrosis is encountered often in tuberculous infection (Fig. 2.5). Earlier the presence of epithelioid granuloma along with caseous necrosis would be

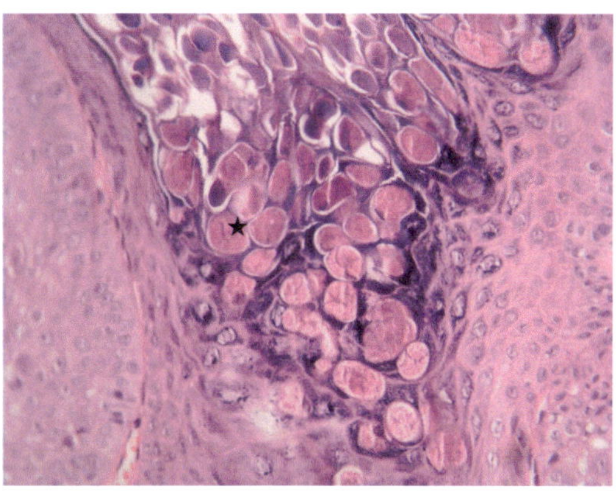

Fig. 2.4 Molluscum contagiosum. Cluster of cells with large intracytoplasmic eosinophilic hyaline inclusions (Henderson-Peterson bodies) (asterix)

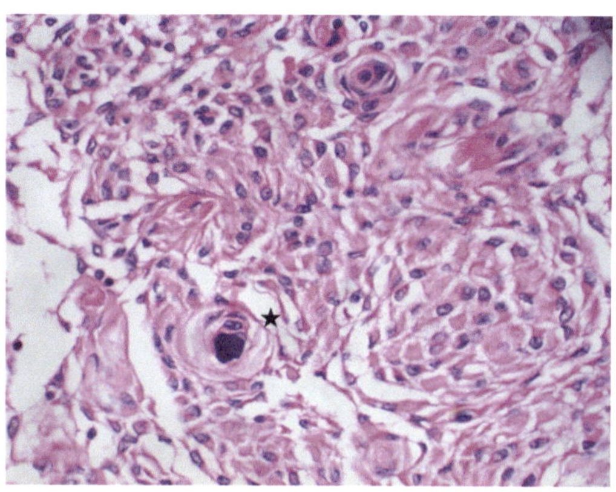

Fig. 2.5 Calcification. Tumor cells of meningioma showing concentric lamellar basophilic calcifications (psammoma bodies)

considered as hallmark of tuberculous infection; however, the evidence for a mycobacterial infection should be documented by the presence of acid-fast bacilli or a molecular diagnosis of Tb by PCR studies. Caseous necrosis is a combination of both coagulative and liquefactive necrosis. On gross examination, foci of caseous necrosis resemble dry cheese and are soft, granular and yellowish. On light microscopy, the center of the necrotic focus contains eosinophilic material having scattered granular debris of disintegrated nuclei. The surrounding tissue shows a granulomatous inflammatory reaction consisting of epithelioid histiocytes and multinucleate giant cells cuffed by mature lymphocytes.

2.4.4.4 Fat Necrosis

Focal fat destruction (e.g., traumatic) occurs due to release of activated lipases [5, 29]. The leaked enzymes liquefy membranes of fat cells (adipocytes) with splitting of triglycerides esters within fat cells. The released fatty acids combine with calcium salts to form macroscopically visible "chalky-white" areas of saponification [5, 23, 29]. Microscopically necrotic foci contain shadowy outlines of necrotic adipocytes surrounded by calcium deposits and inflammatory cells. Common sites of fat necrosis are breast, omentum, and pancreas.

2.4.4.5 Fibrinoid Necrosis

This is a special form of necrosis that occurs following immune reactions (e.g., granulomatosis with polyangiitis) in which antigen–antibody complexes deposit imparting a fibrin-like (fibrinoid) appearance and being PTAH-positives similar to fibrin [5, 29]. Microscopically, it is identified by brightly eosinophilic, hyaline-like deposition. Sometimes, the necrotic focus is surrounded by nuclear debris of neutrophils (leucocytoclasis).

2.4.5 Apoptosis

Apoptosis (falling off or dropping off) is a pathway of cell death in which cells activate enzymes that degrade the cells' own nuclear DNA and nuclear and cytoplasmic proteins [1, 3]. As opposed to necrosis where in the dying cells swell and burst, apoptosis leads to condensation and shrinkage. It is a form of programmed cell death and important in embryologic development, homeostasis, and involution of organs or tissues deprived of hormonal stimulation or growth factors [1, 23, 24].

2.4.5.1 Types of Apoptosis

Physiological Apoptosis

1. Organized cell destruction in sculpting of tissues during development of embryo [1, 30, 31].
2. Physiologic involution of cells in hormone-dependent tissues, for example, endometrial shedding, regression of lactating breast after withdrawal of breast-feeding [24, 32, 33].

Pathological Apoptosis

1. Cell death in tumors after chemotherapy.
2. Progressive depletion of CD4+T cells in the pathogenesis of AIDS [24, 27].
3. Cell death in viral infections, for example, formation of Councilman bodies in viral hepatitis [34, 35].

2.4.5.2 Mechanisms of Apoptosis

Apoptosis is a programmed form of cell death that is regulated by the biochemical pathways that control the balance of death- and survival-inducing signals [1, 3, 5, 24, 36]. Apoptosis proceeds through an *extrinsic pathway* (initiated by the binding of a ligand to its death receptor [DR]) or an *intrinsic pathway* (initiated in mitochondria in response to various stresses or DNA damage) and almost always activates *caspases* [1, 24, 36–40]. Caspases are cysteine proteases that cleave peptides after aspartate residues. The initiator caspases start the process of apoptosis (caspase-8, caspase-9, caspase-2). These activate effector caspase-3, caspase-6, and caspase-7, which then execute apoptosis [24, 31, 36, 38].

2.4.5.3 Morphology of Apoptotic Cells

Apoptotic cells appear as small cells with intensely eosinophilic cytoplasm (mummified cell) containing shrunken or almost-normal organelles [1, 3, 5, 24]. They display condensation and fragmentation of the nucleus (pyknosis and karyorrhexis) with blebbing of the plasma membrane to form membrane-bound apoptotic bodies that contain nuclear fragments, organelles, and condensed cytosol. The plasma membrane that surrounds apoptotic bodies prevents the triggering of inflammation.

Clearing of Apoptotic Cells

The plasma membrane that surrounds apoptotic bodies expresses factors and/or undergoes structural changes so as to emit signals that attract phagocytes and stimulate heterophagy [24, 42, 43].

Other pathways of cell death include *necroptosis,* a regulated form of necrotic cell and *Pyroptosis*, which is a cell death associated with fever [9, 20]. This form of cell death is associated with activation of cytosolic danger-sensing protein complex called *inflammasome*, which in turn leads to caspase activation. Some of these caspases trigger apoptosis, while others induce cytokine production, thus inducing inflammation manifested by fever. Pyroptosis is seen in some microbial infections.

2.4.6 Autophagy

Autophagy (*self-eating*) refers to lysosomal digestion of the cell's own components [5, 9]. It is a cell survival mechanism during ischemia or involution in response to loss of growth factors or hormonal stimuli. Cells consume their own damaged organelles, as a housekeeping function, and cytosolic proteins and carbohydrates, as a source of nutrients.

2.5 Ischemia and Reperfusion Injury

Sometimes, restoration of blood flow to ischemic but otherwise viable tissues may result in increased cell injury [5, 7]. Based on the duration of ischemia, there could be total restoration, partial damage or severe reperfusion injury. Ischemia-reperfusion injury occurs due to excessive accumulation of free radicals or reactive oxygen species (ROS). The mechanism of reperfusion injury is by the cumulative effect of calcium overload, excessive generation of free radicals. Reactive oxygen species may interact with cytoskeletal elements and interfere in mitochondrial aerobic phosphorylation, thus causing ATP depletion.

The body also has antioxidants, which are endogenous and inactivate the free radicals. These include vitamins (E, A, and C), sulfhydryl-containing compounds (e.g., cysteine and glutathione), and serum proteins (e.g., ceruloplasmin and transferrin).

Stress Proteins and Cell Injury

When under stress, cells release of proteins that move molecules within the cell cytoplasm. These *stress proteins* are of 2 types: heat shock proteins (HSPs) and ubiquitin [1, 5]. HSPs are the intracellular carrier proteins present in most cells of the body, which increase in response to stress, for example, toxins, drugs, poisons, ischemia [44]. *Ubiquitin* is another stress protein that directs intracellular molecules for either degradation or for synthesis. The clinical significance of Ubiquitin is that it is involved in a variety of human degenerative diseases such as Alzheimer's disease, Parkinson's disease, etc.

Pathogenesis of Chemical Injury

Chemicals induce cell injury either by direct cytotoxicity, or by conversion of chemicals into reactive metabolites [5].

The direct cytotoxicity does not require metabolic activation, for example, Cyanide. On the other hand, some chemicals may be metabolized to yield a toxic product, for example, Carbon tetrachloride CCl4 that is converted to a highly toxic free radical, CCl 3, which causes liver damage.

2.6 Gangrene

Gangrene is necrosis of tissue associated with superadded putrefaction and can be of two types [1, 3, 5, 45]. Dry gangrene is seen in distal limbs due to ischemic injury. The invading bacteria find it hard to grow; hence, the gangrene spreads slowly upward. The affected part is dry, shrunken, and dark black due to release hemoglobin from lysed RBCs. Microscopically, necrosis is seen with smudging of the tissue. The line of separation consists of inflammatory granulation tissue.

On the other hand, wet gangrene occurs in naturally moist tissues and organs such as the bowel, mouth, cervix, etc., for example, diabetic foot and bed sores [1, 3, 5]. The affected part is stuffed with blood, thus favoring rapid growth of putrefactive bacteria. The toxic bacterial products are absorbed, causing profound systemic manifestations of septicemia and, finally, death. Macroscopically, the affected part is soft, swollen, putrid, rotten, and dark (e.g., gangrene of the bowel due to strangulated hernia, volvulus, or intussusception). It is stained dark black due to the action of bacterial hydrogen disulfide on the hemoglobin released from hemolyzed RBCs.

Histologically, there is coagulative necrosis with intense acute inflammatory exudates and thrombosed vessels (Table 2.2).

Gas gangrene is another form of wet gangrene caused by gas-forming clostridia (e.g., *Clostridium* spp.) [1, 5, 46]. These bacteria gain entry into the tissues, especially muscles, through open contaminated wounds or as a complication of surgeries on tissues, which colonize clostridia. The toxins induce necrosis and edema and also enter blood stream, causing systemic manifestations. Clinically, the affected area is swollen, painful with characteristic crepitations due to accumulation of gas liberated due to fermentation of sugars by bacterial toxins [5, 45]. The tissues become dark foul smelling with colonies of bacteria. At the periphery, a zone of leucocytic infiltration, edema, and congestion are found.

Table 2.2 Dry gangrene versus wet gangrene [3]

Feature	Dry gangrene	Wet gangrene
Site	Usually limbs	Mostly in the bowel
Mechanism	Arterial occlusion	Blockage of both venous drainage and arterial flow
Gross appearance	Organ dry, contracted, & tan	Part moist, soft, expanded, rotten, and dark
Putrefaction	Less due to limited blood supply	Marked due to stuffing of organ with blood
Line of demarcation	Present at the junction between viable and gangrenous tissues	No clear line of demarcation
Bacteria	Bacteria fail to survive	Numerous
Prognosis	Generally better due to inconspicuous systemic toxic manifestations	Generally poor due to marked toxemia and septicemia

2.7 Calcification

This refers to the deposition of calcium salts in tissues other than osteoid or enamel and could present as dystrophic or metastatic calcification based on the serum calcium levels [5, 47, 48]. Dystrophic calcification is due to the deposition of calcium salts in dead or degenerated tissues with normal calcium metabolism and normal serum calcium levels, for example, caseous necrosis, calcification of fat necrosis, calcification of tumors, around dead parasites, atherosclerotic patches, in tumors like meningioma, ovarian cysts (Fig. 2.4) [5, 49].

Whereas Metastatic calcification occurs in apparently normal tissues and is associated with abnormal calcium metabolism and hypercalcemia, for example, excessive mobilization of calcium from the bone in Hyperparathyroidism, Paraneoplastic syndrome Patients with prolonged immobilization. It could also result due to Excessive absorption *of calcium from the gut, for example,* Hypervitaminosis D, Milk-alkali syn-

Table 2.3 Differences between dystrophic and metastatic calcification [1, 3, 5, 49]

Feature	Dystrophic calcification	Metastatic calcification
Definition	Passive deposits of calcium salts in damaged or nonviable tissues	Deposits of calcium salts in normal tissues
Calcium homeostasis	Normal with regular serum calcium levels	Abnormal with elevated serum calcium levels
Organ involvement	Localized process limited to the damaged tissue	Many organ sites may be involved
Reversibility	Usually, irreversible	Reversible upon correction of the underlying metabolic abnormality
Pathogenesis	Increased binding of phosphates with necrotic tissue, which then coheres with calcium forming calcium phosphate precipitates	Precipitation of calcium salts in hypercalcemic state facilitated by alkaline environment in some tissues
Associated diseases	Ehler Danlos syndrome, pseudoxanthoma elasticum, crystal deposition disorder, arteriosclerosis obliterans	Hyperparathyroidism, renal failure, hypervitaminosis D, neoplasms, milk-alkali syndrome, tumoral calcinosis

drome, Idiopathic hypercalcemia of infancy (Williams syndrome), and Renal tubular acidosis [1, 47, 49].

While metastatic calcification may affect any normal tissue of the body, certain tissues are more commonly affected than the others. These include kidneys (especially the basement membrane of tubular epithelium and tubular lumina), lungs (especially in the alveolar walls), stomach (acid-secreting fundal glands), and the blood vessels (internal elastic lamina). Cornea and synovium are other sites where metastatic calcification may occur (Table 2.3).

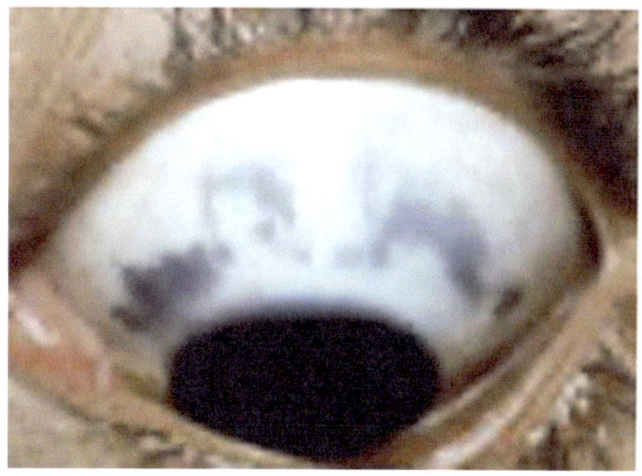

Fig. 2.6 Melanin pigmentation—Ocular melanosis. Brown pigmentation of conjunctiva due to increased melanocytes and melanin

2.8 Intracellular Accumulations

Intracellular accumulation of substances in abnormal amounts can occur within the cytoplasm or nucleus of the cell [5, 8]. It is beyond the scope of this chapter to discuss all types, but some of the important ones are described below.

These accumulations can be constituents of normal cell metabolism produced in excess [3, 5], for example, accumulation of lipids (steatosis), proteins (e.g., Russel bodies, Mallory bodies) and carbohydrates (glycogen); accumulation of abnormal substances, for example, products of abnormal metabolism seen in inborn errors of metabolism. Sometimes, there are accumulation of pigments, for example, hyperpigmentation, hemosiderosis, porphyria, chronic lead poisoning, etc. The endogenous pigments include melanin (Fig. 2.6), Melanin-like pigment (e.g., alkaptonuria, Dubin-Johnson syndrome); Hemoprotein-derived pigments (Hemosiderin, hemozoin, bilirubin, porphyrins) (Fig. 2.7); Lipofuscin.

The exogenous pigments are introduced either by inhalation (coal workers pneumonia); ingestion (lead silver); or inoculation, for example, Tattooing.

Hyperbilirubinemia causes jaundice and may be unconjugated or conjugated. Excessive accumulation of bilirubin pigment can be seen in different body tissues and fluids, especially the hepatocytes, Kupffer cells, and bile sinusoids. Skin and sclerae become distinctly yellow. In infants, rise in unconjugated bilirubin may pro-

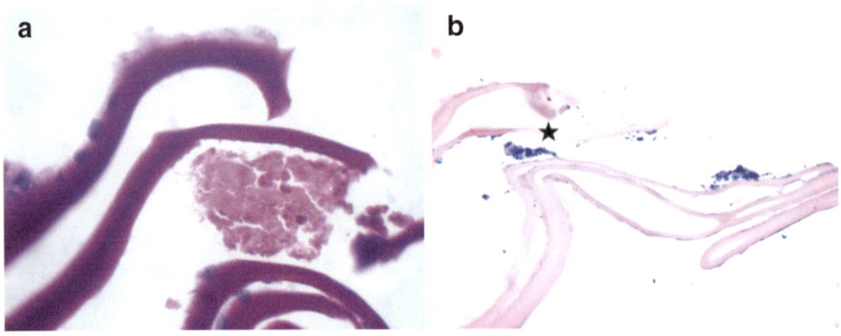

Fig. 2.7 Ocular siderosis. An old case of penetrating eye injury with cataract and brown-colored lens capsule. (**a**) The lens capsule, which stains strongly positive with PAS stain, showing some granular deposits. (**b**) Perls' stain shows blue stained subcapsular deposits confirming hemosiderin

duce toxic brain injury, a condition termed as kernicterus [5, 50].

Inborn abnormality of porphyrin metabolism, resulting from genetic deficiency of one of the enzymes required for the synthesis of hem, results in excessive production of porphyrins [5, 51].

Porphyrias are broadly classified as "erythropoietic" (defective synthesis of heme in the red cell precursors in the bone marrow) and "hepatic" porphyrias (normal erythroid precursors but have a defect in synthesis of heme in the liver).

Lipofuscin (*lipo* = fat, *fuscus* = brown) is yellowish-brown intracellular lipid pigment often found in atrophied cells of old age [5, 52]. It can be seen in the myocardial fibers, hepatocytes, Leydig cells of the testes, and in neurons in senile dementia. It appears coarse, golden-brown granular on microscopy and often accumulates in the central part of the cells around the nuclei. Lipofuscin granules are electron-dense and composed of lipid–protein complexes.

2.9 Adaptations

Adaptations are the adjustments the cells make in response to stresses, which may be for physiologic needs *(physiologic adaptation)* or in response to nonlethal pathologic injury *(pathologic adaptation)* [5, 8]. Such adaptations occur by following processes. Some of the important ones are described below:

2.9.1 Atrophy

Atrophy is the decrease in the number and size of parenchymal cells of an organ or its parts [1, 5]. It is distinct from *hypoplasia* (developmentally small size), and *aplasia* (extreme failure of development so that only rudimentary tissue is present). The *physiologic atrophy* is a normal ageing process, for example, atrophy of lymphoid tissue, thymus, brain, gonads (after menopause), and bones (osteoporosis).

The *pathologic atrophy* occurs in *Starvation atrophy* and cachexia (cancer patients), prolonged *Ischemia*, for example, atrophy of kidney in atherosclerosis of renal artery, *Disuse atrophy*, *Neuropathic atrophy (poliomyelitis), or Endocrine atrophy*, for example, atrophy of thyroid, adrenal and gonads in hypopituitarism; P*ressure atrophy*, for example, sternal erosion in aortic arch aneurysm.

Organ appears shrunken and there is a reduction in cell organelles, notably, the mitochondria, myofilaments, and ER [5, 53]. Autophagic vacuoles are often increased. These vacuoles may persist to form "residual bodies" in the cell cytoplasm.

2.9.2 Hypertrophy

Hypertrophy is an increase in the size of parenchymal cells with resultant enlargement of the organ or tissue, without any change in the number of cells [1, 3, 5].

The *Physiologic hypertrophy* is seen in puberty: for example, enlarged uterus in pregnancy. On the other hand, the *Pathologic hypertrophy* is seen in the heart (Left ventricular hypertrophy) in systemic hypertension, stomach (Hypertrophy of smooth muscle) in cardiac achalasia (in esophagus), and pyloric stenosis (in stomach), Hypertrophy of skeletal muscle in athletes and manual laborers, and Compensatory hypertrophy (and hyperplasia) of nephrons in one kidney when the other is removed (nephrectomy).

The affected organ becomes enlarged and heavy. There is enlargement of muscle fibers as well as of nuclei. Ultrastructurally, there is increased synthesis of DNA and RNA, increased protein synthesis, and increased number of organelles such as mitochondria, endoplasmic reticulum, and myofibrils [5, 53].

2.9.3 Hyperplasia

Hyperplasia is an increase in the number of parenchymal cells resulting in enlargement of the organ or tissue [1, 3, 5]. It occurs due to cell division when stimulated.

Based on the property to divide, the labile cells such as epithelial cells of the skin and mucous membranes; cells of the bone marrow lymph nodes; and stable cells such as parenchymal cells of the liver, pancreas, kidney, adrenal, and thyroid can undergo hyperplasia. The permanent cells such as neurons and cardiac and skeletal muscle have little or no capacity for regenerative hyperplastic growth.

Pathologic hyperplasia usually results from excessive stimulation of hormones or due to excessive growth factors. Examples include endometrial hyperplasia following estrogen excess, formation of granulation tissue in wound healing due to proliferation of fibroblasts and endothelial cells, etc. The affected organ or tissue is enlarged with increase in the number of cells (Fig. 2.8).

2.9.4 Metaplasia

Metaplasia is a reversible change of one type of epithelial or mesenchymal adult cells to another type of adult epithelial or mesenchymal cells, usually in response to abnormal stimuli [1, 5]. Metaplasia often reverts back to normal on removal of stimulus. Persistent or severe stimuli may however cause irreversible metaplasia or progression to dysplasia and, ultimately, cancer [5, 54].

Different types of metaplasia include.

Epithelial Metaplasia

It may be squamous or columnar.

Squamous Metaplasia: It often occurs following chronic irritation. Examples include

(i) Squamous metaplasia in bronchi of chronic smokers
(ii) Squamous metaplasia of the uterine endocervix in uterine prolapse

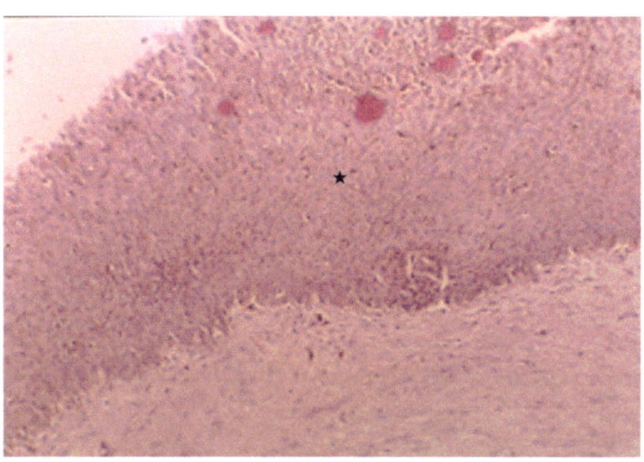

Fig. 2.8 Hyperplasia. Conjunctival mucosa showing increased number of layers. Note that polarity is maintained with normal cellular maturation

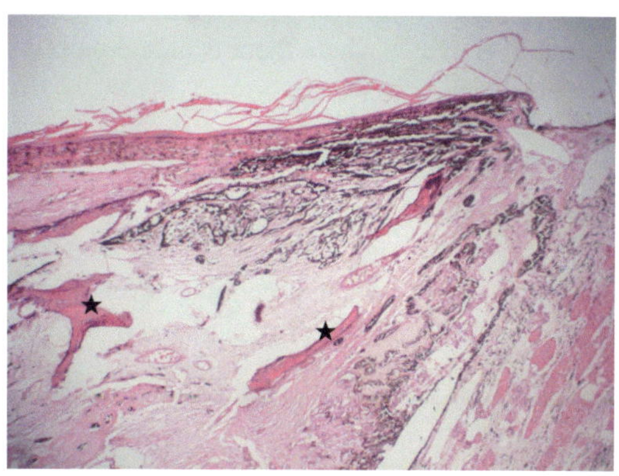

Fig. 2.9 Osseous metaplasia. Bone-like eosinophilic trabeculae (asterix) formed due to metaplasia of connective tissue in long-standing phthisical eye

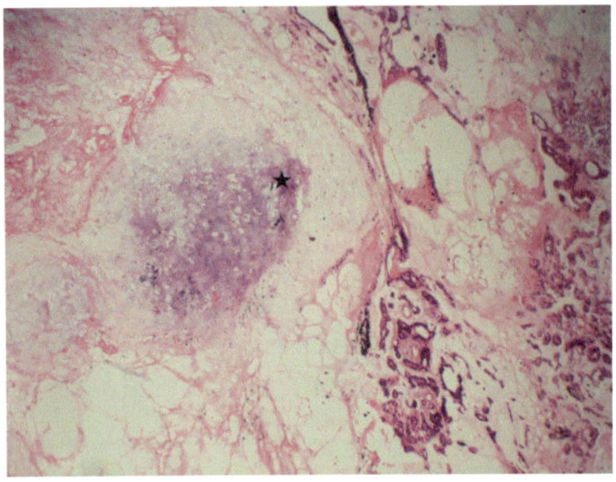

Fig. 2.10 Chondroid metaplasia. Bluish cartilage-like mesenchymal metaplastic tissue formation (asterix) in a phthisical eye

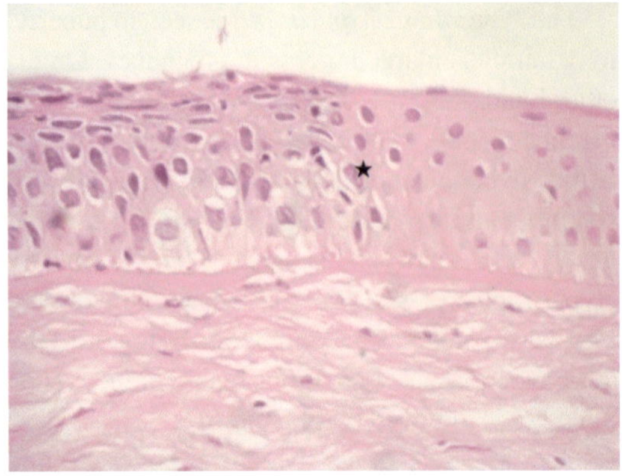

Fig. 2.11 Carcinoma in situ with normal mucosa. The picture shows abrupt transition of normal squamous mucosa (asterix) to full-thickness dysplasia (carcinoma-in-situ) (left side) with hyperplasia, loss of polarity, and nuclear pleomorphism. Basement membrane is intact; so, no invasion is present

(iii) Squamous metaplasia of lacrimal epithelium in chronic dacryocystitis

Columnar Metaplasia

(i) Intestinal metaplasia in healed chronic gastric ulcer
(ii) Barrett's esophagus
(iii) Chronic bronchitis and bronchiectasis

Mesenchymal Metaplasia

Less often, one adult type of mesenchymal tissue transforms to another. Examples include.

Osseous metaplasia seen in the arterial wall in Mönckeberg's sclerosis, soft tissues in myositis ossificans, cartilage of larynx and bronchi in elderly people, in long-standing scars of chronic inflammation (Fig. 2.9), and sometimes in tumors (e.g., leiomyoma).

Cartilaginous metaplasia may occur during healing of fractures where there is undue mobility (Fig. 2.10).

Table 2.4 Features differentiating metaplasia from dysplasia [3]

Feature	Metaplasia	Dysplasia
Definition	Transformation of one type of epithelial or mesenchymal cell to another type	Disordered cellular development associated with loss of polarity
Types	Epithelial (squamous, columnar) and mesenchymal (osseous, cartilaginous)	Epithelial only
Examples of tissues affected	Epithelia like conjunctival mucosa, bronchial mucosa, uterine endocervix; Mesenchymal tissues like cartilage, arterial wall	Epithelial surfaces like conjunctiva, oral mucosa, uterine cervix, bronchial mucosa, etc.
Cellular changes	Mature cellular development	Disordered cellular development (pleomorphism, nuclear hyperchromasia, mitosis, loss of polarity)
Natural history	Reversible on withdrawal of stimulus	Irreversible in higher grade
Outcome	May reverse or progress to dysplasia	Progression to carcinoma in situ or invasive carcinomas

2.9.5 Dysplasia

Dysplasia is a disordered cellular development, which is often preceded or accompanied by metaplasia and hyperplasia [54]; it hence was earlier referred to as atypical hyperplasia. It is characterized by [5]

1. Increased number of layers of epithelial cells
2. Disorderly arrangement of cells from basal layer to the surface layer
3. Loss of basal polarity, that is, nuclei lying away from basement membrane
4. Cellular and nuclear pleomorphism
5. Increased nucleocytoplasmic ratio
6. Nuclear hyperchromatism
7. Increased mitotic activity

Dysplasia is commonly seen the ocular surface (Fig. 2.11), uterine cervix, and respiratory tract. Dysplastic changes often occur due to chronic irritation or prolonged inflammation and may disappear on removal of the inciting stimulus. Sometimes, dysplasia may progress into carcinoma in situ or invasive cancer (Table 2.4).

2.10 Ageing

We age because our cells age. In general, the life expectancy of an individual depends upon *Intrinsic genetic process, Environmental factors*, for example, consumption and inhalation of harmful substances, type of diet, role of antioxidants, etc. It could also be a result of *lifestyle of the individual* such as diseases due to alcoholism (e.g., cirrhosis, hepatocellular carcinoma), smoking (e.g., bronchogenic carcinoma and other respiratory diseases), drug addiction or *Age-related diseases*, for example, atherosclerosis and ischemic heart disease, diabetes mellitus, hypertension, Alzheimer's disease, Parkinson's disease etc. [5, 55]

Cellular ageing results from progressive decline in the life span and functioning of the cells. There is accumulation of mutations in the DNA resulting in decreased cellular replication, which is called as replicative senescence. Therefore, after a fixed number of division cells cannot further replicate. This results from progressive shortening of telomeres with eventual arrest in cell cycle. Telomeres, which are short DNA sequences at the ends of chromosomes, protect the ends from fusion and degradation [1, 3]. Certain proteins bind to this telomeric DNA, thus shielding it and preventing DNA damage response. As cells divide, a part of telomere does not duplicate and thus with every cell division, telomeres shorten. Ends of chromosomes with shortened telomeres cannot be protected; they are sensed as broken DNA and thus follows cell cycle arrest. Telomerase is a specialized RNA–protein complex that maintains the telomerase length by using its own RNA as template for adding nucleotides to chromosomal ends. Telomerase is expressed in germ cells and stem cells but not somatic cells. Hence, as somatic cells mature, telomeres shorten and eventually, cells exit the cell cycle. Ageing is also a result of defective protein homeostasis and persistent inflammation [5, 55].

References

1. Kumar V, Abbas AK, Aster JC. Robbins & Cotran pathologic basis of disease. 9th ed. Philadelphia: Elsevier Saunders; 2015.
2. Galluzzi L, Bravo-San Pedro JM, Kepp O, Kroemer G. Regulated cell death and adaptive stress responses. Cell Mol Life Sci. 2016;73(11–12):2405–10. https://doi.org/10.1007/s00018-016-2209-y. Epub 2016 Apr 5
3. Mohan H. Cellular adapataion and cell injury. In: Textbook of pathology. 8th ed. New Delhi: Jaypee Brothers; 2019. p. 33–69.
4. Cobb JP, Hotchkiss RS, Kearl IE, Buchman TG. Mechanism of cell injury and death. Br J Anaesth. 1996;77:3–10.
5. Miller MA, Zachary JF. Mechanisms and morphology of cellular injury, adaptation, and death. In: Zachary JF, editor. Pathologic basis of veterinary disease. 6th ed. Mosby; 2017. p. 2–43. e19.
6. Hotchkiss RS, Strasser A, McDunn JE, Swanson PE. Cell death. N Engl J Med. 2009;361(16):1570–83.

https://doi.org/10.1056/NEJMra0901217. PMID: 19828534; PMCID: PMC3760419.
7. Kalogeris T, Baines CP, Krenz M, Korthuis RJ. Cell biology of ischemia/reperfusion injury. Int Rev Cell Mol Biol. 2012;298:229–317. https://doi.org/10.1016/B978-0-12-394309-5.00006-7.
8. Fitzpatrick SG, Gordon SC. Cell injury, adaptation, and necrosis. In: Radosevich JA, editor. Apoptosis and beyond: the many ways cells die. New Jersey: Wiley; 2018. p. 83–98.
9. Fink SL, Cookson BT. Apoptosis, pyroptosis, and necrosis: mechanistic description of dead and dying eukaryotic cells. Infect Immun. 2005;73(4):1907–16.
10. Trump BF, Berezesky IK, Chang SH, Phelps PC. The pathways of cell death: oncosis, apoptosis, and necrosis. Toxicol Pathol. 1997;25(1):82–8. https://doi.org/10.1177/019262339702500116. PMID: 9061857.
11. Vardhan P, Goel S, Goyal G, Kumar N. Solitary giant molluscum contagiosum presenting as lid tumor in an immunocompetent child. Indian J Ophthalmol. 2010;58(3):236–8. https://doi.org/10.4103/0301-4738.62652.
12. Ehrenreich T. T1 Histochemistry, Theoretical and Applied A. G. Everson Pearse. (2nd), Boston, Little, Brown and Company, 1960, 998 pp., 10 color plates, 245 black and white illustrations, $20.00. Clin Chem. 1961;7(3):300. https://doi.org/10.1093/clinchem/7.3.300.
13. Li Y, Lip G, Chong V, Yuan J, Ding Z. Idiopathic orbital inflammation syndrome with retro-orbital involvement: a retrospective study of eight patients. PLoS One. 2013;8(2):e57126. https://doi.org/10.1371/journal.pone.0057126.
14. Fu DA, Campbell-Thompson M. Periodic acid-Schiff staining with diastase. Methods Mol Biol. 2017;1639:145–9. https://doi.org/10.1007/978-1-4939-7163-3_14.
15. Mulay K, Menon V, Lahane S, Sharma M, Honavar SG. Endocrine mucin-producing sweat gland carcinoma (EMPSGC) of the eyelid: Clinicopathologic features, immunohistochemical findings and review of literature. Indian J Ophthalmol. 2019;67(8):1374–7. https://doi.org/10.4103/ijo.IJO_1745_18.
16. Al-Osaily AM, Al-Dosari FN, Elewa MA, Butt SA. Extraskeletal myxoid chondrosarcoma of the orbit. Middle East Afr J Ophthalmol. 2016;23(2):232–4. https://doi.org/10.4103/0974-9233.171776.
17. Rao R, Honavar SG, Mulay K, Reddy VAP. Primary orbital low-grade fibromyxoid sarcoma – a case report. Indian J Ophthalmol. 2019;67(4):568–70. https://doi.org/10.4103/ijo.IJO_633_18.
18. Xiao MY, Tang LS, Zhu H, Li YJ, Li HL, Wu XR. Adult nasolacrimal sac mucocele. Ophthalmologica. 2008;222(1):21–6. https://doi.org/10.1159/000109274.
19. Mynatt CJ, Feldman KA, Thompson LDR. Orbital infantile myofibroma: a case report and clinicopathologic review of 24 cases from the literature. Head Neck Pathol. 2011;5(3):205–15. https://doi.org/10.1007/s12105-011-0260-4.
20. Linkermann A, Green DR. Necroptosis. N Engl J Med. 2014;370(5):455–65. https://doi.org/10.1056/NEJMra1310050. PMID: 24476434; PMCID: PMC4035222.
21. Li CJ, Friedman DJ, Wang C, Metelev V, Pardee AB. Induction of apoptosis in uninfected lymphocytes by HIV-1 Tat protein. Science. 1995;268:429–31.
22. Samali AB, et al. Apoptosis: cell death defined by caspase activation. Cell Death Differ. 1999;6:495–6.
23. Kerr JF, Wyllie AH, Currie AR. Apoptosis: a basic biological phenomenon with wide-ranging implications in tissue kinetics. Br J Cancer. 1972;26:239–57.
24. Elmore S. Apoptosis: a review of programmed cell death. Toxicol Pathol. 2007;35(4):495–516. https://doi.org/10.1080/01926230701320337.
25. Galluzzi L, et al. Molecular mechanisms of cell death: recommendations of the Nomenclature Committee on Cell Death 2018. Cell Death Differ. 2018;25(3):486–541. https://doi.org/10.1038/s41418-017-0012-4. Epub 2018 Jan 23. PMID: 29362479; PMCID: PMC5864239.
26. Buja LM, Eigenbrodt ML, Eigenbrodt EH. Apoptosis and necrosis. Basic types and mechanisms of cell death. Arch Pathol Lab Med. 1993;117(12):1208–14.
27. Li Z, Zhou Z. How are necrotic cells recognized by their predators? Worm. 2015;5(1):e1120400. https://doi.org/10.1080/21624054.2015.1120400. PMID: 27073733; PMCID: PMC4805362.
28. Challa S, Chan FKM. Going up in flames: necrotic cell injury and inflammatory diseases. Cell Mol Life Sci. 2010;67:3241–53.
29. Tonnus W, Meyer C, Paliege A, Belavgeni A, von Mässenhausen A, Bornstein SR, Hugo C, Becker JU, Linkermann A. The pathological features of regulated necrosis. J Pathol. 2019;247(5):697–707. https://doi.org/10.1002/path.5248. Epub 2019 Feb 25. PMID: 30714148.
30. Brill A, Torchinsky A, Carp H, Toder V. The role of apoptosis in normal and abnormal embryonic development. J Assist Reprod Genet. 1999;16(10):512–9. https://doi.org/10.1023/a:1020541019347. PMID: 10575578; PMCID: PMC3455372.
31. Voss AK, Strasser A. The essentials of developmental apoptosis. F1000Res. 2020;9:F1000 Faculty Rev-148. https://doi.org/10.12688/f1000research.21571.1. PMID: 32148779; PMCID: PMC7047912.
32. Lund LR, et al. Two distinct phases of apoptosis in mammary gland involution: proteinase-independent and -dependent pathways. Development. 1996;122:181–93.
33. Tilly JL, Kowalski KI, Johnson AL, Hsueh AJ. Involvement of apoptosis in ovarian follicular atresia and postovulatory regression. Endocrinology. 1991;129:2799–801.
34. Santavanond JP, Rutter SF, Atkin-Smith GK, Poon IKH. Apoptotic bodies: mechanism of formation, isolation and functional relevance. In: Mathivanan

S, Fonseka P, Nedeva C, Atukorala I, editors. New frontiers: extracellular vesicles. subcellular biochemistry, vol. 97. Cham: Springer; 2021. https://doi.org/10.1007/978-3-030-67171-6_4.
35. Guicciardi ME, Gores GJ. Apoptosis: a mechanism of acute and chronic liver injury. Gut. 2005;54:1024–33.
36. Locksley RM, Killeen N, Lenardo MJ. The TNF and TNF receptor superfamilies: integrating mammalian biology. Cell. 2001;104:487–501.
37. Brunner T, et al. Fas (CD95/Apo-1) ligand regulation in T cell homeostasis, cell-mediated cytotoxicity and immune pathology. Semin Immunol. 2003;15:167–76.
38. Wajant H. The Fas signaling pathway: more than a paradigm. Science. 2002;296:1635–6.
39. Saelens X, et al. Toxic proteins released from mitochondria in cell death. Oncogene. 2004;23:2861–74.
40. Du C, Fang M, Li Y, Li L, Wang X. Smac, a mitochondrial protein that promotes cytochrome *c*-dependent caspase activation by eliminating IAP inhibition. Cell. 2000;102:33–42.
41. Kischkel FC, et al. Cytotoxicity-dependent APO-1 (Fas/CD95)- associated proteins form a death-inducing signaling complex (DISC) with the receptor. EMBO J. 1995;14:5579–88.
42. Fadok VA, de Cathelineau A, Daleke DL, Henson PM, Bratton DL. Loss of phospholipid asymmetry and surface exposure of phosphatidylserine is required for phagocytosis of apoptotic cells by macrophages and fibroblasts. J Biol Chem. 2001;276:1071–7.
43. Ferraro-Peyret C, Quemeneur L, Flacher M, Revillard JP, Genestier L. Caspase-independent phosphatidylserine exposure during apoptosis of primary T lymphocytes. J Immunol. 2002;169:4805–10.
44. Szyller J, Bil-Lula I. Heat shock proteins in oxidative stress and ischemia/reperfusion injury and benefits from physical exercises: a review to the current knowledge. Oxidative Med Cell Longev. 2021;2021:6678457. https://doi.org/10.1155/2021/6678457. PMID: 33603951; PMCID: PMC7868165.
45. Buttolph A, Sapra A. Gangrene. 2022 Aug 8. In: StatPearls. Treasure Island (FL): StatPearls Publishing; 2023.
46. Mehdizadeh GI, Navarro MA, Li J, Shrestha A, Uzal F, BA MC. Pathogenicity and virulence of *Clostridium perfringens*. Virulence. 2021;12(1):723–53. https://doi.org/10.1080/21505594.2021.1886777. PMID: 33843463; PMCID: PMC8043184
47. Anderson HC. Mechanisms of pathologic calcification. Rheum Dis Clin North Am. 1988;14(2):303-19. PMID: 2845491. Black AS, Kanat IO. A review of soft tissue calcifications. J Foot Surg. 1985;24(4):243–50.
48. Vidavsky N, Kunitake JAMR, Estroff LA. Multiple pathways for pathological calcification in the human body. Adv Healthc Mater. 2021;10(4):e2001271. https://doi.org/10.1002/adhm.202001271. Epub 2020 Dec 4. PMID: 33274854; PMCID: PMC8724004.
49. Black AS, Kanat IO. A review of soft tissue calcifications. J Foot Surg. 1985;24(4):243–250. PMID: 4045112.
50. Creeden JF, Gordon DM, Stec DE, Hinds TD Jr. Bilirubin as a metabolic hormone: the physiological relevance of low levels. Am J Physiol Endocrinol Metab. 2021;320(2):E191–207. https://doi.org/10.1152/ajpendo.00405.2020. Epub 2020 Dec 7. PMID: 33284088; PMCID: PMC8260361
51. Krishnamurthy P, Xie T, Schuetz JD. The role of transporters in cellular heme and porphyrin homeostasis. Pharmacol Ther. 2007;114(3):345–58. https://doi.org/10.1016/j.pharmthera.2007.02.001. Epub 2007 Feb 21. PMID: 17368550.
52. Terman A, Brunk UT. Lipofuscin. Int J Biochem Cell Biol. 2004;36(8):1400–4. https://doi.org/10.1016/j.biocel.2003.08.009.
53. Sartori R, Romanello V, Sandri M. Mechanisms of muscle atrophy and hypertrophy: implications in health and disease. Nat Commun. 2021;12(1):330. https://doi.org/10.1038/s41467-020-20123-1. PMID: 33436614; PMCID: PMC7803748.
54. Giroux V, Rustgi AK. Metaplasia: tissue injury adaptation and a precursor to the dysplasia-cancer sequence. Nat Rev Cancer. 2017;17(10):594–604.
55. López-Otín C, Blasco MA, Partridge L, Serrano M, Kroemer G. The hallmarks of aging. Cell. 2013;153(6):1194–217. https://doi.org/10.1016/j.cell.2013.05.039. PMID: 23746838; PMCID: PMC3836174.

3 Hemostasis

Shilpa Goyal

Contents

3.1 Introduction

One of the common sign and symptoms of any injury is edema and bleeding, which can be seen in any part of the body including different layers of the eye (except cornea, which is avascular) [1]. This is a result of interaction and interplay of different factors affecting the osmolarity, blood vessels, blood components, and the interstitial spaces [2]. In normal conditions, there is a balance between fluid exchange among each compartment (blood vessels and extracellular space), the coagulation pathways, and the pro- and anti-inflammatory cytokines. But when an injury or insult of any kind ensues in our body, these balances tilt and progress from mild reversible changes of edema, congestion, and hemorrhage to severe complications like thrombosis, embolism, and life-threatening conditions including disseminated intravascular coagulation (DIC) and shock. The challenge lies in identifying the underlying etiology and timely manage the patients with minimal complications. Since the clinical presentation is a reflection of the disease process, understanding of the basic processes is very helpful in arriving at an accurate diagnosis.

S. Goyal (✉)
Sattvaguna Lab & Healthcare Private Limited,
Ambala City, Haryana, India

G. K. Vemuganti et al. (eds.), *Ocular Pathology*, https://doi.org/10.1007/978-981-96-8614-8_3

In this chapter, following aspects relating to basic mechanism of hemostasis, the pathobiology of the most common conditions, and their clinical relevance have been dealt with:

Congestion and hemorrhage
Edema
Thrombosis
Embolism
Bleeding disorders
Shock
DIC

3.2 Congestion and Hemorrhage

3.2.1 Congestion

The body's homeostasis aims to provide energy for basic metabolism in resting phase as well as in raised demand by increasing the blood flow through that organ. The process by which our body adjusts blood flow through the organs to fulfill the metabolic need is called hyperemia [3, 4]. Hyperemias are of two types: active hyperemia and passive hyperemia.

Active hyperemia is an increased blood flow to an organ due to increased activity like exercise or inflammation and blushing due to emotional stress or anxiety. The pathophysiology of hyperemia is due to vasodilation, which results in enhanced blood flow to the organ or tissue [3, 4]. This supplies more nutrients and oxygen to provide for the increased energy requirements [5]. The patient presents with redness and increased temperature of that site, and is a common feature of any activity, injury, or inflammation. For example, cheeks become red on blushing or exercise; conjunctivitis clinically presents as a red eye [6, 7], etc. This phenomenon is also of great importance in normal functioning of retina as photic stimulation of retina results in dilatation and hyperemia of the retinal arterioles, and any reduction in this flicker-evoked increase in blood flow (ageing, diabetes) may lead to retinal hypoxia [5, 8–11].

Passive hyperemia occurs due to interrupted blood flow to an organ resulting in local vasodilation, venous stasis, and pooling of blood in organs [4]. These cause accumulation of waste metabolites as occurs in heart failure or deep vein thrombosis (DVT). It is also known as *venous congestion*. Congestion can be localized to a particular organ as lower limb in DVT, or it can be generalized with multiorgan involvement as in heart failure causing chronic venous congestion (CVC) of lungs, liver, kidney, spleen, etc. [2, 4, 12, 13] In eye, chronic congestion of choroidal veins may lead to pachychoroid diseases like central serous chorioretinopathy [14]. Occasional cases of choroidal congestion post trabeculectomy leading to reduced visual acuity have also been reported [15].

3.2.2 Hemorrhage

Hemorrhage is the escape or extravasation of blood from blood vessel externally or into the body cavities [4]. Hemorrhage may be caused due to any injury, inflammatory lesions, vessel wall abnormalities like aneurysms, erosion of the vessel wall by surrounding neoplasms, and elevated blood pressure, which may cause retinal hemorrhages, epistaxis, or other forms of blood loss.

Bleeding from arteries or the arterial hemorrhage is usually caused due to injuries, and presents with rapid and pulsating blood loss. In comparison, venous hemorrhage is steadier, whereas the capillary hemorrhage presents with slow blood ooze and is the most common form of hemorrhage. Petechial hemorrhages are a type of pericapillary bleeding and hemorrhage that occur in a wide variety of disorders like infections, trauma, hematological causes, vasculitis, malignancies, drug reactions, vitamin K deficiency, etc. [16, 17]. They clinically present as pinpoint nonblanching spots, which are usually less than 2 mm in size. Petechial hemorrhages in conjunctiva may be seen in conjunctivitis, trauma, or postmortem in both conjunctiva and eyelids after death due to strangulation [18, 19]. Roth spots in retina are also a result of retinal capillary rupture and intraretinal hemorrhage [20].

While hemorrhage is a surgical and medical disease, there are occasions where old hemorrhage may show varying stages of organization, e.g., breakdown, hemosiderin deposition, calcification, cholesterol clefts, and granulations tissue formation [2, 4].

3.3 Edema

Edema is an accumulation of fluid in the interstitial space. It may occur due to acute conditions like trauma, infection, inflammation, or may be due to more chronic diseases like heart failure, cirrhosis, nephrotic syndrome, etc. [21] Edema occurs from an abnormal expansion in the interstitial fluid volume. The fluid movement between the interstitial and intravascular spaces is governed by the balance between capillary hydrostatic pressure gradient and the oncotic pressure gradient across the capillary [21–24]. The main causes of edema are increased capillary hydrostatic pressure, increased plasma volume, decreased plasma oncotic pressure, or lymphatic obstruction (Fig. 3.1).

Clinically, edema presents as swelling of the area, or of the dependent part like ankle in generalized edema [24, 25]. This swelling may be unilateral, bilateral, generalized, or localized depending upon the etiology. While generalized edema is commonly due to chronic conditions mentioned above, localized edema is generally due to inflammation, trauma, lymphoedema, DVT, or venous insufficiency. Edema due to infections or thrombosis is usually accompanied with rise in temperature and tenderness of that area. The nature of edema fluid also differs according to its etiology and further classified into exudative and transudative fluids.

Depending on the fluid composition, edema fluid can be classified as follows [4]:

- Transudate—is a low protein fluid, which is predominately an ultrafiltrate of blood plasma mainly due to cardiac or renal causes.
- Exudate—a high protein fluid associated with increased vascular permeability due to inflammation.

Diagnosis of edema is made from clinical perspective and thorough history taking. However, some tests can be done to determine the nature and probable cause of edema fluid, which are described in Table 3.1.

The rapid development of edema associated with systemic diseases requires timely diagnosis and management [21]. Acute swelling of a limb within 72 h is more characteristic of deep vein thrombosis, cellulitis, trauma, or drugs, while chronic edema (>3 months duration) is more likely due to systemic conditions like congestive heart failure, renal disease, malignancy, obesity, or hepatic disease [21, 28–30].

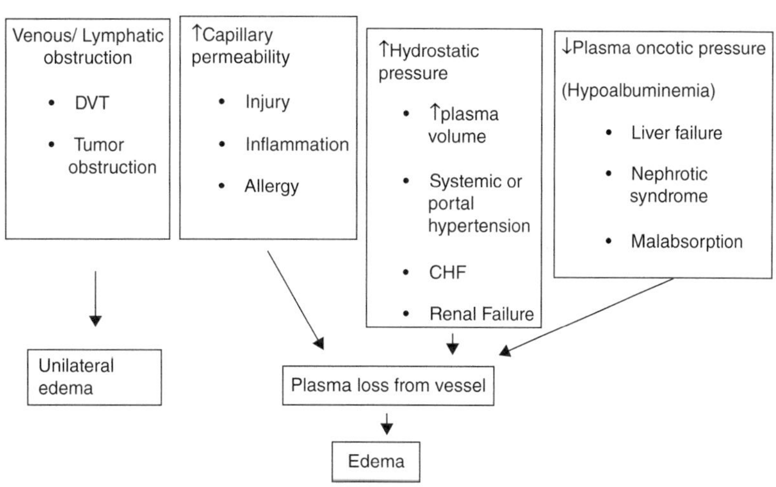

Fig. 3.1 Mechanism of edema. Obstruction of blood flow due to thrombus or tumor is usually localized and causes unilateral edema. Imbalance of hydrostatic and plasma oncotic pressures result in generalized edema

Table 3.1 Lab differences between transudates and exudates [4, 26, 27]

S.No	Lab parameter	Transudate	Exudate
1.	pH	>7.3	<7.3
2.	Specific gravity	<1.015	>1.018
3.	Glucose content	Low	High
4.	Protein content	<1 g/dL	2.5–3.5 g/dL
5.	Fluid protein: Serum protein ratio	<0.5	>0.5
6.	Fluid LDH	<200 U/L	>200 U/L
7.	Fluid LDH: Serum LDH ratio	<0.6	>0.6
8.	Cells	Few cells	Many cells with inflammatory cells

Edema of a single tissue like cornea may occur due to a localized pathology like injury to epithelium, which may result in imbibing of fluid into stroma from the tear film, or due to decompensated endothelium, which in turn is unable to push excess fluid out of stroma into the aqueous, resulting in overhydration of cornea [31–33]. Conjunctival edema in inflammation or trauma occurs mainly due to increased blood flow resulting in elevated hydrostatic pressure.

3.4 Thrombosis

In hemostasis, a plethora of events occurs, which maintain normal blood flow in vessels. This involves a delicate balance among the blood vessels, platelet activation, and blood coagulation [2]. Imbalance of any one of its functions can either lead to localized clot formation known as thrombosis, or alternatively can lead to bleeding due to impaired blood coagulation (Fig. 3.2). Thrombosis can occur in both arteries as well as veins and may have different risk factors for both (Table 3.2) [34].

The pathophysiology of arterial and venous thrombosis is different although they might look the same [36]. The primary trigger for arterial thrombosis is the rupture of atherosclerotic plaque, while venous thrombosis occurs mainly due to blood stasis and hypercoagulability [34].

Arterial thrombosis: The rupture of atherosclerotic plaque results in exposure of its core, which is rich in tissue factor (TF) [36]. TF is an important initiator of the extrinsic pathway of coagulation cascade, the mechanism of which has been explained in detail in Fig. 3.3. Also following a breach in the vascular integrity, the Von Willebrand factor (vWF) circulating in plasma is deposited on the exposed subendothelial collagen, starting platelet rolling, adhesion, activation, aggregation, and platelet plug formation [36, 37]. The thrombi thus formed are rich in platelets and are called the white thrombi.

Sudden arterial thrombosis is the most common cause of acute myocardial infarction (MI) and stroke, and can be prevented or treated with use of antiplatelet drugs like cyclooxygenase inhibitors, ADP receptor antagonists, etc. [34]. For acute arterial obstruction (as in MI, stroke, or CRAO), immediate fibrinolytic therapy using tissue plasminogen activator (t-PA) is given to dissolve the clot and resume the blood flow. Venous thrombosis is the most prevalent vascular event after MI and stroke, and is characterized by two main events—deep vein thrombosis (DVT) and pulmonary embolism (PE) [20] and can be treated with the use of anticoagulant drugs [34, 38].

Venous thrombosis: Rudolf Virchow proposed a triad of factors that contribute to venous thrombosis: stasis, hypercoagulability, and endothelial injury [36–39]. In contrast to the arterial thrombi, venous thrombi lack platelets and are rich in fibrin and trapped red blood cells, and are called red thrombi. Deep vein thrombosis occurs most often in the large veins of the legs causing pain, swelling, or discoloration of the extremity.

The main anticoagulant drugs used in venous thromboembolism are heparins and vitamin K antagonists like warfarin. The main complication of this therapy is bleeding and, therefore, the

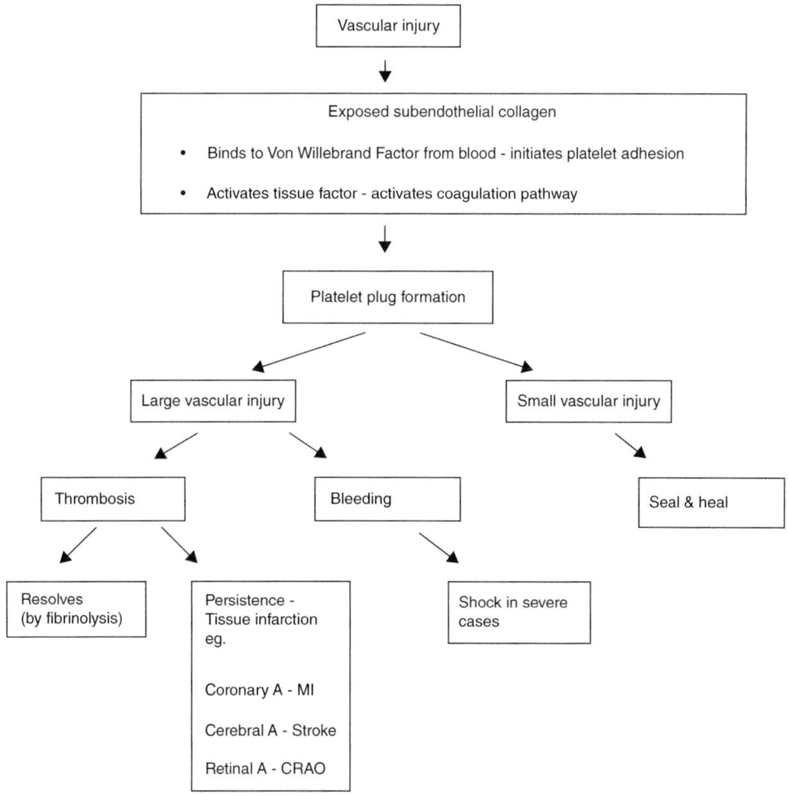

Fig. 3.2 Hemostasis in vascular injury. Any damage to the blood vessel leads to activation of platelets to form a plug and subsequently clot formation, thereby sealing of a small gap. Larger vessel defects may close with a thrombus or alternately may lead to continued bleeding

Table 3.2 Risk factors for thrombosis

Predisposing conditions for arterial thrombosis [35, 36]	Risk factors of venous thrombosis [34, 36]
1. Increasing age 2. Obesity 3. Arterial hypertension 4. Dyslipidemia 5. Diabetes 6. Tobacco consumption 7. Hyperhomocysteinemia	1. Increasing age 2. Congenital deficiencies like that of Protein C, Protein S, antithrombin III, or antiphospholipid antibody syndrome 3. Cancer 4. Obesity 5. Major surgery 6. Pregnancy 7. Increased amount of circulating tissue factor as in cancers, or inflammation 8. Hyperhomocysteinemia

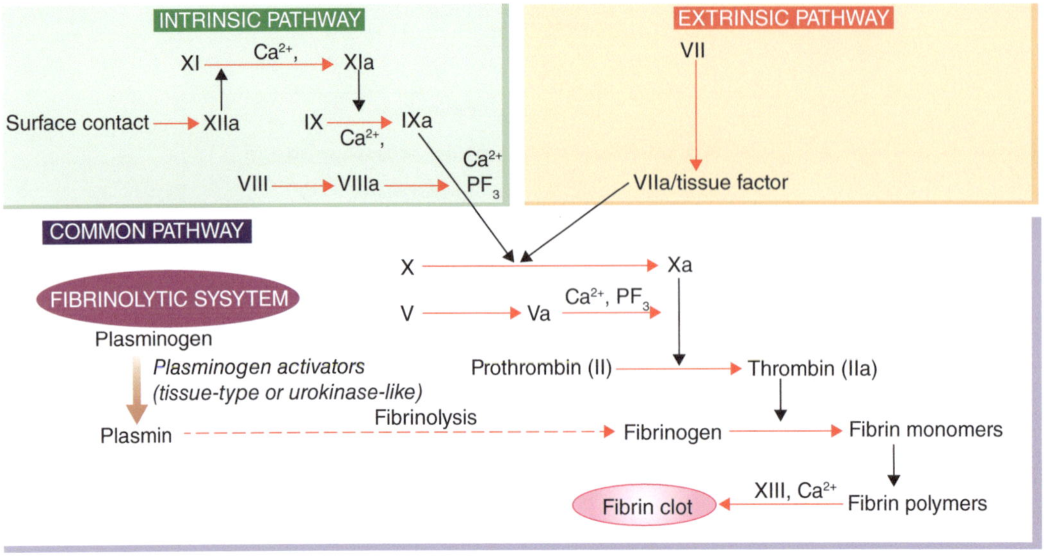

Fig. 3.3 The coagulation pathways. The intrinsic and extrinsic pathways of coagulation have been described here

patients on warfarin need to be monitored regularly with PTI and **international normalized ratio** (INR), while those on heparin are monitored using **activated partial thromboplastin time** (aPTT) or antifactor Xa assays.

3.5 Embolism

The clot or thrombus formed in the blood vessels may get dislodged from the primary site and travel in the vessel. This "free" clot known as embolus may be originated from arteries, venous, or lymphatic channels, and can produce symptoms when it blocks a distal artery [40]. An embolus is usually a clot, but also can be gas (air embolism), amniotic fluid (amniotic fluid embolism), fat globules (fat embolism), or even tumor cells (tumor embolism).

5.i. Arterial emboli—arise from the left side of the heart due to left heart failure, prosthetic valves and fibrillations, or from ulceration of atheromatous plaques in the major vessels like aorta, carotid artery, etc. [40–42]. The thrombi then can travel to any part of the body and produce symptoms of ischemia wherever they get lodged depending on the site of arterial blockage like stroke (cerebral artery), myocardial infarction (coronary artery), CRAO (retinal artery), and limb ischemia (femoral artery).

5.ii. Venous thromboembolism (VTE)—Deep vein thrombosis is the main preceding event here. DVT can get complicated when the thrombus breaks away, travels to the lungs, and gets lodged in pulmonary artery, and this is known as pulmonary embolism [2, 4, 43]. The embolus can completely or partially obstruct the pulmonary blood flow and produce symptoms of dyspnea, chest pain, or even death [43]. In some cases, hypercoagulable states and VTE can also predispose to retinal vein occlusions leading to CRVO [44]. Laboratory tests can be an aid in both diagnosis and as well as in predicting the risk of thrombosis in high-risk patients (Table 3.3).

5.iii. Air embolism—is presence of air in blood vessels. It can arise from infusion drips, surgical procedures, trauma, or due to decompression sickness [51]. Air in circulation can lead to increased vascular permeability, platelet aggregation, clot formation, and more severe systemic

Table 3.3 Laboratory tests in thromboembolism [38, 45–50]

Diagnostic tests
D-dimer test – provides a measure of ongoing fibrinolysis, and is recommended for the diagnosis of VTE and PE,
Protein C, Protein S, antithrombin deficiency, antiphospholipid antibodies, factor V Leiden, and homocysteine levels – in cases of unprovoked and recurrent episodes of VTE or recurrent abortions
Prognostic tests
Fasting lipid profile (predictor of atherosclerosis)
C-reactive protein (risk of future myocardial infarction or peripheral arterial disease)

inflammatory response [51–53]. This in turn may damage the pulmonary vasculature leading to pulmonary edema [51, 54]. Cardiovascular collapse and neurologic deficits followed by shock can occur if the embolus is large enough to block the ventricular outflow [55].

Air bubbles in circulation can arise from simple things like improper needle or mentioned lethal dose of air to be around 3–5 mL/kg [51, 56]. But it also depends on other factors like proximity of the vein to the heart, where the lethal dose is much less. Small amounts of air introduced rarely cause harm, but a few asymptomatic cases of superior ophthalmic vein and right ventricle air emboli have been reported following intravenous injections [55, 57, 58]. Therefore, extreme caution should be observed during routine injections to avoid this condition.

Decompression sickness, also known as the Caisson disease or bends, is an acute neurological emergency caused by release of dissolved nitrogen bubbles in circulation or extravascular tissue, on rapid reduction in environmental pressure (decompression) in divers, astronauts, or in miners [59–61]. The presentation may range from itching, pain, neurological symptoms, cardiovascular collapse, and even death. Eye involvement in such cases is rare, but blurring of vision, choroidal ischemia, and even loss of vision following ophthalmic artery occlusion have been reported in some cases [62, 63].

5.iv. Fat embolism—is a serious complication following bone and blunt trauma, intramedullary procedures, liposuction surgeries, and other inflammatory conditions like pancreatitis [64, 65]. It is characterized by release of fat droplets into the systemic circulation [66]. Fat embolism can lead to obstruction of vascular channels causing thrombocytopenia, anemia, hepatic changes (jaundice), and renal and retinal changes [65]. In eye, occlusion of the ophthalmic artery can lead to transient or permanent visual loss and retinal changes [65, 67]. Diagnosis is dependent on clinical symptoms of dyspnea, petechiae, and cognitive dysfunction following a long bone or pelvic trauma or procedure [64, 66].

5.v. Amniotic fluid embolism—is a rare and dangerous complication of pregnancy in which a breach in amniotic fluid-maternal blood barrier results in entry of amniotic fluid, fetal cells, hair, etc. into the maternal circulation [68]. The patient may present with cough, hypotension, cardiovascular collapse, and fetal bradycardia. A rare presentation in eye may occur in the form of loss of vision due to occlusion of branched retinal arterioles and ischemic retinopathy [69, 70].

5.vi. Tumor embolism—occurs when tumor cells are shed off into circulation from a primary or secondary malignancy [2, 4]. The circulating tumor cells in blood act as a seed to further grow the same tumor wherever they find the right soil and lead to metastasis.

3.6 Bleeding

Bleeding may be caused by a variety of factors. From the hematologic point, we can classify the etiology based on blood vessel, platelet, and coagulopathic causes and this has been elaborated in Table 3.4.

Table 3.4 Causes of bleeding based on etiology [2, 4, 71–73]

Blood vessel	Platelet	Coagulopathic
Trauma to vessel Atherosclerosis and plaque rupture Structural abnormalities Aneurysms Varicosities like piles AV malformations Invasion by a nearby malignancy	Low platelets(<10,000/uL) Platelet destruction, e.g., ITP, dengue Reduced production, e.g., chemotherapy, radiation, bone marrow aplasia Abnormal platelet functions, e.g., Chediak–Higashi syndrome, Von Willebrand disease (vWD) Hypothermia (impairs platelet adhesion and aggregation) Drugs, e.g., Aspirin	Vitamin K deficiency Acidosis (reduces procoagulant act) Excessive fibrinolysis (t-PA administration) DIC Drug induced – heparin, warfarin Factor deficiency – e.g., hemophilia

Table 3.5 Lab diagnosis of bleeding [74]

Primary screening tests for bleeding	Specific confirmatory tests if aPTT is prolonged in presence of normal PT and platelet count
1. Platelet count 2. Activated clotting time (aCT) 3. Prothrombin time (PT) 4. Activated partial thromboplastin time (aPTT) 5. Thrombin time (TT) 6. Serum fibrinogen levels	1. Correction and mixing studies based on aPTT – to distinguish factor deficiency from inhibitor 2. Specific factor assay to determine the deficient factor, e.g., deficient f VIII in hemophilia

A minor bleed is easily compensated by our body's hemostatic mechanisms. However, a major bleed may lead to increased heart rate, low blood pressure, vasovagal syncope, cold extremities, etc. Restoration of body fluid volume along with stoppage of bleed is important to prevent complications like hypovolemic shock. Bleeding without any obvious cause (trauma, surgical, or medical) asks for blood investigations to assess the etiology, treatment, and possible prevention. Blood tests in bleeding start from basic tests like platelet count and involve a stepwise approach from screening to specific tests as discussed in Table 3.5 [68].

Bleeding may be visible externally, like in piles, or it may take place in internal organs. Upper gastrointestinal (GI) bleed may be identified by hematemesis, while lower GI bleed has malena. Joint swelling in hemophilia is indicative of joint bleeds and needs immediate medical measures.

3.7 Shock

Shock is defined as a state of cellular and tissue hypoxia due to reduced oxygen delivery, increased oxygen consumption, inadequate oxygen utilization, or a combination of these processes. In the initial stage of shock, the body compensates and maintains all the vitals [75]. This is the reversible stage, which should be identified and prompt medical treatment be given to prevent the irreversible stage, which is a point of no return with ensuing decompensation and multiorgan involvement. Shock can be classified into different types based on the etiology and pathophysiology, but finally, they all conclude in multiorgan failure due to imbalance in demand and supply of oxygen [76].

Classification of Shock

7.i. Hypovolemic shock

Hypovolemic shock is a condition of inadequate organ perfusion due to blood or fluid loss. The onset of hypovolemic shock may be sudden as in major vessel injury, or more gradual, like in vomiting or diarrhea [75, 77]. Although the response to volume losses is variable individually, but generally, in previously healthy adults, reduction in plasma volume by 25% may occur without producing overt hypotension as the body's compensatory mechanisms come into action [77, 78]. Increased losses in presence of comorbidity like anemia may lead to early hypovolemia, as well as reduced cardiac output and arterial pressures. Low circulating volume leads to decreased organ perfusion, acidosis, and cold extremities (Fig. 3.4). The patients present with hypotension, tachycardia, sweating, pallor, peripheral cyanosis, hyperventilation, oliguria, and clouding of consciousness. Hemo-concentration and decreased organ perfusion lead to end-organ damage in the patients. The blood test results thus observed are mentioned in Table 3.6.

Hypovolemic shock is a component and end-result of all the types of shock, and may finally lead to ischemia and failure of all the organs. Initial stages are reversible and needs correction by fluid replacement and crystalloids. Failure to treat the underlying derangements timely and adequately may commence the beginning of the irreversible stage or the refractory shock, characterized by drug-resistant hypotension and multiorgan failure [79].

7.ii. Cardiogenic Shock

Cardiogenic shock is a disorder of cardiac function in the form of critical reduction of heart's pumping capacity [75, 76]. It is most commonly caused by acute myocardial infarction, which causes reduced ejection fraction, or may also be due to valvular stenosis and pericardial tamponade, which results in inadequate cardiac filling. Other causes are cardiomyopathies, myocarditis, drug toxicity, or trauma to heart.

Improper cardiac function leads to reduced left ventricular stroke volume [75, 76]. Tissue perfusion is reduced, resulting in similar features of cold shock (hypovolemic shock) as described above. However, heart rate is reduced here.

The laboratory findings in cardiogenic shock are both due to damage to heart muscle as well as resulting decreased blood pumping and end-organ damage (Table 3.7). Cardiogenic shock may result in hemodynamic instability, systemic inflammation, or multiorgan failure, and has high mortality. Primary treatment is to remove the cardiac cause of shock by coronary reperfusion and other supportive treatment.

7.iii. Anaphylactic Shock

Anaphylactic shock is characterized by a Type -I hypersensitivity reaction with massive histamine release [2, 4]. The most common trigger is food allergen, or insect venom, drugs, etc. Hypersensitivity reactions are usually IgE dependent and result in large amount of histamine release by the mast cells, resulting in vasodilation and fluid shift to extravascular spaces. The clinical presentation may vary according to the site and dose of allergen inoculation, but patients usually show increased eosinophils and IgE levels in blood.

7.iv. Septic Shock

Sepsis is a life-endangering organ failure caused by dysregulation of a patient's response to infection [80]. Septic shock is a grave complication of sepsis and is characterized by profound circulatory,

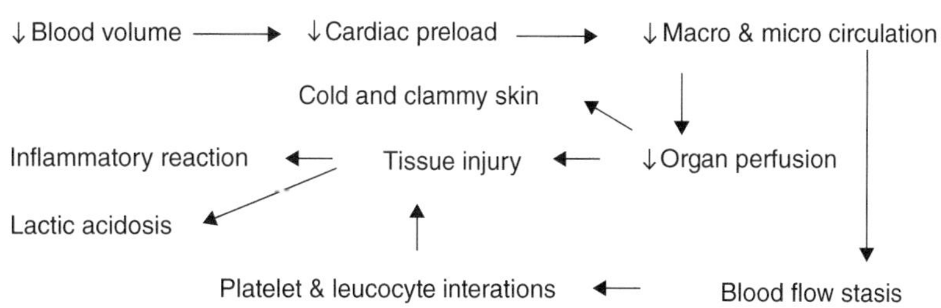

Fig. 3.4 Pathophysiology of hypovolemic shock. Decreased blood volume leads to reduced organ perfusion and blood stasis, precipitating tissue acidosis, inflammation, and injury

cellular, and metabolic abnormalities associated with sepsis. Severe sepsis occurs as a result of both community- and hospital-acquired infections, *Pneumonia* being the most common clinical presentation [81]. Exaggerated inflammatory response to the bacterial pathogens results in tissue damage, coagulopathies, and shock (Fig. 3.5). The symptoms of septic shock may overlap somewhat with those of sepsis, and the patients may present with fever, chills, and malaise due to severe infection. Later due to shock, symptoms of confusion, decreased urination, shortness of breath, and other symptoms of the affected organs may be seen [80]. Diagnosis can be confirmed by clinical conditions correlating with laboratory tests (Table 3.8).

Severe sepsis and septic shock represent one of the most common and challenging medical conditions [81]. Systemic bacterial infection can lead to bacterial infection of the other uninvolved organs. For example, such a patient may present with a red eye, and needs urgent attention as it can lead to metastatic (endogenous) endophthalmitis and subsequent visual loss [82].

Table 3.6 Lab investigations in hypovolemic shock

↑Hemoglobin and PCV
↑BUN, ↑creatinine, electrolyte imbalance
↓urine output, ↑ specific gravity, ↓urinary sodium

Table 3.7 Lab investigations in cardiogenic shock

↑WBC count
↑Cardiac troponins (MI) and/or ↑natriuretic peptides (CHF)
↓spO_2
↑liver transaminases, serum creatinine levels, etc. (later in multiorgan involvement)

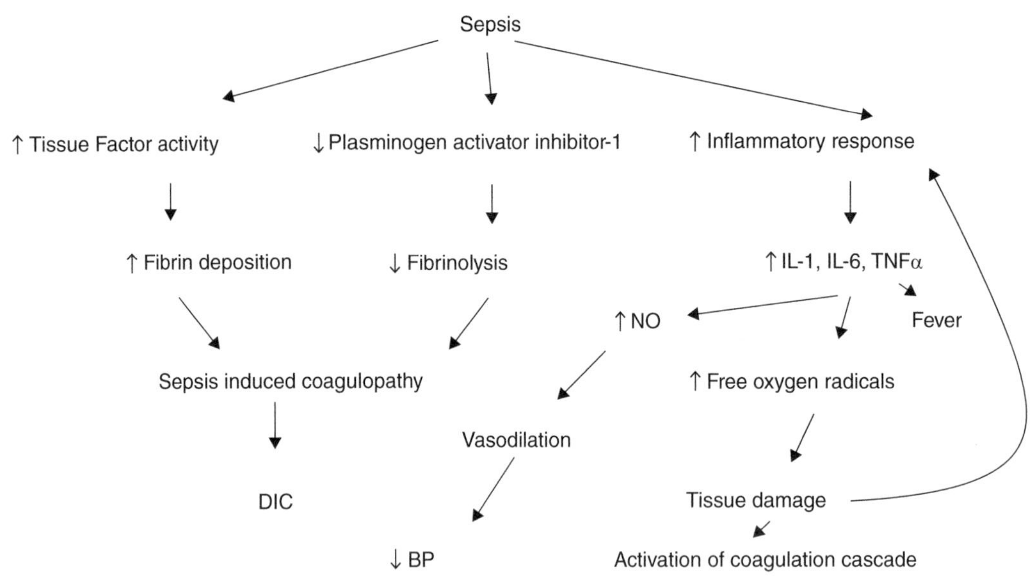

Fig. 3.5 Pathophysiology of septic shock [76, 80]. Severe infection leads to increased expression of tissue factor and reduces the expression of plasminogen activator inhibitor-1, thereby initiating coagulopathy. Also, inflammatory response to sepsis generates free radicals that further damage the tissue

Table 3.8 Laboratory findings in sepsis [75, 76, 80, 81]

1. Blood counts – leucocytosis, leucopenia, ↓ platelets
2. Biochemistry – ↑creatinine, ↑bilirubin, ↑lactate
3. Inflammatory markers – ↑IL -10, ↑↑CRP , ↑procalcitonin
4. Blood culture – positive
5. Sepsis-induced coagulopathy: prolonged PT, aPTT, ↑ D-dimer

3.8 Disseminated Intravascular Coagulation (DIC)

DIC is an acquired, life-threatening syndrome manifesting as extensive and unregulated coagulation activation [83]. It can arise from and damage the microvasculature, which can be good enough to cause the organ dysfunction [84]. Several pathological conditions like sepsis, trauma, pancreatitis, malignancies, liver cirrhosis, snake bites, and obstetric calamities like placenta previa, abortion, abruptio placentae, intrauterine death, etc., may trigger DIC [85].

In DIC, there is increased and widespread clot formation in circulation (Fig. 3.6). Thrombi formed cause microvascular obstruction and organ ischemia, while hemodynamic disturbances and metabolic derangements cause multi-organ dysfunction [83]. This may be manifested according to the organ involved, for example, renal insufficiency, respiratory failure, hypotension, circulatory failure, and impaired cerebral function. It may also present with multiorgan failure and bleeding. Bleeding occurs due to consumption of the clotting factors during excessive coagulation and, therefore, is also known as "consumption coagulopathy."

The diagnosis of DIC is based on clinical condition and the laboratory parameters (Table 3.9). Other causes of bleeding like impaired synthesis of coagulation factors, vitamin K deficiency, anticoagulant therapy, etc. need to be ruled out [83–85].

DIC can affect multiple organs, eye also being the one to face the vascular blockage. Patients with DIC can present with retinal detachment, vacuolar disruption of the pigment epithelium, choroidal hemorrhage, and occlusion of choriocapillaries [88]. A patient with these symptoms, especially if predisposed to DIC (like in eclampsia, abruptio placentae, etc.), should also be suspected and investigated for an early DIC besides treating the ophthalmic condition [89].

Covid-19 infection caused by SARS-COV2 virus usually causes self-limiting illness when the virus propagates down the airways, initiating an immune response, associated with systemic pro-inflammatory cytokines and activated immune cells [90, 91]. However, in about 20% of the patients, the virus may infect distal alveolar cells causing acute lung injury, leading to respiratory deterioration and mortality. Levels of pro-inflammatory cytokines like IL-1 and IL-6 are markedly raised. IL-6 induces increased Tissue Factor expression, consequently causing thrombin generation and coagulopathy. These patients are also found to develop venous thromboembolism and symptoms that *mimic* DIC with thrombocytopenia, elevated D-dimer, prolonged PT, and aPTT.

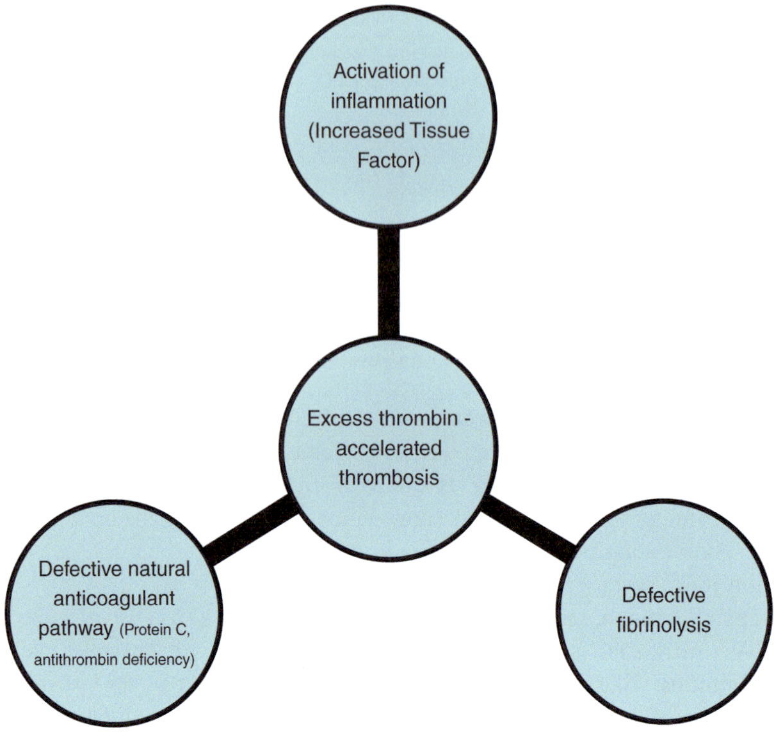

Fig. 3.6 Mechanisms causing accelerated microvascular fibrin deposition in DIC [86, 87]. Increased generation of thrombin, defective anticoagulation, and inadequate clot resolution go hand in hand for excessive clot formation

Table 3.9 Laboratory parameters in DIC

1. Platelet count – reduced
2. Bleeding time / clotting time – prolonged
3. Prothrombin time (PT) – prolonged
4. Activated partial thromboplastin time (aPTT) – prolonged
5. D- dimer levels – elevated
6. Serum fibrinogen levels – reduced

3.9 Summary

It is well known that any imbalance in homeostasis may lead to disturbances in fluid compartment and coagulation pathways in body. Some of the most common clinical conditions resulting from the loss of homeostasis include thrombosis, thromboembolism, edema, and shock. This chapter discusses their pathogenesis and also throws light on how they can affect eyes, with symptoms so vague, which can be easily overlooked until the ophthalmologist is aware of the disease pathogenesis. Laboratory tests to screen for the hemostatic disease and tests to monitor the therapy have also been described.

Acknowledgments I thank my mentors without whom this would not have been possible; Prof Geeta K. Vemuganti for the opportunity, direction, and guidance to write this chapter and also editing it; and Prof Harsh Mohan for great advice and providing the figure on coagulation pathways.

References

1. Klyce SD, Hallak J, Romond K, Azar D, Kim T-I. Corneal physiology: corneal form and function. In: Albert D, Miller J, Azar D, Young LH, editors. Albert and Jakobiec's principles and practice of ophthalmology. Cham: Springer; 2021. p. 1–74. https://doi.org/10.1007/978-3-319-90495-5_203-1.
2. Kumar V, Abbas AK, Aster JC, Perkins JA, Robbins SL, editors. Robbins basic pathology. 10th ed. Philadelphia: Elsevier; 2018.
3. Bliss MR. Hyperaemia. J Tissue Viability. 1988;8(4):4–13.
4. Mohan H. Textbook of pathology. 8th ed. New Delhi: Jaypee Brothers; 2018.
5. Newman EA. Functional hyperemia and mechanisms of neurovascular coupling in the retinal vasculature. J Cereb Blood Flow Metab. 2013;33(11):1685–95. https://doi.org/10.1038/jcbfm.2013.145. Epub 2013 Aug 21. PMID: 23963372; PMCID: PMC3824187.

6. Singh RB, et al. Ocular redness – I: Etiology, pathogenesis, and assessment of conjunctival hyperemia. Ocul Surf. 2021;21:134–44. https://doi.org/10.1016/j.jtos.2021.05.003. Epub 2021 May 16. PMID: 34010701; PMCID: PMC8328962.
7. Dunlop AL, Wells JR. Approach to red eye for primary care practitioners. Prim Care. 2015;42:267. https://doi.org/10.1016/j.pop.2015.05.002.
8. Riva CE, Logean E, Falsini B. Visually evoked hemodynamical response and assessment of neurovascular coupling in the optic nerve and retina. Prog Retin Eye Res. 2005;24:183–215.
9. Werblin FS, Dowling JE. Organization of the retina of the mudpuppy, *Necturus maculosus*. II. Intracellular recording. J Neurophysiol. 1969;32:339–55.
10. Roy CS, Sherrington CS. On the regulation of the blood-supply of the brain. J Physiol. 1890;11:85–108.
11. Arden GB, Sivaprasad S. The pathogenesis of early retinal changes of diabetic retinopathy. Doc Ophthalmol. 2012;124:15–26.
12. Boorsma EM, et al. Congestion in heart failure: a contemporary look at physiology, diagnosis and treatment. Nat Rev Cardiol. 2020;17(10):641–55. https://doi.org/10.1038/s41569-020-0379-7.
13. Dupont M, Mullens W, Tang WH. Impact of systemic venous congestion in heart failure. Curr Heart Fail Rep. 2011;8(4):233–41. https://doi.org/10.1007/s11897-011-0071-7.
14. Kishi S, Matsumoto H. A new insight into pachychoroid diseases: Remodeling of choroidal vasculature. Graefes Arch Clin Exp Ophthalmol. 2022;260(11):3405–17. https://doi.org/10.1007/s00417-022-05687-6. Epub 2022 May 16. PMID: 35575932; PMCID: PMC9581833.
15. Marenco M, Borgia L, Vagge A, Iester M. Choroidal congestion after trabeculectomy. Case Rep Ophthalmol. 2019;10(3):384–90. https://doi.org/10.1159/000504318. PMID: 31824290; PMCID: PMC6902214.
16. McGrath A, Barrett MJ. Petechiae. [Updated 2022 Sep 12]. In: StatPearls [Internet]. Treasure Island (FL): StatPearls Publishing; 2023. Available from: https://www.ncbi.nlm.nih.gov/books/NBK482331/.
17. Jaffe FA, Petechial hemorrhages. A review of pathogenesis. Am J Forensic Med Pathol. 1994;15(3):203–7. https://doi.org/10.1097/00000433-199409000-00004. PMID: 7825548.
18. Azari AA, Arabi A. Conjunctivitis: a systematic review. J Ophthalmic Vis Res. 2020;15(3):372–95. https://doi.org/10.18502/jovr.v15i3.7456. PMID: 32864068; PMCID: PMC7431717.
19. Bockholdt B, Maxeiner H, Hegenbarth W. Factors and circumstances influencing the development of hemorrhages in livor mortis. Forensic Sci Int. 2005;149(2–3):133–7. https://doi.org/10.1016/j.forsciint.2004.05.014.
20. Ruddy SM, Bergstrom R, Tivakaran VS. Roth Spots. [Updated 2023 Feb 12]. In: StatPearls [Internet]. Treasure Island (FL): StatPearls Publishing; 2023. Available from: https://www.ncbi.nlm.nih.gov/books/NBK482446/.
21. Trayes K, Pickle S, Tully A. Edema: diagnosis and management. Am Fam Physician. 2013;88(2):102–10.
22. Braunwald E, Loscalzo J. Edema. In: Longo DL, Fauci AS, Kasper DL, Hauser SL, Jameson JL, Loscalzo J, editors. Harrison's principles of internal medicine. 18th ed. New York: McGraw-Hill; 2018.
23. O'Brien J, Chennubhotla S, Chennubhotla R. Treatment of edema. Am Fam Physician. 2005;71(11):2111–7.
24. Cho S, Atwood J. Peripheral edema. Am J Med. 2002;113(7):580–6.
25. Lent-Schochet D, Jialal I. Physiology, Edema. [Updated 2023 May 1]. In: StatPearls [Internet]. Treasure Island (FL): StatPearls Publishing; 2023. Available from: https://www.ncbi.nlm.nih.gov/books/NBK537065/.
26. Paramothayan N, Barron J. New criteria for the differentiation between transudates and exudates. J Clin Pathol. 2002;55(1):69–71.
27. Light R, Macgregor M, Luchsinger P, Ball W. Pleural effusions: the diagnostic separation of transudates and exudates. Ann Intern Med. 1972;77(4):507–13.
28. Yale S, Mazza J. Approach to diagnosing lower extremity edema. Compr Ther. 2001;27(3):242–52.
29. Ely J, Osheroff J, Chambliss M, Ebell M. Approach to leg edema of unclear etiology. J Am Board Fam Med. 2006;19(2):148–60.
30. Moffatt C, Keeley V, Quere I. The concept of chronic edema-A neglected public health issue and an international response: the LIMPRINT study. Lymphat Res Biol. 2019;17(2):121–6.
31. Feizi S. Corneal endothelial cell dysfunction: etiologies and management. Therap Adv Ophthalmol. 2018;10:1–19. https://doi.org/10.1177/2515841418815802.
32. Maurice DM. The cornea and sclera. In: Davson H, editor. The eye. Orlando: Academic; 1984.
33. Bourne WM. Biology of the corneal endothelium in health and disease. Eye. 2003;17:912–8.
34. Mackman N. Triggers, targets and treatments for thrombosis. Nature. 2008;451(7181):914–8.
35. Carobbio A, et al. Risk factors for arterial and venous thrombosis in WHO- defined essential thrombocythemia: an international study of 891 patients. Blood. 2011;117(22):5857–9. https://doi.org/10.1182/blood-2011-02-339002.
36. Previtali E, Bucciarelli P, Passamonti S, Martinelli I. Risk factors for venous and arterial thrombosis. Blood Transfus. 2011;9:120–38.
37. Koupenova M, Clancy L, Corkrey HA, Freedman JE. Circulating platelets as mediators of immunity, inflammation and thrombosis. Circ Res. 2018;122(2):337–51.
38. Parakh R, Sabath D. Venous thromboembolism: role of the clinical laboratory in diagnosis and management. J Appl Lab Med. 2019;3(5):870–82.
39. Bagot CN, Arya R. Virchow and his triad: a question of attribution. Br J Haematol. 2008;143(2):180–90.

40. Lyaker M, et al. Arterial embolism. Int J Crit Illn Inj Sci. 2013;3(1):77–87.
41. Klein R, Klein B, Jensen SC, et al. Retinal emboli and stroke. The Beaver Dam eye study. Arch Ophthalmol. 1999;117(8):1063–8.
42. Russell R. The source of retinal emboli. Lancet. 1968;2(7572):789–92.
43. Moheimani F, Jackson D. Venous thromboembolism: classification, risk factors, diagnosis, and management. ISRN Hematol. 2011;2011:124610.
44. Chen T, Uppuluri A, Zarbin M, Bhagat N. Risk factors for central retinal vein occlusion in young adults. Eur J Ophthalmol. 2021;31(5):2546–55. https://doi.org/10.1177/1120672120960333.
45. Wells P, Owen C, Doucette S, Fergusson D, Tran H. Does this patient have deep vein thrombosis? JAMA. 2006;295(2):199–207. https://doi.org/10.1001/jama.295.2.199.
46. Van Cott E, Laposata M, Prins M. Laboratory evaluation of hypercoagulability with venous or arterial thrombosis: venous thromboembolism, myocardial infarction, stroke, and other conditions. Arch Pathol Lab Med. 2002;126(11):1281–95.
47. Ridker P, Wells P, Owen C, Doucette S, Fergusson D, Tran H. Does this patient have deep vein thrombosis. JAMA. 2006;295(2):199–207. https://doi.org/10.1001/jama.295.2.199.
48. Danesh J, Whincup P, Walker M, et al. Low grade inflammation and coronary heart disease: prospective study and updated meta-analyses. Br Med J. 2000;321(7255):199–204.
49. Ridker PM, Hennekens CH, Buring JE, Rifai N. C-reactive protein and other markers of inflammation in the prediction of cardiovascular disease in women. N Engl J Med. 2000;342:836–43.
50. Ridker PM, Stampfer MJ, Rifai N. Novel risk factors for systemic atherosclerosis: a comparison of C-reactive protein, fibrinogen, homocysteine, lipoprotein (a), and standard cholesterol screening as predictors of peripheral arterial disease. JAMA. 2001;285:2481–5.
51. Mirski M, Lele A, Fitzsimmons L, Toung T. Diagnosis and treatment of vascular air embolism. Anesthesiology. 2007;106(1):164–77.
52. Takeoka M, Sakai A, Ueda G, et al. Influence of hypoxia and pulmonary air embolism on lung injury in perfused rat lungs. Respiration. 1996;63(6):346–51.
53. Kapoor T, Gutierrez G. Air embolism as a cause of the systemic inflammatory response syndrome: a case report. Crit Care. 2003;7(5):R98–R100.
54. Lam K, Hutchinson R, Gin T. Severe pulmonary edema after venous air embolism. Can J Anesth. 1993;40(10):964–7.
55. Horton J. Air bubbles introduced from peripheral intravenous lines into the cerebral venous system. J Neuroophthalmol. 2019;39(3):437.
56. Toung T, Rossberg M, Hutchins G. Volume of air in a lethal venous air embolism. Anesthesiology. 2001;94:360–1.
57. Le S, Rozans M, Szerlip H. Air embolism after intravenous injection of contrast material. South Med J. 1999;92(9):930–3.
58. Woodring J, Fried A. Nonfatal venous air embolism after contrast enhanced CT. Radiology. 1988;167(2):405–7.
59. Phatak U, David E, Kulkarni P. Decompression syndrome (Caisson disease) in an Indian diver. Ann Indian Acad Neurol. 2010;13(3):202–3.
60. Vann RD, Butler FK, Mitchell SJ, Moon RE. Decompression illness. Lancet. 2011;377(9760):153–64.
61. Howle L, et al. The probability and severity of decompression sickness. PLoS One. 2017;12(3):e0172665.
62. Iordanidou V, , et al. Choroidal ischemia secondary to a diving injury. Retin Cases Brief Rep 2010;4(3):262–265.
63. Omar A, Ibrahim M, Hussein A. Acute ophthalmic artery occlusion in decompression illness with underlying anterior cerebral artery A1 segment hypoplasia. Diving Hyperb Med. 2018;48(2):112–3.
64. Muller C, Rahn B, Pfister U, Meinig R. The incidence, pathogenesis, diagnosis, and treatment of fat embolism. Orthop Rev. 1994;23(2):107–17.
65. Cantu C, Pavlisko E. Liposuction-induced fat embolism syndrome: a brief review and postmortem diagnostic approach. Arch Pathol Lab Med. 2018;142(7):871–5.
66. Parisi D, Koval K, Egol K. Fat embolism syndrome. Am J Orthop (Belle Mead NJ). 2002;31(9):507–12.
67. Putthirangsiwong B, et al. (2021) superior ophthalmic vein embolism following forehead augmentation with autologous fat injection. Aesth Plast Surg. 2022;46(1):450–5. https://doi.org/10.1007/s00266-021-02414-0.
68. Kaur K, et al. Amniotic fluid embolism. J Anaesthesiol Clin Pharmacol. 2016;32(2):153–9.
69. Kim I, Choi J. Occlusions of branch retinal arterioles following amniotic fluid embolism. Ophthalmologica. 2000;214(4):305–8.
70. Fischbein F. Ischemic retinopathy following amniotic fluid embolization. Am J Ophthalmol. 1969;67(3):351–7.
71. Slichter S. Relationship between platelet count and bleeding risk in thrombocytopenic patients. Transfus Med Rev. 2004;18(3):153–67.
72. Wolberg AS, Meng ZH, Monroe DM 3rd, Hoffman M. A systematic evaluation of the effect of temperature on coagulation enzyme activity and platelet function. J Trauma. 2004;56(6):1221–8.
73. Meng ZH, Wolberg AS, Monroe DM 3rd, Hoffman M. The effect of temperature and pH on the activity of factor VIIa: implications for the efficacy of high dose factor VIIa in hypothermic and acidotic patients. J Trauma. 2003;55(5):886–91.
74. Peyvandi F, et al. Laboratory testing in hemophilia. Impact of factor and non-factor replacement therapy on coagulation assays. J Thromb Haemost. 2020;18(6):1242–55.

75. Standl T, et al. The nomenclature, definition, and distinction of types of shock. Deutsch Arztebl Int. 2018;115(45):757–68.
76. Kislitsma O, et al. Shock- classification and pathophysiological principles of therapeutics. Curr Cardiol Rev. 2019;15(2):102–13.
77. Ledingham MCA, Ramsay G. Hypovolaemic shock. Br J Anaestheiol. 1986;58:169–89.
78. Hardaway R. Monitoring of the patient in a state of shock. Surg Gynecol Obstet. 1979;148:339.
79. Bonanno FG. Clinical pathology of the shock syndromes. J Emerg Trauma Shock. 2011;4(2):233–43.
80. Huerta L, Rice T. Pathologic difference between sepsis and bloodstream infections. J Appl Lab Med. 2019;3(4):654–63.
81. Angus D, Poll T. Severe sepsis and septic shock. N Engl J Med. 2013;369:840–51.
82. Khan A, Okhravi N, Lightman S. The eye in systemic sepsis. Clin Med (London, England). 2002;2(5):444–8.
83. Papageorgiou C, et al. Disseminated intravascular coagulation: an update on pathogenesis, diagnosis, and therapeutic strategies. Clin Appl Thromb/Hemost. 2018;24(9S):8S–28S.
84. Wada H, et al. Guidance for diagnosis and treatment of DIC from harmonization of the recommendations from three guidelines. J Thromb Haemost. 2013;11(4):761–7.
85. Okabayashi K, et al. Hemostatic markers and the sepsis-related organ failure assessment score in patients with disseminated intravascular coagulation in an intensive care unit. Am J Hematol. 2004;76(3):225–9.
86. Giles AR, Nesheim ME, Mann KG. Studies of factors V and VIII:C in an animal model of disseminated intravascular coagulation. J Clin Invest. 1984;74(6):2219–25.
87. Gando S, Nanzaki S, Sasaki S, Kemmotsu O. Significant correlation between tissue factor and thrombin markers in trauma and septic patients with disseminated intravascular coagulation. Thromb Haemost. 1998;79(6):1111–5.
88. Cogan DG. Ocular involvement in disseminated intravascular coagulopathy. Arch Ophthalmol. 1975;93(1):1–8.
89. Hoines J, Buettner H. Ocular complications of disseminated intravascular coagulation (DIC) in abruptio placentae. Retina. 1989;9(2):105–9.
90. Levi M, Iba T. COVID-19 coagulopathy: is it disseminated intravascular coagulation? Intern Emerg Med. 2021;16:309–12.
91. Honavar S, Sen M, Sharma N, Sachdev M. COVID-19 and eye: a review of ophthalmic manifestations of COVID-19. Indian J Ophthalmol. 2021;69(3):488–509.

Inflammation and Healing

4

Indranil Chakrabarti

Contents

I. Chakrabarti (✉)
Department of Pathology and Laboratory Medicine,
All India Institute of Medical Sciences,
Kalyani, West Bengal, India

G. K. Vemuganti et al. (eds.), *Ocular Pathology*, https://doi.org/10.1007/978-981-96-8614-8_4

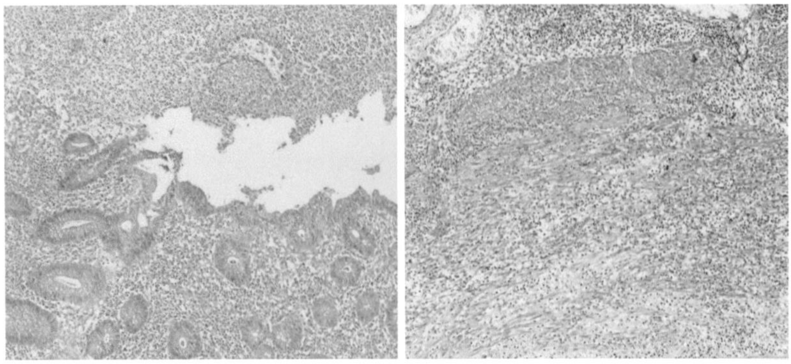

Fig. 4.1 Section from appendix showing ulcerated mucosa and acute inflammatory cells in all the layers in a case of acute appendicitis

4.1 Inflammation

Inflammation is the tissue response of the host to sublethal injury by injurious agents as part of the body's defense mechanism to eliminate the offending agent. The injurious agent is nonself in most of the cases but may rarely be the own cell or tissue of the host, which, being mistakenly treated as nonself, can lead to autoimmune diseases. Though part of the protective mechanism of the body, if unchecked, it may result in severe damage to the host, for example, rheumatoid arthritis, hypersensitivity reactions etc. The inflammation of tissue is denoted by adding "itis" at the end of the inflamed organ, for example, the acute inflammation of the appendix is known as acute appendicitis (Fig. 4.1).

It is important to note the difference between inflammation and infection. Infection is the invasion and growth of microorganisms (bacteria, viruses, viroids, fungus, parasites, etc.) as well as the tissue response against such offending agents or their toxins. Inflammation, on the other hand, can be against infectious or noninfectious agents (e.g., necrotic tissue, foreign bodies like sutures, immunological agents, etc.). Thus, inflammation may be considered a part of infection, but inflammation is not always accompanied by infection. More so, inflammation is a protective response that consists of an early inflammatory response followed by healing, while infection refers to the invasion of microorganisms and its harmful effects only.

4.2 Cardinal Signs of Inflammation [1]

Roman encyclopedist Aulus Cornelius Celsus in first century AD described the 4 cardinal signs of inflammation: Those are

1. Rubor (redness)
2. Calor (heat)
3. Dolor (pain)
4. Tumor(swelling)

The legendary fifth cardinal sign of function laesa or loss of function was promulgated to the tetrad by Rudolf Virchow who is widely regarded as "the father of modern pathology."

4.3 Classification of Inflammation

According to the duration and host defense, inflammation can be divided into the following:

(a) Acute inflammation (a few minutes to less than 48 h)
(b) Chronic inflammation (lasting for days, weeks, years)

However, it must be remembered that inflammation is a dynamic process, the duration and hence the classification depends on several factors like persistence of the inciting agent, host defense capacity, etc.

4.4 Acute Inflammation

Acute inflammation is a rapid onset, early response of the host, which is transient and that lasts for less than 48 h. The common etiological agents include infectious agents, toxins, mechanical, chemical, or physical injury, tissue necrosis, foreign bodies, endogenous products, immunological reactions (hypersensitivity reactions, autoimmune disorders), etc.

Acute inflammation is characterized by the escape of fluid rich in proteins and blood cells from the vascular space to the site of injury (interstitial tissues/body cavity). This process is known as *exudation*. Thus, by definition, an exudate is an extravascular fluid of high specific gravity, rich in protein and cellular debris, which occurs due to increased vascular permeability during inflammation. On the other hand, a transudate is a fluid with low protein and cell content, low specific gravity resulting due to osmotic/hydrostatic pressure imbalance across the vessels with normal vascular permeability. Edema, which refers to excessive accumulation of fluid in interstitial tissue or body cavities, can be either an exudate or transudate [2].

4.5 Pathogenesis of Acute Inflammation [3]

Though acute inflammation is a continuous process, the major events may be divided into

1. Vascular events
2. Chemical events

1. *Vascular Events*:

The earliest changes occur in the microvasculature (arterioles, capillaries, venules) of the host circulation with the main purpose of delivering the protein-rich exudate and circulating cells to the site of injury in an attempt to limit the tissue damage. It can be broadly divided into

(i) Changes in the vessel caliber or hemodynamic changes and
(ii) Cellular changes

(i) *Changes in the Vessel Caliber*:

The earliest reaction to injury or trauma is known as the *triple response* of *Flush, Flare, and Weal.*

Transient vasoconstriction lasting for seconds (earliest vessel response to injury due to neurogenic effect mediated by catecholamines released from sympathetic nerve endings) is followed by persistent.

Vasodilatation of arterioles>capillaries and venules with increased blood flow lasting for about 8 h and responsible for the rubor (redness) and calor (heat) (caused by various vasodilators like histamine, prostaglandins, serotonin, nitric oxide etc. released from various inflammatory cells and damaged tissue).

This is followed by increased vascular permeability of postcapillary venules (mediated by histamine, serotonin, prostaglandins, nitric oxide, bradykinin, Interleukin 1, Tumor necrosis factor (TNF), Interferon γ, C3, C5a fibrin split products etc.)

[Mechanisms involved are contraction of the endothelial lining by various chemical mediators, direct endothelial injury by toxins, physical and chemical agents, burns, etc., injury caused by leucocytes, and leaky new vessel formation by Vascular Endothelial Growth Factors (VEGFs)].

Consequently, there is increase in blood volume with an increase in local hydrostatic pressure resulting in exudation of fluid in the extracellular space along with large protein molecules (exudation causes localized edema or weal of the triple response)

Once there is exudation of fluid from the vascular component, there is an increase in viscosity of blood due to a higher cell: plasma ratio resulting in slowing of blood flow (*STASIS* of blood)

(ii) *Cellular Changes*

The cellular response is a multistep process that includes the recruitment of leucocytes at the extravascular site of injury, their activation to identify the microbes, phagocytosis, and clearing off the offender.

In acute inflammation, the key players are neutrophils supported by mast cells and macrophages, while in chronic inflammation, the major role is played by lymphocytes along with macrophages.

The cellular phase of acute inflammation can be divided into 4 headings:

(a) Exudation of leucocytes
(b) Chemotaxis
(c) Activation of leucocytes
(d) Phagocytosis
(a) *Exudation of Leucocytes*

To effectively control the offending agent, the leucocytes need to escape from the microvasculature to the interstitial tissue. This involves several steps as follows:

- *Margination*: In axial or normal blood flow, the heavier leucocytes move through the center of the blood flow. The lighter RBCs travel more peripherally, close to the cell-free plasmatic zone that flows along the sides of the vascular wall. When stasis occurs and the increased hydrostatic pressure drives out a part of the plasma into the extravascular compartment, the axial flow is disrupted. The RBCs stick together loosely (Rouleaux formation) and displace leucocytes to the periphery along the margins of the vessel wall (known as *Margination*).
- *Rolling and Pavementation*: The marginated leucocytes tumble along endothelial lining (known as *rolling*). At first, the cells attach transiently while eventually they adhere and line the endothelial cells with the help of *adhesion molecules* like the stones in a pavement (known as *pavementation*). The adhesion molecules are present on the surfaces of both leucocytes and endothelial cells, which help the process.

  The *leucocyte adhesion molecules* include *selectins* like *L-selectin* (LCAM/CD62L), which are Sialyl-Lewis-X modified proteins and *integrins* (e.g., B1 integrins VLA-4 binding to VCAM −1 on endothelial cells and B2 integrins like LFA-1 and MAC-1 binding to ICAM-1).

  The *endothelial adhesion molecules* include *selectins* like *E-selectin*, and *P-selectin* (also present on platelets) as well as ligands belonging to the *immunoglobulin G superfamily* (e.g., VCAM-1 and ICAM-1).
- *Transmigration*: After adhesion, the neutrophils throw out their pseudopods from their surface and by active amoeboid movement move out through the gaps between the endothelial cells and pierce through the basement membrane. This process is known as *diapedesis*. The process is mediated by PECAM-1, another molecule belonging to the immunoglobulin superfamily. Along with the neutrophils, some RBCs also passively leave the circulation to the extravascular space giving a hemorrhagic appearance to the exudate.

(b) *Chemotaxis*

Chemotaxis is the process of migration of leucocytes to the extravascular site of injury guided by several chemical molecules and factors known as *chemoattractants*.

The chemoattractants may be exogenous (soluble bacterial and mitochondrial products) or endogenous (components of complement system, for example, C5a, a product of lipoxygenase pathway, for example, Leukotriene B4 or LT4, Cytokines like Interleukin 8, Kallikrein, etc.).

4.6 Steps of Chemotaxis

Step 1: Binding of chemoattractants to the seven-transmembrane G-protein-coupled receptors (GPCRs) on the surface of leucocytes.
Step 2: GPCRs sends activation signals to effector molecules within the leucocytes, which leads to increased cytosolic calcium entry.
Step 3: Entry of calcium leads to cytoskeletal changes resulting in the polymerization of actin and contraction of actin-regulating proteins.
Step 4: Forward movement of leucocytes to the site of injury.

The predominant leucocytes at the epicenter of injury for the first 6–24 h are the neutrophils. These neutrophils disappear after 24–48 h except in *Pseudomonas* infection where the neutrophilic infiltrate is long-lasting. The neutrophilic infiltrate after 48 h is replaced by monocytes. Slowly, if the inflammation persists for a few days, macrophages and lymphocytes are recruited. In viral infections, the lymphocytes predominate from the very beginning, while eosinophils predominate in hypersensitivity reactions and parasitic infections.

(c) *Activation of Leucocytes*

Several receptors exist on the surface of leucocytes that recognize various stimuli (e.g., microbial products/microbes, chemical mediators etc.) once they are at the site of injury. These lead to the activation of leucocytes, which is essential for phagocytosis and the final degradation of injurious agents. The various receptors on the surface, which lead to leucocyte activation include the following:

Toll-like receptors (TLRs), seven-transmembrane G-protein-coupled receptors (GPCRs), cytokine receptors, opsonin receptors, phagocytic receptors, etc.

(d) *Phagocytosis*

Phagocytosis is a property of phagocytes like neutrophils and macrophages in which the injurious agent, dead cells, etc. are recognized, internalized, and degraded. It was first described by *Elie Metchnikoff* in 1882 after experimenting on the larvae of starfish.

The major steps of phagocytosis are as follows:

Opsonization Opsonins are molecules like IgG, C3b, mannose-binding lectin (MBL), etc., which coat the injurious agents and make them "tasty" for the leucocytes to engulf. Leucocytes contain specific receptors (e.g., FcR1, MBL receptors) for opsonins so that they can recognize and bind with the injurious agents. Defect in opsonization result in *Bruton's agammaglobulinemia.*

Engulfment of Injurious Agent The phagocytes by the help of actin filaments create pseudopods in and around the opsonized injurious agent and internalize it completely within an endophagocytic vacuole known as *phagosome.*

Formation of Phagolysosome and Destruction of Injurious Agent The phagosome fuses with lysosome to form the *phagolysosome* within which the neutrophils release the hydrolytic lysosomal enzymes, leading to the degradation of the injurious agent. Defect in phagolysosome formation and defective degranulation of neutrophils cause *Chediak -Higashi syndrome.*

The intracellular microbial killing agents include the following:

(a) Reactive species from oxygen: Oxygen-derived free radicals (ODFRs) such as superoxide ($O^-{}_2$) ions, hydroxyl (OH^-) radicals, and hydrogen peroxide (H_2O_2) (see below)
(b) Reactive species from halides (HOCl, HOI, HOBr)
(c) Nitric oxide
(d) Lysosomal granules (MPO, protease, phospholipase lactoferrin, defensins, DNase, Major basic protein (MBP), etc.)

Phagocytosis stimulates rapid activation of its NADPH oxidase, which results in the following reaction:

$$2O_2 + NADPH \xrightarrow{\boxed{\text{NADPH oxidase}}} 2O_2^- + NADP^+ + H^+$$

$$2O_2^- + 2H^+ \xrightarrow{\boxed{\text{Superoxidase dismutase}}} H_2O_2 \rightarrow OH^- + OH$$

MPO-dependent microbial killing may occur as follows:

$$H_2O_2 \xrightarrow{\boxed{\text{Myeloperoxidase+Chloride}}} HOCl(\text{hypochlorous acid}) + H_2O$$

MPO-independent microbial killing may occur by the following reactions:

$$Fe^{2+} + H_2O_2 \rightarrow Fe^{3+} + OH^- + HO^- \ (\textbf{Fenton reaction})$$

$$\cdot O_2^- + H_2O_2 \rightarrow \cdot OH + OH^- + O_2 \ (\textbf{Haber Heiss reaction})$$

4.7 Chemical Mediators of Inflammation

The various chemical mediators of inflammation may be (a) cell-derived mediators and (b) plasma protein-derived mediators.

4.7.1 Cell-Derived Chemical Mediators

These may be preformed or newly synthesized by cells under some stimulation. These include

(i) Vasoactive amines: Histamine, serotonin (5-hydroxytryptamine), Neuropeptides (Substance P, VIP, somatostatin, etc.).
(ii) Eicosanoids (Arachidonic acid metabolites): They may be cyclo-oxygenase pathway derived (Prostaglandins, Prostacyclins, Thromboxane A_2) or Lipoxygenase pathway derived (Leukotrienes, Lipoxins, 5 HETE).
(iii) Cytokines (Interleukins like IL1, IL-6, IL-8, IL-12,IL-17, TNFα and β, IFNγ, etc.).
(iv) Platelet-activating factor (PAF).
(v) Free radicals (as mentioned above).

4.7.2 Plasma-Protein-Derived Mediators

These are the products derived from

(i) The kinin system (Bradykinin, kallikrein)
(ii) The coagulation pathway (fibrin, etc.)
(iii) The fibrinolytic system (plasmin)
(iv) The complement system (C3a, C3b, C5a, etc.)

4.8 Morphological Patterns of Acute Inflammation [4]

The etiological agent, the duration of inflammation, and the tissue involved dictate the morphological patterns of acute inflammation. The major types are

(a) *Serous inflammation*—Serous (serum-like or watery) fluid exudation with low cellular content in coelomic cavities (e.g., in natural spaces like pleural, peritoneal, and pericardial cavities, synovial spaces, which are known as effusions) and skin (blisters, burns).
(b) *Fibrinous inflammation*—Inflammation in which the fibrin content is very high caused by increased vascular permeability and extravasation of fibrinogen forming an eosinophilic thread-like meshwork in coelomic surfaces or meninges. The "bread and butter pericarditis" in patients with acute rheumatic pericarditis refers to such shaggy, fibrinous pericardial exudates.
(c) *Purulent (suppurative) inflammation*—Formation of creamy pus due to the liquefactive necrosis by pyogenic bacteria like *Staphylococcus aureus* results in abscess formation. The pus contains inflammatory fibrinous exudate with degenerated neutrophils (*pus cells*), bacteria, and cell debris.
(d) *Catarrhal inflammation*—Catarrhal inflammation is characterized by a seromucinous secretion in mucosal surfaces, for example, catarrhal rhinitis in common cold.
(e) *Hemorrhagic inflammation*—It is characterized by blood-tinged discharges resulting from vascular damage, for example, in acute pancreatitis, etc.
(f) *Gangrenous inflammation*—Also known as necrotizing inflammation, this is caused by vascular occlusion, for example, gangrenous appendicitis.
(g) *Pseudomembranous inflammation*—This refers to the formation of a shaggy false or pseudomembrane caused by coagulated plasma along with necrosed epithelium on the denuded mucosal surfaces caused by irri-

tant gases or toxins, for example, pseudomembranous colitis caused by *Clostridium difficile*, pseudomembrane in pharynx and trachea caused by *Corynebacterium diphtheriae*, etc.

4.9 Systemic Effects of Acute Inflammation Include

1. Fever
2. Leukocytosis
3. Rise in acute phase reactants like C-reactive protein (CRP), haptoglobin, fibrinogen, ceruloplasmin, $\alpha 1$ antitrypsin, etc.
4. Lymphangitis and lymphadenopathy
5. Septic shock

4.10 Fate of Acute Inflammation

The fate of acute inflammation may be one of the following:

(a) *Resolution*: Complete restoration to the original, normal state following acute inflammation. This occurs when the injury is short lasting and not severe and the tissue damage is limited.
(b) *Healing by fibrosis*: If the destruction is more extensive and resolution is not possible, the tissue is repaired by fibrosis.
(c) *Suppuration and abscess formation*: Pyogenic bacteria may cause suppuration, that is, formation of pus (vide Purulent inflammation above) in a body cavity forming an *abscess*. The pus accumulating within a hollow viscus like pleural cavity or gall bladder is known as *empyema*.
(d) *Progression to chronic inflammation*: Recurrent or persistent acute inflammation may proceed to chronic inflammation.

4.11 Chronic Inflammation

Chronic inflammation is defined as inflammation of prolonged duration (weeks and months) due to persistent or recurrent injury in which the process of inflammation and healing go on side by side. e.g. chronic cholecystitis (Fig. 4.2).

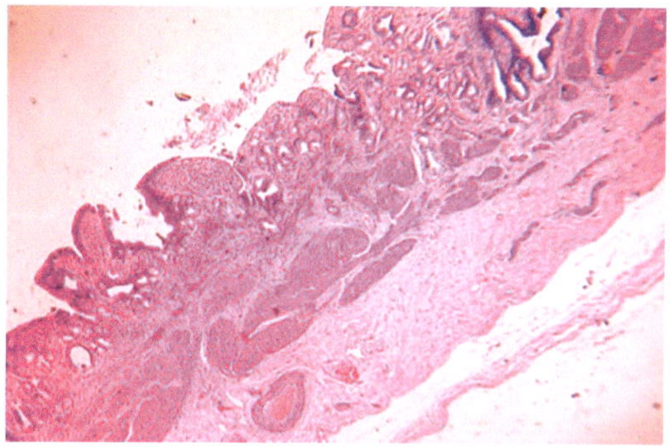

Fig. 4.2 Section from gall bladder wall showing features of chronic cholecystitis

It may be a consequence of acute inflammation, but most cases arise de novo, that is, without preceding acute inflammation.

The common causes of chronic inflammation are as follows:

(a) Progression from acute inflammation: If the injurious agents persist, acute inflammation may give way to a persistent chronic inflammation, for example, peptic ulcer, etc.
(b) Persistent infection: Microorganisms of low virulence, which resist elimination or intracellular microbial killing, may incite chronic inflammation, for example, tuberculosis caused by *Mycobacterium tuberculosis*.
(c) Prolonged exposure to toxic agents: Exposure to irritant gases may cause chronic inflammation of the respiratory tract.
(d) Autoimmune diseases.

4.12 Pathogenesis of Chronic Inflammation

Chronic inflammation is characterized by the following:

1. *Mononuclear cell infiltration*: The cellular hallmark of chronic inflammation is infiltration by lymphocytes and macrophages. The tissue macrophages are believed to be derived from extravasation of blood mono-

cytes. The macrophages and lymphocytes secrete many biologically active molecules and activate each other. They also recruit the antibody-producing plasma cells. Other inflammatory cells like eosinophils, mast cells, and neutrophils also play a part. Following the acute inflammation-induced neutrophilic infiltration, macrophages rush to the site and clear up the dead cells and inflammatory exudate if the inciting agent is removed. If the inflammation progresses to the chronic phase, the macrophage accumulation and proliferation continue and it also regulates the lymphocytic response. The various subtypes of lymphocytes involved are T cells, B cells, and NK cells. The macrophages get activated by toxins, various chemical mediators, IFNγ released by activated T lymphocytes. The activated macrophages secrete various products like cytokines (IL1, IL-6, IL-8, TNFα, etc.), lysosomal enzymes, reactive oxygen and nitrogen species, and growth factors like PDGF, TGFβ, FGF, etc. These substances activate lymphocytes, which in turn activate macrophages, thus perpetuating the inflammatory response till the injurious agent is eliminated. The other factors carry out tissue destruction, granulation tissue formation, and fibrosis.

2. *Tissue Destruction*: This is brought about by various proteases (e.g., elastase, collagenase, metalloproteinases), free radicals, and cytokines secreted by activated macrophages.
3. *Granulation Tissue Formation and Fibrosis*: Following necrosis, there is the formation of neoangiogenesis (formation of new vessels) and proliferation of fibroblasts due to secretion of angiogenic growth factors (e.g., VEGF), fibroblast growth factor (FGF), etc. secreted by activated macrophages, resulting in the formation of *granulation tissue*. This is followed by healing by fibrosis. Several factors like PDGF, EGF, TGF-β, etc. are involved in the recruitment of fibroblasts, which is followed by collagen deposition and early wound healing.

Systemic Effects of Chronic Inflammation Include the Following

1. Fever
2. Leukocytosis—dominated by lymphocytes
3. ESR: ESR is raised
4. Anemia
5. Secondary systemic amyloidosis: in long-standing cases

4.13 Granulomatous Inflammation

Granulomatous inflammation is a specific and distinct type of chronic inflammation against poorly digestible organisms, of which the body cannot get rid of easily or prolonged exposure to various endogenous and exogenous substances or due to immune causes. It is characterized by granuloma along with mononuclear cells like lymphocytes and plasma cells. The various causes can thus be grouped as:

1. *Infectious Causes*: Mycobacterial infections (e.g., *Mycobacterium tuberculosis, Mycobacterium leprae*), syphilis (*Treponema pallidum*), fungal infections (Histoplasmosis, cryptococcosis, coccidioidomycosis), parasitic diseases (schistosomiasis), bacterial diseases (Cat scratch disease).
2. *Prolonged Exposure to Substances* (*endogenous substances* like fat necrosis, uric acid crystals, etc. and *exogenous substances* like surgical suture materials, talc, asbestos fibers, silica, etc.) Such granulomas are also known as foreign body granulomas.
3. *Immune Diseases*: Rheumatoid arthritis, Ulcerative colitis, and Crohn's disease, etc.

4.14 Formation of a Tubercular Granuloma

A tubercular granuloma is a Type IV hypersensitivity reaction of the host against the capsular protein of the persistent tubercular bacilli, which

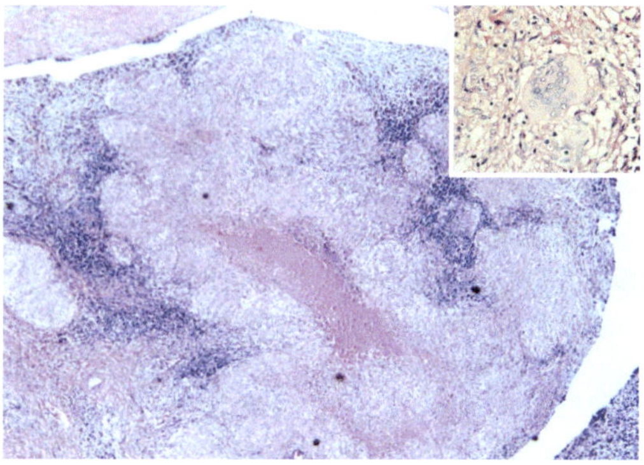

Fig. 4.3 Caseating granuloma with Langhan's giant cell (inset) in a case of tubercular lymphadenitis

the host could not digest. This leads to activation of macrophages resulting in the presentation of antigen to the CD4+ T lymphocytes, which in turn synthesize IL 1, IL 2, TNFα, IFN γ, etc. IFN γ, in turn, transforms the macrophages into epithelioid cells, while IL 1 and 2 recruit more lymphocytes. Thus, a granuloma is a microscopic focus of chronic inflammation composed of epithelioid cells, lymphocytes, plasma cells, and a few multinucleated giant cells (Langhan's type and foreign body type), which is surrounded by fibroblasts or collagen, depending upon the age of the granuloma. Langhan's giant cells are multinucleated giant cells formed by the fusion of macrophages in which the nuclei are arranged at the periphery in a circular fashion like a ring or in a semicircular pattern as a horseshoe. The center of a tubercular granuloma often shows cheese-like necrosis known as caseous necrosis (Fig. 4.3). However, it must be remembered that a tubercular granuloma can be noncaseating as well.

4.15 Fate of Chronic Inflammation

The fate of chronic inflammation is usually healing by fibrosis resulting in the formation of scar tissue, strictures (e.g., Crohn's disease), or adhesions (e.g., constrictive pericarditis).

Healing and Repair

The host tissue tries to come back to normal following inflammation by the process of repair. There are 2 major methods of tissue repair, depending upon the tissue and the severity of the injury.

(i) *Regeneration*: Some tissue has the capacity to revert to the normal state following a superficial injury by a process known as *regeneration*. This is particularly true in the case of the rapidly dividing cells of skin and gut epithelia as well the liver. This occurs by the proliferation of the remaining undamaged cells and from the stem cell pool of the organs.

(ii) *Repair by Connective Tissue Deposition (Scar)*: If the damage is severe enough to destroy the supporting structures of the tissue, there is no scope for regeneration. In those cases, the repair or healing is done by deposition of connective tissue by fibroblasts resulting in the formation of a *scar*. The scarred tissue retains most of the normal functioning of the organ, but extensive fibrosis can compromise the architecture and functioning at times. When the collagen deposition is extensive, the term fibrosis is generally used. If fibrosis occurs in a space that is occupied by inflammatory exudate, it is known as *organization*. Fibrosis can occur in many organs following damage/inflammation, forming definitive disease entities.

However, it must be remembered that in most common injuries, the elements of tissue regeneration and scar formation go hand in hand.

4.15.1 Cell Proliferation and Regeneration

The regeneration of injured tissue depends on the intrinsic proliferative capacity of the cells, the intactness of the extracellular matrix (ECM), and the various growth factors.

The *labile tissue (continuously dividing tissue)* is composed of cells that are continuously lost and rapidly replaced by new cells originating from the stem cells. Examples include bone marrow, columnar epithelia of the gastrointestinal tract, basal cell layer of skin, etc.

The *stable tissue (Quiescent tissue)* consists of cells that enter the G0 stage (quiescent stage) of the cell cycle and have left the proliferating cycle. But in response to loss or injury of tissue, these cells re-enter the cell cycle and start proliferating. Examples include the parenchyma of most solid organs like the pancreas, adrenal, thyroid, lung, and particularly the liver (following hepatectomy).

In *permanent tissue (nondividing tissue),* the cells are terminally differentiated and they do not proliferate even in response to injury and are replaced by scar tissue, for example, neural tissue, skeletal muscle, cardiac muscle, etc.

The regenerating cells are derived from the tissue-specific quiescent stem cells. This is facilitated by the secretion of various growth factors secreted by the macrophages and epithelial and stromal cells near the site of injury. An intact extracellular matrix is also essential for this complex process to occur. Complete restoration is possible only if the residual tissue is intact.

The major growth factors involved in healing are

- Epidermal growth factor (EGF)
- Transforming growth factor-α (TGF α)
- Platelet-derived growth factor (PDGF)
- Transforming growth factor-β (TGF-β)
- Fibroblast growth factor (FGF)
- Transforming growth factor (TGF-β)
- Various cytokines like TNFα, Interleukin 1, etc.

Repair by Fibrosis

Repair of the injured tissue by fibrosis involves the steps of

(i) *Granulation tissue formation*
(ii) *Wound contraction*

4.16 Granulation Tissue Formation

Granulation tissue is soft, pink, healing tissue, which appears granular in appearance. It should not be confused with granulomatous inflammation. While granuloma is a collection of activated epithelioid macrophages, granulation tissue is composed of numerous thin-walled new blood vessels in a loose, edematous stroma composed of plump fibroblasts and a variable population of inflammatory cells (Fig. 4.4).

The process of granulation tissue formation has 4 phases [1]:

(a) *Bleeding Phase*: Following injury, there is bleeding followed by clot formation, which forms a scaffold for inflammatory cell infiltration.
(b) *Inflammatory Phase*: Following clotting, there is infiltration of neutrophils within few hours and phagocytic cells (macrophages, monocytes) within 24 h, which degrades the necrotic tissue, fibrin mesh, clot products, etc. by proteolytic enzymes and then cleared off by the phagocytes.
(c) *Proliferation Phase*: It starts 1–2 days after injury and reaches its peak in 2–3 weeks,

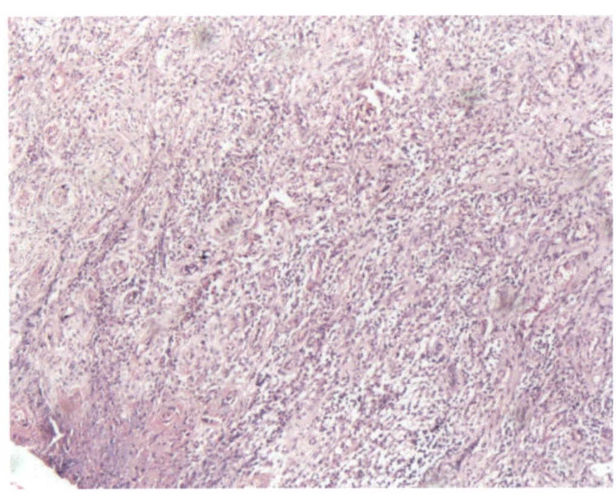

Fig. 4.4 Granulation tissue under a superficial skin ulcer composed of thin-walled blood vessels, plump fibroblasts, mild lymphocytic inflammation in an edematous background

while it takes around 4–6 months to form strong scar tissue. It consists of *2 phases—the phase of angiogenesis (neovascularization)*, that is, the phase in which new vessels are formed first under the influence of angiogenic factors like VEGF, etc. Slowly, these vessels differentiate to capillaries, venules, veins, or arteries. The other phase is the *phase of fibrogenesis* (Scar formation) in which myofibroblasts and fibroblasts proliferate. The initially formed weak Type III collagen is gradually replaced by the stronger type I collagen.

(d) *Remodeling Phases*: It starts in 2–3 weeks and may continue from months to years. In this phase, degradation of the collagen and extracellular matrix (ECM) occurs by metalloproteinases and the formation of new ECM, thus replacing the vascular granulation tissue with avascular, strong scar tissue.

4.17 Wound Contraction

Wound contraction is a dynamic process of healing that starts about 5 days post injury and functions to reduce the size of the tissue defect that needs repair. This response involves the highly contractile myofibroblasts, which are formed from fibroblasts by undergoing a phenotypic transformation by activating the alpha-smooth muscle actin (α-SMA) gene. These myofibroblasts have increased smooth muscle actin expression and pull the newly formed collagen fibers toward the wound center, thereby resulting in the size of the defect that needs to be repaired.

Wound contraction is a dynamic process through which a connective tissue matrix is formed by collagen fibers synthesized by newly migrated fibroblasts. Then, fibroblasts differentiate to myofibroblasts that are responsible for tensile force to pull the wound edges toward the wound center, which results in gradually reducing the wound area. This wound contraction is a very important part of wound healing, leading to 40% reduction in the size of the wound.

4.18 Types of Healing of Skin Wounds

Healing of skin wounds can be of 2 types:

(a) *Healing by First Intention (Primary Union)*, in which there is epithelial regeneration with minimal scarring in cases where the wound edges are approximated (e.g., surgical incisions).
(b) *Healing by Second Intention (secondary union)* refers to a combination of regeneration and scarring that heals the wound from the bottom in cases where there is larger tissue loss and whose edges are not approximated.

4.19 Factors Interfering with Tissue Repair [1]

They may be extrinsic or intrinsic, and systemic or local. The most important factors include:

1. Infection: Most important local factor responsible for the delay in wound healing.
2. Uncontrolled Diabetes Mellitus or other chronic diseases result in poor wound healing.
3. Nutritional status: Deficiencies of Vitamin C, Vitamin A, Zinc, and protein malnutrition delay the process of healing.
4. Use of steroids (Glucocorticoids) is responsible for the delay in wound healing by inhibition of fibrosis. In some conditions like corneal infections, this may be desirable and often glucocorticoids are prescribed with antibiotics to prevent corneal opacity due to collagen deposition.
5. Mechanical factors such as increased local pressure, movement, or trauma may result in a delay in wound healing or wound dehiscence.
6. Poor perfusion, due to arteriosclerosis or from obstructed venous drainage (e.g., in varicose veins), also impairs healing.
7. Foreign bodies such as fragments of steel, glass, or even bone impede healing.

8. The type and extent of tissue injury: Complete restoration is possible in tissue with proliferating cells (labile tissue) even in cases with large tissue defects, while injury to tissues with nondividing cells heals with scarring, for example, myocardial infarct.
9. Therapeutic influences like exercise therapy, electrotherapy, etc. may stimulate wound healing in cases of delayed wound healing.

4.20 Complications of Wound Healing [3, 4]

The complications depend on the tissue injured. The common complications of cutaneous wound are as follows:

(a) *Infection.*
(b) Development of *epidermal (inclusion) cyst.*
(c) *Pigmentation* following wound healing due to deposition of hemosiderin.
(d) *Deficient scar tissue formation*, which may lead to *wound dehiscence* or *development of incisional hernia.*
(e) *Excessive scar tissue formation resulting in hypertrophic scars* or *Keloid.* While hypertrophic scars are formed 1–2 months after injury, composed of bundles of collagen arranged parallel to the upper skin layer and confined to the area of the original wound, the keloid forms months or years after injury and is composed of haphazardly arranged collagen bundles extending beyond the confines of the original wound.
(f) Excessive contraction of the wound may result in various contractures like Dupuytren's contracture (palmer contracture), Ledderhose's disease (plantar contracture), and Peyronie's disease (penile contracture).
(g) Rarely, *neoplasia* may develop, the classic example being squamous cell carcinoma arising in Marjolin's ulcer, which develops following burn injury.

Similarly, the complications of fracture healing include the following:

(a) *Delayed union* may result from increased age of the patient, movement, the distraction of bone fragments, poor nutritional status, systemic or local infections, poor blood supply, comorbid conditions like Diabetes mellitus, etc.
(b) *Nonunion* occurs when the two ends of the fracture fail to unite even after 6 months. It may be of atrophic or hypertrophic types. Factors causing nonunion include infection at the fracture site, the interposition of soft tissue between the bone ends, inadequate immobilization that disrupts callus formation, impaired blood supply, resulting in avascular necrosis.
(c) *Fibrous union* may result in case there is inadequate immobilization of fractured bone and as a consequence of nonunion. In the case of persistent, mobile nonunion, the fibrous tissue at the fracture site may form a "false joint" or pseudarthrosis.

References

1. Mohan H. Inflammation and repair. In: Mohan H, editor. Textbook of pathology. 8th ed. Jaypee Brothers; 2019. p. 70–120.
2. Kumar V, Abbas AK, Aster JC. Inflammation and repair. In: Kumar V, Abbas AK, Aster JC, editors. Robbins basic pathology, Robbins pathology. 10th ed. Philadelphia: Elsevier – Health Sciences Division; 2017. p. 57–96.
3. Mandal AK, Choudhury S. Inflammation. In: Mandal AK, Choudhury S, editors. Textbook of pathology for MBBS. 1st ed. Avichal Publishing Company; 2017. p. 51–67.
4. Kamal V. Inflammation, tissue healing and repair. In: Kamal V, editor. Textbook of pathology. 1st ed. CBS Publishers & Distributors; 2017. p. 51–133.

Pathology of Ocular Infections

5

Saumya Jakati, Sanchita Mitra,
and Somasheila Murthy

Contents

S. Jakati (✉)
Ophthalmic Pathology Laboratory, Kallam Anji Reddy Campus, L V Prasad Eye Institute, Hyderabad, Telangana, India
e-mail: saumyajakati@lvpei.org; saumya.jakati@gmail.com

S. Mitra
Jhaveri Microbiology Centre, Kallam Anji Reddy Campus, L V Prasad Eye Institute, Hyderabad, Telangana, India
e-mail: sanchita.mitra@lvpei.org

S. Murthy
Specialist in Corneal Diseases, Uveitis, Cataract and Refractive Surgery
Shantilal Shanghvi Eye Institute, Mumbai, Maharashtra, India

G. K. Vemuganti et al. (eds.), *Ocular Pathology*, https://doi.org/10.1007/978-981-96-8614-8_5

5.1 Introduction

Microorganisms are ubiquitous in nature and have developed complex interactions over time [1].The term "ocular microbiome" encompasses all the microorganisms colonized in the eye and ocular adnexa. A few of the resident flora, such as *Staphylococcus* species, *Corynebacterium* species, and *Propionibacterium* species [2], are normal residents of the conjunctival fornix and are nonpathogenic. The anatomy of the ocular surface together with the ocular microbiome has a unique defense mechanism against pathogenic microbes [3, 4]. Any alteration in these defense mechanisms leads to infection by colonization by the pathogenic microbes [4].

Ocular Infections can be categorized based on

1. Duration—acute or chronic
2. Origin of infection—endogenous or exogenous
3. Location—focal or diffuse
4. Various categories of microbes—Bacterial, fungal, viral, and parasitic
5. The type of inflammatory reaction—granulomatous or nongranulomatous
6. Site of infections:
   (a) Orbital soft tissue—orbital cellulitis, dacryocystitis
   (b) Eyelids—blepharitis, folliculitis, meibomitis
   (c) Ocular surface—conjunctivitis, keratitis, and scleritis
   (d) Intra-ocular—iridocyclitis, uveitis, vitritis, retinitis, chorioretinitis, endophthalmitis, and pan-ophthalmitis
   (e) Optic nerve—optic neuritis

5.2 Demography and Significance of Infection

The geographical distribution of infections shows an uneven distribution worldwide with a denser incidence in the Asian and African countries. Risk factors, such as age, sex, race, and socioeconomic status, are most linked to ocular infections. Factors predisposing the eye to infections can be categorized into

- Local: trauma, corneal anesthesia, nasolacrimal duct obstruction, dry eye syndrome, exposure keratitis
- Systemic: malnutrition, immunodeficiency syndrome, immune-suppressive state, malignancies, burns, and injuries
- Environmental factors:exposure to extreme temperatures, ultraviolet light, and irritant substances

5.3 Pathogenesis

To combat infections caused by microbes, various contributors of the human defense system, such as inflammatory cells and mediators, are released from the vascular compartment into the tissues, which generate a reaction to kill or restrict the offending pathogen. Inflammatory cells comprising neutrophils, lymphocytes, eosinophils, plasma cells, mast cells, and macrophages play a major role in the course of the disease. The interplay of various cytokines released by these inflammatory cells contributes to tissue reaction and damage. If this inflammation is not mitigated immediately, it can obscure the visual axis by scarring, which might lead to partial or complete vision loss [5].

5.3.1 Routes of Infection, Spread, and Transmission

Microbes primarily enter the eye through two major routes:

5.3.1.1 Direct Implantation

Upper and lower eyelids are natural barriers and act as a shield to protect the cornea, conjunctiva, and sclera. Tears form the first line of defense and protect the ocular surface by forming a thick layer that constantly nourishes and lubricates the eye. The ocular microbiome is the recent focus in microbiology to understand the microbiological interactions and the pathogenesis of infections in the ocular milieu [6]. Infections in the eye are a sequential process of exposure to the microbe, epithelial adhesion, invasion of the epithelium, colonization, and production of toxic substances, which lead to tissue damage and disease. Traumatic implantation, chronic mechanical irritation of the eye, and penetrating injuries allow the entry of organisms into the eye.

5.3.1.2 Hematogenous Route

Endogenous infection elsewhere in the body or neighboring ocular structures acts as a source of infection and reaches the eye through a hematogenous route.

5.3.2 Host–Pathogen Interactions

Host–Pathogen Interactions are categorized under the following headings:host defense, immune evasion, injurious effects, and immunodeficiencies.

5.3.2.1 Host Defense

The host immune responses are primarily responsible to determine the intensity of infection by invading the pathogen. Defense systems include physiological barriers and the host immune system (both innate and adaptive). The role of innate defense mechanisms is ambiguous and includes protective mechanisms such as defensins over the ocular surface, lactoferrin in tear fluids, Immunoglobin A (IgA), and lysozyme [3].

5.3.2.2 Immune Evasion

Immune evasion in microbial pathogens is caused by various mechanisms including.

Antigenic Variation

Antigenic variation—periodic change of surface protein (such as in *Spirochetes*), alterations in the genome, and high mutation rate (viruses).

Antimicrobial Resistance

Antimicrobial resistance—resistance to peptides such as defensins and cathelicidins.

Resistance to Phagocytosis

Resistance to phagocytosis—dense carbohydrate capsule, expression of proteins, which bind to the "Fc" portion of an antibody.

Evasion of Apoptosis

Evasion of apoptosis—viruses, fungi, bacteria, and protozoa that proliferate in the cell generate factors that alter the autophagy process.

Resistance to Host Defense

Resistance to host defense—viral factors that block actions of various cytokines and signaling cascade.

Evasion of Recognition by T-Cells

Evasion of recognition by T-cells—viruses bind or alter the localization of major histocompatibility complex (MHC)- class I or generate MHC class-II homologs to evade recognition by CD4+ and CD8+ T cells.

Downregulation of Antimicrobial T-Cell Responses

Downregulation of antimicrobial T-cell responses—T-cell exhaustion due to upregulation of immunoinhibitory T cell pathway.

Injurious Effects

The immune cells of the host cause cytolytic effects on the infected cells causing deleterious effects leading to cell death. The microbes do not carry any active oncogenes; however, they might initiate a chronic inflammatory cascade leading to oncogenesis, for example, Hepatitis B or Hepatitis C infection [7].

5.3.2.3 Immunodeficiencies

Individuals with innate or acquired immune deficiencies have damage in single or multiple components of the immune system. These deficiencies include antibody deficiencies, complement deficiencies, inability to form a phagolysosome, toll-like receptor deficiency (pathway deficiency), and T-helper cell defects [8]. Each of these defects makes the individual susceptible to various bacterial and viral infections.

5.3.2.4 Host Damage

Microbial pathogens cause host cell/tissue damage by 3 basic mechanisms.

- Direct cell death or change in cellular metabolism
- Release of toxins, which damage the tissue
- Stimulate host response, which indirectly causes tissue damage

5.3.3 Tissue Inflammatory Response

Tissue inflammatory response can be broadly categorized into five basic histologic patterns including.

3.3.1. Suppurative inflammation
3.3.2. Granulomatous inflammation
3.3.3. Cytopathic-cytoproliferative reaction
3.3.4. Tissue necrosis
3.3.5. Chronic inflammation and scarring

5.3.3.1 Suppurative Inflammation

Suppuration is due to dense leukocytosis predominantly by neutrophils and increased vascular permeability due to the release of chemo-attractants from the microbes. Pus is the collection of liquified and devitalized tissue cells along with dead neutrophils. Small neutrophilic collections also termed microabscesses are noted in corneal infections. *Staphylococcus* spp., *Streptococcus* spp., *Pseudomonas* spp., and fungal infections are some of the organisms, which cause suppuration.

5.3.3.2 Granulomatous Inflammation

This is a chronic inflammatory response characterized by cell-mediated immunity caused due to persistent antigenic stimulation. It is characterized by the formation of granulomas, which are an accumulation of modified or activated histiocytes, also known as epithelioid cells (has classic slipper-shaped nuclei). Epithelioid cells are noted in the center of the lesion surrounded by lymphocytes and plasma cells followed by fibrosis. Granulomas are described as discrete (seen separately) or coalescent (fused), well-defined or ill-defined, with or without cuff of surrounding lymphocytes and plasma cells, and presence or absence of central necrosis.

5.3.3.3 Cytopathic-Cytoproliferative Reaction

These reactions are often seen with viral infections. Viral cytopathic effects include nuclear margination, nuclear molding, and nuclear multinucleation, which occurs due to the multiplication of viral particles in the host nucleus.

5.3.3.4 Tissue Necrosis

Tissue necrosis is due to cytolytic enzymes released by the microbe or by the occlusion of the vascular supply causing infarction.

5.3.3.5 Chronic Inflammation and Scarring

Scarring is a result of prolonged and sustained chronic inflammation, which is characterized by the proliferation of fibroblasts. Scarring in the cornea can cause serious visual morbidity.

5.4 Classification of Pathogens

Classification of all the pathogens causing infection in the eye and ocular adnexa is listed in Table 5.1.

Table 5.1 Classification of ocular pathogens (Basic course 2020–2021)

Condition	Virus	Bacteria	Fungi	Parasites
Dermato-blepharitis	HSV *Varicella-zoster* virus	*Staphylococcus aureus* *Streptococcus* spp.	-*Trichophyton rubrum* *Candida* spp	–
Blepharitis	HSV *Molluscum contagiosum*	*Staphylococcus aureus* CONS *Corynebacterium* spp. *Moraxella* spp.	*Pityrosporum ovale*	*Phthirus pubis* *Pediculosis capitis* *Demodex folliculorum* *D. brevis*
Conjunctivitis	*Adenovirus* HSV Varicella zoster *Picornavirus EV70* *Coxsackievirus A24* *SARS-CoV 2 coronavirus*	*Chlamydia trachomatis* *Staphylococcus aureus* *Streptococcus* spp. *Neisseria gonorrhoeae* *Hemophilus influenzae* *Moraxella* spp.	-*Candida* spp. (*C. albicans, C. tropicalis, C. parapsilosis)* *Paracoccidiodes brasileinsis,* *Coccidioides imitis* *Blastomyces dermatitidis* *Rhinosporidium seeberi*	-*Trypanosoma brucei*
Keratitis	HSV Cytomegalovirus Ebstein Barr virus Varicella zoster virus	*Pseudomonas aeruginosa* *Staphylococcus aureus* *Staphylococcus epidermidis* *Streptococcus pneumoniae* *Moraxella* spp.	Hyaline molds like *Fusarium* spp. and *Aspergillus* spp. Dematiaceous molds like species of *Curvularia, Alternaria, Lasiodiplodia, Bipolaris, Exserohilum,* Yeasts like *Candida* spp., *Trichosporon* spp.	*Acanthamoeba* spp. *Microsporidia*
Dacryoadenitis	Epstein Barr virus Mumps virus Herpes simplex virus Adenovirus Varicella zoster virus Rhinovirus Cytomegalovirus	*Staphylococcus aureus* *Streptococcus pneumoniae*	Rarely: *Aspergillus* spp. *Histoplasma capsulatum* *Blastomyces dermatitidis*	Rarely: *Cysticercus cellulosae*
Canaliculitis	HSV	*Actinomyces* spp. *Nocardia* spp. *Streptococcus* spp. *Staphylococcus* spp.	*Candida* spp. *Aspergillus* spp. *Malassezia furfur*	–
Dacryocystitis	Rarely: Ebstein Barr virus	*Staphylococcus* spp. *Streptococcus* spp.	*Candida* spp. *Aspergillus* spp. *Fusarium* spp. Mucorales	*Rhinosporidium seeberi* *Leishmania* spp.

5.5 Clinical Presentation

Symptoms of ocular infection include swelling of the lids and adnexa, discharge, blurred vision, pain, photophobia, corneal opacity, or hypopyon [9]. Systemic symptoms can be noted such as fever or based on the comorbid systemic infections. Infections can also be categorized by age as a denominator as follows:

Children: varicella conjunctivitis and keratitis, active inflammatory trachoma in children.

Middle-aged: infections include Herpes zoster ophthalmicus (HZO), cicatricial trachoma, and fungal infections.

5.6 Diagnosis

Early and precise diagnosis of these infections is essential and can help in targeted medical intervention with appropriate antimicrobials. Although histopathology helps partially in the identification or the presence or absence of micro-organisms in tissues, direct identification of the pathogens by standard microbiological techniques such as culture and microscopy remains the gold standard. Further, antibiotic susceptibility testing helps in delineating the antibiotic of choice. Newer diagnostic modalities such as in vivo confocal microscopy hasten the diagnosis of fungal and acanthamoeba keratitis [10]. Advanced molecular techniques such as conventional and real-time polymerase chain reaction (RT-PCR) and sequencing techniques such as next-generation sequencing (NGS) have high sensitivity and specificity of microbial detection even from a minimal volume of the sample, for example, in samples obtained from vitreous biopsy for diagnosis of endophthalmitis [10, 11].

5.7 Histopathology of the Cases

Diagnosis of infection on histopathology is always confirmatory and is essential in smear and culture-negative cases (if the infection is in the posterior cornea). Hematoxylin and eosin (H&E) staining is appended by a battery of special histochemical stains (Table 5.2). Limitation of histopathology includes species identification and antibiotic susceptibility. Specific diagnosis of the pathogen is essential while the ocular tissue is still salvageable. Most of the time, samples for histopathology can be obtained only after complete excision of the tissue: for example, in therapeutic keratoplasty or after complete removal of the eyeball such as in enucleation or evisceration.

Table 5.2 Basic stains used in the diagnosis of ocular infections

Stain	Organism—color
Ziehl–Neelsen stain (20% AFB stain)	*Mycobacterium tuberculosis*—red Hydatid hooklets—red
Fite-Farraco stain (5% AFB stain)	*Mycobacterium leprae*—red
Kinyoun stain (1% AFB stain)	*Nocardia*—red Microsporidia—red
Gomori or Grocott methanamine silver stain	Fungus—black Microsporidia—black Ectocyst of *Acanthamoeba*—black *Pythium*—black
Brown and Brenn stain or Brown and Hopps	Gram-positive organism—blue Gram-negative organism—red
Giemsa	*Acanthamoeba*, chlamydia, cysts of toxoplasma—blue
Per-iodic acid Schiff's stain	Fungus—magenta *Pythium*—variable magenta Parasite cuticle—magenta *Acanthamoeba*—magenta colored
Alcian blue	Capsule of cryptococcus—blue

5.7.1 Bacterial Infections

A direct smear of samples from infected sites, followed by general stains like Gram stain and microscopy, aids in the detection of the bacteria; Gram-positive bacteria stains blue and Gram-negative stain red. Exogenous bacterial colonization and infection occurs due to alteration of the structure of the corneal surface due to ulceration following trauma or due to decreased tear film formation. Dense infiltration of polymorphonuclear leukocytes from the adjacent limbal vessels is noted. This infiltrates the stromal lamellae leading to formation of abscesses. The karyorrhectic debris released from the inflammatory cells gives a basophilic hue to the background stroma. Stromal necrosis, which occurs because of collagenolysis by enzymes released by the microbes and inflammatory cells, is noted in the background. Stromal edema is also noted in a few cases. Features of bacterial keratitis include surface ulceration with dense stromal infiltrates predominantly of neutrophils and stromal necrosis which is due to the release of collagenolytic enzymes from the injured cells. Extensive stromal necrosis often leads to perforation of superficial layers of the eye like cornea, thereby transmitting the infection to inner cavities leading to infections like exogenous or traumatic endophthalmitis [5].

The etiological cause for endophthalmitis is either exogenous or endogenous [5].

Salient Points

- Bacteria can often be confused with the uveal pigment, which is round, larger, and brown colored.
- Bacteria are more likely to be detected in the center of the abscess and areas of injury.

Case Illustration 1

An 82-year-old male presented with a 5-day duration of history of watering and redness of the right eye days. Examination revealed a perforated corneal ulcer. Imaging (ultrasound B-scan) showed features suggestive of vitreous opacities, membranes, and choroidal detachment. As there was complete loss of vision, eye salvage was not possible and evisceration surgery was performed (Fig. 5.1).

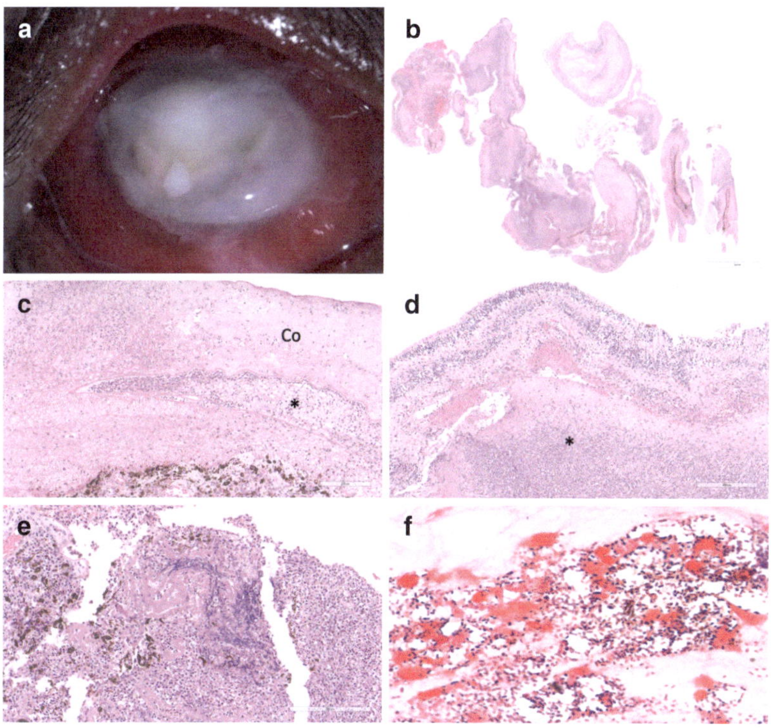

Fig. 5.1 (**a**) Clinical image showing corneal perforation with diffuse and dense infiltrates with congested sclera. (**b**) Scanner view of the eviscerated contents (Hematoxylin and eosin; scanner view). (**c**) perforated and necrosed cornea (Co) with dense diffuse infiltrates (asterisk) and adherent iris tissue. (Hematoxylin and eosin; 10× original magnification). (**d**) Necrosed retina with intravitreal pyogenic abscess (asterisk) (Hematoxylin and eosin; 10× original magnification). (**e**) Higher magnification of the neutrophilic infiltrates admixed with basophilic stained bacterial colonies. (Hematoxylin and eosin; 20× original magnification). (**f**) Clusters and singly scattered Gram-positive bacilli are noted admixed with infiltrates (Gram's stain; 100× original magnification)

5.7.2 Fungal Infections

5.7.2.1 Fungal Keratitis

Fungal keratitis, also known as keratomycosis, is more common in the Indian subcontinent, and frequently occurs due to trauma or injury with vegetable matter [12]. Clinically, the infiltrates have feathery edges, with deep stromal involvement and satellite lesions [12]. Though fungal infections are caused by both yeasts and molds, in our country, the hyaline fungi, *Aspergillus* and *Fusarium*, are the most common offending fungal pathogens. [13] On histopathology, fungal hyphae are seen in the anterior stroma or ulcer bed and can penetrate deep into the stroma up to the Descemet's membrane (DM). Fungal hyphae can be seen admixed with infiltrates posterior to DM, forming microabscesses and within multinucleate giant cells (Fig. 5.2).

Fungal granulomas of sino-orbital location tend to show extensive granulomatous inflammation with foreign-body type of multinucleate giant cells and dense fibrosis (Fig. 5.3).

Salient Points

- Histopathologically, fungal hyphae are usually seen away from the inflammatory infiltrates and are often found at the edge of the necrotic stroma.
- They can be located deep in the posterior stroma, while anterior stroma may be relatively less involved.
- They can also invade the intact DM.

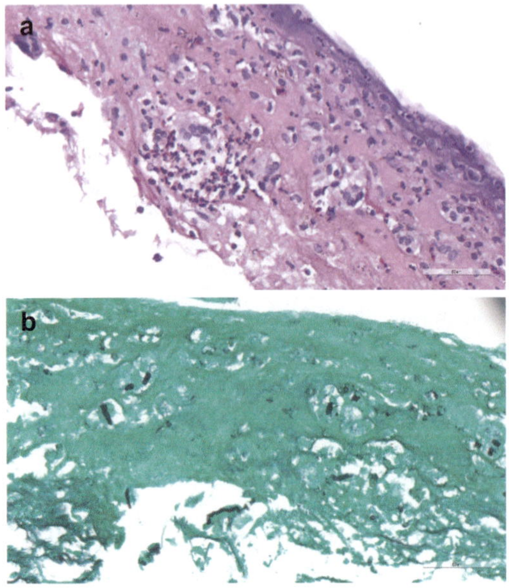

Fig. 5.2 Photomicrographs highlight (**a**) Microabscess and multinucleate giant cell reaction in the corneal stroma (H&E;30× original magnification). (**b**) Fungal hyphae seen within the cytoplasm of the giant cells (GMS; 30× original magnification)

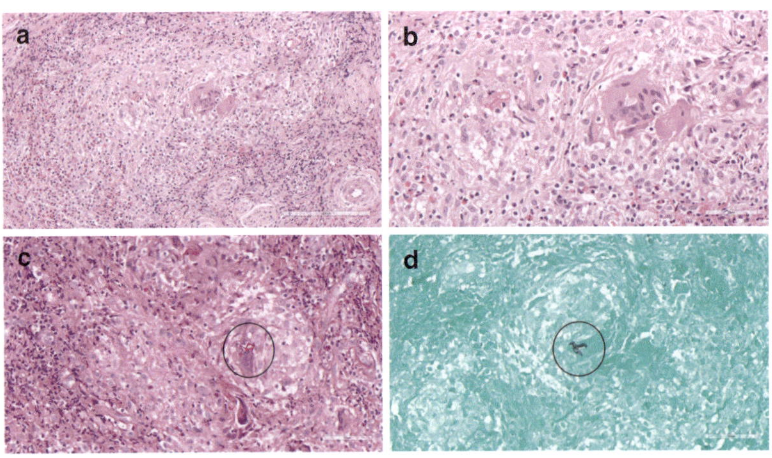

Fig. 5.3 Fungal granulomatous inflammation of the orbit—(**a**) Low magnification of the orbital fibroadipose tissue densely infiltrated by the chronic inflammatory cells, epithelioid cells, and multinucleate giant cells. (**b**) Granuloma with refractile structures in the multinucleate giant cells surrounded by lymphocytes, eosinophils, and plasma cells. (**c** and **d**) Fungal hyphae are highlighted on Periodic acid Schiff (PAS) and Gomori methenamine silver (GMS) stains (PAS and GMS; 40× original magnification)

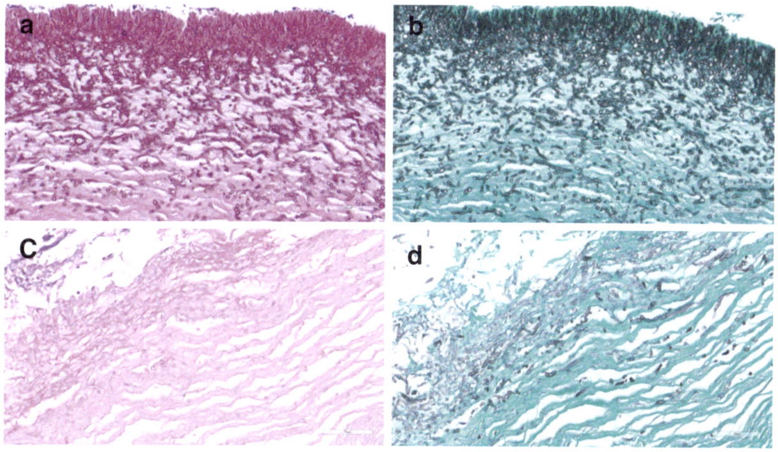

Fig. 5.4 Differentiating features between fungal and pythium keratitis: (**a** and **c**) Fungal filaments show bright magenta-colored filaments in comparison to variable to negative staining pythium filaments (PAS; 30× original magnification). (**b** and **d**) Both fungal and *Pythium* filaments are positive on GMS stain (GMS; 30× original magnification)

5.7.2.2 Pythium Keratitis

Pythium insidiosum is a recently discovered plant pathogenic fungi, seen infecting humans. *Pythium* as seen microscopically appears typically broad, ribbon-like, folded onto itself, and aseptate or sparsely septate. The cell wall contains chitin instead of the ergosterol (which is present in fungus). Histopathology of the corneal button reveals refractile fungal-like filaments, which are negative or variably stained on Periodic acid Schiff (PAS) stain, unlike fungi, which stain brilliant magenta colored and are further highlighted on Grocott methenamine silver (GMS) stain (Fig. 5.4) [14].

Cellulose is part of the cell wall of *Pythium* and is a complex carbohydrate. Cellulose is oxidized by a strong oxidizing agent as chromic acid in GMS stain. Periodic acid Schiff's stain is a weak oxidizing agent. Hence, it cannot reduce cellulose. These filaments stain blue on Iodine Potassium Iodine-Sulfuric acid (IKI-H_2SO_4) staining [14]. The importance of early diagnosis of *Pythium insidiosum* lies in the fact that it is nonresponsive to antifungals (most of the antifungals act on fungal cell wall ergosterol) and instead responds to antibacterials. The growth on culture is also different from the regular molds: it grows as an adherent carpet-like layer, much faster on blood or chocolate agar, than on Sabouraud or potato dextrose agar (specific fungal media). Also, it reproduces by the formation of zoospores in special induction media in the lab, which are then utilized for testing drug susceptibility to various antibacterials.

Salient Points

- *Pythium* is a fungus-like pathogen, with aseptate filaments with ribbon-like folds.
- It is nonresponsive to antifungal medication.
- Histopathologically, it is identified by special stains (IKI-H_2SO_4).

5.7.2.3 Dematiaceous Fungi

Clinically, this infection is associated with prolonged/insidious history and on examination, the fungal ulcer appears pigmented. On histopathology, the fungal hyphae appear brown (often referred to as "copper penny appearance") on H&E staining. The filaments appear tightly packed together as a colony (corresponding to the plaque observed clinically). On culture, these fungi typically grow as pigmented colonies, mostly dark brown, to gray to black, and take longer to sporulate compared to their hyaline counterparts and thus longer for species identification. Masson Fontana stain can be used for the diagnosis of these fungi in cases of dilemma [13].

Salient Features

- The filaments are pigmented both in vivo and on histopathology.
- They take longer to sporulate and have a prolonged clinical course.

5.7.2.4 Mucormycosis

Mucormycosis is encountered frequently in the elderly, immunocompromised hosts and diabetics and is often referred to as black fungus. A steep rise in cases was reported during the COVID-19 pandemic. A comprehensive diagnostic approach was implemented during the pandemic, which included histopathology, direct microscopy, culture, and PCR assays [15].These fungal hyphae are broad, aseptate, with right-angle to obtuse angle branching. They are known to cause hemorrhagic and infarcted necrosis as the fungal hyphae block the blood flow in the vessels. Both perivascular and perineural invasion are noted with Mucormycosis.

Salient Features

- It is encountered frequently in immune-weakened status such as elderly and diabetics.
- IKI-H_2SO_4 stain can help in differentiating *Pythium* sp. and *Mucor* sp. as well.

5.7.3 Viral Infections

Viral infections in the eye are mainly caused by a few genera of which Herpes viral infections dominate. Herpes simplex virus (HSV), Herpes zoster, and Cytomegalovirus (CMV) are known to involve the posterior segment of the eye causing progressive outer retinal necrosis, retinal necrosis, and retinopathies. Human immunodeficiency virus is usually seen in immunocompromised individuals. Other sets of viruses like the measles virus are known to infect the pediatric population. There are few case reports of viral infection due to rabies, Ebstein-Barr virus, and the Chikungunya virus. Dengue virus has also been reported to cause ocular infections either directly or by immune alterations leading to secondary infections.

Viral keratitis is most often caused by HSV-1 virus. The most common presentation is a "dendritic ulcer," which appears like a branching pattern. The virus remains latent in the trigeminal ganglion, and reactivation of the virus leads to a recurring course. Corneal scraping might reveal the characteristic Cowdry "A" type of inclusions in the epithelial cells. On cytopathology, the triad of nuclear margination, nuclear molding, and multinucleation is the classic feature for the identification of viral infection. Intranuclear inclusions are also noted. Viral stromal keratitis can be classified into (A) Immune keratitis (B) Nonimmune stromal keratitis. Chronic stromal keratitis cases usually undergo penetrating keratoplasty and usually show scarring and vascularization on histopathology [15]. Inflammatory infiltrates are usually minimal in these cases and are composed of lymphocytes, plasma cells, histiocytes, and epithelioid cells. Multinucleate giant cells are noted close to or clinging to Descemet's membrane. This is highly suggestive of viral keratitis (Fig. 5.5).

Perforation can occur in these corneas with progressive stromal loss due to repeated episodes of scarring [16]. Herpes zoster also causes dendritic ulcer similar to HSV and has a very indolent course. Viral PCR from the corneal scraping and aqueous humor serve as the diagnostic samples. Adenovirus is another common virus that causes an epidemic form of kerato-conjunctivitis. HSV, CMV, and measles virus (rubeola and rubella) can cause acute retinal necrosis. A vitreal or retinal biopsy would be a diagnostic sample; this is usually sent for histopathology and microbiology [17].

- *COVID-19*:

  One of the most recent emerging pathogens causing mass fatalities was COVID-19 [18].

  Ocular involvement was noted in diabetic patients, especially during the second wave of the virus. The spectrum of manifestations included mild conjunctivitis, hyper-reflective lesions on the retina, cotton wool spots, and micro-

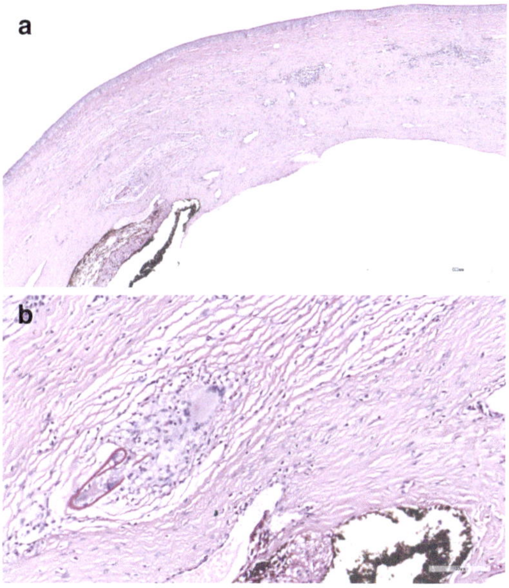

Fig. 5.5 Viral keratitis: Photomicrographs show (**a**) scarred and vascularized cornea with anterior synechiae. Perivascular chronic inflammatory infiltrates are seen. (H&E; 4× original magnification) (**b**) Multinucleate giant cells seen clinging to the fragmented Descemet's membrane incarcerated into the posterior stroma. (H&E; 40× original magnification)

hemorrhages [19].The ocular surface acted as a reservoir for many organisms and also for COVID-19; therefore, the virus has been detected in the tears of the affected patients [18].

Case Illustration
A 54-year-old male presented with unilateral proptosis in his right eye and fullness of sinuses. The patient was a known diabetic with a history of COVID-19 infection 2 months back. The smear from the nasal swab showed hyphae of *Mucor*. Exenteration was performed. On gross morphology, a necrotic area was noted in the posterior inferior quadrant of the eye adjacent to the optic nerve. Histopathology sections of the necrotic areas showed infarcted necrosis with fungal hyphae that are broad, aseptate, and right-angled branched (Fig. 5.6).

Molluscum Contagiosum: (Fig. 5.7)
Molluscum contagiosum is a common condition especially in the pediatric population, which is a viral infection caused by a double-stranded poxvirus (DNA) virus. The virus replicates in the cytoplasm to form the characteristic intracytoplasmic eosinophilic inclusions also known as Henderson-Paterson bodies [17]. Clinically, whitish, irregularly rounded sessile lesion is noted on the lid margins, which spreads by self-contact. These lesions are benign, self-limiting, and are not associated with any complications.

5.7.4 Parasitic Infections

Ocular parasitic infections are caused by unicellular (protozoal) or multicellular organisms (like cestodes, trematodes, and nematodes like helminths). Common protozoal organisms encountered are sporozoans like *Microsporidia* and *Acanthamoeba*, which are known to cause corneal infection and the multicellular organism is nematodes like *Dirofilaria*, *Taenia*, and *Echinococcus* are usually noted to involve posterior compartments of the eye.

5.7.4.1 Parasitic Keratitis

Microsporidia
Microsporidia sp. are spore-forming obligate intracellular parasites infecting the eye, sinuses, gastrointestinal, renal, pulmonary, and muscle.

Microsporidial ocular infections are known to occur both in immunocompromised individuals as keratoconjunctivitis and as stromal keratitis in immunocompetent individuals [20]. It infects corneal epithelium, and stroma with or without involving the adjacent conjunctiva. The patient presents with a history of redness and pain. *Microsporidia* can be easily detected on calcofluor white staining of corneal scraping. However, deep stromal keratitis is difficult to detect; hence, corneal biopsies serve as the crucial diagnostic samples. *Microsporidia* are seen interlamellar in location and appear as small, oval, refractile, 1% acid-fast-stain-positive bodies and also stain with Kinyoun stain [20, 21]. They cannot be cultured in conventional media (but need cell lines); hence, direct microscopy of infected samples or direct observation in tissues by in vivo confocal

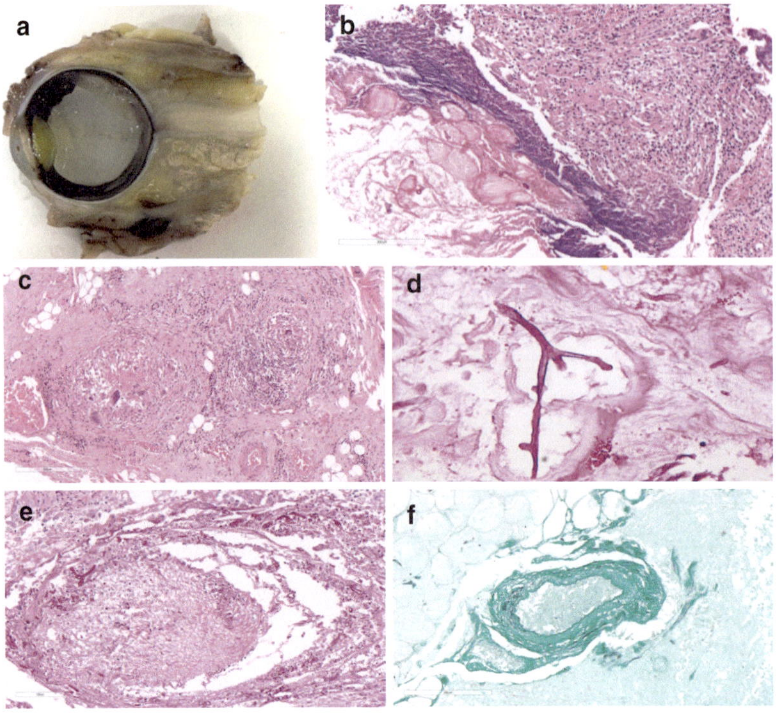

Fig. 5.6 Mucormycosis—(**a**) Cut section of the formalin fixed exenterated specimen showing the area of necrosis in the posterior inferior orbit (**b**) Areas of infarction with adjacent chronic inflammation (H&E; 10× original magnification). (**c**) Areas of granulomatous inflammation (H&E; 10× original magnification). (**d**) Fungal hyphae, which are magenta colored, broad, aseptate, and right angle branched in the background of necrosis (PAS; 40× original magnification). (**e**) Perineural invasion (PAS; 20× original magnification). (**f**) Perivascular invasion (GMS; 20× original magnification)

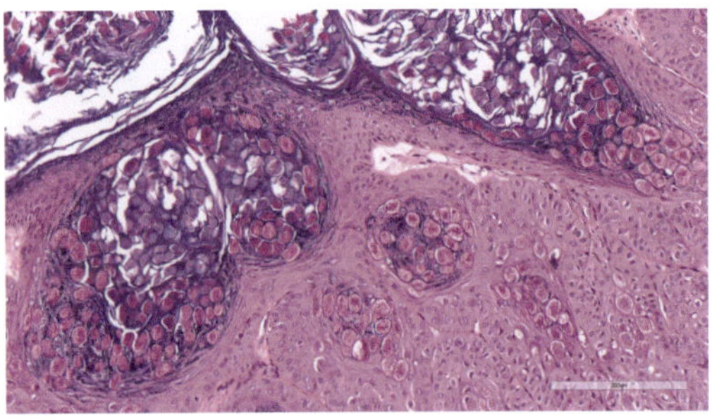

Fig. 5.7 Molluscum contagiosum—Photomicrograph shows markedly hyperplastic keratinized stratified squamous epithelium with inverted nodules containing molluscum bodies or Henderson-Paterson bodies. These inclusions are eosinophilic at the base of the lesion and turn hematoxyphilic at the surface (H&E; 20× original magnification)

microscopy or histopathology forms the backbone of identification.

Acanthamoeba

Acanthamoeba is a free-living freshwater protozoan that is known to cause severe pain and infection and was associated with contact lens users but is also reported frequently in agrarian populations. Prior history of swimming wearing contact lenses or using contaminated water, trauma with vegetative matter is noted in most of the cases. Ring infiltration is characteristically seen in these eyes [22].

On light microscopy, histology of the corneal button shows intact or denuded epithelium. The striking feature here would be minimal stromal infiltrates and the absence of necrosis, unlike other forms of infectious keratitis. Cysts of *Acanthamoeba* are hexagonal to round and contain an inner endocyst and outer exocyst (hence appear as double-walled on microscopy), which stain with PAS, GMS, Giemsa stains and fluoresce when examined under fluorescent light using calcofluor white, fluorescent stain. Rarely, trophozoites (which are the active motile forms of the parasite) can be seen, which often may be confused with macrophages. In microbiology, these are detected on calcofluor white stain [23]. Presence of mannose-binding protein indicates a major virulence factor. They are culturable on nonnutrient agar layered with heat-inactivated *E.coli* bacteria.

5.7.4.2 Cestodes

Cysticercosis: *Taenia solium* is the causative cestode. The patient usually presents with loss of vision, periorbital pain, scotoma, and photopsia. Neurocysticercosis must be ruled out in these cases.

5.7.4.3 Nematodes

Loa loa: this is another filarial parasite that is endemic to the African continent. Hence, travel history to African countries must be ruled out. These worms migrate in the subconjunctival plane causing severe itching, pain, and foreign body sensation. It causes characteristic "Calabar swelling," which is due to the local tissue reaction. A dead worm may show features of vitritis with hazy vitreous and iridocyclitis. It can also cause intravitreal hemorrhage, retinal detachment, neovascularization, and subretinal exudates.

Case Illustration 3

A 36-year-old female presented with left upper eyelid swelling for the past 6 months. A history of waxing and waning of the swelling is noted. On examination, the cyst measures about 3 × 2 mm in size and is firm on palpation. Histopathology revealed fragmented worms with adjacent tissue reactions. The worm is covered by a thick cuticle with spinous processes and an inner integument. Internally, it contains two gravid uterus and intestines (Fig. 5.8).

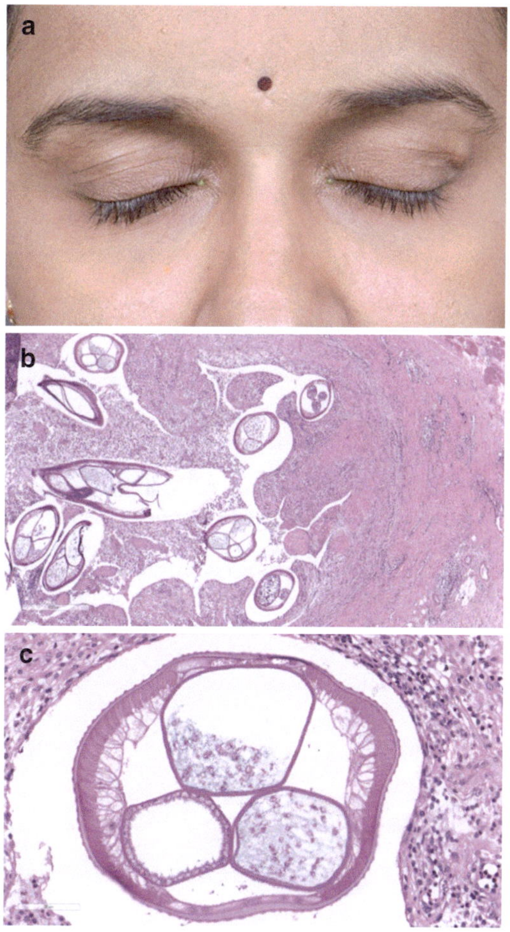

Fig. 5.8 Dirofilariasis—(**a**) Clinical image of the left upper eyelid cyst. (**b**) Cut section of the parasite with adjacent tissue reaction showing chronic inflammatory infiltrates (H&E; 4× original magnification). (**c**) Cross-section of the worm showing cuticle with ridges and integument, two uteri and intestinal canal (H&E; 30× original magnification)

Case Illustration 4

A 7-year-old male child presented with a reddish mass arising from the inner side of the right eyelid for 2.5 months. On examination, a reddish pedunculated soft tissue lesion measuring 1 cm was noted arising from the fornical conjunctiva. An excision biopsy was performed with a provisional diagnosis of pyogenic granuloma (Fig. 5.9).

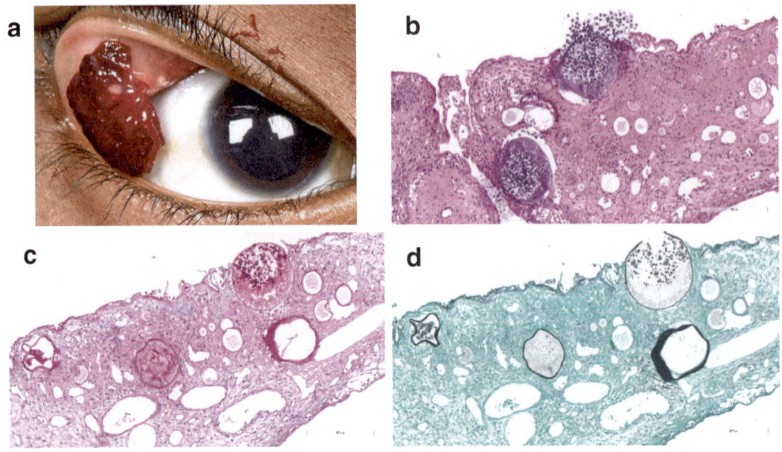

Fig. 5.9 Rhinosporidiosis—(**a**) Clinical image showing characteristic reddish polypoidal growth arising from the tarsal conjunctiva. (**b**) Section shows variable sized sporangia with numerous endospores and chronic inflammation in the conjunctiva and underlying stroma. (H&E; 20× original magnification). C&D) The endospores highlighted on PAS stain (periodic acid Schiff's stain; 20× original magnification) and GMS stain (Gomori methenamine silver; 20× original magnification)

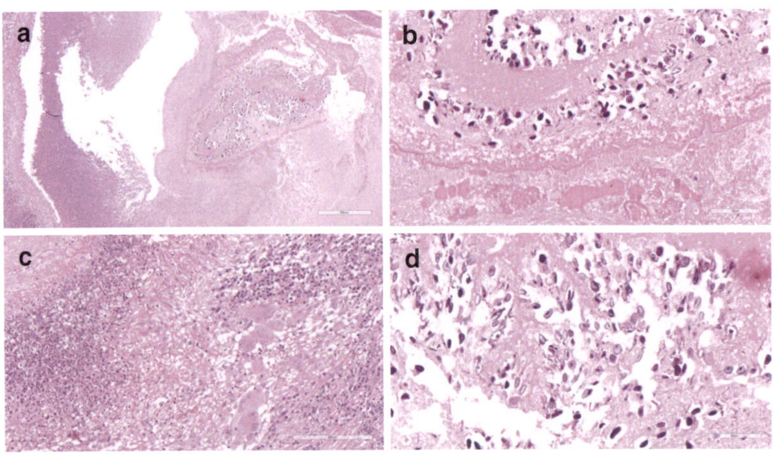

Fig. 5.10 Calcified parasitic cyst—(**a**) Section shows calcified cysts with adjacent large areas necrosis and dead parasite outlines (H&E; 2× original magnification). (**b**) Higher magnification of the calcified concretions and adjacent Splendore–Hoeppli phenomenon (H&E; 30× original magnification). (**c**) Chronic inflammation with multinucleate giant cell reaction (H&E; 20× original magnification). (**d**) Higher magnification of the calcified concretions with endocyst (H&E; 40× original magnification)

Case Illustration 5

A 50-year-old female presented with complaints of lower lid swelling in her right eye, not associated with pain or diplopia. On examination, the mass was nodular, soft to a firm consistency, and the posterior extent was not palpable. Localized lymphadenopathy was not seen. Computed tomography showed a well-defined heterogenous lesion in the inferior and lateral quadrants of the right orbit with intralesional hypodensities (Fig. 5.10).

Financial Disclosures None for all authors.

Funding Funding by Hyderabad Eye Research Foundation, Hyderabad, Telangana, India.

References

1. Fierer J, Looney D, Pechère JC. Nature and Pathogenicity of Micro-organisms. Infect Dis. 2017:4–25.e1. https://doi.org/10.1016/B978-0-7020-6285-8.00002-2. Epub 2016 Aug 12. PMCID: PMC7173513.
2. Sharma S. Diagnosis of infectious diseases of the eye. Eye (Lond). 2012;26(2):177–84. https://doi.org/10.1038/eye.2011.275. Epub 2011 Nov 18. PMID: 22094299; PMCID: PMC3272189.
3. Ueta M, Kinoshita S. Innate immunity of the ocular surface. Brain Res Bull. 2010;81(2–3):219–28. https://doi.org/10.1016/j.brainresbull.2009.10.001. Epub 2009 Oct 12. PMID: 19828129.
4. Deepthi KG, Prabagaran SR. Ocular bacterial infections: pathogenesis and diagnosis. Microb Pathog. 2020;145:104206. https://doi.org/10.1016/j.micpath.2020.104206. Epub 2020 Apr 21. PMID: 32330515.
5. Durand ML. Bacterial and fungal Endophthalmitis. Clin Microbiol Rev. 2017;30(3):597–613. https://doi.org/10.1128/CMR.00113-16. PMID: 28356323; PMCID: PMC5475221.
6. Bu Y, Chan YK, Wong HL, Poon SH, Lo AC, Shih KC, Tong L. A review of the impact of alterations in gut microbiome on the Immunopathogenesis of ocular diseases. J Clin Med. 2021;10(20):4694. https://doi.org/10.3390/jcm10204694. PMID: 34682816; PMCID: PMC8541376.
7. Kew MC. The hepatitis-B virus and hepatocellular carcinoma. Semin Liver Dis. 1981;1(1):59–67. https://doi.org/10.1055/s-2008-1063930.
8. Friedlaender MH, Masi RJ, Osumoto M, Smolin G, Ammann AJ. Ocular microbial flora in immunodeficient patients. Arch Ophthalmol. 1980;98(7):1211–3. https://doi.org/10.1001/archopht.1980.01020040063004. PMID: 7396772.
9. Watson S, Cabrera-Aguas M, Khoo P. Common eye infections. Aust Prescr. 2018;41(3):67–72. https://doi.org/10.18773/austprescr.2018.016. Epub 2018 Jun 1. PMID: 29922000; PMCID: PMC6003010.
10. Austin A, Lietman T, Rose-Nussbaumer J. Update on the management of infectious Keratitis. Ophthalmology. 2017;124(11):1678–89. https://doi.org/10.1016/j.ophtha.2017.05.012. Epub 2017 Sep 21. PMID: 28942073; PMCID: PMC5710829.
11. Ma L, Jakobiec FA, Dryja TP. A review of Next-Generation Sequencing (NGS): applications to the diagnosis of ocular infectious diseases. Semin Ophthalmol. 2019;34(4):223–31. https://doi.org/10.1080/08820538.2019.1620800. Epub 2019 Jun 6. PMID: 31170015.
12. Bourcier T, Sauer A, Dory A, Denis J, Sabou M. Fungal keratitis. J Fr Ophtalmol. 2017;40(9):e307–13. https://doi.org/10.1016/j.jfo.2017.08.001. Epub 2017 Oct 4. PMID: 28987448.
13. Mahmoudi S, Masoomi A, Ahmadikia K, Tabatabaei SA, Soleimani M, Rezaie S, Ghahvechian H, Banafsheafshan A. Fungal keratitis: an overview of clinical and laboratory aspects. Mycoses. 2018;61(12):916–30. https://doi.org/10.1111/myc.12822. Epub 2018 Jul 27. PMID: 29992633.
14. Permpalung N, Worasilchai N, Chindamporn A. Human pythiosis: emergence of fungal-like organism. Mycopathologia. 2020;185(5):801–12. https://doi.org/10.1007/s11046-019-00412-0. Epub 2019 Dec 16. PMID: 31845178.
15. Song G, Liang G, Liu W. Fungal co-infections associated with global COVID-19 pandemic: a clinical and diagnostic perspective from China. Mycopathologia. 2020;185(4):599–606. https://doi.org/10.1007/s11046-020-00462-9. Epub 2020 Jul 31. PMID: 32737747; PMCID: PMC7394275.
16. Lobo AM, Agelidis AM, Shukla D. Pathogenesis of herpes simplex keratitis: The host cell response and ocular surface sequelae to infection and inflammation. Ocul Surf. 2019;17(1):40–9. https://doi.org/10.1016/j.jtos.2018.10.002. Epub 2018 Oct 11. PMID: 30317007; PMCID: PMC6340725.
17. Vemuganti GK, Murthy SI, Das S. Update on pathologic diagnosis of corneal infections and inflammations. Middle East Afr J Ophthalmol. 2011;18(4):277–84. https://doi.org/10.4103/0974-9233.90128. PMID: 22224015; PMCID: PMC3249812.
18. Bertoli F, Veritti D, Danese C, Samassa F, Sarao V, Rassu N, Gambato T, Lanzetta P. Ocular findings in COVID-19 patients: a review of direct manifestations and indirect effects on the eye. J Ophthalmol. 2020;2020:4827304. https://doi.org/10.1155/2020/4827304. PMID: 32963819; PMCID: PMC7491448.
19. Ozturker ZK. Conjunctivitis as sole symptom of COVID-19: a case report and review of literature. Eur J Ophthalmol. 2021;31(2):NP161–6. https://doi.org/10.1177/1120672120946287. Epub 2020 Jul 24. Erratum in: Eur J Ophthalmol. 2020 Aug 27;:1120672120956486. PMID: 32703010; PMCID: PMC7383095.
20. Joseph J, Vemuganti GK, Sharma S. Microsporidia: emerging ocular pathogens. Indian J Med Microbiol. 2005;23(2):80–91. https://doi.org/10.4103/0255-0857.16045.
21. Joseph J, Vemuganti GK, Garg P, Sharma S. Histopathological evaluation of ocular microsporidiosis by different stains. BMC Clin Pathol. 2006;6:6. https://doi.org/10.1186/1472-6890-6-6. PMID: 16792818; PMCID: PMC1513581.
22. Frangie JP, Moore MB. Parasitic infection including Acanthamoeba. In: Leibowitz HM, Waring GO, editors. Corneal disorder: clinical diagnosis and management. 3rd ed. Philadelphia: W.B. Saunders Company; 1988. p. 719.
23. Das D, Ramachandra V, Islam S, Bhattacharjee H, Biswas J, Koul A, Deka P, Deka A. Update on pathology of ocular parasitic disease. Indian J Ophthalmol. 2016;64(11):794–802. https://doi.org/10.4103/0301-4738.195590. PMID: 27958200; PMCID: PMC5200979.

Neoplasia 6

Indranil Chakrabarti

Contents

6.1 Introduction

Neoplasia means "new growth" (Ancient Greek; *neo* = new, *plasma* = creation) and has been defined by Willis as "an abnormal mass of tissue, the growth of which exceeds and is uncoordinated with that of the normal tissues and persists in the same excessive manner after cessation of the stimuli which evoked the change." Thus, neoplasia is an irreversible process, unlike hyperplasia and metaplasia. A common term that is used for all malignant tumors is cancer. Hippocrates (460–370 BC) used the term *karkinos*, the Greek word for crab, to several types of cancers as the cut surface of the solid malignant tumors grossly resembled that of a crab. Celsus (25 BC–50 AD) coined the term cancer (from karkinos), which is the Latin word for crab, that is, cancer. The word *Oncology* (Greek *oncos* = tumor, *logos* = study)

I. Chakrabarti (✉)
Department of Pathology and Laboratory Medicine, All India Institute of Medical Sciences, Saguna, Kalyani, West Bengal, India

G. K. Vemuganti et al. (eds.), *Ocular Pathology*, https://doi.org/10.1007/978-981-96-8614-8_6

refers to the study of tumors or neoplasms. The original term "tumor," which was used to denote swelling in inflammation, has gone into disuse and is presently used only to represent neoplasia.

Broadly speaking, tumors can be benign or malignant. Benign tumors are slow-growing, do not invade adjacent tissue, and do not spread to other sites (metastasis). On the contrary, malignant tumors tend to grow rapidly with invasion to the adjacent tissue and distant spread.

The suffix "-oma" usually refers to the tumor, more so a benign neoplasm, for example, lipoma, fibroadenoma (Fig. 6.1), etc.

However, there are certain malignant tumors like seminoma, dysgerminoma, and astrocytoma, which end with "-oma." For this reason, some of the tumors ending with "-oma" had an additional qualifier as malignant, for example, malignant melanoma, malignant lymphoma, etc., though nowadays, melanoma and lymphomas are considered malignant even without this qualifier.

A *hamartoma* (Greek hamartia = fault, defect) is a tumor-like malformation formed by the disorganized overgrowth of normal mature tissue indigenous to the particular organ. It may sometimes mimic a neoplasm. For example, Juvenile polyp of the colon, Peutz-Jegher's polyp, pulmonary hamartoma, etc., A *choristoma* is a tumor-like mass formed by normal cells in an abnormal or foreign location. For example, middle ear choristoma, salivary gland choristoma, etc., *Heterotopia* refers to finding normal tissue in abnormal location, but when it forms a mass-like lesion, it is generally referred to as choristoma. Examples of heterotopia include gastric tissue or pancreatic tissue in Meckel's diverticulum.

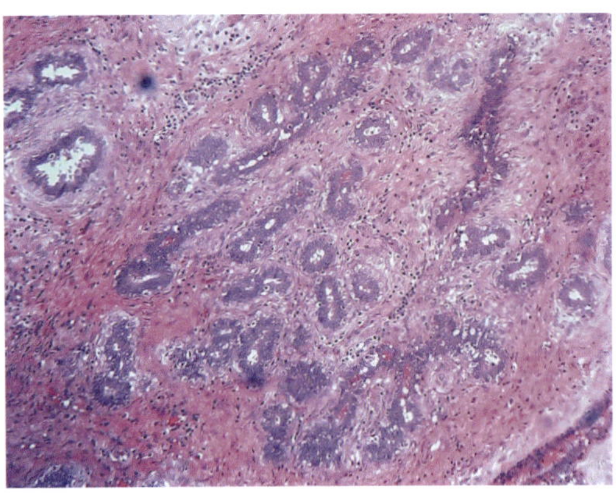

Fig. 6.1 Section showing the fibroadenoma of breast

6.2 Classification of Tumors

A. *Based on histogenesis*: The malignant tumors that originate from the parenchymal or epithelial tissue are known *carcinomas,* while those arising from mesenchymal tissue are referred to as *Sarcomas*. The major differences between carcinomas and sarcomas are highlighted in Table 6.1.

All tumors, benign or malignant, have 2 components:

(a) *Clonal neoplastic cells*, which constitute their parenchyma and determine the biological behavior of the tumor
(b) *Reactive stroma,* which is made up of connective tissue, blood vessels, and variable number of macrophages and lymphocytes and provides support to the tumor

Desmoplasia is defined as the dense, fibrous stroma around the invading cells in infiltrating carcinomas, for example in stomach carcinoma, pancreatic carcinoma, breast carcinoma (Fig. 6.2), collecting duct carcinoma of kidney, and desmoplastic tumors like desmoplastic small round cell tumors (DSRCTs), desmoplastic basal cell carcinoma (BCC), trichoepithelioma, etc.,

Benign tumors of squamous epithelium are papillomas (Fig. 6.3) while adenomas are benign tumors of glandular epithelium.

Malignant tumors of squamous epithelium are called squamous cell carcinomas (Fig. 6.4), while those of glandular epithelium are called adenocarcinomas.

Tumors may include malignancies of more than one epithelium, for example, adenosquamous carcinoma of the cervix in which both the squamous and glandular components are malignant and are mixed with each other.

Certain benign tumors known as *mixed tumors* display a combination of both epithe-

Table 6.1 Differences between carcinomas and sarcomas

	Carcinoma	Sarcoma
Histogenesis	Malignant tumor of epithelial tissue	Malignant tumor of mesenchymal tissue
Incidence	Much common	Relatively rare
Age	Common in middle-age and older age groups	Common in younger age groups, some are even common in children (e.g., rhabdomyosarcomas)
Rate of growth	Relatively slow	Rapid growth
Preferred route of metastasis	Lymphatic spread Late spread occurs through the hematogenous route.	Hematogenous spread
Response to chemotherapy	More responsive	More resistant
In situ phase	Common	Absent
Microscopic examination	Malignant cell clusters separated and well supported by reactive stroma Hemorrhage, necrosis less common except poorly differentiated tumors	Diffuse, infiltrative growth of malignant mesenchymal cells with poorly formed tumor stroma Hemorrhage, necrosis more common

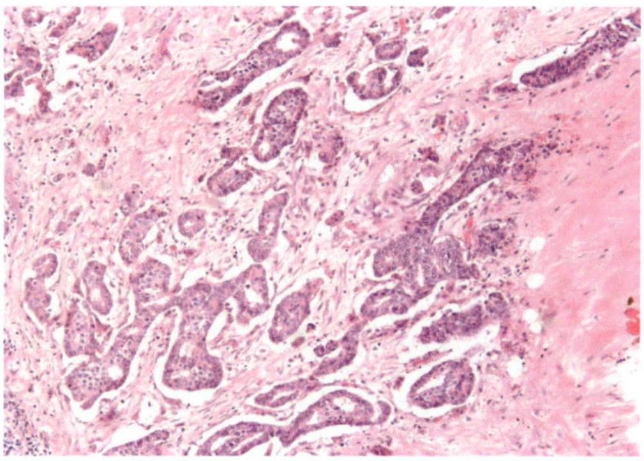

Fig. 6.2 Section from invasive breast carcinoma showing desmoplastic stroma

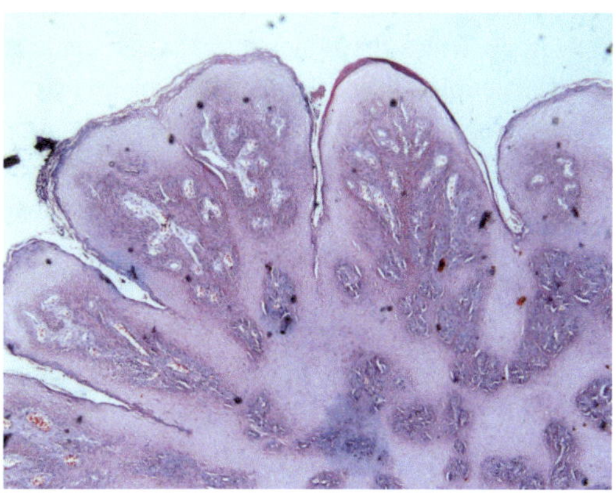

Fig. 6.3 Section from a squamous papilloma showing finger-like projections

lial and mesenchymal tissues, for example, pleomorphic adenoma of salivary glands (Fig. 6.5). Similarly, some malignant tumors known as *carcinosarcomas* refer to malignant tumors that are formed of carcinomatous as well as sarcomatous elements, for example, malignant mixed Mullerian tumors (MMMTs) in the uterus.

Collision tumors are neoplasms that show 2 distinct neoplastic cell populations, which do not intermingle with each other and maintain distinct borders. They may be formed by 2 benign tumors, 1 benign and 1 malignant tumor, or 2 malignant tumors for example, collision tumor of gastric carcinoma with neuroendocrine tumors.

The malignancies of the hematopoietic system include *leukemias* (arising from blood cells), *lymphomas* like Hodgkin lymphoma, non-Hodgkin lymphoma (arising from lymphoid tissue), *multiple myeloma* (arising from plasma cells), etc.,

Teratomas are germ cell tumors composed of a mixture of different tissue types arising from the three germ cell layers (ectoderm, mesoderm, endoderm) They may arise from testis (Fig. 6.6), ovary mediastinum, retroperitoneum, sacrococcygeal region, head and

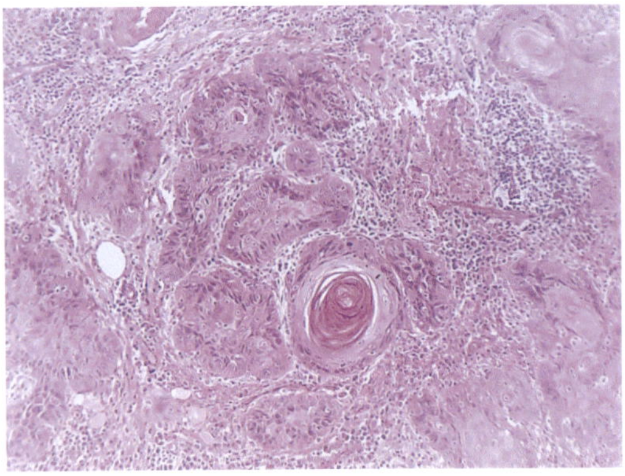

Fig. 6.4 Section showing well-differentiated squamous cell carcinoma with prominent squamous pearls

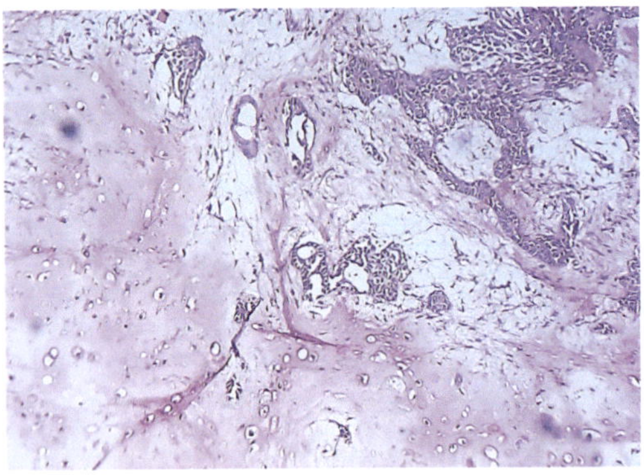

Fig. 6.5 Section from pleomorphic adenoma of salivary glands showing myoepithelial cells and epithelial cells with chondromyxoid matrix

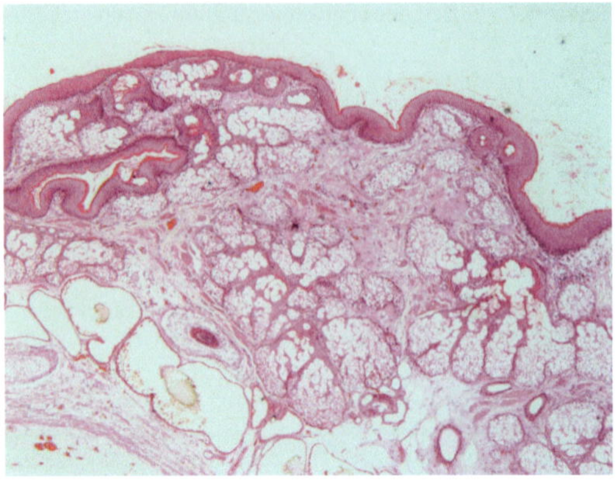

Fig. 6.6 Mature teratoma lined by keratinizing squamous epithelium and skin adnexal structures

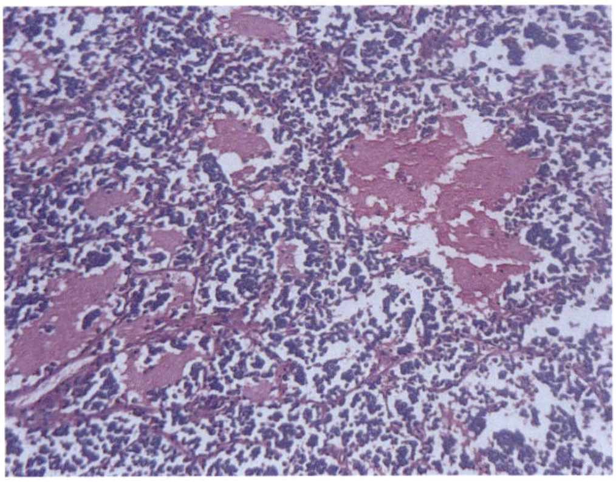

Fig. 6.7 Section showing Ewing's sarcoma from the tibia of a 13-year-old boy

neck, central nervous system, etc., They may be benign (mature) or malignant (immature).

Blastomas are a group of malignant tumors usually arising in childhood from the embryonal cells or immature cells of that organ, for example, hepatoblastoma (liver), nephroblastoma, or Wilm's tumor (kidney) neuroblastoma (adrenal glands), retinoblastoma(retina), etc., These tumors are also included in the group of *small round cell tumors* (SRCTs).

Neuroectodermal tumors are tumors arising from the neuroectoderm and usually affect the central and peripheral nervous systems.

They belong to 2 groups: Group I includes tumors with epithelial differentiation and cytokeratin positivity (e.g., the neuroendocrine tumors, pituitary adenoma/carcinomas). Group II are the nonepithelial neuroectodermal neoplasms with cytokeratin negativity and more neural features (e.g., Granular cell tumor, paraganglioma, olfactory neuroblastoma, Ewing's family of tumors (Fig. 6.7), primitive neuroectodermal tumor (PNET), etc.,)

Neuroendocrine tumors are tumors arising from neuroendocrine cells, and they may be well differentiated (typical and atypical carcinoid) or poorly differentiated (small cell carcinomas and large cell neuroendocrine carcinoma) depending on mitosis and/or Ki67 index (proliferation marker) and morphology (cytology, architecture, necrosis, etc.,); they may be functional (producing hormones) or nonfunctional. *Mixed neuroendo-*

crine nonneuroendocrine neoplasms (MiNENs) are neoplasms that show both neuroendocrine and nonneuroendocrine components, each ≥30% of the tumor

B. *Based on biologic Behavior:*

The neoplasms, based on their biologic behavior, can be broadly divided into benign and malignant neoplasms. The basic differences are highlighted in Table 6.1

6.3 Microscopic Features of Neoplasia

Microscopic features of neoplasms are important for the recognition, categorization, and prognostication of tumors. The major important features of benign and malignant tumors are highlighted in Table 6.2.

It is worthwhile to elaborate 2 important terminologies: Differentiation and Anaplasia.

Differentiation is defined as the extent of the resemblance of a neoplasm, both histologically and functionally, to the normal cells of that organ ranging from none to close resemblance. This scheme of differentiation into well, moderate, and poorly differentiated/undifferentiated tumors are used for the grading of tumors.

Anaplasia (meaning "to form backward") is a term to denote the lack of differentiation and is the hallmark of malignancy.

Anaplasia is often associated with the following:

Table 6.2 Differences between benign and malignant tumors

	Benign	Malignant
Clinical and gross features		
Boundaries	Encapsulated/well circumscribed	Irregular margins/poorly circumscribed
Adjacent tissue	Often compressed	Invades the adjacent tissue
Secondary changes like hemorrhage, infarction, ulceration, necrosis, etc.,	Not common	Usually present
Microscopic features		
Pattern	Resembles cell of origin	More often shows poor resemblance to tissue of origin or cellular differentiation
Basal polarity	Retained	Usually lost
Pleomorphism	Usually absent	Usually present
N:C ratio	Normal or slightly increased (1:4 or 1:6)	High (1:1)
Nuclear features	Usually normal	Hyperchromasia present with irregular outlines, pleomorphism, anisonucleosis, and multiple nucleoli
Mitoses	May be increased but no atypical forms present	Increased with atypical mitotic figures
Tumor giant cells	Rare; if present no nuclear atypia	Often present with atypical nuclei; usually multinucleated, may have single nuclei
Biological behavior		
Rate of growth	Usually slow growing	Rapid
Local invasion	Compresses adjacent tissue without invasion/infiltration	Invades and infiltrates adjacent tissue
Metastasis	Uncommon (rare examples include leiomyoma, cardiac myxoma, salivary adenoma, etc.,)	Frequently present (exceptions include basal cell carcinoma, which is locally invasive, giant cell tumor of bone, etc.,)
Prognosis	Good, easily resectable, local complications only	Usually poor with local and systemic complications (due to metastasis)

- Loss of polarity
- Pleomorphism
- N:C ratio
- Abnormal nuclear features
- Mitosis
- Tumor giant cells
- Other changes

Loss of Polarity: This refers to the loss of normal orientation of cells. Normally, the cells of any epithelium are arranged along the basement membrane, which is known as *basal polarity*. In malignancies, this orientation is disrupted and after a breach of the basement membrane, the tumor cells infiltrate the subepithelium in sheets or singles.

Pleomorphism: This refers to variation in size and shape of the tumor cell. The more anaplastic tumors are more pleomorphic.

Nuclear: Cytoplasmic ratio (N/C): The nuclei are enlarged disproportionately compared to the cell size resulting in high nuclear: cytoplasmic ratio (N:C ratio) approaching 1:1 from the normal 1:4–6.

Abnormal Nuclear Features: Nuclear hyperchromasia with irregular nuclear outlines, clumped coarse chromatin distributed along the nuclear membrane, anisonucleosis, and multiple nucleoli are some of the abnormal nuclear features of anaplastic cells.

Mitosis: Increased mitosis signifies increased cellular proliferation, which may be seen in actively proliferating cells, hyperplastic tissue as well as benign and malignant neoplasms. However, atypical, bizarre mitotic figures with tripolar, quadripolar, or multipolar spindles indicate malignancy.

Tumor Giant Cells: May be present in benign neoplasms but without any nuclear atypia. Malignant tumors show tumor giant cells, more often multinucleated, with atypical nuclei.

Other Changes: In rapidly growing tumors, the central area may undergo ischemic necrosis when the neoangiogenesis cannot keep up with the demand for blood supply.

Two other similar-sounding terms that need to be differentiated from neoplasia are metaplasia and dysplasia.

Metaplasia is defined as a reversible process of replacement of one adult cell type with another better-suited adult cell type by reprogramming of stem cells in response to tissue damage, repair, or regeneration. For example, chronic irritation of the squamous lining of the lower part of the esophagus by gastric acid due to gastroesophageal reflux leads to its replacement by glandular (gastric or intestinal) epithelium, which is better suited to withstand an acidic environment. This is known as *Barret esophagus*, which may be a site for dysplasia and subsequently adenocarcinoma.

Dysplasia is a term that means "disordered proliferation" and may be considered a precursor to malignancy, but at the same time, it must be borne in mind that all cases of dysplasia do not progress to malignancy and many may be completely reversible. The changes are usually seen in epithelial tissue, and dysplastic cells may exhibit many of the above-mentioned features of anaplasia. The extent of this disordered proliferation is graded as mild, moderate, and severe dysplasia or low-grade and high-grade dysplasia depending upon the tissue. Mild and moderate dysplasia may revert back completely on the removal of the inciting stimulus, while severe or full-thickness dysplasia (also known as carcinoma in situ) may eventually after several long years breach the basement membrane leading to invasive malignancy.

6.4 Invasiveness or Spread of Tumors

An important aspect of neoplasms is invasiveness, which may be of 2 types:

(a) Local invasion and b) Distant spread (metastasis)

(a) *Local Invasion:* Local invasion or infiltration into the adjacent tissue is the feature of malignant neoplasm. Benign neoplasms are slow-growing tumors that develop a capsule and are well circumscribed. The capsule separates the tumor from the adjacent tissue, which may be subjected to compression by the expans-

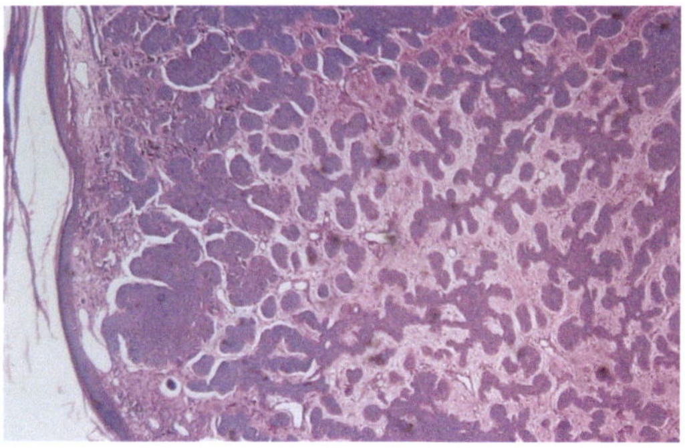

Fig. 6.8 Section showing presence of basal cell carcinoma of skin

ile growth. On the contrary, malignant tumors most often lack such a capsule and the tumor cells tend to infiltrate and invade the surrounding tissue, making them difficult to resect or unresectable.

(b) *Metastasis:* Metastasis, which is the hallmark of malignancy, is defined as the spread of tumor cells to sites that are physically discontinuous with the primary tumor. However, there are certain malignant tumors that are locally invasive, but they rarely metastasize, for example, basal cell carcinoma of the skin (Fig. 6.8). On the other hand, there are rare examples like metastasizing pleomorphic adenoma and benign metastasizing leiomyoma, which are characterized by metastasis of benign tumors to distant sites.

Metastasis in malignant tumors indicates poor prognosis and poor response to treatment. Liquid tumors (leukemias and lymphomas) are almost always disseminated and considered malignant at diagnosis. Metastasis remains the major cause of cancer deaths.

6.4.1 Pathways of Metastasis

The 3 most common pathways of tumor spread or metastasis are as follows:

(i) Direct spread
(ii) Lymphatic spread
(iii) Hematogenous spread

Another important but rare mode of tumor spread is iatrogenic or surgical implantation caused by surgical intervention.

Direct Spread: Also known as the local spread, this refers to the spread of tumor cells through the path of least resistance, be it tissue planes or natural cavities (like peritoneal, pleural, pericardial cavities, and spaces like subarachnoid and joint spaces). This spread, through natural body spaces/cavities, is also known as *tumor seeding or transcoelomic spread* and is more common in malignancies of organs, which are in close proximity to these natural spaces.

Pleural cavity may be affected by tumor cells from peripherally located lung carcinomas, breast carcinomas, lymphomas, mesotheliomas, etc., resulting in malignant pleural effusion. Microscopic examination of pleural fluid by diagnostic thoracentesis reveals malignant cells in such cases.

Subarachnoid space invasion may be seen in glioblastoma multiforme, medulloblastoma, ependymoma, metastatic tumors, etc., which can spread through CSF.

Lymphatic Spread/Metastasis: This is a very important and common mode of metastasis mostly seen in carcinomas and only a few sarcomas like synovial sarcoma, rhabdomyosarcoma, epithelioid sarcoma, clear cell sarcoma, angiosarcoma, etc., In a tumor specimen or lymph node dissection, meticulous microscopic examination of the subcapsular space of submitted lymph nodes is warranted to detect any metastasis. After partial/complete replacement, the tumor cells move further to involve the next node. Figure 6.9 shows metastatic deposits of squamous cell carcinoma in lymph node.

The metastasis of a tumor through lymphatics follows the natural route of lymphatic drainage starting with *regional lymph nodal metastasis*. The first lymph node in the regional lymph nodal basin that receives the lymph flow and hence the metastasis from the primary tumor is known as the *sentinel lymph node*.

These sentinel lymph nodes can be identified by the injection of blue dyes or radiolabeled tracers and examined on frozen sections under a microscope intraoperatively by the pathologist to

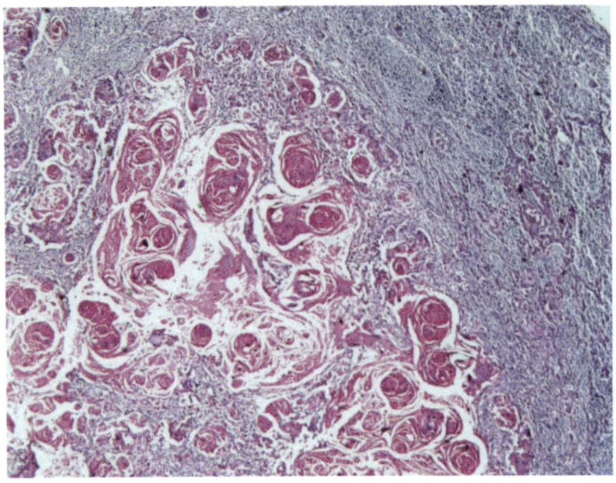

Fig. 6.9 Metastatic deposits of well-differentiated squamous cell carcinoma in cervical lymph node

look for the involvement of tumor cells. If uninvolved, it is unlikely that other lymph nodes further down the line will be involved. This will guide the surgeon to refrain from extensive lymph nodal exenteration, thus considerably reducing the postsurgical morbidity of the patient. Sentinel lymph node mapping is also done for other tumors like melanomas and colonic cancers.

Sometimes, the tumor cells may skip or bypass the nearest lymph node and involve other lymph nodes, a phenomenon known as *skip metastasis*.

Retrograde Metastasis: Sometimes due to tumor cell permeation of lymphatics, the lymphatic flow gets blocked and starts to flow in reverse direction, thus carrying the tumor cell in a retrograde fashion to unusual sites. This is known as *retrograde metastasis* and is seen in metastasis of gastric carcinoma in the left supraclavicular lymph node or *Virchow's node*. This clinical finding is known as *Troisier's sign*.

Lymph node enlargement due to other causes needs to be ruled out.

Hematogenous Spread/Metastasis: This route is generally preferred by sarcomas, but there are certain carcinomas that spread through blood vessels like renal cell carcinoma, hepatocellular carcinomas, adrenocortical carcinoma, etc., Arteries, because of their thick walls, are less commonly permeated by tumor cells as compared to the venous channels. Of particular importance is the renal cell carcinoma, which involves the renal vein and, through it, reaches the inferior vena cava and even the right side of the heart, growing in a snake-like pattern. Such spread upstages the tumor and indicates a poor prognosis.

The blood-borne metastasis is more common in the lung, liver, bones, brain, kidneys, and adrenals where the blood flow is sluggish. But this alone does not explain the common sites of metastasis or the preference of certain tumors to metastasize in certain organs. This organ tropism of tumors can be partly explained by the fact that tumor cells express certain adhesion molecules whose ligands are expressed in their preferred sites of metastasis and partly by the fact that tumor cells express receptors for chemokines, which are secreted in abundance in the preferred organs for metastasis and/or endothelial cells of those organs may express ligands for adhesion molecules that are expressed in tumor cells [1].

6.5 Epidemiology of Cancers

Despite various successful treatment breakthroughs, cancer is still a leading cause of death worldwide, accounting for nearly ten million deaths in 2020. It has been projected that by 2030, the estimated number of cancer cases and cancer deaths will increase to 21.4 million and 13.2 million, respectively. In India, there have been 1.32 million new cases of cancer and 8.5 lakh cancer deaths in 2020 (source Globocan 2020) [2].

The 3 major causes of cancer and cancer-related deaths throughout the world are breast cancer, lung cancer, and colorectal cancer in women, and lung cancer, prostate cancer, and colorectal cancer in males. In India, aerodigestive cancers in men and cervical carcinomas in females cause a major burden in addition to the tumors mentioned above. In children, the common cancers are leukemias and brain tumors followed by lymphomas, bone sarcomas, and soft tissue sarcomas.

Though neoplasia is now known to be multifactorial, there are certain modifiable risk factors like smoking, fibrepoor diet, etc., that can be taken care of by public awareness strategies.

Various screening programs, for example, pap smears for cervical cancers, upper gastrointestinal endoscopy for gastric carcinoma, mammography for breast cancers, etc., have been started in many countries as per the prevalence of specific cancers in that population, which has led to early detection and, hence, a decline in the number of advanced cases.

The various epidemiological factors responsible for neoplasia may be grouped into

(a) Environmental factors
(b) Age
(c) Acquired predisposing factors
(d) Genetic predisposition

Environmental Factors: Genetics and environmental parameters are the two most important factors responsible for most cancers. The most established environmental factors include

- *Infectious Agents*: About 15% of all cancers are estimated to be caused, directly or indirectly, by infectious agents, particularly in developing countries: for example, HPV, EBV, HTLV, etc.,
- *Smoking*: Cigarette smoking is one such modifiable risk factor, the cessation of which can result in the decline of the vast majority of cancers. It contains several mutagenic as well as tumor-promoting substances that are responsible for cancers of the lung, upper aerodigestive tract, esophagus, pancreas, and bladder [1].
- *Alcohol*: Alcohol works in synergy or independent of smoking to cause multiple types of cancers. Alcohol consumption is implicated in cancers of the liver (hepatocellular carcinomas), esophagus, oropharynx, and larynx. Growing evidence also links it to colorectal carcinomas and breast carcinomas [3]. The production of acetaldehyde (as a metabolite), increase in oxidative stress, inhibition of absorption of important nutrients like folate, and causation of inflammation are some of the ways in which alcohol acts as a carcinogen. Together, alcohol and tobacco cause a super-additive effect resulting in an elevation of cancer risk particularly those of the oral cavity, oropharynx, larynx, and digestive tract. It is generally believed that alcohol can act as a solvent, thus promoting the entry of carcinogenic substances of cigarette smoke into the tissues.
- *Diet:* Dietary factors have been found to be associated with cancers of the colorectum, stomach, prostate, and breast. A Western dietary pattern characterized by low fiber intake, high fat consumption, and associated obesity is considered a major contributing factor in most cases. High consumption of smoked foods, salted food, food rich in nitrosamines, etc., lead to an increased risk of gastric carcinomas. On the other hand, a high intake of fresh fruits and vegetables rich in Vitamin C, selenium, lycopene, etc., may reduce the risk. Aflatoxin B produced by *Aspergillus flavus* in stored grains is an established risk factor for hepatocellular carcinomas [1].
- *Obesity:* Overweight and obesity appear to be a significant contributor to the incidence of cancers particularly seen in developed countries and is attributed to the type of diet and sedentary lifestyle in addition to genetic factors [1].
- *Reproductive History:* An early menarche, the timing of pregnancy, and late menopause may influence the cumulative estrogen exposure, which, when unopposed by progesterone, can lead to cancers of the breast and endometrium. Similarly, patients receiving hormone replacement therapy have an increased risk of endometrial and breast carcinomas and, to some extent, ovarian carcinomas. Again, ladies with early age of first intercourse and multiple sexual partners suffer from an increased risk of developing HPV-induced cervical carcinomas [1].
- *Environmental Carcinogens:* We are constantly exposed to the environment around us, be it indoors or outdoors, which is laden with an endless list of carcinogens, for example, Ultraviolet rays, arsenic, benzene, hydrocarbons, polyvinyl chloride, etc., The occupational environment may expose us to harmful

agents by inhalation, ingestion, or direct dermal content: for example, asbestos (may cause mesotheliomas, lung carcinomas), aromatic amines (bladder cancer), arsenic (skin cancer, lung cancer), cadmium (prostrate carcinomas), ionizing radiation(leukemias, breast cancer), vinyl chloride (hepatic angiosarcoma, brain tumors, leukemias), etc., [1].

Age: Common childhood tumors include leukemias (also called liquid cancers), lymphomas, brain tumors, neuroblastoma, nephroblastoma (Wilm's tumor), retinoblastoma, rhabdomyosarcomas, teratoma, etc., Carcinomas affect middle-aged and elderly individuals, while sarcomas occur in all decades sometime with bimodal peaks.

Acquired Predisposing Factors: The common acquired predisposing factors may be grouped under precursor lesions, benign tumors, chronic inflammatory conditions, and immunodeficiency states.

Precursor lesions are lesions that result from chronic irritation/inflammation due to certain injurious agents or increased proliferation due to growth-promoting stimuli and may progress to cancers particularly if the stimuli are not removed. For example *Barret esophagus* (metaplastic columnar epithelium in distal esophagus secondary to chronic gastric reflux), which may lead to adenocarcinoma of the esophagus, *squamous metaplasia of bronchial epithelium* (chronic irritation by smoking) leading to squamous cell lung carcinomas, *leukoplakia* of oral cavity leading to squamous cell carcinomas, *endometrial hyperplasia* (sustained estrogenic stimulation), which may lead to endometrial carcinomas, etc., (Table 6.3).

Benign tumors sometimes act as precursor lesions that may undergo malignant transformation over the course of time. However, it must be remembered that most of the benign tumors do not turn malignant. The classical example of neoplastic precursor lesions is the colonic adenoma turning into colonic carcinoma by the adenoma-carcinoma sequence (explained later in this chapter). Other rare examples include pleomorphic adenoma of salivary glands undergoing malignant transformation (carcinoma, ex pleomorphic adenoma) etc.

Table 6.3 Some common precursor lesions of malignancies

Precursor lesion	Associated malignancy
Leukoplakia of tongue	Squamous cell carcinoma of the tongue
Barret esophagus	Adenocarcinoma of esophagus
Endometrial hyperplasia	Endometrial carcinoma
Adenomatous colonic polyp	Colon carcinoma
High-grade squamous intraepithelial lesion (HSIL)	Squamous cell carcinoma of the cervix

Chronic inflammatory conditions result in increased cell turnover and exposure to various cytokines and oxidative stress, which may cause several mutations that the cells accumulate over time to develop neoplasia: for example, chronic gastritis (by *H. pylori* infection) may develop into gastric adenocarcinoma or MALT lymphoma, ulcerative colitis (a form of inflammatory bowel disease) may develop into colorectal carcinoma, chronic hepatitis may develop into hepatocellular carcinoma, etc.,

Immunodeficiency states: Immunodeficient states particularly those affecting T cell immunity are prone to developing cancers. For example, patients infected with HIV develop several malignancies like Kaposi's sarcoma, aggressive B cell non-Hodgkin lymphomas, cervical cancers, head and neck cancers, etc.,

Genetic Predisposition: Genetic and epigenetic alterations lie at the heart of carcinogenesis. Genetic predisposition is seen in familial cancer syndromes. Individuals who inherit germline mutations from their parents have a greater risk of developing cancer. Such cancers usually manifest earlier than the sporadic cases and may affect multiple sites. However, how and when this cancer will manifest depends upon multiple factors like genetic polymorphisms, epigenetic factors, nongenetic factors, etc., Ladies who inherit mutations in the breast cancer susceptibility tumor-suppressor genes BRCA1 and BRCA 2 have about fivefold higher risk of developing breast carcinoma and about 10–30 times the risk of developing ovarian cancers. They also have a higher risk of developing pancreatic cancers. Men who inherit these mutations have an increased risk of developing breast cancer, prostatic carcinomas, and pancreatic cancers. Patients who suffer from familial adenomatous polyposis (FAP) have inherited mutations in the APC gene at Chromosome 5q21, which results in numerous colorectal adenomatous polyps (often exceeding 100) at an early age and have a 100% lifetime risk of developing colorectal carcinomas without any surgical intervention.

6.6 Molecular Basis of Cancer

It is now known that the changes in genes form an essential part of how a normal cell transforms into a neoplastic cell. With the advent of newer technologies, it has been possible to find out some of many changes while the rest are being discovered with each passing day. In recent years, epigenetic changes, which in turn may alter the expression of various changes, have caught considerable attention and have been a target for therapeutic intervention. However, to understand the molecular basis of carcinogenesis, the following points need to be remembered:

(a) *Nonlethal Mutation of the Gene of the Cell Is the Essential First Step for Carcinogenesis*: A normal cell needs to undergo a change in its DNA (mutation) to be transformed into a precursor cell and set foot on its path to carcinogenesis. However, such initial damage should be nonlethal for the cell, for understandably, if the cell dies as a result of mutation, it cannot continue to undergo further changes and ultimately give rise to neoplasia.

Such initiating mutations can be inherited (known as *germline mutations*) or acquired (either due to various endogenous or exogenous *environmental factors* or *spontaneous and random* without any possible explanation). Such mutagenesis can be large scale (amplifications, duplications, large-scale deletions, inversions, etc.,) and small scale (substitutions, insertions, deletions affecting one or few nucleotides of the gene) or may be influenced by epigenetic modifications like histone modification or DNA methylation, which result in heritable changes affecting gene expression without changing the basic DNA sequence.

(b) *Clonal Proliferation of the Single Precursor Cell, Which Has Undergone the Initial Mutation*: Though this may appear as an oversimplification, various studies have shown that clonality is a quintessential component of neoplasia. The cell carrying the initial mutation gives rise to daughter cells with the same heritable mutation. Subsequent generations go on accumulating further mutations and ultimately give rise to neoplasia, but they all originate from the clonal proliferation of the precursor cell and carry the same mutation. For example, in multiple myeloma, which is a malignancy of the plasma cells, it can be demonstrated by light chain restriction studies that there is a clonal proliferation of a particular type of plasma cell producing only a specific type of immunoglobulin and producing a monoclonal or "M" spike on serum electrophoresis.

(c) *Mutations Occur in One or More of the Four Regulatory Genes Essential for Normal Growth and Proliferation*: In normal cell growth, the 4 types of regulatory genes involved are.
   (i) *Proto-oncogenes*: These are growth-promoting, that is, they cause cellular proliferation.
   (ii) *Tumor-Suppressor Genes*: Growth-inhibiting genes, that is, they check cell proliferation.
   (iii) *Apoptosis Regulatory Genes*: Genes that increase or check apoptosis, which is a programmed cell death.
   (iv) *DNA Repair Genes*: Genes that repair any mutation that may arise due to nor-

mal cell proliferation (mitosis) or acquired due to various causes.

During normal state, the cell proliferation is tightly regulated by the interactions among these 4 types of regulatory genes. However, the gain of functions of growth-promoting oncogenes or apoptosis-suppressing genes results in an increase in cell numbers forming a tumor mass. Similarly, loss of function of growth-inhibiting tumor-suppressor genes or apoptosis-promoting genes and/or DNA repair genes will contribute to cell accumulation.

(d) *Carcinogenesis Is a Multistep Process as a Result of the Accumulation of Complementary Mutations over Time:* It must be remembered that though the initiating mutation in the first precursor cell has set the ball rolling, it is thankfully not enough to cause cancer. Though the proliferating cells of subsequent generations all harbor that mutation, they, over time, gradually accumulate further mutations in a step-wise manner, which results in genomic instability and evolution of the precursor cell with mutator phenotype. Those mutations confer a clonal growth advantage and result in the development of a malignant phenotype (abnormal excessive growth independent of inciting stimulus, invasiveness, metastasis, etc.,) and are known as *driver mutations*. The mutations that do not do so but are still present in larger numbers are known as *passenger mutations*. Cancer genome analysis aims at identifying the driver mutations, which thankfully appear clustered in a subset of genes. Passenger mutations, on the other hand, are more randomly distributed.

(e) *Emergence of Subclones and Tumor Progression:* As the tumor evolves, subclones emerge with potential growth advantages following the Darwinian theory of "survival of the fittest" by the subsequent accumulation of genetic driver mutations and epigenetic modifications. The more malignant subclones sideline and replace the less malignant ones as the tumor becomes more and more aggressive. This phenomenon is known as *tumor progression* which is the final stage of tumor development.

6.6.1 Molecular Hallmarks of Cancer

These are the advantageous characteristics acquired by the phenotypically normal cells which change or transform them into malignant cells and promote their progression at the cost of the host tissue. The molecular hallmarks of cancer as described by Hanahan and Weinberg in 2000 were updated in 2011. The same was reviewed by Fouad and Aanei [4] who came up with a more updated and organized scheme. These 7 fundamental hallmarks are as follows: (Fig. 6.10)

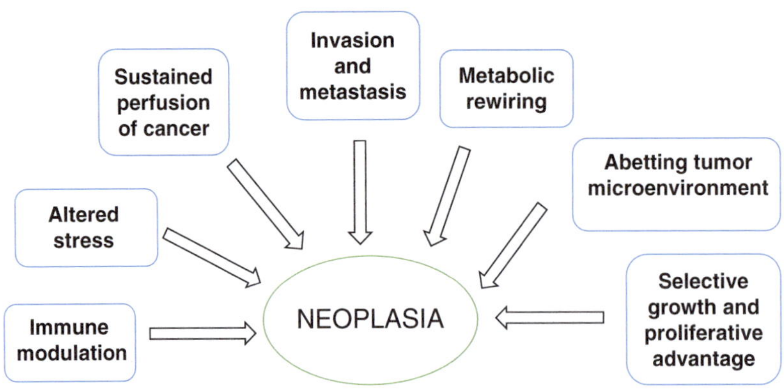

Fig. 6.10 Schematic diagram showing the molecular hallmarks of neoplasia

1. *Selective Growth and Proliferative Advantage:*
   (a) *Self-sufficiency of Growth-Promoting Oncogenes:* Oncogenes are the accelerators of cell proliferation, which, by virtue of "gain of function" mutations, become insensitive to their inciting stimulus, thus becoming self-sufficient and remaining in the "on" state *(full throttle).*
   (b) *Refractoriness to the Growth-Inhibiting Tumor-Suppressor Genes:* Tumor-suppressor genes, which act as the brakes to cell proliferation, during the evolution of malignancy, fail in their duty to control cell proliferation due to "loss-of-function" mutations *(failing brakes).*

   Thus, with failing brakes and full throttle, the car moves forward in an uncontrolled manner, waiting for the accident to happen. A list of oncogenes and tumor-suppressor genes is provided in Table 6.3.
2. *Altered Stress Response Favoring Overall Survival of Cells:*

   The path of the malignant cell is no less hazardous. It has to overcome many obstacles in its transformation from a normal cell to a malignant cell. Immunovigilance, growth disadvantage, DNA damage, lack of oxygen and nutrients, anticancer therapy—the list is endless. However, it shows immense adaptive capabilities to overcome all odds. One of the major mechanisms is the metabolic rewiring or the Warburg effect, which is discussed as an independent hallmark. The other important stress responses are as follows:
   (a) *DNA repair*
   (b) *Apoptosis*
   (c) *Autophagy*
   (d) *Senescence*

DNA repair: DNA damage and mutations accumulate at a frequency of 10^{-6} to 10^{-8} per cell per generation [5]. In addition, other endogenous causes of DNA damage include hydrolytic reactions with water and oxidative reactions with reactive oxygen species (ROS), etc., Exogenous factors such as environmental factors like various physical, chemical, and biological agents cause further genetic and epigenetic alterations. However, fortunately enough, DNA damage response (DDR) pathways are in place to tackle the situation. However, if the DDR system is faulty either due to germline or acquired mutations, the mutational damage is passed on to the progeny, and the integrity of the genome is compromised. For example, in xeroderma pigmentosum due to germline defect in the nucleotide excision repair (NER) pathway, there is an accumulation of unrepaired damaged DNA caused by exposure to the harmful effects of UV rays, resulting in an increased risk of skin cancers, brain cancers etc.,

Lynch syndrome, initially known as hereditary nonpolyposis colon cancer (HNPCC), is the most common hereditary colorectal carcinoma syndrome caused by germline mutations in the mismatch repair (MMR) genes, which usually are involved in the repair of DNA damage in the microsatellite region of the chromosomes. Other than colorectal carcinomas, patients with Lynch syndrome have an increased risk of endometrial and ovarian carcinomas along with other cancers of the brain, gastrointestinal tract, and upper urinary tract.

Apoptosis: The normal homeostasis depends upon the balance between cell proliferation and cell death. The evasion of apoptosis, as noted in several cancers, results in the building up of damaged cells, which pass on the mutations to their progenies. Under normal circumstances, the guardian of the genome, p53, senses the DNA damage, arrests the cell cycle, and activates mechanisms of cell repair. However, if the repair mechanisms fail to repair the damage, the cell is destined to die by apoptosis. However, it also must be remembered that p53-independent pathways for apoptosis are also present.

The 2 major pathways are the *extrinsic pathway* and the more relevant *intrinsic or mitochondrial pathway,* both of which ultimately converge to the executioner caspase 3, which cleaves the DNA and other substrates, resulting in cell death. It is by the intrinsic pathway predominantly that the DNA-damaged cells are pushed down the apoptotic pathway by upregulation of the proapoptotic genes and increase in the mitochondrial outer membrane permeabilization (MOMP) as well as downregulation of the antiapoptotic genes. BAK and BAX are the proapoptotic BH proteins, while BCL-2, BCL-XL, and MCL-1 are the antiapoptotic proteins that act by inhibiting the proapoptotic proteins. BH3-only proteins like BAD, BID, and PUMA sense the DNA damage, activate the proapoptotic molecules, and neutralize the actions of antiapoptotic proteins, thus acting as arbiters of apoptosis. Apoptosis, under normal circumstances, is kept in check by some other antiapoptotic mechanisms like inhibitors of apoptosis proteins (IAPs) like Smac/Diablo, which inhibit the action of Caspases.

The tumor cells evade apoptosis in several ways:

(a) Loss of p53, which prevents the activation of proapoptotic genes
(b) Upregulation of antiapoptotic genes like BCL-2, BCL-XL, and MCL-1, which act by decreasing the mitochondrial outer membrane permeabilization (MOMP) and preventing the release of cytochrome c from mitochondria to cytosol, which normally activates the initiator Caspase 9
(c) Loss of apoptotic peptidase-activating factor 1 (APAF 1)
(d) Upregulation of inhibitors of apoptosis proteins (IAP)
(e) Reduced CD 95/Fas (surface receptor molecule; important in Extrinsic pathway)
(f) Inactivation of death-induced signaling complex (important in Extrinsic pathway)

However, it must be remembered that not all cells in a tumor are resistant to apoptosis and many anticancer drugs act on tumors by inducing apoptosis.

Autophagy: Autophagy is an adaptive survival mechanism seen in unicellular as well as mammalian cells in which a cell eats its own cellular contents in stressful situations like nutrient deprivation. It is of 3 types—macroautophagy (the major form), microautophagy, and Chaperon-mediated autophagy. The macroautophagy, hereafter referred to as autophagy, involves the stages of initiation (formation of an isolation membrane or phagophore), nucleation (of phagophore), and elongation (of phagophore) followed by the formation of autophagosome containing the sequestrated organelles, which subsequently fuse with the lysosome, are degraded and digested essential metabolites are recycled. Autophagy is seen in many physiological as well as pathological states, for example, cancers, neurodegenerative disease, inflammatory bowel disease, etc., Autophagy is known to have a tumor-suppressor effect by removing misfolded, overexpressed, or abnormal proteins, damaged mitochondria, and acting against oncogenic bacteria and viruses. However, autophagy is now known to be upregulated in certain tumors, thus helping tumor survival in harsh conditions like hypoxia, nutrient deprivation, etc., and secreting tumor microenvironment (TME)-reshaping proteins.

Senescence: Senescence is a permanent state of cell cycle arrest, which marks an irreversible exit of the cell from the cell cycle. Shortening of the telomere, nontelomeric DNA damage, hypoxia, or any other oncogenic stress result in p53 accumulation, which may arrest further cell proliferation and force the cell to enter a state of senescence in which the abnormal cell cannot further proliferate to give rise to neoplasia. However, in recent years, this simplistic view has been challenged and further research is under process regarding the exact role of senescence in cancers.

3. *Sustained Perfusion of Cancer: Vascularization* tumors depend upon vascular supply for survival, growth, and metastasis. The major form of vascularization is tumor angiogenesis, while some other mechanisms of perfusion also exist.
   (a) *Tumor Angiogenesis*: A tumor cannot grow beyond 2–3 mm^3 unless it can induce angiogenesis. Tumor neovascular-

ization occurs by the sprouting of new vessels from pre-existing vessels. While on one hand, the new vascular channels supply nutrients, and oxygen as well as remove waste products, the proliferating endothelial cells secrete several molecules like PDGF, IGF, etc., which promote tumor growth.

Tumor angiogenesis, again, involves an interplay between various pro-angiogenic and anti-angiogenic factors.

(i) *Promoters of Angiogenesis*: Vascular endothelial growth factor (VEGF) and basic fibroblastic growth factor (bFGF) are proangiogenic factors, the transcription of which is triggered by HIF1α (hypoxia-inducible transcription factor α), which is, in turn, induced by hypoxia. Other angiogenic switches include acidic tumor microenvironment (TME), mechanical stress, inflammatory cells, etc.,

(ii) *Antiangiogenic Factors:* Thrombospondin 1, angiostatin, endostatin, and vasculostatin are antiangiogenic factors that are downregulated in many cancers, thus promoting angiogenesis and tumor growth.

When the balance tips in favor of proangiogenic factors, tumor angiogenesis starts. VEGF, the most potent angiogenic factor, is overexpressed in various malignancies and is presently a potential candidate for targeted therapy. The newly formed vessels are dilated, tortuous, and faulty with increased leakiness, thus impeding the drug delivery to the tumor cells.

(b) *Nonangiogenic Mode of Tumor Vascularization*:

This form of nonangiogenic vascularization mechanism includes

(i) *vascular co-option*
(ii) *intussusceptive microvascular growth (IMG) and*
(iii) *vasculogenic/vascular mimicry (VM)*

Vascular co-option is the process by which tumor cells hijack the existing vasculature of the tissue to feed themselves. Although the process is believed to involve angiogenic factors like VEGF, the co-opted tumor cells have shown to be refractory to antiangiogenic therapy.

Intussusceptive microvascular growth (also known as nonsprouting or splitting angiogenesis) is another additional process that occurs by splitting existing vessels by transluminal pillars or transendothelial bridges to form daughter vessels. The added advantage is that the newer vessels develop faster and are less leaky than the sprouting vessels of neoangiogenesis.

Vasculogenic mimicry or vascular mimicry is another tumor blood supply system independent of angiogenesis and even endothelial cells. This is seen mostly in tumors with high tumor grade and is associated with poor prognosis. By this mechanism, the tumor cells form de-novo vascular networks which are lined by the tumor cells covered by glycoprotein. VM has been described in most major types of malignancies particularly melanoma, glioblastoma, breast cancer, lung cancer, hepatocellular carcinoma etc.

4. *Spread of Cancer: Invasion and Metastasis*

A malignant tumor is best characterized by invasion of the surrounding tissue and spread to distant sites or metastasis. Metastasis is responsible for most cancer-related deaths. It involves several steps:

(i) Clonal proliferation of primary tumor.
(ii) Evolution of metastatic subclone.
(iii) Loss of tumor cell-to-tumor cell and tumor cell-to-extracellular matrix (ECM) adhesions.
(iv) Degradation of ECM and interstitial connective tissue by matrix metalloproteinases (MMPs).
(v) Attachment to novel ECM components and migration or invasion through the degraded basement membrane and ECM. The immotile epithelial cells acquire some mesenchymal phenotype known as an epithelial-mesenchymal transition (EMT), which helps in the movement of the tumor cells.

(vi) Intravasation through the walls of blood vessels to form tumor embolus or circulating tumor cells (CTCs), which can be detected by liquid biopsy.

(vii) Vascular dissemination, extravasation, and homing in a distant site. Some cancers prefer certain metastatic sites over others (organotropism), which can partly be explained by the "seed and soil" hypothesis and partly by the "anatomical mechanical" hypothesis (passive arrest of tumor cells).

(viii) Survival of tumor cells in the secondary site forming micrometastasis, which depends not only on the inherent property of the tumor cell but also on the microenvironment of the secondary site, the angiogenesis, infiltrating immune cells, etc.,

(ix) Clonal expansion and tumor progression to form clinically relevant macrometastasis (colonization).

5. *Metabolic Rewiring*

In the initial phase of growth and expansion, the tumor cells need a supply of both energy and building blocks for the production of new cells. The two most important constituents in this phase are glucose and glutamine. It has been demonstrated that tumor cells prefer anaerobic glycolysis over the more efficient Kreb's Cycle even in the presence of ample oxygen. This is known as the Warburg effect as it was described by Otto Warburg who received the Nobel Prize in 1931 for this discovery. The Kreb's cycle produces 36 molecules of ATP from one molecule of glucose, while glycolysis generates only 2 molecules of ATP per molecule of glucose. But the metabolic intermediates in glycolysis generate 2 more molecules of ATP and more importantly provide carbon moieties for the synthesis of protein, lipids, and nucleic acids, which is necessary for giving rise to two daughter cells. This advantage is lacking in mitochondrial oxidative phosphorylation. The uptake of glucose is guided by several mechanisms, one of which is via the glucose transporter (GLUT) proteins, which is upregulated in many cancers. This "glucose hunger" of the tumor cells is utilized in a very important nuclear medicine procedure in cancer patients, the Positron emission tomography or PET scan. In this, patients are being injected intravenously with a radiopharmaceutical (the glucose derivative ^{18}F-fluorodeoxyglucose-FDG), which is preferentially taken up by the tumor cells and actively dividing tissues (e.g., bone marrow). The radiation emitted is then sensed by external detectors.

Compared to glucose, the mechanism of glutamine uptake is less clear. Some studies show the role of MYC and RB in the transport of glutamine across the membrane. Other methods of acquisition include micropinocytosis, entosis, or phagocytosis of extracellular proteins and apoptotic products.

6. *Tumor Microenvironment*

A continuous paracrine cross-talk between the tumor cells and the various members of the tumor microenvironment (TME) helps in carcinogenesis, progression, metastasis, and drug resistance. The components of TME include cellular as well as noncellular modified stroma. Such aiding and abetting microenvironment also protects the tumor cells from the various chemotherapeutic agents and may be partly responsible for the minimum residual disease (MRD) as seen in some cancers, particularly some leukemias.

7. *Immune Modulation*

The presence of cancer immune surveillance is now a well-accepted occurrence, and various mechanisms for this have been proposed. It is believed that the immune system continuously hunts for any emergence of malignant cells and tries to annihilate them. Some cancer cells express a variety of antigens that can stimulate the host immune machinery and at times may even promote tumor growth. Tumor cells may present products of oncogene or mutated tumor-suppressor genes, mutated self-proteins, overexpressed or aberrantly expressed self-proteins, oncogenic viruses, etc., to the immune system of the body, which does not recognize them as self. These neoantigens are presented in the context of the MHC class 1 molecule to the CD8+ T cells, which become activated to give rise to active cytotoxic T lymphocytes (CTLs) and destroy the tumor cells presenting these neoantigens. A variety of tumors show an increase in tumor-infiltrating lymphocytes (TILs), which is associated with a somewhat better prognosis. Other than CTLs, NK cells and macrophages are also involved in antitumor activity. However, this mechanism of immune surveillance is, understandably, not foolproof.

The tumor cells devise various mechanisms of immune evasion. Cancer immunoediting is the ability of the immune system of the body to select the tumor subclones that are capable of avoiding host immunity. Since CTLs are an important part of immunosurveillance, most of the mechanisms are devised by the tumor cells to ward off the attack of the T cells. There may be a selection of subclones with reduced/absent expression of neoantigens, acquired mutation of β2-microglobulin which prevent the assembly of the MHC 1 class of molecules necessary for presenting the neoantigens to the CTLs or producing proteins that activate the immune checkpoints like PD-L, etc., thus shutting off the antitumor activity of the CTLs.

Of recent interest is the PD-L1 (programmed cell death ligand 1), a protein that is increasingly expressed on the surface of the tumor cells. This attaches with its receptor PD-1 on the CTLs and inactivates their antitumor activity. This immune checkpoint inhibition is utilized for the development of immunotherapy in which monoclonal antibodies (mAbs) have been designed as drugs against the PD-L1/PD-1 checkpoint. Pembrolizumab, Nivolumab, and Cemiplimab are some of the anti-PD-1 mAbs injected intravenously, while Atezolizumab, Avelumab, and Durvalumab are anti-PD-L1 agents, which are used in various types of cancers with fairly encouraging results. Cancers of the lung, bladder, melanoma, and Hodgkin lymphoma are some of the tumors that have shown promising results with immune checkpoint therapy.

Similarly, CTLA4 on T cells binds to CD80 and CD86 (also called B7–1 and B7–2 respectively) on antigen-presenting cells and shuts off the antitumor activity of the CTLs. Drugs like Ipilimumab have been developed to target this immune checkpoint in patients with melanoma.

Another breakthrough in immunotherapy is the development of CAR T-cell therapy in which the patient-derived CTLs are genetically engineered to express chimeric antigen receptors (CARs). These CAR T cells bind to specific antigens on the tumor cells and mediate MHC-unrestricted tumor cell killing. CAR T cell therapy with Tisagenlecleucel in patients of B cell acute lymphoblastic leukemia in the younger age group has produced long-term remissions.

Apart from these, there are two enabling factors for carcinogenesis.

These are:

(a) *Genomic Instability* caused by defects in the various DNA repair mechanisms like base excision repair, mismatch match repair, nucleotide excision repair, nonhomologous end joining repair, etc.,
(b) *Tumor-Enabling Inflammation* that helps in the release of proliferation-promoting factors, removal of growth suppressors and play an important role in invasion, metastasis, angiogenesis, and evasion of immune destruction.

6.6.2 Model of Multistep Carcinogenesis

As mentioned earlier, no single mutation is enough to cause cancer. Multiple mutations in a step-wise and complementary manner are required for carcinogenesis. The mutations can either be driver mutations, that is, drive the process of carcinogenesis or mere passenger mutations. The best molecular model in support of this concept is the adenoma-carcinoma sequence in the evolution of colorectal carcinoma through various driver mutations occurring sequentially in the APC, KRAS, SMAD4, and TP53 genes.

The germline mutation (inherited cases) or somatic or acquired mutation (sporadic cases) in the tumor-suppressor gene APC at chromosome 5q21 acts as the **"first hit,"** which makes the normal colonic mucosa more liable to develop neoplasia.

The **"second hit"** is produced with further inactivation of the remaining normal allele of the APC gene resulting in the commencement of adenoma formation, which goes on accumulating mutations resulting in the activation of proto-oncogene KRAS located at chromosome 12p12. Further homozygous loss of TP53 (Chromosome 17p13) and loss of heterozygosity at 18q21 result in the formation of carcinoma from the adenoma.

However, this model is a simplified way of explaining the mechanism of carcinogenesis: it does provide valuable insight into the process. It must be remembered that all the changes may not be present in each tumor or may not appear in the same temporal sequence as mentioned, but the presence of dysplasia ultimately evolving into neoplasia with further mutations does point in favor of this model of multistep carcinogenesis.

It must also be remembered that other than the chromosomal instability (CI) pathway, as discussed, there are other mechanisms like microsatellite instability pathway (MSI) and CpG island methylator phenotype (CIMP) that are involved in subsets of colorectal carcinoma.

Micro-RNAs and Cancer:
Small RNA molecules called Micro-RNAs (miRNAs) are relatively short, noncoding single-stranded RNAs (22 nucleotides on average) that control normal cell growth, differentiation, and cell survival. They usually participate in post-translational silencing of gene expression.

Altered expression (from deletions/amplifications) can lead to neoplasia.

In cancer, miRNAs regulate the expression of several genes, thus having functions like oncogenes or tumor-suppressor genes.

Oncogenic MicroRNAs (OncomiRs): Overexpression of OncomiRs inhibits tumor-suppressor genes and promotes cell proliferation. For example, increased expression of mi155 upregulates MYC in B cell lymphomas, thus promoting cell proliferation.

Overexpression of miR-200 helps in promoting EMT and thus contributes to invasiveness and metastasis of tumors.

Overexpression of miR221 is seen in triple-negative breast cancers.

Tumor-Suppressive MicroRNAs (miRs):
The most notable examples of tumor-suppressive miRs are deletions affecting miR-15, 16, which upregulate the antiapoptotic BCL2 protein in cases of Chronic Lymphocytic Leukemia (CLL).

Tumor-Suppressive Properties of MiR Processing Factors:
DICER protein encoded by the DICER1 gene acts as a riboendonuclease, which helps in the processing of miRNAs from primary transcript microRNAs (pri-miRNA) and long double-stranded RNAs (dsRNAs) resulting from the transcription of miRNA genes. Germline defects in DICER result in pleuropulmonary blastoma and some unusual neoplasms of the ovary and testis.

6.6.3 Chemical Carcinogenesis

Exposure to harmful chemicals can induce carcinogenesis and this also supports the model of multistep carcinogenesis. Certain carcinogens induce a permanent change in the DNA of the cell, which initiates the process of carcinogenesis (*initiators*) and some others enhance the cell proliferation, resulting in further accumulation of mutations and finally neoplasia (*promoters*).

For example, scrotal skin cancers in chimney sweepers. Since then, hundreds of chemical agents have been shown to have carcinogenic potential. Experimental models have shown that initiators cause DNA damage (mutation), which is permanent, rapid, and long-lasting but cannot go all the way to cause tumors. Promoters, on the other hand, although nontumorigenic by themselves, can induce cell proliferation in the initiated cells, resulting in neoplasia.

The initiators can be either directly acting or indirectly acting agents. The directly acting agents need not be metabolized further for inducing carcinogenesis although they are weak carcinogens. Examples include *alkylating agents, acylating agents,* etc., (Table 6.4) [6].

Table 6.4 Common chemical carcinogens

Initiators	
Directly acting carcinogens	*Alkylating agents*, e.g., various anticancer drugs (e.g., cyclophosphamide, chlorambucil, nitrosourea, etc.,), β-propiolactone, epoxides
	Acylating agents, e.g., acetyl imidazole, dimethyl carbamyl chloride
Indirectly acting carcinogens (procarcinogens)	*Polycyclic aromatic hydrocarbons, e.g.,* anthracenes (benza-, dibenza-, dimethyl benza-), benzapyrene, methylcholanthrene
	Aromatic amines and azo-dyes (b-*naphthylamine, benzidine, azo-dyes)*
	Naturally occurring products aflatoxin B1, actinomycin D, mitomycin C, safrole,betel nuts
	Miscellaneous: Nitrosamines and nitrosamides, vinyl chloride monomer, asbestos, etc.,
Promoters	
	Phorbol esters (tetradecanoyl phorbol acetate)
	Phenols
	Hormones (diethylstilbestrol, endogenous hormones)
	Drugs

The indirectly acting agents (known as "pro" carcinogens), on the other hand, need to be metabolized to electrophilic intermediates, which bind with DNA to form adducts and induce permanent DNA damage (mutation).

Since metabolism pathways are involved, polymorphisms of endogenous enzymes such as cytochrome P-450 may influence carcinogenesis by altering the conversion of indirect-acting agents to active carcinogens. The notable examples include *Polycyclic and Heterocyclic Aromatic Hydrocarbons, Benzopyrene, Aromatic Amines, Amides, Azo Dyes, and natural Plant and Microbial Products* (Aflatoxin B1 causing hepatocellular carcinoma, betel nuts causing oral squamous cell carcinoma) (Table 6.4).

Both directly as well as indirectly acting carcinogens target the usual important oncogenes and tumor-suppressor genes like TP53, RAS, etc.,

The promoters are nonmutagenic and include hormones, phorbol esters, phenols, drugs, etc., which cause cell proliferation, particularly clonal expansion of the mutated or initiated cell, gathering further mutations and ultimately developing neoplasia.

6.6.4 Physical Carcinogenesis

Physical agents causing cancer can be broadly be divided into (i) Radiation carcinogenesis and (ii) nonradiation carcinogenesis.

For example, Cancers following Hiroshima and Nagasaki and the Chornobyl disasters, secondary tumors, for example, thyroid tumors after receiving head and neck irradiation.

Radiation can broadly be divided into two types:

(a) *Nonionizing* (e.g., UV rays, Infrared rays, Microwaves, Sound waves)
(b) *Ionizing* –
  (i) Electromagnetic (X-rays, Gamma rays)
  (ii) Particulate (α and β particles, neutrons)

Of particular importance are the UV rays in sunlight, which induce the formation of pyrimidine dimers within the DNA, causing mutations that give rise to various skin cancers like squamous cell carcinoma, basal cell carcinoma, and melanomas of the skin. While cumulative UV exposure seems more important in the pathogenesis of squamous cell carcinomas and basal cell carcinoma, intermittent intense exposure to sunlight (like sunbathing) appears to be important in causing melanomas of the skin. The fair-skinned individuals are more susceptible to these UV-ray-related skin cancers.

Normally, the pyrimidine dimer formation is repaired by the nucleotide excision repair (NER) pathway, but with excessive exposure, even this repair pathway gets overwhelmed and gives way to skin cancers.

Xeroderma pigmentosum is an autosomal-recessive disorder in which there is a germline mutation in the genes involved in the NER pathway, leading to increased predisposition to skin cancers (even in children) in addition to cataracts, neurological problems, brain tumors, etc.,

6.6.5 Microbial Carcinogenesis

Several microbes (virus, bacteria, parasites etc.,) are now known to cause cancers.

Viral Carcinogenesis:
Many DNA and RNA viruses have from time to time been implicated in causing cancers.

Among the various oncogenic RNA viruses, Human T-cell leukemia virus type 1 (HTLV-1) is now known to cause adult T-cell leukemia/lymphoma (ATLL) after a long latent period following the infection of T cells. Hepatitis C virus is a single-stranded RNA virus that has been associated with hepatocellular carcinoma.

Among the DNA viruses, the five most common ones implicated in causing cancers are Human Papilloma Virus (HPV), Epstein-Barr virus (EBV), Human herpesvirus-8 (HHV-8), Merkel cell virus, and Hepatitis B virus (HBV).

HPV and Cancer
Of these, the association of cervical cancer with HPV infection is most well elucidated. The low-risk HPV strains 6 and 11 cause genital warts, which rarely develop into cancers, while the high-risk strains 16,18, and 31 are often associated with cervical cancers and squamous cell carcinomas of the anogenital region. A significant number of oropharyngeal cancers, penile, anal, vulvar, and vaginal cancers are also caused by these high-risk HPVs.

The pathogenesis of cervical carcinoma has been extensively studied. The products of the two viral genes E6 and E7 influence various stages of the cell cycle and help in carcinogenesis.

The E6 protein results in the degradation of p53 and also causes telomerase activation by stimulating the expression of the TERT gene, which helps in the synthesis of one subunit of telomerase, the enzyme which allows repeated cell divisions without cell death.

The E7 protein binds to the RB protein and displaces the E2F transcription factor, which activates the transcription of the S phase gene and ultimately progresses the cell cycle. E7 also inactivates the Cyclin-Dependent kinase 4 (CDK4) inhibitors like p21 and p27, thus resulting in the increased formation of CDK4/Cyclin D, progression of the cell cycle, and, hence, increased cell proliferation. The integration of the viral DNA into the host cell DNA contributes to the genomic instability of the cells, which go on acquiring subsequent mutations, thus resulting in the development of cancer.

Nowadays, vaccines against the various HPV strains have been developed, all of which offer protection against strains 16 and 18. They have considerably high preventive rates against cervical and anogenital squamous cell carcinomas as well as HPV-positive oropharyngeal squamous cell carcinomas.

Epstein-Barr Virus (EBV) and Cancer
EBV is the first virus that has been known to cause human cancers. It has been implicated in Burkitt lymphoma, particularly the endemic (African) form, nasopharyngeal carcinoma, lymphomas associated with immunosuppression, a subset of T cell and NK cell lymphomas, Hodgkin lymphomas, plasmablastic lymphomas, primary effusion lymphomas, gastric adenocarcinomas, leiomyosarcomas, etc.,

The EBV attaches to and infects the B cells with the help of complement receptor CD21. The infection is latent, and they produce various oncoproteins, which virtually render the B cells virtually immortal in vitro. Latent membrane Protein 1 (LMP1) is an EBV gene that acts as an oncogene that promotes autonomous B cell proliferation by stimulating the JAK/STAT and NF-κβ pathways and inhibiting cell death by apoptosis. This is true for EBV-induced nasopharyngeal carcinomas as well.

In Burkitt lymphoma, EBV induces polyclonal B cell proliferation, which sets the stage for the characteristic t(8;14) translocation and other related mutations, which results in MYC activation and cell proliferation.

Hepatitis B Virus (HBV) and C virus (HCV) and Hepatocellular Carcinomas (HCCs)
Though the causation of HCC by HBV and HCV is multifactorial, the 3 major factors in the pathogenesis are

(a) Widespread hepatocyte death (necrosis) due to viral hepatitis followed by regeneration of hepatocytes and propensity of genomic damage.
(b) Immunologically mediated chronic inflammation.
(c) HBx protein produced by the HBx gene activates various transcription factors and signal transduction pathways.

The first two factors produce an environment that is rich in proliferating cells in a background of chronic inflammation along with several growth factors, reactive oxygen species, cytokines, chemokines, etc., which are mutagenic and can cause irreversible DNA damage, finally resulting in hepatocellular carcinoma.

Oncogenic Bacterium: *Helicobacter pylori*, which has long been known to cause chronic gastritis and peptic ulcer, is also associated with gastric adenocarcinomas and gastric lymphomas. Again, the pathogenesis of gastric carcinoma is multifactorial, but just like HBV-induced HCC, here also the proliferation of reparative gastric cells in the background of chronic inflammation plays an important role.

H. pylori strains that harbor the Cag A pathogenicity gene (cytotoxin-associated gene A) stimulate growth factor pathways and contribute to carcinogenesis.

Chronic gastritis also results in *H pylori*-reactive T-cell-mediated polyclonal B cell proliferation followed by accumulation of various mutations leading to MALT lymphomas.

Parasites Causing Cancers: Parasites such as Schistosoma haematobium, Opisthorchis viverrini, and Clonorchis sinensis have been linked to specific cancers—for example, Schistosoma haematobium is associated with squamous cell carcinoma of bladder , while Opisthorchis viverrini and Clonorchis sinensis are implicated in the development of cholangiocarcinoma.

6.7 Clinical Aspects of Neoplasia

(a) *Clinical Effects of the Tumor on the Host:* The cancer is a leading cause of patient morbidity and mortality. Understandably, the effects of malignant tumors are far more sinister than those of benign ones. The effects can be grouped under:
 (i) *Local Effects:*
  (a) *Compression:* The compressive effects of a growing tumor depend upon the location of the tumor. Benign tumors usually cause cosmetic problems, but an increase in size may lead to compressive effects. But even a small pituitary adenoma can compress and destroy the surrounding pituitary gland and cause hypopituitarism.
  (b) *Mechanical Obstruction:* A small benign tumor at the ampulla of Vater can cause biliary obstruction. Both benign and malignant tumors of the gut can cause intestinal obstruction.
  (c) *Tissue Destruction:* Malignancies (primary or secondary/metastasis) often destroy vital structures.
  (d) *Infarction, Secondary Infection, Ulceration, Hemorrhage:* These are secondary changes that may occur, more commonly in malignant tumors.
 (ii) *Systemic Effects:*
  (a) *Hormonal Effects:* A beta cell tumor despite being benign and of small size can cause fatal hypoglycemia by producing large amounts of insulin. Nonendocrine tumors can also secrete hormones or hormone-related peptides that cause endocrine effects on other organs (a type of paraneoplastic syndrome).
  (b) *Cancer Cachexia:* Patients with advanced malignancies suffer from

loss of lean body mass and fat (emaciation), weakness (asthenia), anemia, anorexia, elevated basal metabolic rate, and evidence of systemic inflammation together referred to as *cancer cachexia*. Though the exact mechanism of this complex interaction between host factors and tumor cells is not known, it appears to be an interplay between various factors like TNF α (cachectin), IFNγ, IL1, anemia-inducing substance (AIS), Macrophage inhibitory cytokine-1, etc.,

(c) *Paraneoplastic Syndromes:* (PNS) This includes a constellation of signs and symptoms occurring as a result of altered immune response of the host to the malignancy, that cannot be attributed to the anatomic distribution (primary or metastasis) of the tumor or by the hormones normally produced by the tissue from which the tumor arose. About 10–15% of malignancies show features of paraneoplastic syndromes. They are important to recognize, because they may appear even before the cancer is diagnosed, thus confounding diagnosis or may mimic metastasis, thereby confounding management. Often, they cause significant morbidity and mortality. Some of the notable PNS include Cushing syndrome in small cell carcinoma lung, pancreatic carcinoma, etc., (due to secretion of ACTH or ACTH-like substances), Syndrome of inappropriate antidiuretic hormone secretion (SIADH) in Small-cell carcinoma of the lung; intracranial neoplasms due to secretion of Antidiuretic hormone or atrial natriuretic hormones, hypercalcemia in ovarian carcinomas, polycythemia in renal cell carcinoma, hepatocellular carcinoma, Myasthenia gravis in thymic neoplasms, Trousseau syndrome (superficial migratory thrombophlebitis) in pancreatic cancers, etc.

(d) *Fever:* Tumor-associated fever may occur in Hodgkin disease, osteosarcoma, etc., though the exact causal mechanism is unknown. Patients may also develop fever due to infections (pneumonia, urinary tract infection, sepsis, etc.,)

(e) *Anemia:* Patients may develop anemia due to blood loss (colorectal and gastric cancers), folate deficiency due to rapid tumor growth or myelophthisic anemia secondary to bone marrow metastasis

(f) *Tumor Lysis Syndrome:* This refers to a constellation of metabolic disturbances like hyperuricemia, hyperphosphatemia, hyperkalemia, and hypocalcemia due to release of cellular contents of a large number of tumor cells following their lysis, either spontaneously or as a result of therapy. This usually occurs following the therapy of lymphomas and leukemias.

6.8 Grading and Staging of Tumors

The apparent biological behavior of a tumor, its prognosis, and treatment response can be predicted with a certain degree of confidence by certain gross and microscopic features of the tumor.

Grading of a tumor is done on the basis of cytologic appearance, its degree of differentiation, and in some tumors based on mitosis, necrosis, or architecture. The well-differentiated tumors are believed to have a better prognosis than the poorly differentiated or undifferentiated ones.

Staging of tumors is more important in predicting the prognosis and treatment response. It can be done based on clinical examination, by imaging (CT, MRI, PET), or by pathological examination of resected tissue, the latter being known as pathological staging.

Previously, various staging systems were used for different organs, but now the most widely used system for almost all sites is the TNM system, which is based on T for the primary tumor, N for lymph nodal involvement, and M for metastasis. For each component, a number is assigned, which corresponds to the extent of involvement. For example, T0 to T4, No to N3, and M0 to M2, which is followed by the AJCC (American Joint Committee on Cancer).

6.9 Pathological Diagnosis of Tumors [7, 8]

A wide variety of diagnostic modalities have been developed and have resulted in early diagnosis of tumors, which, in turn, have reduced the morbidity and cancer-related deaths.

The most widely used methods are as follows:

(a) *Histopathology*: The biopsy may be of several types—incisional biopsy, excision biopsy, endoscopic biopsy, core-needle biopsy, etc., This is routinely done by formalin-fixed paraffin embedding (FFPE) section stained by Hematoxylin and Eosin, aided by special stains and immunohistochemistry. For urgent intraoperative diagnosis, the frozen section (cryosection) helps in determining the diagnosis and also the extent of tumor spread, which guides the surgeon to carry out the surgery accordingly.

(b) *Cytopathology:* The common cytological methods of diagnosis are
   (i) *Exfoliative Cytology*: Cervicovaginal smears stained by Papanicolaou stain (better known as Pap smears) used for cervical cancer screening, examination of sputum, bronchial washings, body fluids (pleural, peritoneal, pericardial fluid, etc.,), cerebrospinal fluid (CSF) are all based on microscopic examination of exfoliated cells.
   (ii) *Fine-Needle Aspiration Cytology (FNAC)*: In this method, with the help of a fine-needle fitted to a syringe, cytological material is aspirated by giving negative suction from superficial or deep-seated lesions, either under direct vision or image guidance (Ultrasound/Computed tomography guided). The smears prepared from the aspirates are air-dried or alcohol fixed and stained with appropriate stains.
   (iii) *Cell Blocks*: This is a method in which the aspirated cytological specimen is processed by special techniques and processed as a routine histopathological tissue. The added advantage is that along with cytological details, the architecture of the lesion can be appreciated and immunohistochemical stains can be performed with good results (Fig. 6.11).

(c) *Electron Microscopy:* Though helpful in certain conditions like evaluation of microvilli, dense bodies in cytoplasm, etc., and differen-

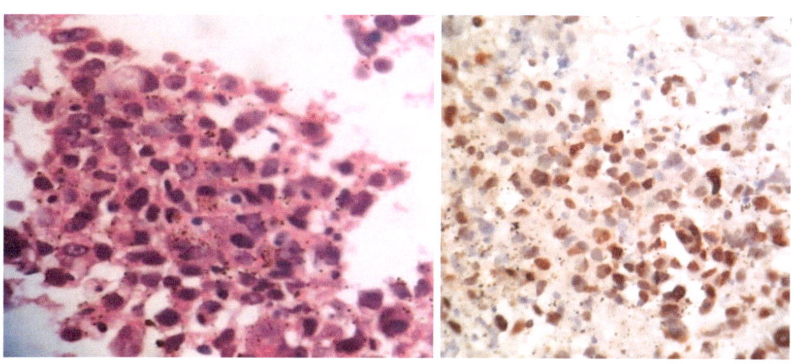

Fig. 6.11 Cell block preparation from a case of breast carcinoma (left) with immunohistochemistry for estrogen receptors (ERs) performed on cell block (right)

tiating among carcinoma, sarcoma, and lymphoma in some cases. In routine cancer diagnosis, electron microscopy is not commonly used. In electron microscopy, 2% buffered glutaraldehyde is used as a fixative.

(d) *Serum Tumor Markers:* Biochemical assay of tumor products in blood or body fluids can aid in tumor diagnosis—these are known as tumor markers. They include cell surface antigens (*oncofetal antigens*), enzymes, hormones, etc., Two of the best-characterized tumor markers are (i) *Alpha foetoprotein (AFP)*, which is elevated in hepatocellular carcinoma and yolk sac tumors as well as few nonneoplastic conditions and (ii) *Carcinoembryonic antigen (CEA)*, which is elevated in colorectal carcinoma, tumors of the pancreas, stomach, breast as well as nonneoplastic conditions. Though they cannot be used for definitive diagnosis of malignancy, they are a useful adjunct to diagnosis as well as treatment monitoring and detection of relapse.

(e) *Flow Cytometry:* It is now widely used in lymphomas and leukemias both from aspirates and blood. Fluorescent-labeled monoclonal antibodies against specific cell surface antigens are used to determine the immunophenotype of the tumor cells.

(f) *Liquid Biopsy:* Also known as fluid phase biopsy, this test is done on a sample of blood to look for circulating tumor cells (CTCs) or pieces of circulating DNA (ctDNA) from tumor cells in a patient. This is a minimally invasive, rapid method and can be used to monitor treatment response and detect relapse of malignancy. Tests have been approved for patients having tumors of the prostate, breast, lung, etc.,

(g) *Fluorescent In Situ Hybridization (FISH):* FISH is often used to diagnose translocations like t(9;22) for the Philadelphia chromosome in Chronic Myeloid Leukemia (CML) and N-MYC amplification in neuroblastoma.

(h) *Molecular Methods:* This refers to various methods in which DNA/RNA is extracted from tumor cells and analyzed by different methods, for example, DNA analysis by Southern blot, RNA analysis by Northern Blot, and Polymerase chain reaction (PCR).

DNA microarray analysis is a method of molecular profiling in which the expression of thousands of genes can be measured simultaneously. Next-Generation sequencing (NGS) allows whole-exome sequencing (WES), large-scale whole-genome sequencing (WGS), target sequencing epigenetic factor analysis, etc., by involving massive parallel sequencing.

The diagnostic tools are becoming more and more precise and with the emergence of targeted therapy, we have now entered the era of personalized medicine, which is now more popularly known as precision medicine.

References

1. Kumar V, Abbas AK, Aster JC. Robbins basic pathology. In: Robbins pathology. 10th ed. Philadelphia: Elsevier – Health Sciences Division; 2017.
2. https://gco.iarc.fr/today/data/factsheets/populations/356-india-fact-sheets.pdf accessed on 22/01/2022
3. Oyesanmi O, Snyder D, Sullivan N, Reston J, Treadwell J, Schoelles KM. Alcohol consumption and cancer risk: understanding possible causal mechanisms for breast and colorectal cancers. Evid Rep Technol Assess (Full Rep). 2010;197:1–151. PMID: 23126574; PMCID: PMC4781486.
4. Fouad YA, Aanei C. Revisiting the hallmarks of cancer. Am J Cancer Res. 2017;7(5):1016–36.
5. Chatterjee N, Walker GC. Mechanisms of DNA damage, repair, and mutagenesis. Environ Mol Mutagen. 2017;58(5):235–63.
6. Mohan H. Textbook of pathology. 8th ed. India: Jaypee Brothers; 2019.
7. Mandal AK, Choudhury S. Textbook of pathology for MBBS. 1st ed. India: Avichal Publishing Company; 2017.
8. Kamal V. Textbook of pathology. 1st ed. India: CBS Publishers & Distributors; 2017.

Inherited Metabolic Disorders

7

Triveni Bandi

Contents

T. Bandi (✉)
Government Medical College, Maheshwaram,
Hyderabad, Telangana, India

G. K. Vemuganti et al. (eds.), *Ocular Pathology*, https://doi.org/10.1007/978-981-96-8614-8_7

7.1 Introduction

Metabolic syndrome or disorders are a cluster of conditions that result in defective metabolism in our body. Metabolism is the complex set of chemical reactions that our body uses to maintain normal life that includes energy production. It refers to all the chemical reactions taking place in our body to convert or use energy. The term "Inborn errors of metabolism" was first described by Sir Archibald Garrod in 1902—to describe those diseases caused by a block in a metabolic pathway due to deficient activity of a specific enzyme [1].

Special enzymes are needed to either break down food or certain chemicals so that our body can use them immediately as fuel or store them. In addition, certain chemical processes break down substances that our body no longer needs. When such chemical processes are hampered due to lack of hormone or enzyme deficiency, a metabolic disorder occurs. It could be due to a single enzyme, which is not produced by the body or is produced in a defective form. Depending on the function of the enzyme or chemical, its defect or absence means toxic chemical may build up or an essential product may not be produced.

7.1.1 Etiopathogenesis

Metabolic disorders are primarily inherited disorders and most of them inherit 2 defective copies of the genes, one from each parent, and both of them happen to be carriers of the defective gene.

Since the parents carry one defective or mutated gene, their enzyme levels are usually within normal limits; hence, they are asymptomatic with normal metabolism. However, the child with 2 defective genes cannot produce enough of the effective enzyme and, therefore, develops the genetic metabolic disorder. This form of genetic transmission is called Autosomal-Recessive (AR) inheritance. Many IMDs have AR inheritance; a few are X-linked.

Since these are inherited, they are also be called as "Inborn errors of metabolism" (IMDs). IMDs are disorders in which there is a block at some point in the normal metabolic pathway (Fig. 7.1).

Therefore, IMDs are a heterogenous group of genetic conditions mostly occurring in childhood. They are individually rare but collectively numerous, causing substantial morbidity and mortality [2].

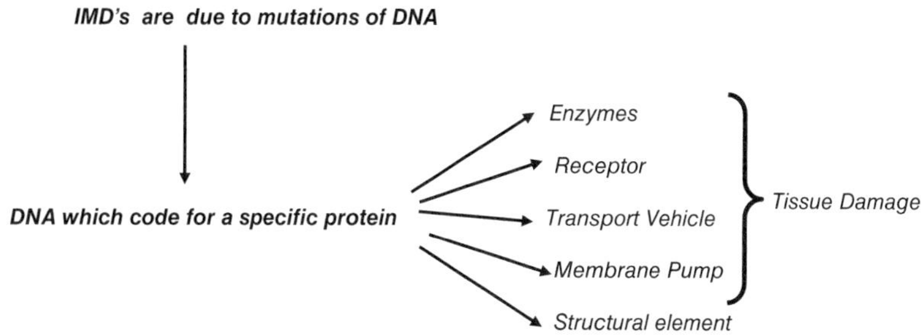

Fig. 7.1 Inherited metabolic disorders' etiological mechanisms

7.1.2 Incidence

There are many, over 3500 inherited metabolic disorders and the number is increasing with more widespread use of whole-gene exome sequencing in diagnosis of such disorders. Each of them is quite rare in the general population—affecting 1 in 1000–2500 newborns. However, in certain ethnic populations like Ashkenazi Jews—Jews of Central / Eastern Europe, the rate of inherited metabolic disorders is high [3].

7.1.3 Types

Inherited metabolic disorders (IMD) fall into different categories, depending on the specific substances and whether it builds up in harmful amounts (because it cannot be broken down) or it is too low or totally missing in the body.

Several informal systems of classifications currently exist. IMDs can be classified according to the Organ involved, such as neurological/ hepatic; to Organelles involved, such as Mitochondrial, peroxisomal, or lysosomal disorders. Disorders can also be classified according to the age of presentation ranging from neonatal, juvenile to adult onset. Because each of these approaches may depend upon the actual setting, no single classification is universally applied [4].

Effects of IMDs: As mentioned above, Inherited Metabolic Disorders (IMDs) result in abnormalities in the synthesis or catabolism of carbohydrates, proteins, fats, or nucleic acids. Many of them are due to a defect in an enzyme or transport

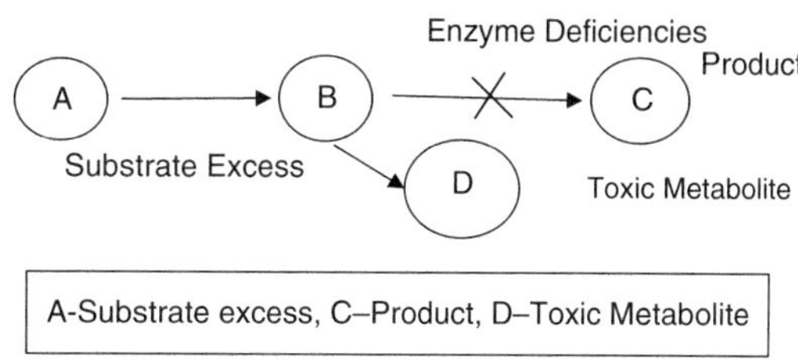

Fig. 7.2 Garrod's Hypothesis

protein, which results in a block in the respective metabolic pathway, leading to toxic accumulation of substrates before the block, intermediate from alternative metabolic pathway, and defects in energy production and utilization, which is caused by a deficiency of products beyond the block. This above process can be categorized under *Garrod's Hypothesis* [5] (Fig. 7.2).

Although there is an extensive understanding of many inborn errors of metabolism at the biochemical, molecular, and metabolic levels, little is known about their exact pathogenesis, especially as to how some of these systemic metabolic diseases contribute to ocular defects [41]. Ocular involvement is probably due to similar basic pathogenesis of IMD (*Garrod's Hypothesis*) [5] direct toxic mechanisms of abnormal metabolic products, or accumulation of normal metabolites by error of alternate pathways or by deficient energy metabolism. Therefore, definite diagnosis of IMD needs a multidisciplinary approach.

Most of the above-mentioned inherited metabolic disorders are very rare and their detailed description is better relegated to specialized text books and reviews. In this chapter, we shall study the basic concepts, genetic basis, and metabolic consequences and mention their ocular relations of the few of the more common conditions.

Disorders of carbohydrate metabolism are the most common IMDs. Some of them shall be discussed here.

7.2 Lysosomal Storage Defects: [6, 7–11, 12]

Lysosomes are key components of the intracellular digestive system, which contain a battery of hydrolytic enzymes that function in an acidic milieu of lysosomes. These enzymes are synthesized in the Endoplasmic reticulum and transported to the Golgi apparatus in which they undergo a variety of modifications, which help in its normal function, that is, degradation of a complex macromolecular substrate into soluble end products. If there is a deficiency or malfunction of one of the enzymes, then catabolism is incomplete and insoluble intermediates accumulate in the lysosomes and in intracellular organelles.

The complex macromolecules may be derived from metabolic turnover of intracellular organelles (autophagy) or they may be acquired from outside the cells by phagocytosis (heterophagy). Therefore, an inherited deficiency of a functional lysosomal enzyme gives rise to pathologic consequences as follows:

A. Due to lack of Catabolism of the macromolecule due to missing enzyme, they get accumulated within lysosomes, which in turn enlarge and interfere with normal cell function. This causes defective degradation of intracellular organelles, leading to accumulation of toxic proteins and subsequent induction of cell damage and cell death. In addition, accumulation of toxic proteins within the cells causes secondary storage, in turn disturbing the normal cell function.
B. There is a tight link among autophagy, mitochondrial functions, and lysosomes. Autophagy is essential for turnover of mitochondria whereby dysfunctional mitochondria are degraded. But due to dysfunctional lysosomes, the dysfunctional and leaky mitochondria persist, which in turn generate free radicals and release molecules that trigger the intrinsic pathway of apoptosis and cause cell death.

   The impaired autophagy gives rise to secondary accumulation of autophagic substrates (α—alpha synculin and Huntington protein), which provides a molecular link between several neurodegenerative disorders and lysosomal storage diseases.

In general, the distribution of the stored material and organs affected is determined by 2 interrelated factors.

1. The tissue where most of the material is degraded and
2. The site where this degradation normally occurs.

The cells of mononuclear phagocytic system are particularly rich in lysosomes; therefore, reticuloendothelial organs with many phagocytic cells like the liver and spleen are most commonly involved in lysosomal storage diseases.

The lysosomal storage diseases can be divided into categories based on the biochemical nature of the accumulated metabolite.

Example: Glycogenosis, Sphingolipidoses, Mucopolysaccharidoses, Mucolipidoses. Most of these conditions are very rare. Only few of these important disorders are discussed below:

Gaucher's disease, Tay Sach's disease, and Niemann pick disease, all of which have an autosomal-recessive inheritance.

7.3 Gaucher's Disease: [8, 9, 10]

It is the most common lysosomal storage disorder, caused due to defect in the enzyme glucocerebrosidase, which normally cleanses—glucosoceramide, a glycolipid, to ceramide and glucose. More than 150 mutations have been identified in this gene, and it is commonly seen in Jewish population, and 1 in 40,000 in Non–Jewish population.

7.3.1 Etiopathogenesis

Glucocerebrosides are continuously formed from the catabolism of glycolipids, derived from cell membranes of senescent leukocytes and red blood cells. Due to the deficiency of the enzyme glucocerebrosidases, glucerebrosides accumulate principally in phagocytes and also in central nervous system in phagocytes in some subtypes. The pathologic changes in Gaucher's disease are caused due to the burden of storage of chemicals along with byproducts formed due to activation of macrophages and the consequent release of cytokines interleukin (ILI), IL-6, and tumor necrosis factor (TNF).

There are 3 subtypes of Gaucher's disease.

Sub Type I: It is the most common (99%) and is the Chronic-Non-Neuronopathic type. It has glucocerebrosides stored only in the mononuclear phagocytes. It involves spleen and skeletal system, and it causes bone destruction. Brain is not involved. It is seen mostly in Jews of European origin. In this condition, there is decreased level of glucocerebrosidase activity.

Sub Type II: It involves brain and is also called Acute Neuronopathic Gaucher's disease. Has progressive central nervous system involvement, leading to death at an early age. (within 2 years of life) This infantile form has no predilection to Jews. In this condition, there is virtually no detectable glucocerebrosidase activity.

Sub Type III: It has features of both the above subtypes. Systemic involvement along with progressive central nervous system involvement and is seen in adolescence or early adulthood.

7.3.2 Clinical Features

Gaucher's disease has a range of diverse clinical manifestations that have been well documented in literature (ref. [9–13]), and clinical features depend on the subtype. In sub type I, the features are seen in adults due to splenomegaly or skeletal bone fractures. Pancytopenia is seen secondary to hypersplenism. Though it is a progressive disease, it is compatible with long life. In subtypes II and III, the features of central nervous system dominate viz. convulsion, progressive mental deterioration, and organomegaly (liver, spleen, lymph node) that is also seen in some.

Patients with Gaucher's disease have a higher risk for development of Parkinson disease due to the reciprocal relationship between the level of the enzyme glucocerebrosidase and aggregation of α—alpha synuclein, the protein which is involved in the pathogenesis of Parkinson disease.

Histologically,—in phagocytic cells, glucocerebrosides are seen throughout the body, depending on the subtypes. The distended phagocytes are the Gaucher's cells and are seen in organs—spleen, liver, bone marrow, lymph nodes, tonsils, thymus, Peyer's patches, lung, and in the brain-Virchow—Robin spaces and in arterioles. Bone destruction occurs due to release of cytokines, whereas neurons appear shriveled and are progressively destroyed. Gaucher's cell appears large and are 20–100 μm microns in diameter with fibrillary type of cytoplasm, which has *crumpled tissue-paper*-like appearance and has 1–2 dark eccentric nuclei. Rarely, these cells appear vacuolated. Special stain PAS (Periodic Acid Schiff) is strongly positive and with electron microscope, the fibrillary cytoplasm has elongated distended lysosomes with intracytoplasmic inclusion bodies, having stored lipid in stacks of bilayers.

Molecular diagnosis is possible by molecular tests to detect mutations and by the measurement of glucocerebrosidase activity in peripheral blood leucocytes or in extracts of cultured skin fibroblasts [14].

Therapy involves replacement of enzymes, along with allogenic hematopoietic stem cell transplantation. Correction of the enzyme defect by transfer of normal glucocerebrosidase gene into patient's hematopoietic stem cells is also being evaluated.

7.4 Tay-Sach's Disease: (GM_2_Gangliosidoses) [15, 45]

GM_2_Gangliosidoses are a group of 3 lysosomal storage diseases caused due to deficiency of the enzyme—hexosaminidase (HexA)—and has autosomal inheritance [45]. It results in inability to catabolize GM_2 gangliosides.

7.4.1 Etiopathogenesis

Tay-sach's disease is the most common form of GM_2 Gangliosidoses, and it is prevalent among Jews (Ashkenazic) who seem to have a carrier rate of 1 in 30. The enzyme defect results from mutation in the alpha α-sub unit locus on chromosome 15, resulting in severe deficiency of hexosaminidase Alpha, leading to progressive destruction of nerve cells in the brain and spinal cord. The exact molecular basis of such neuronal injury is not fully understood. However, more than 100 mutations have been described in the α-sub unit gene, resulting in misfolding of the mutant proteins, which are unstable and undergo proteosomal degradation, leading to accumulation of toxic substrates and intermediates within neuron.

It has been found that hexosaminidase A is absent from virtually all tissues—heart, liver, spleen, and nervous system, especially involved are neurons in the central and autonomous nervous system and retina, which dominate the clinical scenario.

7.4.2 Clinical Features

There are 3subdivisions of Tay Sachs Disease. 1. Infantile, 2. Juvenile, and 3. Late-onset. Most common is the infantile form. Infants appear normal at birth, but slowly around 6 months of age, they manifest features of motor and mental maldevelopment leading to motor incoordination, intellectual disability, and muscular flaccidity, which eventually lead to blindness. On examination, the characteristic cherry-red spot appears in the macula of the eye in almost all patients. Slowly the neuronal function deteriorates within 1 or 2 years followed by death at the age of 2 to 3 years.

Antenatal diagnosis and carrier detection are possible by enzyme assays and DNA-based analysis. This disorder has also spurred clinical trials of Molecular Chaperone Therapy, for some variants of later onset of Tay-Sach's and other Lysosomal storage diseases. Such therapy involves the use of synthetic substitute, which can cross blood-brain barrier, bind to the mutated misfolded protein, so that it enables proper folding, thereby enough functional enzyme can be saved to ameliorate the effects of the inborn error.

On histologic examination, the neurons appear ballooned-up with cytoplasmic vacuoles, which represent distended lysosomes filled with gangliosides. There is progressive destruction of neurons, proliferation of microglia, and accumulation of complex lipids in phagocytes within brain. The ganglion cells in retina are also swollen, particularly at the margin of the macula, causing accentuation of the normal color of the macular choroid and pale swollen ganglion cells giving it a *cherry-red-spot* in the macula—characteristic feature of Tay-Sach's disease and other storage disorders affecting the neurons.

7.5 Neimann–Pick Disease [16, 17, 43, 44]

It is another lysosomal storage disorder, due to lack of enzyme sphingomyelinase and results in the accumulation of sphingomyelin, a phospholipid, which is a structural component of cell membrane and influences integral membrane proteins and ion channels. Therefore, the deficiency of the enzyme blocks degradation of lipids and results in their accumulation within lysosomes, especially within various tissues of the body, especially in cells of phagocyte system.

7.5.1 Etiopathogenesis

The gene for this enzyme maps to chromosome 11 and is expressed from maternal chromosome with an epigenetic silencing of the paternal gene. More than 180 mutations are found in the sphingomyelinase gene. This disorder is also common in Ashkenazi Jews.

There are 3 types of Niemann Pick disease: Type A, B, and C. *Type A* affects infants in a severe form and has extensive and diffuse neurologic and visceral involvement of spleen, liver, lymph nodes, bone marrow, tonsils, gastrointestinal tract, and lungs.

Type B disease has predominantly visceral involvement with organomegaly but no central nervous system involvement. Niemann Pick diseases type A and B are now considered a distinct disorder called Acid sphingomyelinase deficiency [17, 43].

Type C is distinct at the biochemical and genetic levels, compared to types A and B and is the more common type. It is due to the mutations in 2 related genes NPC_1 and NPC_2, which are involved in transport of free cholesterol from the lysosomes to the cytoplasm [44]. Therefore, type C disease is due to defect in nonenzymatic lipid transport.

7.5.2 Clinical Features

Manifestation may be present at birth with organomegaly especially hepatosplenomegaly or become evident by 6 months of age with enlarged other organs—lymph nodes. There would be vomiting, fever, and progressive deterioration of psychomotor functions. Type C may present as hydrops fetalis and stillbirth. Death usually occurs within first or second year of life. Diagnosis is possible by biochemical analysis of Sphingomyelinase activity in leukocytes or bone marrow biopsy material or by DNA analysis.

7.5.3 Morphology

As with other lysosomal storage disorders, cells of mononuclear phagocyte system are affected, which become enlarged up to 90 µm microns in diameter due to accumulation of sphingomyelin and cholesterol in the lysosomes. Many uniform small vacuoles are seen in the cytoplasm, which appears foamy. Electron microscopy confirms the engorged vacuoles, which contain membranous cytoplasmic bodies and resemble concentric lamellated myelin figures called the *Zebra Bodies.* These lipid-laden phagocytic foamy cells cause organomegaly, especially splenomegaly.

Involvement of the neurons causes vacuolation, and ballooning appearance leads to cell death and loss of brain substance. Similar to Tay—Sachs disease, a *cherry-red spot* is seen in the retina.

7.6 Mucopolysaccharidoses (MPS) [18, 19, 47, 48]

These are a group of disorders resulting due to mutations of enzymes involved in degradation of mucopolysaccharides (glycosaminoglycans—GAGs) [48]. These mucopolysaccharides are complex carbohydrates, which are linked with proteins to form proteoglycans.

They are found in the extracellular matrix, joint fluid, and connective tissue. The different mucopolysaccharides that accumulate in different tissues are dermatan sulfate, heparan sulfate, keratan sulfate, and chondroitin sulfate.

7.6.1 Etiopathogenesis

Seven types of MPS are known due to 11 different enzyme deficiencies. MPS II is the only one with X-linked inheritance, while all other MPS have an autosomal-recessive transmission. Each MPS shows a wide spectrum of phenotypic variability from most severe form to milder form, due to different residual enzyme activities. Molecular basis of such differences remains unknown.

These enzymes are involved in the degradation of the molecules, which cleave the terminal sugars from the polysaccharide chains that are disposed along a polypeptide or core protein. Therefore, in the absence of the prime enzymes, all these chains accumulate within lysosomes in various tissues and organs of the body especially in the mononuclear phagocytic cells, endothelial cell, intimal smooth muscle cells, and fibroblasts. Other common organs are spleen, liver, bone marrow, lymph nodes, blood vessels, and heart. Therefore, MPS are genetic, progressive Lysosomal storage disorders affecting virtually all organs and systems. The first MPS was clinically identified about 100 years ago [18].

7.6.2 Clinical Features

Of the many clinical variants of MPS, 2 are important.

1. Hurler's syndrome MPS-I.
2. Hunters syndrome MPS-II. All the variants are inherited as autosomal-recessive trait, except Hunters syndrome, which is an X-linked recessive trait. These differences result in different clinical picture. Many of these variants have communicating hydrocephalus [47].

Hurler Syndrome, also called as MPS-I-H, results due to deficiency of apha-L-idouronidase, and is one of the severe forms of MPS. Children appear normal at birth, but by 6–24 months develop hepato-splenomegaly, coarse facial features, corneal clouding, and skeletal deformities with distinct coarse facial features. Their growth is retarded and death occurs by age of 6–10 years due to myocardial infarction and cardiac decompensation.

Hunter syndrome has no corneal clouding, is milder in course, and has longer survival and almost always occurs in boys.

Morphology: As mentioned earlier, the common sites involved are spleen, liver, bone marrow, tonsils, lymph nodes, blood vessels especially coronary arteries, valvular lesions of heart, and brain having mononuclear phagocytic cells.

Affected cells are distended like balloons with clear cytoplasm, are positive with PAS stain (Periodic Acid Schiff), and appear as finely granular cytoplasm. Under electron microscopy, these vacuoles are resolved as numerous lysosomes. Similar changes are seen in the neurons and some may also have *lamellated Zebra bodies*. Similar to Neiman-Pick disease, *Cherry-Red Spot* is also seen in the retina.

7.7 Glycogen Storage Diseases (Glycogenosis) [20, 21, 22, 23, 46]

Glycogen is a storage form of glucose, the synthesis of which begins with the conversion of glucose to glucose-6-phosphate and is as follows [21, 22].

A large polymer is built up by addition of linked glucose molecules, which is mediated by glycogen synthetases. There are many branching and debranching enzymes which degrade glucose residues. If the lysosomes are deficient in the enzyme, acid alpha glucosidase the glycogen contained within them is not accessible to degradation by cytoplasmic enzymes such as phosphorylases.

On the basis of pathophysiology and specific enzyme deficiencies, glycogenosis can be divided into *3 major subgroups of GSDs*

I. Hepatic type GSD
II. Myopathic type GSD
III. Miscellaneous type GSD

I. *Hepatic Type Glycogenosis:* The liver is important in the metabolism of glycogen as it contains various enzymes needed. An inherited deficiency of hepatic enzymes, which are involved in degradation of glycogen, leads to accumulation of glycogen in the liver, causing hypoglycemia due to its reduction in blood glucose. Deficiency of enzymes Glucose-6-Phosphatase results in Von-Gierke disease or Type I Glycogenosis, which is an important example of Type I Glycogen storage disease.
II. *Myopathic Type GSD*

    Glycogen is used predominantly as a source of energy during physical activity by the skeletal muscle. ATP is generated by glycolysis which ultimately lead to formation of lactate thereby primarily impairing muscle activity and energy production. Important enzymes that are deficient in this condition are muscle phosphorylase and muscle phosphofructokinase. There arc several forms of these disorders.

Examples are (A) Mc Ardle Disease or Type V Glycogenosis (B) Type VII GSD is due to Muscle Phosphofructokinase.

III. *Miscellaneous types of GSD*: GSD, which does not specifically fit into the above two—hepatic / myopathic types, is due to deficiency of acid alpha glucosidase (acid maltose): this causes Pompe's disease, a Type II GSD having cardiomegaly as its prominent feature. Eye changes include multiple, bilateral, punctate, and peripheral opacities in the lens [23].

7.7.1 Clinical Features

Clinical features vary in the different types. *Hepatic type* presents with stunted growth, organomegaly of both heart and kidney and hypoglycemia leads to convulsions. Some present with bleeding tendency due to platelet dysfunction, gouty arthritis and skin xanthomas due to hyperlipidemia and hyperuricemia.

Many of them have stunted growth due to failure to thrive.

In the Myopathic type, onset is usually in the adulthood with severe painful cramps associated with strenuous exercise, myoglobinura in 50% cases, and elevated serum creatine kinase levels. The miscellaneous type of GSD is predominantly associated with massive cardiomegaly with hypotonia of muscles and often cardiorespiratory failure within 2 years. However, with treatment, most of these patients survive and are compatible with normal longevity.

7.7.2 Morphology

Most of the organs are enlarged with special mention of few organs in the respective types of GSD.

Hepatic Type: Have enlarged kidneys and liver. Microscopically, there are intracytoplasmic vacuoles due to accumulation of glycogen and lipids and intranuclear glycogen accumulation in the liver, whereas in kidneys, the cortical tubular epithelial cells have more intracytoplasmic glycogen accumulation.

Myopathic Type: Subsarcolemmal accumulation of glycogen predominates in the skeletal muscles.

Miscellaneous Type: Changes are seen in liver, heart, and skeletal muscle, seen as ballooning of lysosomes with glycogen and creating a lacy intracytoplasmic pattern in liver and within sarcoplasma and membrane bound in cardiac muscle and skeletal muscles.

7.8 Phenylketonuria (PKU): [24, 25, 26, 27, 42]

Phenylketonuria is a historically significant Inborn error of metabolism. It was first described by Asbjorn Folling—one of the first Norwegian Physicians in 1934. [42] It is also an autosomal-recessive disorder caused due to deficiency of the enzyme phenylalanine hydroxylase (PAH). This causes an increase in phenylalanine, an amino acid, which cannot be converted to tyrosine, which is an important component of neurotransmitters (Epinephrine, norepinephrine, and dopamine) and skin pigment melanin.

7.8.1 Etiopathogenesis

More than 950 (PAH) gene variants have been identified in people with PKU [25]. Incidence is variable: 1 in 10,000 affected infants belong to the Caucasian population, especially of Scandinavian origin. Affected infants are normal at birth but soon start to develop changes in brain development,(severe intellectual disability), which becomes evident by 6 months of life. In normal children, about half of the dietary intake of phenylalanine is necessary for protein synthesis and the rest gets converted to tyrosine by phenylalanine hydroxylase system. Due to the deficiency of this enzyme phenylalanine hydroxylase, other minor shunt pathways come into play, releasing certain metabolites, which get excreted in large amounts in the urine and sweat, giving a strange odor-musty or mousy odor. These metabolites also cause brain damage. And lack of tyrosine, which is also a precursor to melanin, results in physical change in hair and skin (a lighter shade).

As mentioned earlier, over 950 mutant alleles of PAH gene are identified and the clinical presentation depends on the severity of mutation: 98% of PKU is attributed to mutation of PAH gene, whereas about 2% of PKU seem to occur because of abnormalities in the synthesis or recycling of the intermediate cofactor tetrahydrobiopterin BH_4. This recognition is important in the treatment modalities, as dietary restriction may help overcome or avoid intellectual disability. Due to oxidative stress, there seems to be disruption of pro-oxidants / antioxidants balance in PKU [26].

It is found that many female PKU patients if treated with dietary restriction with high proteins and aspartame, an artificial non-saccharide sweetener, early in life, can reach child-bearing age and remain clinically asymptomatic.

7.8.2 Clinical Features

Clinical features depend upon the severity of the disease. Classic PKU is marked, with brain damage and leads to marked intellectual disability within few months of life, whose pathomechanisms are poorly understood [27]. A dangerous build-up of phenylalanine can develop when a child ingests protein-rich foods such as milk, cheese, nuts, or artificial sweeteners like aspartame.

Patients may develop musty odor in their breath, skin, or urine. Neurological problems like seizures and, tremors later on develop marked intellectual disability, behavioral and emotional problems. Skin rashes (eczema), light colored skin and hair (Blond hair), along with eye abnormalities - blue eyes and corneal opacities may also be present. There is no cure for PKU; however, normal growth can be achieved in less severe cases through dietary restriction.

7.9 Galactosemia: [28]

Galactosemia is a rare autosomal-recessive disorder of carbohydrate (Galactose) metabolism that results in inability to convert galactose to glucose. There are 2 variants of this disorders. The most common variant results due to total lack of the enzyme galactose-1-phosphate uridyl transferase (GALT) and the rare variant, which is the milder form, is due to the lack of the enzyme galactokinase (GALK) or uridine diphosphate galactose 4 epimerase (GALE) [16].

7.9.1 Etiopathogenesis

Normally, lactose, which is a major carbohydrate in mammalian milk, is split into glucose and galactose in the intestinal microvilli, galactose is later converted to glucose through several steps in metabolism. But due to lack of these enzymes, especially GALT, glucose-1-phosphate gets accumulated in different tissues. In addition, alternative metabolic pathways get activated, resulting in by-products, namely, galactitol and galactonate, which also get accumulated in various tissues and in blood, resulting in tissue damage. Liver, eyes, and brain bear the brunt of the tissue damage. However, there is still no clear understanding of the exact mechanism of damage to liver and brain .

7.9.2 Clinical Features

Clinical picture depends on the intensity of mutations and varies from child to child. Infant may appear normal at birth and later show changes within few days or weeks. Initial features may be vomiting, lack of energy, diarrhea, within few days of ingestion of milk, and, later, refusal of milk, followed by jaundice and hepatomegaly.

Accumulation of galactose and galactose-1-PO4 in kidney impairs amino-acid transport, resulting in aminoaciduria. Cataract develops within few weeks to few months. Hemolysis and bleeding diathesis can occur in some.

The disease leads to severe weight loss and struggle to grow and becomes susceptible to infections. Some children have ill-developed motor skills and gonadal failure especially in girls.

Dietary restrictions, by early removal of galactose from diet for at least the first 2 years of life, help children survive into adulthood and prevent cataract and liver damage. Antenatal diagnosis is possible to assess GALT activity in amniotic fluid. Newborns are regularly screened in some countries. Infants must be treated promptly by removing lactose from the diet, and children with special diet usually show satisfactory growth.

Some other IMD disorders as the ones described in the following texts also have Ophthalmologic effects, but are rarely seen.

7.9.3 Morphology

Major organs affected are liver, eye (cataract) gliosis of cerebral cortex, edema, and loss of nerve cells, especially in cerebellum and dentate nuclei. Other organs involved are cardiac muscle, spleen, and kidneys, due to impaired amino-acid transport, leading to amino aciduria. Microscopically, Fatty change is predominant in Liver.

7.10 Metal Metabolic Disorders

Inherited metabolic disorders like these can result in protein malfunction and toxic accumulation of metals in the body. Two most common diseases are (**A**) Wilson's disease and (**B**) Hemochromatosis.

7.10.1 Wilson's Disease: [29, 30, 31]

It is also an autosomal-recessive disorder, resulting in defective copper metabolism, causing impaired copper excretion into bile and accumulation of copper into many tissues leading to copper toxicity. Prevalence of this disease is 1 in 30,000.

7.10.1.1 Etiopathogenesis

Wilson's disease is due to the result of mutation of the ATP7B gene, with more than 300 sequence variations identified, which encodes the transmembrane copper-transporting ATPase, which normally is expressed on the hepatocyte canalicular membrane. The deficiency of ATP7B decreases copper transport into bile. It also impairs the copper incorporation into ceruloplasmin and inhibits ceruloplasmin secretion into the blood, thereby causing decrease in circulating ceruloplasmin and accumulation of copper especially in hepatocytes and other tissues.

Mechanism of copper toxic injury is mainly due to 3 causes: (A) promotion of free radicals formation by Fenton reaction, (B) binding to sulfhydryl groups of cellular proteins, and (C) displacing other metals from hepatic metalloenzymes.

The hepatocyte injury causes non-ceruloplasmin-bound copper to be spilled into blood and accumulate in other tissues, especially the basal ganglia of the brain and cornea along with an increase in urinary excretion of copper.

7.10.1.2 Clinical Features

There is a great variation in the clinical presentation with age range of 6–40 years. Some patients also present features of with acute on chronic liver disease, neurologic features of tremors, poor coordination, and some may also have psychiatric symptoms. Hemolytic anemia is seen in some due to red cell membrane damage. Classic Kayser–Fleischer rings are seen in the outer rim of cornea.

7.10.1.3 Morphology

Hepatic changes are variable ranging from mild to severe damage: Fatty change (Steatosis) with focal hepatocyte necrosis causing acute liver failure. Chronic hepatitis changes are seen causing moderate-to-severe portal inflammation, hepatocyte necrosis fatty change, and steatohepatitis (ballooned hepatocyte), mallory hyaline bodies, and perisinusoidal fibrosis, eventually resulting in cirrhosis. Corneal lesions are seen as green-brown deposits in descements membrane in the limbus of cornea called the *KF rings* (*Kayser–Fleischer rings*) [31]. Neurologic involvement is seen in all patients of toxic brain injury.

7.10.1.4 Diagnosis

Biochemical diagnosis is based on decreased serum ceruloplasmin levels, increased urinary excretion of copper, and increased hepatic copper content, which is the most accurate and sensitive test. Slit-lamp examinatio, demonstrates the K-F ring and sequencing (NGS) of ATP7B gene is now available.

7.10.2 Hemochromatosis [32, 33]

Hemochromatosis is caused due to excess iron absorption, despite normal intake, which gets deposited in parenchymal cells of different organs, especially in liver and pancreas, followed by heart, joints, and endocrine organs. Iron is predominantly a direct hepatotoxin.

7.10.2.1 Etiopathogenesis

It is classified into 2 types

1. *Hereditary Hemochromatosis* is due to mutations of the gene encoding HFE, transferrin receptor 2 (TFR_2) or hepcidin and HJV (Hemojuvelin, Juvenile).
2. *Secondary Hemochromatosis* occurs as a consequence of parenteral administration of iron.

   Hepcidin a small circulating peptide protein, which binds to the cellular iron efflux channel ferroportin (FPN), causing its internalization and proteolysis, and inhibits the release of iron from intestinal cells and macrophages. Decreased synthesis or activity of hepcidin may be caused by mutations in the genes HAMP, HJV, TFR_2, and HFE resulting in either the Juvenile or adult form of hemochromatosis.

   The disease gets manifested after accumulation of 20 gms of stored iron. In the severe form of this disorder, total body iron pool may exceed 50 gms, more than 1/3rd of which get accumulated in the liver.

   The mechanism of liver injury includes (1) stimulation of collagen formation by activation of hepatic stellate cells, (2) lipid peroxidation, and (3) interaction of reactive oxygen species and iron with DNA, leading to lethal cell injury, especially the 2 main organs—liver and pancreas.

7.10.2.2 Clinical Features

The characteristic triad of features are pigmentary liver cirrhosis, diabetes mellitus, and skin pigmentation, along with cardiac dysfunction and gouty arthritis. Visual changes could be diminished due to changes in cornea and retina and macular degeneration. The link between hemochromatosis and the wet form of macular degeneration leading to blindness is being pursued.

7.10.2.3 Morphology

Changes are especially seen in liver and pancreas. In the liver, iron is seen as cytoplasmic granules, which are positive, appear blue on Prussian blue stain, seen initially around periportal area, later became generalized, making it appear large and chocolate brown color, becoming black and ultimately resulting in micronodular cirrhosis. Pancreas too becomes pigmented and affects acinar and islet cells and produces diffuse fibrosis and atrophy leading to diabetes mellitus. Skin pigmentation due to increased epidermal melanin production gives a slate grey color. The above 2 features of skin and diabetes mellitus are also called as "*Bronzed diabetes.*"

Other organs that show morphologic changes are cardiomegaly, later become fibrotic acute synovitis causing pseudogout. Pituitary involvement leads to testicular atrophy leading to reduced levels of hormones (testosterone and gonadotropin).

7.10.2.4 Diagnosis

Hemochromatosis may be identified because of abnormal blood test done for other reasons or from screening of family members of people diagnosed with the disease. Two key tests to detect iron overload done on fasting are as follows:

1. Sr. transferrin saturation
2. Sr Ferritin levels and the diagnosis is confirmed by the below third test
3. Tests for gene mutation for HFE gene

7.11 Leukodystrophies [34]

Leukodystrophies are also a group of Lysosomal storage disorders. They are very rare—progressive, metabolic genetic diseases that affect brain, spinal cord, and often the peripheral nerves. There are many types and each type is caused by a specific gene abnormality that causes abnormal development or *destruction of the myelin sheath* of the brain. Normal brain function depends on the integrity and connection between neurons; therefore, any damage to the myelinated axons has serious consequences.

Some of these disorders are as follows:

I. *Krabbe Disease: (Globoid Cell Leukodystrophy [GLD])*

It is an autosomal-recessive disorder, resulting from a deficiency of the enzyme galactocerebroside β-galactosidase, which is required for the catabolism of galactocerebroside to ceramide and galactose. This deficiency leads to activation of an alternative catabolic pathway, converting galactocerebroside to galactosphingosine.

Elevation of this substance (galactosphingosine) is toxic to astrocytes, oligodendrocytes, and peripheral nerves, especially causing loss of oligodendrocytes. Neurons and axons are relatively spared. Myelin—the protective coating of nerve cells in brain and throughout nervous system—gets destroyed.

Clinical Features

Young patients with seizures, loss of developmental abilities, and constricted muscles, mostly, die before 2 years of age. If it develops in older children, signs and symptoms vary—progressive loss of vision, ataxia, decline in thinking skills, muscle weakness, etc.

Morphology

Mostly affects the white matter giving it a gray / yellow color. *Microscopically,* there are aggregation of swollen macrophages with vacuolated cytoplasm—called the *globoid cells*—seen perivascularily and in the brain parenchyma.

II. *Metachromatic Leukodystrophy (MLD).* It is also an autosomal-recessive disorder caused due to deficiency of lysosomal enzyme arylsulfatase, which degrades sulfate-containing lipids (sulfatides) into sulfate and other products. Thus, the deficiency of this enzyme leads to cytoplasmic binding of sulfatides within macrophages resulting in vacuolated macrophages and increase in cerebroside sulfate, which is toxic to white matter. Symptoms include muscle wasting, weakness, muscle rigidity, developmental delay, progressive loss of vision, leading to blindness and most of them die by age of 5.

Morphology

Vacuolated Macrophages are scattered throughout white matter. These sulfatide-containing macrophages when bound to certain dyes, such as toludine blue, form granules that are described as metachromasia, which is seen in brain peripheral nerves and in the urine.

Unlike the above 2 disorders, Adrenoleukodystrophy differs & is as follows:

III. *Adrenoleukodystrophy: It has several clinically and genetically distinct forms.* It also has an x-linked form and is associated with mutation in ALD gene on chromosome Xq28. This results in abnormality in the transport of fatty acids into peroxisomes, leading to increased serum levels of these very-long-chain fatty acids (lipids), affecting central nervous system, peripheral nerves, and adrenals, especially in boys.

Clinical Features

These leukodystrophies have an insidious onset and have progressive loss of cerebral function. Age of onset is a key factor: early the appearance, faster the progress. Infants have a life expectancy of 2–8 years, whereas adults survive for a decade after onset. Features include loss of motor skills, walking, swallowing, stiff rigid muscles, poor muscle function, loss of bowel and bladder functions, loss of sensation to touch, pain, heat, and sound, and the varied ocular manifestations.

Morphology

Like the other 2 disorders, it affects white matter, causing gliosis and marked lymphocyte infiltration. Adrenal cortical atrophy is an additional feature of this disorders. *Ocular manifestations* include retinal changes, loss of retinal nerve fiber, ganglion cell layer, optic nerve degeneration, and inclusion in retinal pigment epithelial cell macrophages of retina and optic nerve.

Eye as a Window To IMD!!

As has been learnt in the above discussion of inherited metabolic disorders (IMDs), *ocular manifestations* occur in various disorders. Although there seems to be an extensive understanding of these disorders at the biochemical, molecular levels, little is known about their exact pathogenesis, especially how these contribute to ocular defects!! [41].

The occurrence of eye abnormalities includes disorders of any part of the eye, extra-occular muscles, and visual pathways leading to optic neuropathy, retinopathy, lens, opacification and cataracts, corneal clouding, various, keratopathies, etc., The ocular effects could be due to direct toxic mechanism of abnormal metabolic products or accumulation of normal metabolic products or accumulation of normal metabolites by error of synthetic / alternate pathways—Garrod's Hypothesis. Therefore, awareness of the potential ophthalmic effects of IMDs is important for any clinician and should ideally be carried out by a combination of specialists including neonatologists, pediatricians and a detailed ophthalmologic examination by ophthalmologists who may happen to see patients with their initial presentation or as a subsequent disease—course with eye-related features of a specific IMD and needs to correlate with a Biochemist and a Medical Geneticist.

Hence, an IMD should be considered in the differential diagnosis of the eye condition, alongside common acquired or other nonmetabolic genetic causes.

It has been found in IMDs that it is symmetrical bilateral involvement of eyes and severe visual impairment is more common around 2 months of age, when eye contact develops in most children. Often anomalies of the eyes are easily recognized, some may need advanced studies like electro-retinogram and visual-evoked responses related with fundic examination [35].

7.12 Approach to IMD: Ophthalmologist Way [36]

Basically, identification of an IMD needs a high degree of clinical suspicion. A thorough clinical history, namely, age, appropriate growth or any history of failure to thrive, recurrent vomiting, prolonged Jaundice, family history (unexplained neonatal / childhood death), recurrent miscarriages, and, in many cases, eye involvement can be the primary presenting feature of an IMD.

As has been noted in the above earlier detailed discussions on the various IMDs, the following discussion now aims to offer a summary of eye involvement in the different IMDs, which helps assist in the early recognition and diagnosis of IMDs that can facilitate earliest treatment. Some of the common Ophthalmic manifestations are described below and in Table 7.1.

Ophthalmoplegia:

IMD happens to be one of the differential diagnoses. Strabismus is a feature of the commonest

Table 7.1 Eye and IMD

Presenting feature	Type of IMD	Remarks
Abnormal eye movements Ptosis	Pompe disease (glycogen storage disease type-III), mitochondrial disorders	Refer discussion below.
Cornea		Corneal changes could be either due to defective carbohydrate, lipid, or protein metabolism.
Keratitis	Tyrosinemia Type II, Fabry's disorder	
Corneal Clouding/ Opacities	Mucopolysaccharidosis (I, IV, VI) Galactosialidosis	MPS causes severe opacification
Ophthalmoplegia	Gaucher's disease Type III, Nieman Pick Type—C, Early mitochondrial disorders, Late-onset GM2 gangliosidosis, Wilson's disease.	Refer discussions below.
Lens		Homocystinuria-displaces lens inferiorly. Early detection helps in the prevention of complication.
(a) Ectopia Lentis	Homocystinuria	
(b) Cataract	Congenital cataract—Cockayne Lowe syndrome. Neonatal- Galactosemias Infancy—Sialidosis Childhood—Wilson's disease Later / Adult—Fabry's Disease, Homocystinuria, Glycogen storage disease type—I & III	MPS—Have significant lens opacification.
Glaucoma	Mucopolysaccharidosis	Increase intraocular pressure.
Retina		
Retinitis pigmentosa	a. Congenital disorders of glycosylation. (a) Refsum disease. (b) Galactosialidosis GM1, GM2 gangliosidosis, Nieman Pick disease type A & B	Retinitis Pigmentosa is the most common defect in MPS.
Cherry-red spot	Metachromatic leukodystrophy Sialosis Tay Sach's disease Sandhoff's disease	Cherry-red spot is mostly seen in neurometabolic disorders of IMD
Optic atrophy	Metachromatic leukodystrophy	Seen in mitochondrial inherited degeneration of retinal ganglion cells

form of Congenital Disorders of Glycosylation (CDG), a multisystem disorder, which includes nystagmus with or without visual impairments. Mitochondrial disorders (Leigh & Leigh-like Syndrome) can present with squint and usually follows a minor febrile illness. Some of these Mitochondrial disorders can present later in life with primary ocular motor defects.

Some LSDs, like Gaucher's disease, have specific eye movements abnormalities—horizontal supranuclear gaze palsy, whereas Nieman Pick disease Type C (NDC) with its very wide age of presentation has typical eye movement defect—vertical supranuclear gaze palsy.

PTOSIS:

Ptosis has many differential diagnoses and of the IMDs, Mitochondrial disorders can present with ptosis, which gets worse with fatigue. Of the metabolic myopathies, Pompe disease (Glycogen storage disease Type II) may have progressive ptosis, along with generalized motor and respiratory myopathy.

Corneal Pathology:

Tyrosinemia Type II: It is a rare amino-acid disorder, and causes painful keratitis, which results in photophobia, lacrimation, and burning pain. Slit-lamp examination may reveal bilateral herpetic- like lesions with neovascularization, if untreated can result in corneal scarring.

Fabry's disease, an X-linked LSD, which is a multisystem disease, may be detected incidentally in a presymptomatic stage by finding of corneal whorling—Cornea Verticallate, which manifests as corneal opacification at a later stage.

Corneal Clouding/Opacification:

This is a feature of several IMDs, especially some of the progressive LSD conditions. For *example,* Cystinosis has deposits of cysteine, which gets accumulated within stroma of the cornea, Iris, Lens, and retina and manifests as photophobia with visual defect. In other LSDs that present with corneal clouding include MPS I, IV, VI. In some of these, Ocular Manifestations may be the initial presenting feature.

Lens Pathology:

Cataract: Many IMDs present with Cataracts and the age that cataract develops can help in the differential diagnosis, especially seen in Peroxisomal disorders. Cataract can be seen in birth—Cockayne Syndrome. Neonatal onset cataract is a feature of Galactose metabolism disorders.

Juvenile / Adult-onset Cataract is seen in Cerebrotendinous Xanthomatosis *(CTX)* and Wilson's disease, which present as "Sunflower Cataracts" and the classical Kaiser–Fleischer rings.

Late-onset (adult) cataracts may be seen in Ornithine amino transferase deficiency.

Glaucoma: Raised intraocular pressure may be seen as Secondary feature in several IMDs.

For example, Glycosylation and MPS.

RETINA: Retinitis pigmentosa is seen in & as part of many IMDs.

For example, Mitochondrial Disorders.

Cherry-Red Spot:

Cherry-red spot is detected on fundoscopy as a deep red circular area, Temporal to the optic disc at the Centre of Macula, and surrounded by a pale halo. Several LSDs are associated with this feature, which is due to accumulation of intracellular storage material.

Optic Atrophy:

It is the degeneration of the retinal ganglion cells with optic nerve pallor, due to deterioration of optic nerve, which is seen in many IMDs, especially seen in Mitochondrial disorders, LSD—Krabbe's disease and Metachromatic Leukodystrophy.

Salient Clinical Features of IMD:

- Some General Features of IMD include the following:
  - Deafness, abnormal hair, Lethargy, Hydrops
  - Failure to gain weight, growth, developmental delay
  - Organomegaly- Spleen, Liver
- Gastrointestinal—Poor feeding, Abdominal pain, recurrent vomiting,
  - Weight loss, Jaundice

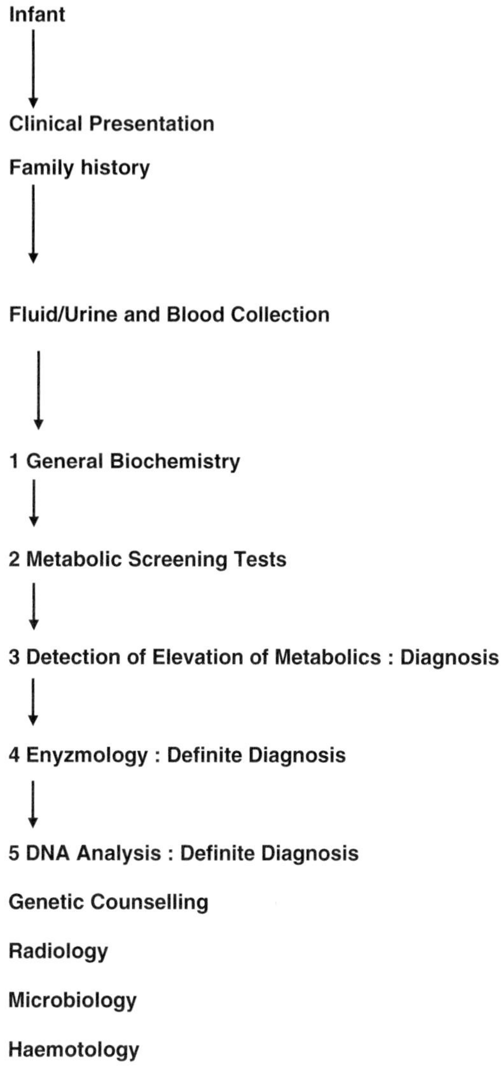

Fig. 7.3 Laboratory Investigation of infants suspected of having an inherited metabolic disease. Tests 1 and 2 can be carried out in most biochemistry laboratories, while 3 to 5 require more sophisticated equipment, facilities, and expertise

- Eyes—Cataract, Cherry-Red Spot, Dislocated Lens, Glaucoma, Neurologic—Hypotonia, Hypertonia
  - Seizures, or coma

  Others—Abnormal odor of urine, breath, sweat, or saliva.
- Symptoms may come as suddenly or progress slowly. Symptoms may be brought on by food, medication, dehydration, minor illness, or other factors.
- Signs and symptoms may appear within few weeks after birth in many conditions. However, some IMDs may take years to develop.

Diagnostic Approach to IMD [37, 38, 39]:
Classic features are often present at birth and some are detected on routine screening. Many States in the USA test newborns for PKU & Galacotosemia. If an IMD is not detected at birth, it is often not diagnosed until symptoms appear. However, once symptoms develop, specific blood or DNA tests are available to diagnose most genetic metabolic disorders. As mentioned, clinical analysis remains the prime modality of suspicion of identification of IMD, followed by planning of specific investigations based on specific pattern of suspicious features.

In general, Metabolic testing will include—General Biochemistry Parameters (Eg., Renal & Liver function Tests, Cholesterol, Creatinine kinase, uric acid estimation). Specific metabolic testing on blood and urine samples (plasma amino acids, urine organic acids, urine glucosamine—glycogens) and later, Confirmatory Diagnostic Tests include specific enzyme assays done on blood samples or on tissues—such as cultures, skin fibroblasts, muscle / liver biopsies,

Table 7.2 Summary of investigations in IMD

Disorder	Sample: Urine	Blood	Other
Lysosomal storage	1. Glycosaminoglycanes	1.Enzyme assays	Histopathology
	2. Sialic acids	2.Vacuolated lymphocytes & electron microscopy	
	1. Glycosaminoglycans	1. Enzyme assays	
	2. Sialic acids	2.Vacuolated lymphocytes & electron microscopy of buffy coat	
	3. Oligosaccharides	3. DNA	
Mitochondrial disorders	1.Urine organic acids 2. Renal tabular markers	1. Lactate 2. Plasma amino acids. 3. DNA (nuclear genes, mitochondrial (mt (DNA))	Muscle biopsy (Histopathology, respiratory chain enzymology)
Peroxisomal disorders	–	1. Very-long-chain fatty acids. 2. Phytanate, pristanate. 3. Red cell plasmalogens 4. DNA	Skin fibroblasts studies
General metabolic screening	Urine organic acids	1. Plasma amino acids. 2. Acylcarnitine profile 3.DNA	
Galactose / Polyols	Urine polyols	1.Gal-1- P Uridyltranserferase 2.Red cell galactose—1-phosphate (GAL1P) 3. DNA epimerase/ galactokinase enzymology	

etc., Fig. 7.3 gives the flow chart for investigations for infants with suspected IMDs. Table 7.2 summarizes the investigations required in the diagnosis IMD.

7.13 Screening Tests for Inherited Metabolic Disease (IMD): [40, 19, 35]

Accurate diagnosis is important for medical management, prognosis, and for genetic counselling. Population screening has the potential to reduce diagnostic delays significantly, which allows early intervention and prevention of irreversible organ damage. As mentioned earlier, there are New born screening (NBS) and screening of high-risk populations. Metabolic screening test in blood, Dried blood spots (DBS) [40], and urine are used to detect many of these disorders [19, 35]. Often a diagnosis is suggested by the pattern of abnormalities on screening with more specific diagnoses made through DNA-based or specific enzyme testing.

Molecular Genetic Testing: Next-Generation Sequencing (NGS) panels for genes causing specific lesions helps us to identify specific or at times unexplained IMDs. Necessary precautions in collecting samples in a suspected case may help arrive at the correct diagnosis with the appropriate samples: For example, Galactose–/ Lactose-free feeds in a neonate at risk for Galactosemia. Recent advances in the diagnosis and treatment of IMDs have improved the prognosis for many of these conditions.

7.14 Conclusions

There is no one-size-fits-all approach to the diagnosis!! . Each disorder is specific and needs a dedicated multidisciplinary approach in all aspects—Clinical examination (General and

Specialists), diagnosis, investigations, overall monitoring, and treatment, to ensure success in patient care. Improvement in screening programs, disease awareness, diagnostic tests, and therapeutic interventions in IMD have led to an increased patient survival and a better prognosis.

References

1. Guerrero RB, Salazas D, Tanpaiboon P. Ann Transl Med. 2018;6(24):470.
2. Sanderson S, Green A, Preece MA, Burton H. The incidence of inherited metabolic disorders in the West Midlands UK. Arch Dis Child. 2006;91(11):896–9.
3. Clarke JT. A clinical guide to inherited metabolic diseases. 2nd ed. New York: Cambridge University Press; 2002.
4. Lanpher B, Brunetti-Pierri N, Lee B. Inborn errors of metabolism: the flux from Mendelian to complex diseases. Nat Rev Genet. 2006;7:449–60.
5. Kumta NB. Inborn errors of metabolism. Indian J Pediatr. 2005;72:325–32.
6. Ramiez AM, Coll MJ, Chabas A, Azhar NB, Ghio AB, Kramer RD. Gene symbol: IDS, Disease mucopolysacharidosis. Hum Genet. 2002;123(5):545.
7. Verma PK, Ranganath P, Dalal AB, Phadke SR. Spectrum of lysosomal storage disorders at a medical genetics center in Northern India. Indian Pediatr. 2012;49:799–804.
8. Stirnemann J, Belmatong, et al. A review of Gaucher disease, pathophysiology, clinical presentation and treatment. Int J Mol Sci. 2017;18(441):1.
9. Sidransky E. Gauchers disease. Complexity in a simple disorder. Mol Genet Metabol. 2004;83:6–15.
10. Kaplan P, Anderson HC, Kancena KA, Yee JD. The Clinical 7 demographic characteristics of non neuronopathic Gauchers disease. Arch Pediatr Addes Med. 2006;160:603–8.
11. Kanli R, Zaizov R, Lazar L, Pertzelan A, Laron Z, Galatzer A, Phillip N, Yaniv Y, Cohn IJ. Delayed growth and puberty in patients with Gauchers disease type 1, Natural history & effect of splenectomy &/or enyme replacement therapy. Isr Med Assoc J. 2000;2:158–63.
12. Vellodi A. Lysosomal storage disorders. Br J Haematol. 2004;128:413.
13. Mento A, Kuter DJ, Salak SS, Belmatong N, Bembi B, Bright J, Vom Dahl S, Deodata F, Rocco MD, Goker-Alpah O, Huges DA, et al. Presenting signs & patient co-variables in Gauchers disease: outcome of the Gaucher earlier diagnosis consensus (GED-C). Delphi initiative. Int Med J. 2019;49:578–91.
14. Verma J, Thomas DC, Kasper DC, Sharma S, Puri RD, Bijarnia-Mahay S, Mistry PK, Verma IC. Efficacy of enzyme assays on Dried blood spots for the diagnosis of Lysosomal Storage Disorder. JIMD Rep. 2017;31:15–27.
15. Breiden B, Sandhoff K. Ganglioside metabolism and its inherited diseases. Methods Mol Biol. 2018;1804:97.
16. Schuchman EH, Desnick RJ. Types A and B, Neiman pick disease. Mol Genet Metab. 2017;120(1–2):27.
17. Schuchman EH. The pathogenesis and treatment of acid sphingomyelinase—deficient Neiman Pick Disease. J Inherit Metab Dis. 2007;30:654.
18. Parini R, Biondi A. Ital J Pediatr. 44. 2018.
19. Filocano M, Tomanin R, Bertola F, Morrone A. Biochemical and molecular analysis in mucopolysacharidosis: what a pediatrician must know. Ital J Pediatr. 2018;44(2):129.
20. Weinstein DA, Stenerward U, Desouza CFM, et al. Inborn errors of metabolism with hypoglycemia: glycogen storage diseases and inherited diseases of gluconeogenesis. Pediatr Cli North Am. 2018;65(2):247.
21. Hers H, et al. Glycogen storage diseases. In: The metabolic basis of inherited disease. 6th ed. New York; 1989.
22. The metabolic basis of inherited disease. 6th ed. NewYork: McGraw Hill; 1989. p. 425.
23. Allegrini D, Antelltano A, Fogagnolo P, De Cilla S, Piozzi P, Mazza M, Paci S, Montanari C, Riva E, Rossetti L. Lens opacities in glycogenoses types I and III. Can J Opthalmol. 2015;50(6):480–4.
24. Scriver CR. The PAH gene, phenylketonuria and a paradigm shift. Hum Mutat. 2007;28:831.
25. Blau N. Genetics of phenylketonuria: then and now. Hum Mutat. 2016;37(6):508–15.
26. Vargas CR, Wajner M, Sitta A. Oxidative stress in phenylketonuria patients. Mol Genet Metab. 2011;104:S97.
27. Ribas GS, Sitta A, Wajner M, Valgas CR. Oxidative stress in PKU. What is the evidence ? Cell Mol Neurobiol. 2011;31(5):653–62.
28. Ferrairaa CR, Gahlc WA. Lysosomal storage disease. Transl Sci Rare Dis. 2017;2(1):1–71.
29. Rosencrantz R, Scilsky M. Wilsons disease: pathogenesis and clinical consideration in diagnosis and treatment. Semin Liver Dis. 2011;31:245.
30. Ala A, Walker AP, Ashkank, Dooley JS, Schilsky ML. Wilsons disease. Lancet. 2007;369:397–408.
31. Amalnath DS, Subramanyam DK. Occular signs in Wilsons disease. Ann Indian Acad Neurol. 2012;15(3):200–1.
32. Pietrangelo A. Genetics, genetic testing and management of Haemochromatosis. 15 years since hepacidin. Gastroenterology. 2015;149(5):1240–51.
33. Pietrangeto A. Hereditary Hemochromatosis. Ann Rv Nutr. 2006;26:25.
34. Van der Knaap MS, Bugiani M. Leukodystrophies. Acta Neuropathol. 2017;134:351.
35. Sinnott Armstrong N, Tanigawa Y, Amar D, Mars N, Benner C, Aguirre M, Venkataramana GR, Wainberg M, Ollila HM, et al. Genetics of 35 blood and urine biomarkers in UK BioBank. Nat Genet. 2021;53:185–94.

36. Davidson JE. Ther Adv Opthalmol. 2020;12:1–20.
37. Applegath DA, Dimmeck JE, Toone JR. Laboratory detection of metabolic disease. Pediatr Clin North Am. 1989;36:49–65.
38. Blan N, durran N, Blaskovies ME, Gibson KM. Physicians guide to laboratory diagnosis of metabolic disorders. 2nd ed. New York: Springer; 2003.
39. Gary SE, Ryan E, Steward AM, Sidransky E. Recent advances in the diagnosis and management of Gauchers Disease. Expert Rev Endocrinol: Metab. 2018;13:107–18.
40. Yoshida S, Kido J, Matsumoto S, Momosaki K, Mitsubuchi H, Shimazu T, Suguwere K, Endo F, Nakamora K. Prenatal diagnosis of Gauchers disease using next generation sequencing. Pediatr Int. 2016;58:946–9.
41. Rajappa M, Goyal A, Kaur J. Inherited metabolic disorders involving the eye: nA Clinico-biochemical perspective. Eye (Lond). 2010;24(4):507–18.
42. Centerwall SA, Centerwall WR. The discovery of phenylketonuria. Pediatrics. 2000;105:89–103.
43. Schuchman EH, DeSnick RJ. Type A, B Neiman pick Disease. Mol Genet Metab. 2017;120(1-2):27–30.
44. Dardis A, Stefania Z, Gallera CZ, Carrozo R, Catharossi S, Peruzza P, Dariol R, et al. Type C Neiman Pick Disease. J Clin Med. 2020;9(3):679.
45. Chen H. Atlas of Genetic Diagnosis & Counselling. 2nd ed. Springer; 2012. p. 1973–9.
46. Kanungo S, Wells K, Tribett T, Gharbawy AE. Glycogen metabolism & glycogen storage disorders. Ann Transl Med. 2018;6(24):474.
47. Fowler GW, Sukoff M, Hamilton A, William JP. Communicating hydrocephalous in children with genetic inborn errors of metabolism. Childs Brain. 1975;1(4):251–4.
48. Pierzynowska K, Gaffke L, Podlacha M, Węgrzyn G. Genetic basis of behavioral disorders in mucopolyscaharidosis transcriptional studies. Int J Mol Sci. 2020;21:1156.

Routine investigations and their interpretation

8

Dilip K. Mishra and Geeta K. Vemuganti

Contents

D. K. Mishra (✉)
Ophthalmic Pathology Laboratory, Kallam Anji Reddy Campus, LV Prasad Eye Institute, Hyderabad, Telangana, India
e-mail: dilipkumarmishra@lvpei.org

G. K. Vemugantı
School of Medical Sciences, University of Hyderabad, Gachibowli, Hyderabad, India
e-mail: gkvemuganti@gmail.com

G. K. Vemuganti et al. (eds.), *Ocular Pathology*, https://doi.org/10.1007/978-981-96-8614-8_8

8.1 Introduction

Clinical pathology, or laboratory medicine, is a branch of pathology that mainly supports the diagnosis of a disease using laboratory tests of blood and body fluids. While the conduct of all the tests, analysis, and reporting is the responsibility of the pathologist, this clinical branch contributes significantly to the interpretation of the investigations, arriving at a diagnosis, evaluating the progress of the disease, thus contributing to the management of the patient [1]. Different studies reported that about in two-third of cases medical decisions are based on laboratory results [2]. Laboratory tests not only provide data to screen early risk factors; but it also helps in opting of noninvasive or less invasive procedure and monitoring the disease process by a physician [3].

Even though the disease may be local, we are aware that there is a strong communication between various systems of the body; hence, the evaluation of the blood, urine, and other body fluids would reflect the ongoing pathologic conditions, stage of the disease. Yet, there is no single test that would give all the information of the disease occurring in a patient. Hence, the routine investigations form the part of the workup of patients at early stage of the disease, and the clinicians top it up with advanced investigations based on the progress of the disease. Some of the investigations contribute to pathognomonic diagnostic criteria of a disease: for example, identification of a malarial parasite in blood, blast cells in leukemia, or identification of sugar in urine in diabetes, [4, 5] while other tests aid in ruling in or ruling out the provisional diagnosis made by the clinician who is examining the patient: for example, high WBC count in infections, low Hb in anemia etc. This chapter provides a brief overview of the routine investigations as well as some of the advanced investigations commonly used in ophthalmic pathology laboratories. Some of the other divisions of pathology, which deal with investigations of body fluids are blood bank, microbiology, immunology and serology, toxicology, etc., Some of the advanced investigations are described along with the diagnostic criteria of the disease in the corresponding chapter.

In brief, the main functions of clinical pathology or laboratory testing are the following:

- In evaluating the severity of diseases
- In monitoring the disease progression or response to therapy
- For the confirmation or rejection of the provisional diagnosis
- Screening of the diseases

The clinical pathology begins with the test advised by the clinician for the confirmation or rejection of the provisional diagnosis, and after the prescribed test, patient identification and preparation are important steps to get the expected result.

8.2 Steps in Patient Identification

Patient identification is the most important step before the collection of specimens, because incorrect patient identification leads to incorrect specimen collection for the test and misdiagnosis, which results in incorrect treatment or, in some cases, the death of a patient if the treatment is given based on the test report.

To prevent this misshaping in a lab, patient identification nowadays is done either by generating a unique registration number or by using a color-coded armband against the name of each patient.

8.3 Patient Preparation

Most of the laboratory tests are done in the morning hours, predominantly between 7 a.m. and 9 a.m. and preferably 10–12 hours of fasting is required [6] in most of the disease conditions, like lipid profile tests for cardiac disease or hyperlipidemia and fasting glucose tests for diabetes. During the fasting period, only water consumption is allowed. [7]

8.4 Specimen Collection and Routine Investigations of Blood

The natural property of blood is to be always in fluid state while in circulation and progresses to form a clot during stasis or exposed to any external agent. Due to this property of blood to coagulate or to form clots, precautions must be taken during blood collection.

Collection of blood is done depending on the type of investigation required and blood collection samples are mainly of 3 types, namely, capillary, venous, and arterial blood [8], and depending on nature of specimen blood collection samples are plasma, serum, buffy coat, or whole blood. The routine blood examination starts from collection to preservation of blood samples. Collection of blood specimens [9] mostly need to be carried out by trained phlebotomists who have training to collect blood from blood vessels, and they are adequately trained to avoid discomfort or compromising the quality or quantity of the sample during the collection.

8.5 Blood Collection Types

The procedure of collecting blood depends on the site and type of investigations required and these are [10]

Venous Blood Venous blood is the most common form of blood collection as it provides flexible and larger amounts as required and is obtained from antecubital fossa (cephalic vein, basilic vein, and median cubital vein).

Capillary Blood In adults, it is collected from palmer surface of distal digit of ring or middle finger of nondominant hand and ear lobe, avoiding excess squeezing of the finger to avoid dilution with the tissue fluids. In infants (< 3 months), the preferred site is lateral and medial aspects of plantar surface of heel, not the great toe.

Arterial Blood Arterial blood collection is not commonly used practice for the normal routine investigation, and its collection is usually done by a specialized medical personal under supervision for the arterial gas analysis (ABG) and to know the pH balance.

(a) *Preservation of blood*

After collection of blood from various methods, blood is preserved in color-coded tubes. Preservation of blood is most essential process to get the accurate result after the investigation. For the blood preservation, various tubes with color-coded caps are in use and these were first invented by Joseph Kleiner and Becton Dickinson [11] in 1949; the colored rubber stopper is used for the evacuated blood collection tube, which is a sterile glass or plastic test tube that creates vacuum and helps in collecting desired amount of blood.

Most blood collection tubes contain an additive, which are either clot activators that fasten the clotting of the blood and anticoagulant to prevent the blood from clotting. The blood collected with additive is centrifuged and the tube containing clot activator will produce serum and tube containing anticoagulant will produce plasma from blood after centrifugation. Depending upon the type of blood test advised by a physician, the sample requires either serum, plasma, or whole blood preserved in color-coded tubes as described in Table 8.1.

The below table shows the type of blood and specimen types.

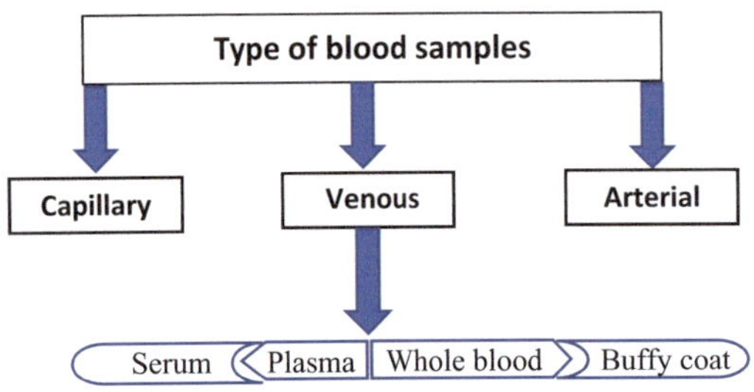

8.5.1 Various Methods of Examination of Blood

Blood is defined as fluid connective tissue in which blood-formed elements, namely, red blood cells (R.B. Cs), white blood cells (W.B.Cs), and platelets, are suspended in plasma. From the collected blood of a person or patient, numerous tests can be done and its results reflect the health status of that person.

Hence, blood investigation is most common tool and investigation, which is routinely done for the screening or diagnosis or prognosis of the disease. The common indication of doing blood examination in ophthalmology field is to rule out blood malignancies, mainly acute leukemia, which can present as orbital swelling or bleeding disorder, or to do platelet count, because low platelet count presents as low or loss of vision due to vitreous hemorrhage. Like wise to rule out sickle cell anemia or chronic myeloid leukemia in patients of retinal disease as this disease blocks the small vessels of retina and can cause disturbance in vision [12].

The most common tests, which are performed through the blood, are as follows:

8.5.2 Hemogram Test /Complete Blood Count (CBC)

The most performed blood test for a patient or in a person is complete blood cell count or hemogram. This test includes hemoglobin, white blood cell count, and platelet count. In addition, detailed red blood cell indices, such as hematocrit (PCV), mean corpuscular volume (MCV), and mean corpuscular hemoglobin concentration (MCHC), are also the part of CBC.

Table 8.1 The most used blood collection tubes

Cap Color of the tube	Additive for the preservation of blood/plasma	Function of the additive	Common laboratory tests indicated
Gray	Sodium fluoride, and sodium or potassium oxalate	Fluoride inhibits the enolase and prevents glycolysis, and oxalate prevents clotting by precipitating calcium.	Blood alcohol, lactic acid, glucose
Green	Sodium or lithium heparin with or without gel	Prevents clotting by inhibiting thrombin and thromboplastin.	Lithium heparin tubes immediately form the clot and make it an ideal tube for STAT procedures and routine biochemistry
Lavender or pink	Potassium EDTA	Binds with calcium and prevents clotting.	Hematology and blood bank
Light-blue	3.2% Sodium citrate	Binds with calcium and prevents clotting.	Coagulation
Red or gold	Serum tube with or without clot activator or gel	Glass or silica particles act as clot activator and promote blood clotting. Gel separates serum from cells.	Chemistry, serology, immunology

This can be done both by manual methods or by coulter counter (Fig. 8.1), which gives a quantitative as well as semiqualitative analysis of all parameters. Hemogram test is necessary for the diagnosis of types of anemia, hematological malignancies, allergic disease, hemorrhagic disease, infections, and immunodeficiencies [13].

Table 8.2 refers to the normal range of all the parameters (CBC) in males and females [14].

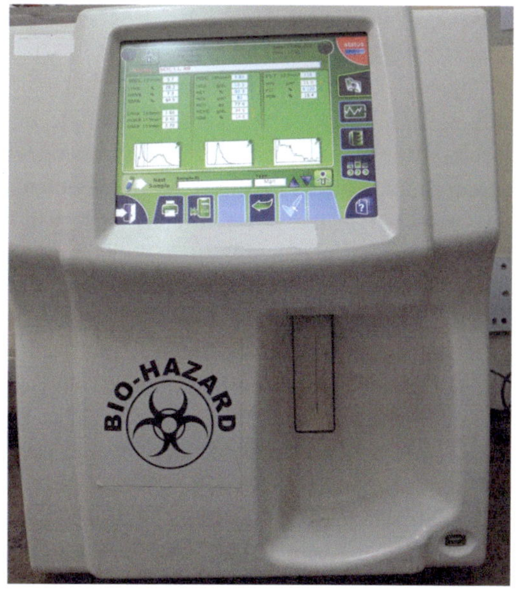

Fig. 8.1 Image of hematology analyzer or cell counter equipment for the complete blood count (CBC)

Table 8.2 Normal range of all the parameters in males and females

Blood component	Abbreviation used	Reference range	SI Reference range
White blood cells	WBC	4500–11,000/mm^3 Neutrophils: 50–70% Eosinophil: 1–3% Lymphocytes: 25–35% Monocytes: 4–6% Basophils: 0–1%	4.5–11.0 × 10^9/L
Red blood cells	RBC	Male: 4.3–5.9 million/mm^3 Female: 3.5–5.5 million/mm^3	Male: 4.3–5.9 × 10^{12}/L Female: 3.5–5.5 × 10^{12}/L
Hemoglobin	HGB	Male: 13.5–17.5 g/dL Female: 12.0–16.0 g/dL	Male: 2.09–2.71 mmol/L Female: 1.86–2.48 mmol/L
Hematocrit	HT	Male: 41–53% Female: 36–46%	Male: 0.41–0.53 Female: 0.36–0.46
Mean corpuscular volume	MCV	80–100 μm^3	80–100 fl
Mean corpuscular hemoglobin	MCH	25.4–34.6 pg/cell	0.39–0.54 fmol/cell
Mean corpuscular hemoglobin concentration	MCHC	31–36% Hb/cell	4.81–5.58 mmol Hb/L
Platelets	Platelets	150,000–400,000/mm^3	150–400 × 10^9/L

8.6 Peripheral Blood Smear Test (PBS)

A peripheral blood smear test is a simple but extremely useful test that provides vast amount of information on all the three cellular elements of the blood, namely, red blood cells, white blood, cells and platelets (Fig. 8.2). This test is inexpensive and has a high diagnostic value, and it is performed by making blood smear on the slide collected from finger or heel prick [13]. Unlike some of the blood tests, which are analyzed by a machine, PBS analysis is done by examining the blood smear under a microscope preferably by a pathologist or health-care worker.

Peripheral blood smear examination along with results of peripheral blood counts and red blood cell indices is an integral part for the initial evaluation of all patients with hematologic disorders. The examination of blood films stained with Romanowsky stain is commonly used for the PBS, and it provides important clues in the diagnosis of anemias and various disorders of leukocytes and platelets.

The information obtained on the peripheral smear includes the following:

RBC: The mean diameter of RBC is about 7.5 μm, and they are smaller than small lymphocytes having biconcave shape (diskocytes). The central pallor of RBC is due to absence of nuclei, and they make 30–45% of diameter of cells with peripheral localization of hemoglobin. The cells, which are normal in size and hemoglobin contents, are designated as normocytic and normochromic cells, whereas macrocytes are larger than normal RBCs and their diameter is more than 9 μm. Microcytes are defined when the diameter of RBCs is less than 6 μm [15].

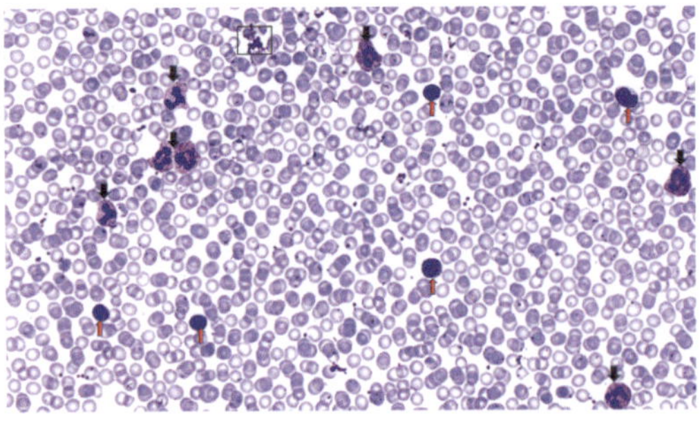

Fig. 8.2 Peripheral blood smear (PBS) showed neutrophils (black arrows), lymphocytes (red arrows), and cluster of platelets (black square); Leishman's stain; ×400

Abnormalities of RBC shape and size that are identified on the peripheral smear include sickle cell anemia/diseases, thalassemia [15]. Anemia is graded as hypochromic and normochromic depending on the central pallor of RBCs. If the central pallor is greater than 50% of the diameter, then the cells are called as hypochromic cells. Similarly, abnormal variation in size is termed as anisocytosis and unusual variation in shape is defined as poikilocytosis. Polychromatophilic RBCs appears in severe degree of anemia and it reflects the bone marrow responsiveness and it is defined as blue-gray hue of the erythrocytes cytoplasm [15]. HB aggregates, inclusion bodies, and parasites can also be identified in PBS examination.

WBC: Numerous morphological changes occur in granulocytes due to infection or disease process such as toxic granules that are increased in numbers and dark blue staining of the cytoplasmic granules of neutrophils, whereas Dhole bodies are light blue 1–2 μm sized inclusion in the cytoplasm. Left shift can also be seen as precursor or immature cells of leucocytes appear in the blood. Hypersegmented neutrophils are found in megaloblastic anemia and have six or more lobes. Reactive lymphocytes are larger than small lymphocytes and may contain cytoplasmic vacuolation and irregular nuclear membrane or bean-shape nuclei [15]. Blast cells count equal to or more than 20% indicates acute leukaemia [16].While the differential counts can be obtained by the coulter counter, absolute values may also be required; for example, absolute eosinophil count in allergic conditions [17].

Platelets: Platelets size varies from 1 to 3 μm in peripheral blood and presence of more than 3 μm diameter size platelets are designated as mega platelets. Presence of a clump and an estimated of number of approximately 10,000 per platelet is usually considered as adequate count in PBS. References state that platelet count in PBS, anywhere from 8 to 25 per oil-immersion field (OIF), correlates with a normal platelet count [18, 19].

Abnormalities of size and shape both could be clubbed into one. According to red cell sizes, RBCs can be macrocytic, microcytic, and normocytic based on MCV mentioned in Table 8.3.

Platelet: Increased platelets are described as thrombocytosis, and decreased count is called thrombocytopenia. Causes of thrombocytosis/thrombocytopenia are described in Table 8.4.

8.6.1 Erythrocytes Sedimentation Rate (ESR)

It is one of the commonly used tests to monitor an increase in inflammatory activity within the body, for example, autoimmune disease, infections, or tumors.

Normally, RBCs carry negative charges on the outside of the cells due to which they repel each other. However, in the blood, many plasma proteins carry a positive charge, which neutralize the negative charge of the RBC and cause them to clump or form a stack called as Rouleaux formation. The sample principle is evaluated in the laboratory through the ESR test where the anticoagulated blood is allowed to stand in vertical tubes undisturbed and the rate at which the RBCs sediment is measured in mm. This process occurs in 3 stages:

1. Stage 1: Rouleaux formation—First 10 minutes.
2. Stage 2: Stage of sedimentation or settling—40 mins.
3. Stage 3: Stage of packing—10 minutes, sedimentation slows, and cells start to pack at the bottom of the tube.

Any condition or disease that causes an increase in plasma proteins, for example, inflammatory conditions, results in an increase in rouleaux formations, which settle more readily than single red blood cells, thus raising the ESR [20].The settling of the rouleaux aggregates in the Westergren tube occurs at a constant rate [21].Therefore, the ESR is not the measure of a single marker but a physical process that is due to increased proteins in the plasma.

The tubes in which the test done are called Westegren or WIntrobe named after the hematologist who discovered the technique [22].

Westergren method is a standard method of measuring ESR and normal values using this method are mentioned below: [23, 24]:

Table 8.3 Type of Anemia based on mean corpuscular volume

Macrocytic (>101 fl)	Microcytic (<80 fl)	Normocytic (83–101 fl)
Megaloblastic anemia nonmegaloblastic causes: Liver disease, hypothyroid	Iron deficiency anemia, thalassemia, sideroblastic anemia, anemia of chronic disease	Hemorrhage, aplastic anemia, and anemia of chronic illness

Table 8.4 Causes of thrombocytosis/thrombocytopenia

Thrombocytosis	Inflammation, myeloproliferative disorder	
Thrombocytopenia	Hematological malignancies, connective tissue disease, idiopathic thrombocytopenic purpura	
Positive acute-phase reactant	Upregulated their concentrations increase during inflammation	Procalcitonin, C-reactive protein, ferritin, fibrinogen, hepcidin, serum amyloid A
Negative acute-phase reactants	Downregulated their concentrations decrease during inflammation	Albumin, prealbumin, transferrin, retinol-binding protein, antithrombin

- Male <50 years old ≤15 mm/hr.
- Female <50 years old ≤20 mm/hr.
- Male >50 years old ≤20 mm/hr.
- Female >50 years old ≤30 mm/hr.
- Child ≤10 mm/hr [25].

Factor increasing ESR—Anemia, pregnancy, old age, high fibrinogen, macrocytosis.

Factors decreasing ESR—Polycythemia, Macrocytosis, increase TLC, low fibrinogen.

8.7 Other Tests for Blood Disorders or Diseases

Once the Hb and the peripheral smear evaluation is suggestive of abnormality in any or all the 3 cellular elements, for example, anemia, polycythemia, leukopenia, leukocytosis, thrombocytosis, or thrombocytopenia, then further special tests are done to evaluate the exact cause of the cytopenia or cytolysis in the respective lineage. They include reticulocyte count, irons stains, serology tests for autoantibodies, coagulation profile, and bone marrow examination.

8.8 Special Investigations

8.8.1 Bone Marrow Examination

8.8.1.1 Bone Marrow Aspiration

Bone marrow contains hemopoietic stem cells, and all the three cellular elements of the blood, that is, RBC, WBC, and platelets, are produced from stem cells and precursor cells located in the spongy tissue of red part of the bone marrow. Since the blood cells have a limited life span, for example, average life span of RBCs are 120 days, and this value may vary between 70 and 140 days for red blood cells [26], the bone marrow stem cells of all the 3 lineages continue to proliferate to maintain the homeostasis in the blood. So, any abnormal reduction or abnormal increase in the blood cells would raise the need to evaluate the function of the bone marrow as part of the investigations.

8.9 Indication of Bone Marrow Aspiration (BMA)

- Pyrexia of unknown etiology.
- Unexplained anemia, leucopenia, thrombocytopenia, or pancytopenia.
- Leucocytois, Acute leukemia, myelodysplastic syndrome suspects.
- Plasma cell dyscrasia.
- Suspected infiltrative disorders.
- Part of work of Malignancy to rule out marrow infiltration, for example, lymphoma, childhood tumors, Retinoblastoma, etc.
- To monitor response to therapy and assess remission or relapse.

8.9.1 Bone Marrow Aspiration

In addition to the bone marrow aspiration, a piece of bone, that is, bone marrow biopsy is indicted where the architectural pattern of bone marrow needs to be studied (Fig. 8.3). This is specifically indicated when the bone marrow tap is negative.

8.9.1.1 Other Indications Include the Following

Grading of lymphoma (The most common indication in ophthalmic pathology)

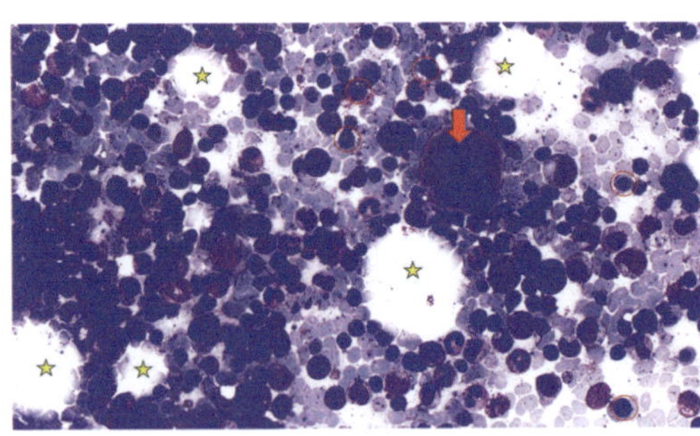

Fig. 8.3 Bone marrow aspirate showed megakaryocyte (thick red arrow), fat spaces (asterisks) in the background of different stages of maturation of R.B.Cs (normoblasts, black circles); Leishman's stain; ×400

- Myeloproliferative disorder.
- Myelodysplastic syndrome.
- For the diagnosis and prognosis of malignancies.
- To know the effectiveness of chemotherapy.

Sites of Bone marrow are posterior superior Iliac spine, manubrim sterum, and tibia in infants under 1 year.

Procedure: Under local anesthesia in lateral keen elbow position, Salah and Klima or Jamshidi needle is used for both aspiration and biopsy. Length of BMB should be at least 2 cm. Specimen is fixed in 10% neutral buffered formalin and sent to lab for processing and reporting. Biopsy is decalcified in nitric acid, EDTA.

The aspirate obtained is collected into a container with anticoagulant. The particles of the marrow are picked up on the glass slides, and crushed gently to make thin smears. The marrow smears stained with Romansky stains are then evaluated for cellularity, normal maturation of all the 3 cellular elements, myeloid to erythroid ratio, and presence of any abnormal cells—native or infiltrative type, parasites, etc., Since the marrow is a store house for hematopoetic regeneration and also the iron turnover, irons stains are performed to evaluate the state of iron stores: that is, whether they are deficient, adequate, or in excess.

Screening for autoimmune diseases: the presence of antibodies toward self-antigens is evaluated further by special tests, a summary of which is provided, the detail of each test is beyond the scope of this chapter.

8.10 Other Investigations Used in Ophthalmic Pathologies

Other common investigations used in eye pathology are acute-phase reactants like C-reactive protein and erythrocyte sedimentation rate that are classical and common markers for the inflammation and can be used as a measure of "sickness index" for the infectious and noninfectious conditions.

8.10.1 Acute-Phase Reactants (APR)

Acute-phase reactants (APRs) are inflammation markers that exhibit significant changes in serum concentration during inflammation. These are also important mediators produced in the liver during acute and chronic inflammatory states. Interleukin-6 (IL-6) is the primary cytokine responsible for inducing the production in the liver. IL-1, tumor necrosis factor-alpha (TNF-alpha), and interferon-gamma (IFN-gamma) can also induce the production of acute-phase reactants. Acute-phase reactants cause several adverse effects. These include fever, anemia of chronic disease, anorexia, somnolence, lethargy, amyloidosis, and cachexia (fat and muscle loss, anorexia, weakness) [27].

Acute-phase reactants can be classified as positive or negative, depending on their serum concentrations during inflammation. Classification of acute-phase reactions is dependent on the change in APP concentration: A 10–100-fold elevation is considered major; a 2–ten-fold elevation is considered moderate; and a less than two-fold elevation is considered minor.

Types of APRs upregulated and downregulated in inflammatory condition are summarized in Table 8.5.

8.10.2 C-Reactive Protein(CRP)

Tillett and Francis [28] in 1930 discovered C-reactive protein (CRP). The name CRP was derived from the "c" carbohydrate antigen of the

Table 8.5 Types of Acute-phase reactants

Positive acute phase reactant	Upregulated Their concentrations increase during inflammation.	Procalcitonin, C-reactive protein, ferritin, fibrinogen, hepcidin, serum amyloid A
Negative acute phase reactants	Downregulated Their concentrations decrease during inflammation	Albumin, prealbumin, transferrin, retinol-binding protein, antithrombin.

capsule of *Pneumococcus* in the serum of patients who suffered acute inflammation due to *Pneumococcus* infection.

CRP is formed by liver in response to inflammation and infections. This protein helps in the diagnosis and monitoring of the progression of infection, autoimmune disease, and treatment's effectiveness.

- During inflammation, it rises early among all acute-phase reactants and rapidly subsides following therapy.
- CRP is not affected by hormones and drugs.
- It is a more sensitive and specific test to detect inflammation.

Less than 6 mg/L (0.3 mg/dL) Normal CRP range is seen in healthy people [28].

A high-sensitivity C-reactive protein (hs-CRP) is more sensitive than standard CRP and this hs-CRP is used for determining the development of coronary heart disease.

8.11 Collagen Vascular Profile

Collagen vascular or connective disorders are autoimmune diseases in which autoantibodies are formed against our own body. Ocular or eye inflammation is seen as part of a number of systemic connective tissue disorders and can affect any part of the eye. Anteriorly, it can affect cornea and posteriorly, it can affect retina, uvea, and sclera. Uveitis or scleritis is the common eye manifestation and sometimes, it needs an aggressive immunosuppressive therapy [29].

Collagen vascular diseases, which commonly affect eyes, are listed below:

8.11.1 Rheumatoid Arthritis (RA)

Rheumatoid arthritis (RA) is an inflammatory arthritis of autoimmune etiology and has three times higher incidence in females than males. RA has genetic predisposition and more than 90% patients carry HLA -DR4 and DR1 genes [30]. Dry eye syndrome is the commonest, and scleritis and episcleritis are the second most common ocular manifestations of rheumatoid arthritis. [29] Peripheral ulcerative keratitis (PUK) is also associated with scleritis of RA origin due to activation of collagenase enzyme, which causes digestion of corneal stroma [31].

8.11.2 Behçet's Disease (BD)

Behçet's disease (BD) is a multiorgan occlusive vasculitis affecting the venules more than the arteries [32]. Uveitis is the commonest ocular manifestation and occurs in more than 50–80% of patients affected with this disease [33]. Like other autoimmune diseases, BD also has a genetic association and human leukocyte antigens (HLA-) B51 and HLA-A26 have been identified as predisposing factors associated with BD-related uveitis, which mostly affects males [34].

8.11.3 Systemic Vasculitides

This systemic disorder mainly consists of microscopic polyangiitis (MPA), granulomatosis with polyangiitis (GPA instead of Wegener's), and eosinophilic granulomatosis with polyangiitis (EGPA instead of Churg-Strauss Syndrome); these three autoimmune disease are components of antineutrophil cytoplasmic antibody (ANCA)-associated vasculitis [35]. Conjunctivitis, episcleritis, and scleritis are the most common presentations of this disease and occur due to inflammation of small- and medium-sized blood vessels.

8.11.4 Systemic Lupus Erythematosus (SLE)

Systemic lupus erythematosus (SLE) is an immune-complex-mediated tissue damage of autoimmune etiology that affects multiorgans. [36] Gender plays a key role in SLE manifestation, because females are more susceptible to

SLE than males, that is, females have 9 times higher incidence of SLE than the males and more common in Asians and African women, especially in their reproductive age groups. [37]

Dry eye syndrome is the most common presentation, retina is the second commonly involved structure, and one-third of patients developed retinal involvement in SLE. In retina vascular thrombosis caused by disease process leads to significant visual morbidity [38].

SLE can cause scleritis and episcleritis; in addition, it causes chiasmopathy, ischemic optic neuropathy, and optic neuritis, and is also seen in about 1% of patients of SLE [39].

8.11.5 Systemic Sclerosis

Systemic sclerosis is a rare connective tissue disorder that is characterized by abnormal proliferation of fibroblast leading to deposition of extracellular matrix in the skin, blood vessels, and viscera.

As this disease also has an autoimmune etiology, this disease is more common in females and the affected female-to-male ratio is 8: 1 [40]. Eye lid stiffness is the commonest manifestation of this disease and seen in more than 50% of the cases and results from deposition of type I collagen in the dermis and keratoconjunctivitis sicca is the second most common presentation. Conjunctivitis, episcleritis, anterior uveitis, and hypertensive retinopathy have also been reported in sclerosis. [41]

8.11.6 Polymyositis and Dermatomyositis

Polymyositis and dermatomyositis are a group of autoimmune diseases characterized by inflammation of the skeletal muscles and skin. This autoimmune disease has a genetic predisposition and is associated with human leukocyte antigens HLA-B8 and DR3 and DR52 [42, 43].

Purplish discoloration or heliotrope rash of the eyelid is the most common ocular manifestation associated with dermatomyositis. Retinal vasculitis is also reported in dermatomyositis of pediatric patient [44].

8.11.7 Sjogren's Syndrome

Sjögren's syndrome is an autoimmune disease characterized by chronic inflammatory cell infiltrates, predominantly lymphocytes on histopathological examination in exocrine glands that clinically present as dry eyes (keratoconjunctivitis sicca) and dry mouth (xerostomia) [45].

Sjögren's syndrome is primary Sjögren's syndrome (pSS) when it occurs alone or secondary Sjögren's syndrome when it is as a part of other chronic inflammatory diseases.

The most common ocular manifestations of pSS are keratoconjunctivitis sicca (KCS), episcleritis, anterior uveitis, lacrimal gland enlargement, and retinal vasculitis [46].

Name of collagen vascular disease and autoantibody tested to confirm the diagnosis of these disease are enumerated in Table 8.6.

8.11.8 Examination of Cerebrospinal Fluid (C.S.F)

The role of CSF examination in eye pathology is limited and mostly done to know the deposits from retinoblastoma, acute lymphoblastic lymphoma, primary central nervous system, or intraocular lymphoma. Rarely, this one is advised in

Table 8.6 Name of collagen vascular disease and the autoantibody

Disease name	Test name (antibody)
Rheumatoid arthritis	RF, Anti-RA33
Behçet's disease	(HLA-) B51 and HLA-A26
Systemic vasculitides	C-ANCA
Systemic lupus erythematosus	Anti-dsDNA, Anti-SM
Systemic sclerosis	Anti-Scl70, Anti centromere
Polymyositis and dermatomyositis	Anti Jo-1
Sjogren's syndrome	Anti-Ro (SS-A), Anti-La (SS-B)

Table 8.7 Normal composition of cerebrospinal fluid

Opening pressure	90–180 mm of water
Color	Colorless
Appearance	Crystal clear
Total leucocyte count	0–5 cells/ microliter in adult 0–30 cells/ microliter in neonates
Mononuclear cell	< 5/ cubic mm
Polymorphonuclear leucocytes	0
Total protein	15–45 mg/dl (1% of plasma protcin)
Glucose	1. 50–80 mg/dl, i.e., 60% of plasma value.

inflammatory or infectious conditions of eye and orbit.

Cerebrospinal fluid (CSF) is formed by choroid plexus in ventricles of brain.

CSF is collected by lumbar puncture at L3–L4 or L4–L5 position from subarachnoid space.

Indication of Lumbar Puncture

- Central nervous system (CNS) infections like meningitis.
- Leukemia or malignancy infiltration.
- Neoplasm of CNS.
- To reduce CSF pressure in psedotumor cerebri.
- Administration of medication.

The normal composition of CSF [47] is shown in Table 8.7.

References

1. Koneman EW, Reiquam CW, Brimhall BB. Clinical pathology. In: Access science. McGraw-Hill Education; 2019. https://doi.org/10.1036/1097-8542.141100.
2. Silverstein MD. An approach to medical errors and patient safety in laboratory sciences—A White Paper, Atlanta, Quality Institute Conference; 13–15 April, 2003. p. 1–23.
3. Molinaro RJ, Winkler AM, Kraft CS, Fantz CR, Stowell SR, Ritchie JC, et al. Teaching laboratory medicine to medical students: implementation and evaluation. Arch Pathol Lab Med. 2012;136:1423–9.
4. Good Clinical diagnostic practice, WHO regional publications. Eastern Mediterranean series 27 Cairo. 2005.
5. Bain BJ. Diagnosis from the blood smear. N Engl J Med. 2005;353:498–507.
6. Kackov S, Simundic AM, Gatti-Drnic A. Are patients well informed about the fasting requirements for laboratory blood testing? Biochem Med. 2013;23(3):326–31.
7. Guder WG, Narayanan S, Wisser H, Zawta B. Samples: from the patient to the laboratory. 3rd ed. Weinheim: Wiley-VCH Verlag GmbH & Co. KgaA; 2003.
8. https://www.neoteryx.com/microsampling-blog/the-best-way-to-collect-a-blood-sample-3-methods-examined
9. Vaught JB. Blood collection, shipment, processing, and storage. Cancer Epidemiol Biomarkers Prev. 2006 Sep;15(9):1582–4.
10. WHO guidelines on drawing blood: best practices in phlebotomy. Geneva: World Health Organization; 2010. Introduction. Available from https://www.ncbi.nlm.nih.gov/books/NBK138675/.
11. Bush V, Cohen R. The evolution of evacuated blood collection tubes. Lab Med. 2003;34(4):304–10.
12. Awuah A, Asiedu K, Adanusa M, Ntodie M, Acquah E, Kyei S. A case of leukemic retinopathy mimicking common ischemic retinopathies. Clin Case Reports. 2016;4(2):133.
13. Celkan TT. What does a hemogram say to us? Turk Arch Pediatr. 2020;55(2):103.
14. Dean L, Dean L. Blood groups and red cell antigens. Bethesda: NCBI; 2005.
15. Walker HK, Hall WD, Hurst JW. Clinical methods: the history, physical, and laboratory examinations.
16. DiNardo CD, Garcia-Manero G, Pierce S, Nazha A, Bueso-Ramos C, Jabbour E, Ravandi F, Cortes J, Kantarjian H. Interactions and relevance of blast percentage and treatment strategy among younger and older patients with acute myeloid leukemia (AML) and myelodysplastic syndrome (MDS). Am J Hematol. 2016;91(2):227–32.
17. Lalrinpuia B. Study on absolute eosinophil count correlation with severity of bronchial asthma.
18. Stiene-Martin EA, Lotspeich-Steininger CA, Koepke JA. Clinical hematology. 2nd ed. Philadelphia: J.B. Lippincott-Raven; 1992. p. 337.
19. Mogadam L. Application of the Miller's disc for the estimation and quality control of the platelet count. Lab Med. 1980;11:131.
20. Abramson N. Rouleaux formation. Blood. 2006;107(11):4205.
21. Hashemi R, Majidi A, Motamed H, Amini A, Najari F, Tabatabaey A. Erythrocyte sedimentation rate measurement using as a rapid alternative to the Westergren method. Emerg (Tehran). 2015;3(2):50–3.
22. Taneja N. Erythrocyte sedimentation rate - is there a need for a fasting blood sample? Med J Armed Forces India. 1997;53(1):72.

23. Brigden ML. Clinical utility of the erythrocyte sedimentation rate. Am Fam Physician. 1999;60(5):1443–50.
24. Böttiger LE, Svedberg CA. Normal erythrocyte sedimentation rate and age. Br Med J. 1967;2(5544):85–7.
25. Al-Marri MR, Kirkpatrick MB. Erythrocyte sedimentation rate in childhood tuberculosis: is it still worthwhile? Int J Tuberc Lung Dis. 2000;4(3):237–9.
26. Cohen RM, Franco RS, Khera PK, Smith EP, Lindsell CJ, Ciraolo PJ, Palascak MB, Joiner CH. Red cell life span heterogeneity in hematologically normal people is sufficient to alter HbA1c. Blood. 2008;112:4284–91.
27. Ceron JJ, Eckersall PD, Martynez-Subiela S. Acute phase proteins in dogs and cats: current knowledge and future perspectives. Vet Clin Pathol. 2005;34:85–99.
28. Nehring SM, Goyal A, Bansal P, et al. C reactive protein. In: StatPearls [Internet]. Treasure Island: StatPearls Publishing; 2020. Available from https://www.ncbi.nlm.nih.gov/books/NBK441843/.
29. Choudhary MM, Hajj-Ali RA, Lowder CY. Gender and ocular manifestations of connective tissue diseases and systemic vasculitides. J Ophthalmol. 2014;2014
30. McDermott M, Mcdevitt H. The immunogenetics of rheumatic diseases. Bull Rheumat Dis 1988;38(1):1–0.
31. Foster CS, Forstot SL, Wilson LA. Mortality rate in rheumatoid arthritis patients developing necrotizing scleritis or peripheral ulcerative keratitis: effects of systemic immunosuppression. Ophthalmology. 1984;91(10):1253–63.
32. Kontogiannis V, Powell RJ. Behçet's disease. Postgrad Med J. 2000;76(900):629–37.
33. Kang EH, Kim JY, Takeuchi F, Kim JW, Shin K, Lee EY, Lee YJ, Lee EB, Park MH, Song YW. Associations between the HLA-Apolymorphism and the clinical manifestations of Behcet's disease. Arthritis Res Ther. 2011;13(2):1–9.
34. Kang EH, Park JW, Park C, Yu HG, Lee EB, Park MH, Song YW. Genetic and non-genetic factors affecting the visual outcome of ocular Behcet's disease. Hum Immunol. 2013;74(s):1363–7.
35. Watts RA, Carruthers DM, Scott DG. Epidemiology of systemic vasculitis: changing incidence or definition?. In: Seminars in arthritis and rheumatism. 1995 (Vol. 25, No. 1, pp. 28–34). WB Saunders.
36. D'Cruz DP, Khamashta MA, Hughes GR. Systemic lupus erythematosus. Lancet. 2007;369(9561):587–96.
37. Costenbader KH, Feskanich D, Stampfer MJ, Karlson EW. Reproductive and menopausal factors and risk of systemic lupus erythematosus in women. Arthritis Rheum. 2007;56(4):1251–62.
38. Ushiyama O, Ushiyama K, Koarada S, Tada Y, Suzuki N, Ohta A, Oono S, Nagasawa K. Retinal disease in patients with systemic lupus erythematosus. Ann Rheum Dis. 2000;59(9):705–8.
39. Frohman LP, Frieman BJ, Wolansky L. Reversible blindness resulting from optic chiasmitis secondary to systemic lupus erythematosus. J Neuroophthalmol. 2001;21(1):18–21.
40. Zulian F, Vallongo C, Woo P, Russo R, Ruperto N, Harper J, Espada G, Corona F, Mukamel M, Vesely R, Musiej-Nowakowska E. Localized scleroderma in childhood is not just a skin disease. Arthritis Rheum. 2005;52(9):2873–81.
41. David R, Ivry M. Focal chorioretinitis and iridocyclitis associated with scleroderma. Ann Ophthalmol. 1976;8(2):199–202.
42. Love LA, Leff RL, Fraser DD, Targoff IN, Dalakas M, Plotz PH, Miller FW. A new approach to the classification of idiopathic inflammatory myopathy: myositis-specific autoantibodies define useful homogeneous patient groups. Medicine. 1991;70(6):360–74.
43. Garlepp MJ. Genetics of the idiopathic inflammatory myopathies. Curr Opin Rheumatol. 1996;8(6):514–20.
44. Whitaker JN, Engel WK. Vascular deposits of immunoglobulin and complement in idiopathic inflammatory myopathy. N Engl J Med. 1972;286(7):333–8.
45. Jonsson R, Brokstad KA, Jonsson MV, Delaleu N, Skarstein K. Current concepts on Sjögren's syndrome–classification criteria and biomarkers. Eur J Oral Sci. 2018;126:37–48.
46. Lim R, Gunasekeran D, Kam J, Thong B, Agrawal RV. Ocular involvement in Sjogren's syndrome–the Singapore Sjogren's syndrome study. Invest Ophthalmol Vis Sci. 2016;57(12):3879.
47. Martín-Ancel A, García-Alix A, Salas S, del Castillo F, Cabañas F, Quero J. Cerebrospinal fluid leucocyte counts in healthy neonates. Arch Dis Child Fetal Neonatal Ed. 2006;91(5):F357–8.

Part II

Ocular Pathology

Handling and Processing of Ocular Tissues

9

Geeta K. Vemuganti and Dilip K. Mishra

Contents

9.1 Introduction

Ophthalmic pathology, like all branches of pathology, is a field, which provides the final diagnosis to the patient based on the interpretation of the changes that occur in the tissues with respect to the structural and functional changes during the disease process. As it is said, the tissues do not lie. Hence, the study provides understanding of the disease process, which has occurred in the patient, and provides information regarding the etiology, pathogenesis, morphology of the lesion, and the effect that the lesion has on the surrounding structures. This is crucial to understand the pathobiology of the disease as well as identification of any precursor lesion, prognosis, and possible complications that could occur and possibly predict response to treatment to a certain extent. The tissues removed during any surgical procedure are obviously a storehouse of information. It is there-

G. K. Vemuganti (✉)
Distinguished Pathologist and Scientist, LVPEI, School of Medical Sciences, Hyderabad, Telangana, India

School of Medical Sciences, University of Hyderabad, Hyderabad, Telangana, India
e-mail: gkvemuganti@gmail.com

D. K. Mishra
Ophthalmic Pathology Laboratory, L V Prasad Eye Institute, Hyderabad, Telangana, India
e-mail: deanmd@uohyd.ac.in

G. K. Vemuganti et al. (eds.), *Ocular Pathology*, https://doi.org/10.1007/978-981-96-8614-8_9

fore important for the ophthalmologist to communicate with the pathologists before, during, and after surgical procedure so that a good clinicopathologic correlation is established and the pathologist is able to provide the most accurate interpretation of the tissue submitted. Most of the aspects of the diseases are covered in various chapters of this book, and it is beyond the scope of this chapter to include pathology details of individual diseases. This chapter gives a brief and simple description of the routine and special techniques adopted by most of the ophthalmic pathology laboratories. This covers the techniques of fixation, gross examination and cutting, tissue processing, embedding, cutting, and staining. It also covers the techniques adopted by the pathologist in providing a rapid intraoperative diagnosis of the lesion. The aim of this chapter is to provide practical tips and solutions to the ophthalmologists and students on how to examine the tissues removed, interpret the histologic findings of different types of tissues, and also meaningfully interpret and understand the report provided by the pathologist. The tissues routinely submitted to any ophthalmic pathology lab include tissues removed from the eye and orbit for diagnostic or therapeutic purposes (e.g., cornea, conjunctiva, lid, orbit, intraocular structures), and fluid samples like aqueous and vitreous taps and aspiration from cystic lesions.

9.2 Histopathology

This is a study of disease process based on the histologic interpretation of the tissues removed. The tissues removed from the body are finally cut into thin sections and stained appropriately so that they can be interpreted by the pathologist so as to arrive at a morphologic diagnosis of the lesion. To facilitate this, the tissues are subjected to a series of procedures that include fixation, processing, embedding, cutting, staining, and mounting, which are discussed in brief in the following sections.

1. *Tissue Fixation*: Fixation is a complex series of chemical events that aims at preventing the tissues from autolysis and bacterial attack, and at the same time maintaining them in a state as close to their living state as possible with no loss of molecules. Different tissues require different fixatives and as such, there is no ideal fixative. The practical approach is to fix the proteins in the tissues, which is the most common substance in tissues. The practical approach is to fix the proteins in the tissues, which is the most common substance in tissues. The aldehyde fixatives, used in the laboratory, produce cross-links between proteins, thereby forming a gel, thus maintaining all tissues in its near native state and organization. Thus, soluble proteins are fixed to "structural proteins" so that it can withstand subsequent steps of processing. These reactions are largely reversible by washing in excess of water. Some of the common fixatives are given in Table 9.1

   The most common fixative used in histopathology is 10% buffered formalin (the commercially available 40% Formaldehyde solution is considered as 100%), which stabilizes the protein, oil, and the carbohydrate [1–4]. For electron microscopy, 2% glutaraldehye or a 4% formaldehyde-gluataraldehyde mixture is preferred [4]. Penetration of fixatives into the tissues is variable and depends on the size of the tissue: for example, small biospies can be fixed within a few hours, but the eyeball requires 24 hours fixation before it can be cut open for further fixation. Nowadays, microwave energy is being used to hasten various procedures involved in histopathology, including the process of fixation. Use of microwave energy interacts with dipolar molecules causing their oscillation, thus increas-

Table 9.1 Types of fixatives used for different procedures

Type of Fixative	Indications
Formaldehyde (10%)	Routine processing
Glutaraldehyde	EM
Formal/gluataraldehye	EM
95% ethyl alcohol	Smears
Tissue culture media/ RPM	Karyotyping, tissue cultures
Fresh	Frozen sections IO cytology

ing the thermal energy of water molecules and polar chain of proteins in the tissues; this results in denaturation of the proteins [5].

Corneal buttons could also be fixed in a fixative called "Perenyi's fluid" (A 100 ml of Perenyi's fluid is prepared by mixing of 40 ml of 10% nitric acid, 30 ml each of absolute alcohol, and 0.5% chromic acid.)

2. *Grossing*

   Macroscopic examination of ocular tissue before submitting the tissues for processing is very important [6]. A brief description of the techniques is given below

   (a) Corneal button: The excised corneal tissues could be extracted either from the surgical procedure of evisceration, full-thickness penetrating keratoplasty, lamellar keratoplasty, or a corneal biopsy. The examination of the cornea includes evaluation of cornea from its convex side for its size, thickness, surface and margins for irregularities, translucency, perforation, presence of blood vessels, areas of thinning, and destruction of any opacities. The concave surface, that is, the endothelial side, is examined for the presence of adherent uveal tissue, membranes, or exudates. The full-thickness cornea is processed with the endothelial surface up, bisecting it into half using a sharp blade. It is then embedded in a process similar to that adopted for handling of all epithelial or skin tissues, that is, by edgeembedding the half cut surface so that the orientation of epithelium and underlying stroma is well visualized. The rest of the tissues are usually preserved for future studies as required. In cases of therapeutic keratoplasty, which requires the identification of the pathogenic organisms, it is a practice to submit half of the tissues for microbiologic studies and other half is processed for histologic examination. In case of eviscerated specimens, the corneo- scleral rims are processed in a similar manner. With regards to corneal biopsy and lamellar keratoplasty specimens, the entire tissue is processed following the same principles of edge embedding of the tissues for proper orientation.

   (b) Lid biopsy: The full-thickness lid biopsy is examined for the lesion. It is preferable to process the surgical margins and the main lesion in separate blocks after noting down the details of the specimen. All fresh specimens could be painted with India Ink preparation before fixing so that the surgical margin involvement by the disease process can be commented upon on all sections. The recommended method of grossing is given in Fig. 9.1.

   (c) Grossing an eye: Examination of the eyeball is one of the important aspects in ophthalmic pathology. Identify the side of the eyeball (Fig. 9.2) A thoroughly and systemic examination of the eyeball at various stages is very important to the pathologist and the clinician [7–9]. It involves the following steps:

      1. Fix the intact ocular globe in formalin for 24 hours before sectioning. Do not open the globe, cut windows in sclera or inject fixative into the vitreous. Wash in running water for one or more hours, or place the eyeball in 60% ethyl alcohol for a few more hours.
      2. Review the summary of the clinical history and the results of the ophthalmic examination prior to opening of the globe, because the physician grossing this tissue may be the only

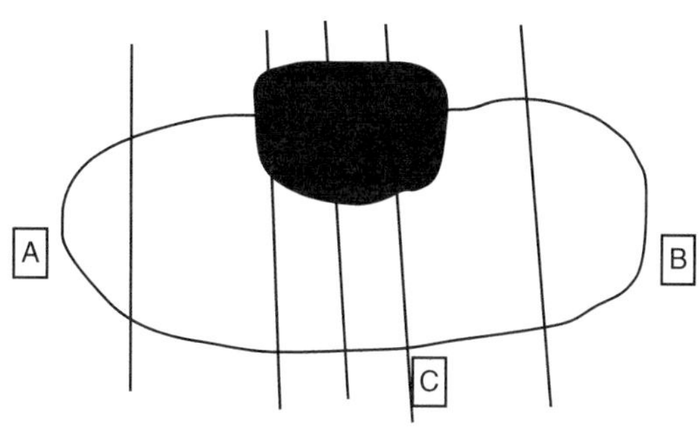

Fig. 9.1 Schematic picture of the lid showing a lesion at the mucocutaneous junction (black fill). The surgical margins **a** & **b** and the main lesion **c** should be proceeded as different blocks

observer ever to have an opportunity to examine the opened eye.

3. Measure the dimensions in the following order: Eye, AP × horizontal × vertical: cornea, horizontal × vertical; Optic nerve, length attached to the globe (Fig. 9.3). Identify the significant external markings like scars; corneal leukomas; staphylomas; areas of unusual pigmentation; distinct, abnormal shadows on transillumination, etc.
4. Transillumination: Before an eye is opened, it is to be transilluminated (Fig. 9.4). The normal eye transmits light well except at the ciliary body/iris and at any optic nerve of significant length. Abnormal shadows should be described.
5. If a choroidal melanoma is suspected, sample at least one of the vortex veins from each of the four quadrants.
6. Opening the eye in an "P-O" means "pupil-optic nerve," choosing any meridian that gives most possible additional information to the P-O section. With the eye held in one hand, cornea down on a moistened towel, and holding the razor knife between thumb and finger or in the blade handle. Use a sawing motion to make the first cut and then the second.
7. Examine the intraocular structures without manipulation and take a gross photographs whenever indicated (Figs. 9.5 and 9.6a).
8. Ideally, the gross description of each and every eye [7, 8] should mention the following structures, in this order:
   (a) Corneal thickness, depth of anterior chamber, configuration of anterior chamber angle.
   (b) Condition of iris, ciliary body, lens.
   (c) Condition of choroid, retina, vitreous body, sclera, optic disk and

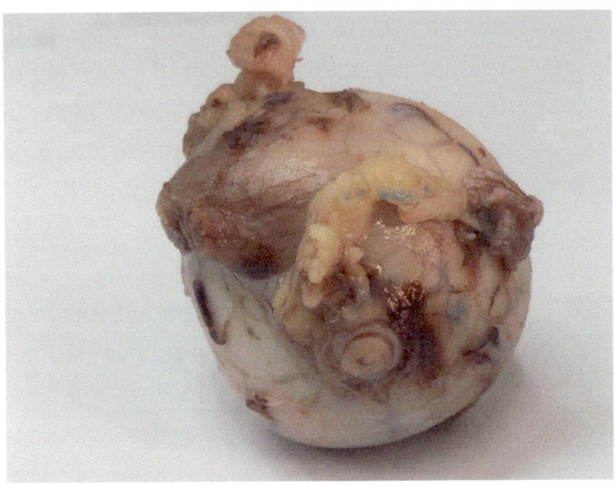

Fig. 9.2 The posterior surface of the eyeball showing the prominent landmarks, which help in identifying the side of the eye ball

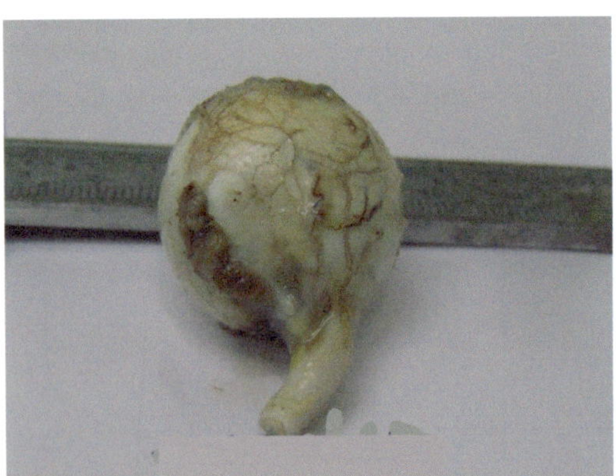

Fig. 9.3 The picture shows an enucleated eyeball along the optic nerve . Measurements of the eyeball should be taken in anterio-posterior, horizontal, and vertical planes. The length of the optic nerve and the diameter without sheath should be measured separately

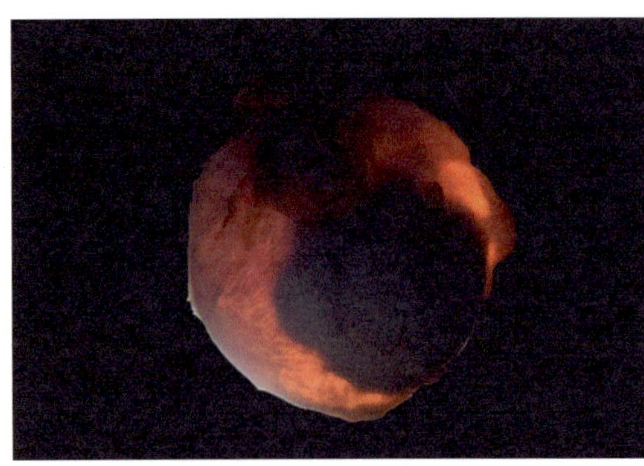

Fig. 9.4 The pictures show transillumination of the globe showing a shadow in the region of the tumor while the surrounding area shows illumination of the sclera. It was a case of choroidal melanoma

optic nerve. Further details, such as particular reference to the iris pigment epithelium, the lens capsule, etc., also need to be noted.

(d) If tumor is present: location, size, color, edges, consistency, presence of hemorrhage or necrosis, ocular structures involved, extension into optic nerve.

9. Sections for histologic examination should include the entire eyeball, abnormal area (Fig. 9.6b) cross section of optic nerve in case of retinoblastoma and sample of at least one of the vortex veins from each of the four quadrants.

(d) Exenterated specimen:

Fix the specimen overnight. Take surgical margins separately form cutaneous, soft tissues, and optic nerve. Measure the specimen, the skin. Cut the specimen through skin, soft tissues, and ocular globe.

Examine and describe the specimen in the following manner:

(a) Skin: shape and length, appearance of lesions present—their size shape, depth of invasion, color, etc.
(b) Soft tissues for the tumor: size, shape, contour
(c) Ocular globe: same as done for enucleated eye ball
   A. Sections for histology should include tumor, cutaneous and soft tissue surgical margins, globe with tumor (Fig. 9.7), orbital soft tissues adjacent to tumor, and surgical margin of optic nerve

3. *Tissue Processing*: The term tissue processing refers to the treatment of tissues necessary to impregnate them with a solid medium to facilitate the production of sections for microscopy [10, 11]. The other method to cut tissues is to freeze them and then cut them in a freezing microtome or a cryostat [12]. The most satisfactory embedding material for routine histology is paraffin wax. The fixed tissues, which are in an aqueous state, before being embedded in paraffin wax, must be subjected to the following: 1. Completion of fixation. 2. Gentle and gradual, but complete dehydration. 3. Clearing with substance, which is totally miscible with both the dehydration agent, which precedes it and the embedding agent, which follows it. The tissue processing

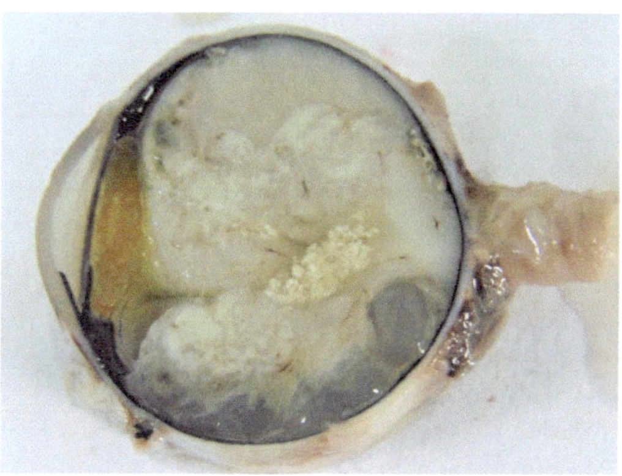

Fig. 9.5 The cut section of the eyeball showing a soft gray white fluffy tumor filling the entire vitreous cavity

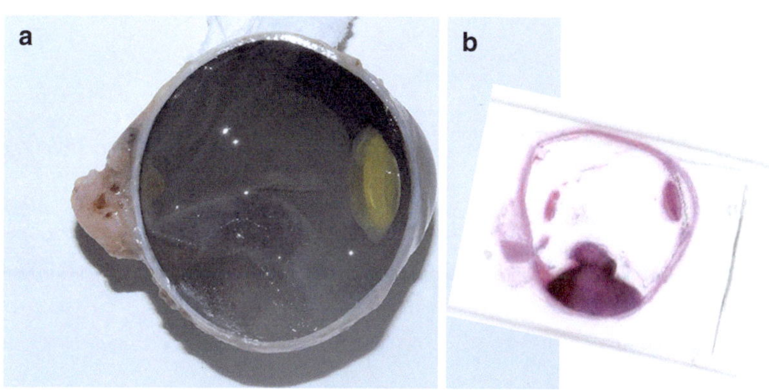

Fig. 9.6 (**a**) The picture shows a central calotte of an eyeball with a polypoidal-shaped melanoma. The whole mount preparation for the section taken from the same block shows the tumor and the eyeball (**b**)

involves embedding that is mostly done by an automated tissue processor and the process includes gradual dehydration through graded alcohol, two bath of clearing agents to remove all traces of alcohol, two baths of melted paraffin at 56 degree C.

4. *Tissue Embedding and Cutting*. The tissues infiltrated with wax are then embedded in molds in an appropriate orientation depending on the type of specimen and then made into blocks that are properly labeled [9] (Fig. 9.8a). Paraffin-embedded tissues are cut on a rotary microtome using blades. The sections cut from these blocks are usually 3–6 microns thick. Serial sections of small tissues can be studied for further details. Care should be taken to ensure that the complete section of the tissue embedded is seen on the glass slides (Fig. 9.8b). If sections thinner than this are required, then the tissues are embedded in plastic resins and can then be cut up to 1micron for semithin sections and 0.2 microns for ultrathin sections that have to studied using an electron microscope.
5. *Staining*: Routinely a combination of two stains- basic and acidic dyes are used to stain the nucleus and the cytoplasm [13]. Hematoxylin (blue or voilet) being a basic dye stains the nucleus while the eosin stain (pink or liliac) stains the cytoplasm (Table 9.2). In addition periodic acid Schiff's

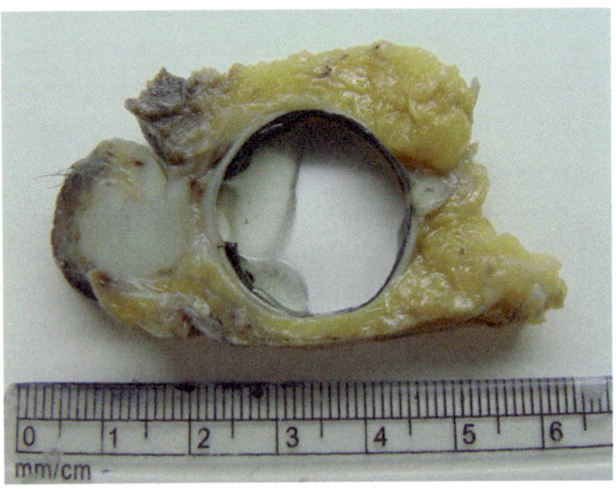

Fig. 9.7 Pictures show one of the slices of the exenterated specimen with a large tumor covering the ocular surface. The entire slice should be submitted for processing so as to examine the entire tumor and the eyeball in their location

Table 9.2 Procedure of routine hematoxylin and eosin staining

Hematoxylin And Eosin Staining procedure	
Xylene	3 changes 2 minutes each
100% Alcohol	10 dips
95% Alcohol	10 dips
Waterwash	
Hematoxylin	10 minutes
Waterwash	2–5 minutes
1% acid alcohol	3 dips
Waterwash	1 minute
Eosin	5 dips
80% alcohol	10 dips
95% alcohol	10 dips
100% alcohol	10 dips
Xylene	2 changes
Mounting	

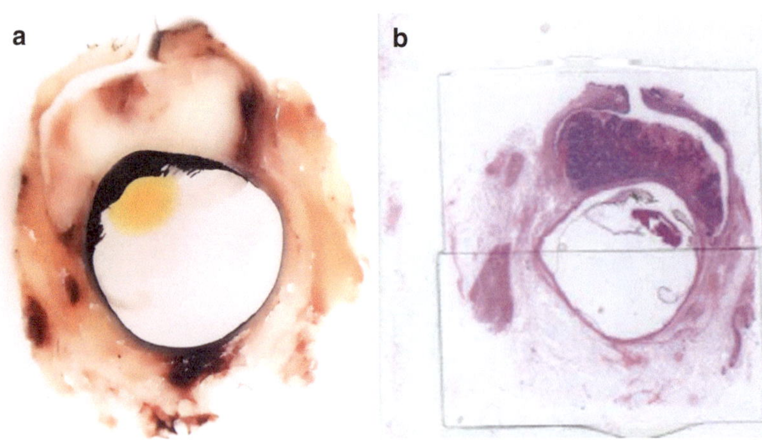

Fig. 9.8 (**a**) The picture shows a block of the exenterated specimen embedded in paraffin wax. (**b**). The whole mount picture of the same block shows a tumor covering the ocular surface with intraocular extension

Table 9.3 Periodic acid Schiff's(PAS) staining

Xylene	3 changes 2 minutes each
100% Alcohol	10 dips
95% Alcohol	10 dips
Waterwash	
Periodic acid	5 minutes
Rinse in distilled water	1 min
Place in Schiff reagent	15 minutes
Wash in tap water	10 minutes
Counter staining in hematoxylin	15 minutes
Wash in tap water	5 minutes
80% alcohol	10 dips
95% alcohol	10 dips
100% alcohol	10 dips
Xylene	2 changes
Mounting	

stain (Table 9.3) is done to stain the basement membranes, glycogen, mucins, fungal filaments and other substances that are not well distinguished with the Hematoxilin and Eosin (H &E) staining.

9.3 Special Stains

In many instances, special stains have to be used on the section to identify or confirm the presence of various types of deposits, microorganisms, and other abnormal changes [13, 14]. The common special stains used in the ophthalmic pathology lab include those done for orbital and lid tumors, corneal dystrophies, etc., The different stains done on corneas to distinguish various types infections and corneal dystrophies are listed in Tables 9.4 and 9.5.

Table 9.4 Special stains for identification of microorganisms in ocular tissues

Microorganism	Stain
Bacteria	Grams
Fungus	PAS, GMS, CFW
Acanthamoeba	Acridine O, PAS, GMS, CFW, Masson's trichrome
Acid-fast *Bacilli*	Ziehl Neelson stain, Fite stain, (hot and cold stain)
Microsporidia	AFB, Grams, modified trichrome stain,

Table 9.5 Special stains for diagnosis of corneal dystrophies

Stromal dystrophy	Special stain
Granular	Mason's trichrome, Wilder's reticulin
Avellino	Congo red [a]stain
Lattice dystrophy type I	Congo red[a]
Lattice dystrophy type II	Congo red[a]
Macular dystrophy	Alcian blue, Colloidal Iron
Fleck dystrophy	Alcian blue, colloidal iron, and lipid stains

[a]Confirmation of amyloid deposits is by the congophilic nature, diachorism, and apple green birefringence when observed under polarized filters

9.4 Electron Microscopy

Transmission electron microscopy is used selectively; it has been supplanted by immunohistochemistry that is cheaper, faster, and less labor intensive. It is used as a tool to identify the basic ultrastructural features of the cells and tissue and has been well established for ocular tissues [15]. It is specifically employed to confirm the nature of the lesion based on the presence of structures within the cell that are identified only by ultrastructure eg the neurosecretory granules of neuroendocrine tumors, the tennis racket shaped body in Langerhan cell histiocytosis, etc. In tumor pathology, it is useful in determining the histogenesis (or differentiation) of various tumors but unfortunately have not shown consistent differences between benign, reactive and malignant tumors of the same cell types. Though the role of EM has decreased with the advent of immunohistochemistry and other techniques, the diagnostic utility of EM includes the following:

1. Differential diagnosis between a carcinoma, melanoma, and sarcoma
2. Differential diagnosis between adenocarcinoma and squamous cell carcinoma
3. Differential diagnosis of round cell tumors—Ewings sarcoma, rhabdomyosarcoma, malignant lymphoma, and neuroendocrine tumors
4. Differential diagnosis of spindle cell tumors of orbit

In ocular pathology, EM is used to characterize the native cells as well to confirm the nature of tumors [16].

9.5 Immunologic and Molecular Techniques

Diagnosis of lesion is usually made on the basis of morphology. However, in many instances, it has to be aided by immunodiagnosis wherein the diagnosis is made based on the property of the given tissue/cell to express specific antigens. These antigens are detected by using a set of antibodies that bind to specific antigens and are labeled either directly or indirectly with the help of secondary antibodies that are attached to a chromogen or a detecting system [17–19]. Some of the commonly used antibodies for diagnosing orbital tumors are given in Tables 9.6, 9.7. The procedure of immunohistochemistry using peroxidas-antiperoxidase method for paraffin sections is described in brief:

1. Prewarm all slides including the positive and negative control for 10 minutes in 60 °C oven.
2. Dewax slides(3 × 5 minutes in Xylene, 1 × 5 minutes in absolute alcohol, 1 × 5 minutes 80% alcohol, 1 × 5 minutes in 75% alcohol).
3. Rinse in distilled water.
4. Wash sections for 5 minute in wash buffer.
5. Block endogenous peroxidase for 30 minutes in methanol/H_2O_2 solution.
6. Wash slides in wash buffer for 15 minutes.
7. Incubate sections in enzyme solution for 10–15 minutes (Pepsin, trypsin, pronase).
8. Wipe around each section separately. Drain off as much buffer as possible but do now allow sections to dry out at any stage after this. Place slides in humidity chamber.
9. Apply 100 Microliter of nonimmune serum (horse, goat, swine in 1: 50 dilutions) for 30 minutes.
10. Drain off the drop of serum, wipe around the section carefully without touching the section. Apply 100 Mic of diluted primary antibody and incubate overnight at 4 0 c.
11. Wash with wash buffer for 10 minutes × 2 changes.
12. Wipe around sections again, apply 100 M second antibody for 30 minutes (anti mouse/anti rabbit, antiswine in 1in 100 dilutions).
13. Wash for 15 minutes in wash buffer.
14. Wipe around sections. Apply 100 M of PAP complex for 45–60 minutes in 1: 50 dilutions.
15. Wash for 15 minutes in wash buffer.
16. Color determination step: Incubate in freshly prepared DAB/H_2O_2 solution at room temperature for 5–10 minutes.
17. Wash for 5 minutes gently in running tap water.

Table 9.6 Immunohistochemical pattern of small cell undifferentiated tumors

NEOPLASM	LCA	Keratin	NSE	NF	Desmin
Lymphoma	+	–	–	–	–
Leukemia	+	–	–	–	–
Neuroblastoma	–	–	+	+	–
Retinoblastoma	–	–	+	+	–
Rhabdomyosarcoma	–	–	–	–	+
Ewing's sarcoma	–	–	–	–	–
Wilms' tumor	–	+	–	–	+/–
Small cell carcinoma	–	+/–	+/–	+/–	–

Table 9.7 Immunohistochemistry for spindle cell tumors

Neoplasm	Vimentin	M Actin	SM actin	Desmin	S-100	F VII Ag	Keratin	Myoglobin
F. Histio	+	±	±	–	–	–	–	–
RMS	+	+	–	+	–	–	–	±
Leiomyo	+	+	+	–	–	–	–	–
Liposa	+	–	–	–	±	–	–	–
HPC	+	–	–	–	–	–	–	–
Angio sa	+	–	–	–	–	+	–	–
Sch/NF	+	–	–	–	+	–	–	–
Chondro	+	–	–	–	±	–	–	–
Spin C Ca	±	–	–	–	–	–	+	–

M Actin muscle actin, *SM actin* smooth muscle actin, *FVIII* factor VIII antigen, *HPC* hemangiopericytoma, *Chondro* chondrosarcoma, *Spind C Ca* Spindle cell carcinoma

18. Counterstain with Harris hematoxylin.
19. Wash till blue and dehydrate, clear and mount.

In addition to academic interest, the common indication for IHC is in diagnosing different types of round cell tumors, for example, differentiating lymphoma from Rhabdomyosarcoma, (Fig. 9.9) amelanotic melanoma from carcinoma (Fig. 9.10) and glioma from other spindle cell tumors (Fig. 9.11).

6. *Molecular Diagnostic Tools*
   1. In many instances, in addition to the tissue or cytology diagnosis, further information is required at DNA, RNA, antigen expression, or identification of organisms at molecular level. In such instances, various molecular techniques are applied to augment the diagnostic accuracy. With the advancing techniques, it is now possible to determine the actual presence or absence of a segment on gene using appropriate molecular tools and primers. In recent times, the most commonly employed technique is the polymerase chain reaction (PCR), which involves the denuturation, annealing and extension. The sequence involves process of first segregating the two strands of DNA in the sample, then amplifying the single strand of nucleic acid to thousand folds so that it can be made visible and measured, thus making it possible to interpret the presence or absence of the test antigen or DNA in the sample [20, 21]. PCR can now be employed on DNA extracted from formalin-fixed and paraffin-embedded tissues, thus making it more feasible to use archived tissues [22, 23]. Another technique that helps to identify the text DNA/gene or organism is the in situ hybridization technique [24, 25]. This involves the use of labeled nucleic acid probes whose sequences are complementary to the DNA of the organism or the gene sought: for example, detection of Human papilloma virus in conjunctival tumors [26, 27]. The labeling of probes could be done by either

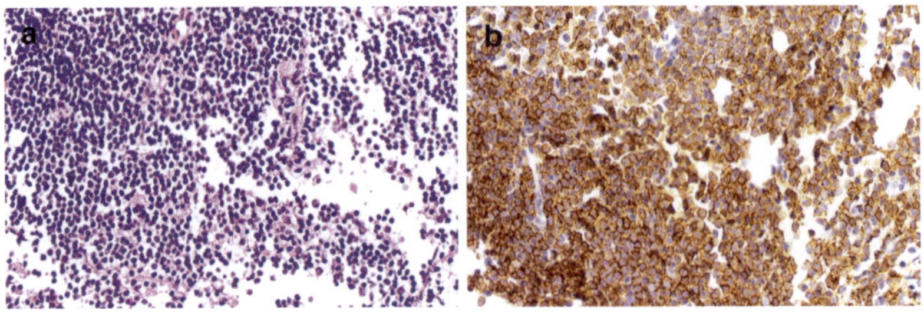

Fig. 9.9 (**a**) Section of an orbital lymphoma showing monotonous population of round cells with scant rim of cytoplasm and basophilic nuclei, which is highly suggestive of lymphoma (hematoxylin & eosin, × 400). (**b**) The clonal nature of the tumor cells is confirmed in this case by immunopositivity to B cell markers (DAB, × 200)

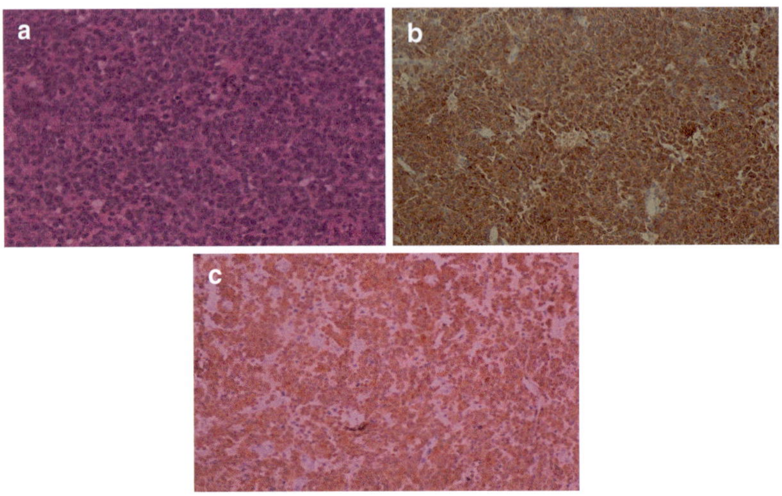

Fig. 9.10 (**a**)The section from a nonpigmented conjunctival tumor showing large epitheloid cells with vesicular nucleus and prominent nucleoli, highly suggestive of amelanotic melanoma (hematoxylin & eosin, × 400). (**b**) Immunohistochemistry using Melan-A and (**c**) HMB-45 shows positive staining, confirming the diagnosis of a melanoma and ruling out a large cell lymphoma (DAB, × 400)

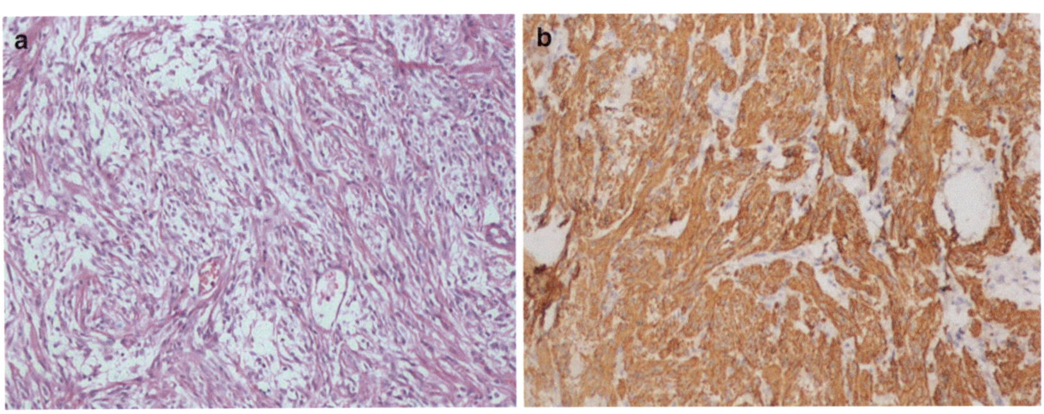

Fig. 9.11 (**a**) The spindle cell tumor of the optic nerve shows elongated spindle cells with ill-defined cell margins and fibrillary background (hematoxylin & eosin, × 200). (**b**) The tumor cells show immunoreactivity to Glial fibrillary acidic protein, thus confirming a glioma of the optic nerve (DAB, × 200)

radioactive substances or biotin and bromodeoxyuridine. The advantage of in situ hybridization is that it allows the visualization of cellular DNA or RNA in the tissue sections, single cells, or chromosome preparation. In situ hybridization [28] can be done using an isotope or nonisotope method. In brief, it involves choosing the appropriate probes specific to detect the test DNA, labeled probes, detection system (streptavidin-alk phosphatase or anti-digoxygenin conjugates), incubating the enzyme-treated sections with test probes, and then heating to denature both the tissue and probe DNA. Hybridization is done in the optimum temperature and medium and the end product is stained for visualization. The main use of this technique is in the detection of microbes (mycobacteria, viruses) and oncogenes.

(a) *Principle of Polymerase Chain Reaction*

The polymerase chain reaction, invented by Kary B. Mullis, is a technique that exponentially amplifies the small unidentifiable quantity of a specific nucleotide sequence. This is done in the presence of template sequence, two oligonucleotide primers that hybridize to opposite strands and flank the region of interest in the target DNA, and a thermostable (taq) DNA polymerase. The reaction is repeated or cycled involving template denaturation, primer annealing, and the extension of the annealed primers by DNA polymerase until enough copies are made for further analysis, hence the term polymerase chain reaction.

In order to accomplish this, it is necessary to know at least some of the DNA sequence flanking the region to be assayed before amplification can be carried out. The brief protocol involves addition of a buffer, forward and reverse primer, appropriate template DNA, and subjecting it into thermocycler with addition of enzyme (*Taq, Tli, Pfu*, etc.) and a few drops of mineral oil. The PCR cycles are run for 29 cycles, each containing steps of denaturation, annealing, and extension. The final product is then run on a gel for confirmation. This protocol can be further modified based on the nature of the primers and test sample. In ophthalmic practice, it has been applied to diagnose various infections from ocular samples: to detect the presence of virus in corneal tissues and in tumors [22, 23, 26, 27]. For tissues already processed and embedded in paraffin blocks, the unstained sections form the basis of extracting the DBA. After deparaffinization, the tissues are digested using Proteinase K . Then the DNA is isolated by phenol-chloroform extraction and ethanol precipitation followed by similar steps of amplification using primers specific for different DNA sequences of the test sample.

(b) *Flow Cytometry*

Flow cytometry is used for simultaneous measurement of several parameters while a suspension of cells flows through a beam of light past stationary detectors [29–31]. The instrument allows analysis of 5000–10,000 cells per second of information on parameters like cell size, cytoplasmic granules, cell viability, cell cycle time, DNA content, surface marker phenotype, and enzyme content. One of the main limitations is that the cells should be in single-cell suspension. This requirement can be achieved in blood, fluids, fresh tissues, needle aspirates, and now nuclear suspension recovered from thick sections for routine formalin-fixed, paraffin-embedded tissues. The current clinical uses include the following: 1. support a diagnosis when the morphological changes are equivocal, 2. subclassification of lesions of borderline malignancy; 3. prognostic markers, independent of stage and grade; 4. monitor response to therapy; and 5. establish development of tumor relapse. In ocular tissues, it has been used to diagnose lymphoproliferative lesions of orbit and conjunctiva [32, 33].

(c) *Tissue Culture and Karyotyping*

Though tissue cultures have been performed in nonocular tumors [34], a few studies have been done on cultures of retinoblastoma tumors, melanoma, and lacrimal gland tumor [35–37]. The rationale behind tissue culture is to demonstrate the differentiation of the tumor cells in ex-vivo conditions, undertake karyotyping, immunocytochemistry, or ultrastructural studies. The culture conditions could be modified based on the objectives of the study. The diagnostic utility of tissue cultures is however practically nonexistent, but it has however contributed extensively as a research tool, including pharmacokinetic studies on drug resistance and may possibly pave way for development of treatment protocols and vaccines [38, 39].

9.6 Special Procedures in Ophthalmic Pathology

Eye and orbital lesions remain an enigma and pose a challenge to the most experienced ophthalmologist with its diverse etiology. In this section, a simple strategy is provided for making cytologic and histologic diagnosis of the eye and orbital lesions. The tissue diagnosis in most instances is the final diagnosis. After coming to a presumptive clinical diagnosis of orbital lesions based on the clinical and radiologic features, a decision needs to be made regarding the procedure to be adopted to confirm the nature of the lesion. The methods of tissue diagnosis include preoperative fine-needle aspiration cytology (FNAC) or biopsy (FNAB) or a routine tissue diagnosis after a surgical biopsy [40], and have been well established in ophthalmology for orbital lesions [41–43]. A preoperative diagnosis is indicated in situations when a suspected tumor can be treated by other medical or conservative methods, and does not require a surgical intervention e.g., rhabdomyosarcoma, sarcoidosis, metastatic tumors, reactive lymphoid hyperplasia, lymphoma, sclerosing orbititis, and infections. It is also indicated to plan the extent of surgery. The decision for the type of biopsy would depend on the size, site, shape, circumscription, encapsulation, consistency, approximation to the neighboring structures, and the accessibility of the lesion from surgical point of view.

(a) *Preoperative Diagnosis*

Fine-needle aspiration/sampling technique:

While in some cases, the tissues are obtained by direct surgical procedures, in many instances, there is a need for a preoperative diagnosis, which can then influence the type and nature of surgery or management that needs to be undertaken. One of the well-established techniques is fine-needle aspiration biopsy or cytology. In this process, the clinician or pathologist or radiologists introduces a needle into the lesion and harvests biological samples for cytologic analysis. For visible lesions or tumors, it is directly done under vision, whereas for deep-seated lesions, it is usually done using the guidance of ultrasound or CT [43]. Usually, it can be performed without the use of any local anesthesia injection except in children where a general anesthesia may be preferred. The technique of obtaining the material could be a "sampling technique" as against the omission of the syringe for aspiration. When performed using 23/24 gauge needle introduced into the lesion and pushed in various directions within the lesion, it facilitates the movement of the cells into the needle (Fig. 9.12) [44, 45]. By the capillary action, the cells are drawn into the needle. The advantage of this technique is it is easy, simple, less hemorrhagic, and causes less apprehension to the patient. For aspiration technique, a syringe is attached to the needle so as to create a negative pressure. To obtain the greater possible yield, the needle could be moved back and forth within the

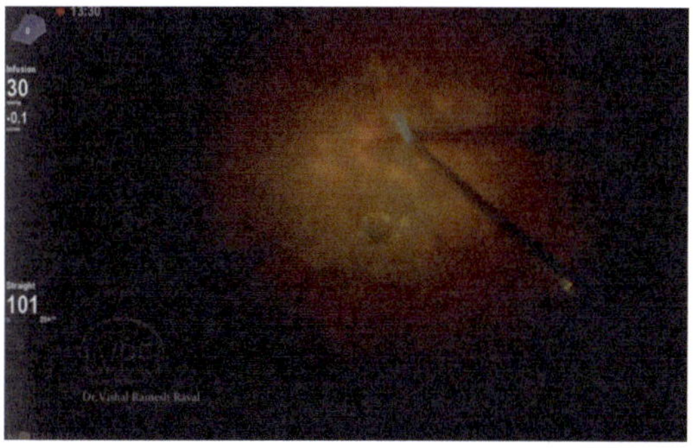

Fig. 9.12 The figure shows the subretinal biopsy. The specimen is collected from the thickest part or active lesion. The collected fluid from the lesion is centrifuged and the sedimented material (ie the pellet), is submitted for the preparation of cell block(paraffin block), from which sections can be made. The sections from the cell block can then be used for routine or special stains, as required for the diagnosis

lesion along the same track with negative pressure maintained. It is important to release the negative pressure while removing the needle from the lesion so as to avoid contamination with the cells along the track. . Two different methods of fixation and staining are used in FNA cytology: air-drying followed by staining with a hematologic stain such as MGG, Jenner-Giemsa, Wright's stain, or Diff-Quik, and alcohol fixation and staining with Pap or H & E [13, 14]. Both techniques are complementary to each other.

The main advantage of this procedure is obtaining an early cytological diagnosis of the lesion. It may be done as an outpatient procedure with avoidance of anesthesia or orbitotomy. A few disadvantages include inadequate material, hemorrhagic aspirate, and bleeding at the site of FNAC [46, 47]. At our center, FNAC has yielded diagnostic yield in more than 90% of cases, while Tijl et al. report the diagnostic yield of orbital FNAB combined with clinical and radiological features as 80% [48]. Very rare potential complications are globe penetration, retrobulbar hemorrhage, diplopia, and ptosis.

(b) *Intraoperative-Operative Diagnosis*

There is often a need for a reliable intraoperative diagnosis, specifically in situations where a definitive preoperative tissue diagnosis is lacking and where the tissue diagnosis is likely to influence the immediate surgical management [49]. It should be remembered that it is not indicated merely to satisfy the curiosity of the surgeon. The established methods of intraoperative diagnosis include frozen section diagnosis and intraoperative cytologic diagnosis, each of which has its own merits and demerits. In general, a complete excision of the mass (excisional biopsy) is indicated for all cystic, well-circumscribed, and encapsulated lesions, easily accessible lesions, and all suspected benign lesions [50]. For the lesions that are suspected to be malignant, with infiltrative margins, solid consistency, and have a complex surgical approach, an incisional biopsy may be indicated.

In an *incisional biopsy*, only a portion of the lesion is removed to provide a sample for diagnosis. The best place to sample the tissue is at the periphery, always including normal tissue for easier interpretation. The center of the tissue should not be biopsied, especially if there is central ulceration.

A. *Frozen Sections*:

Frozen section is one of the most important procedures that requires experience, knowledge of clinical medicine, pathology, good judgment, conservative approach, and a capacity to make quick decision under pressure. It is generally indicated to determine the nature of the lesion, if the resection margins are free from tumor or if the surgeon has biopsied representative material [51, 52]. The fresh unfixed tissue is embedded in a freezing media (OCT/ water) using a block holder. The sections are then cut with the help of a cryostat and are stained with a rapid hematoxylin and eosin technique. Interpretation can be done within 6–10 minutes per block. The advantages of this technique are that it gives good architectural details and are extremely useful to comment on nature of the lesion, surgical margins of malignant lid tumors, and to differentiate between in situ or invasive lesions. The disadvantages, however, include the frozen section artifacts produced in the sections, which most of the pathologists are familiar with. This technique requires a special cryomicrotome, a technician, and a pathologist trained for frozen section reporting. It is not very useful for small tissue, fatty tissues, or bony lesions.

B. *Squash or Imprint Cytology:*

The utility of imprint cytology in eye lesions was first described by Fuchs for uveal melanoma in 1988 [53]. Imprint cytology of fresh unfixed tissue specimens and squash cytology of central nervous system lesions have been extensively used in the last few decades, but have recently been introduced to ophthalmic pathology practice [54, 55]. It can be utilized for the following indications:

1. Infiltrative lesions, suspected malignant lesions, or deeply located lesions where a preoperative tissue diagnosis was not available
2. Discrepancy between a preoperative clinical diagnosis and the intraoperative findings
3. Unusual clinical presentations with diagnostic dilemma

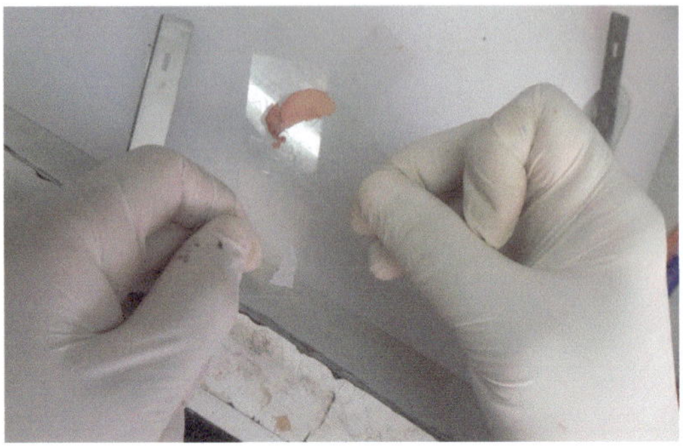

Fig. 9.13 Picture shows the technique of doing imprint cytology on a fresh specimen. Clean glass slides are touched to the freshly cut surface for the tumor and gently pressed so as to get the cells onto the glass slide

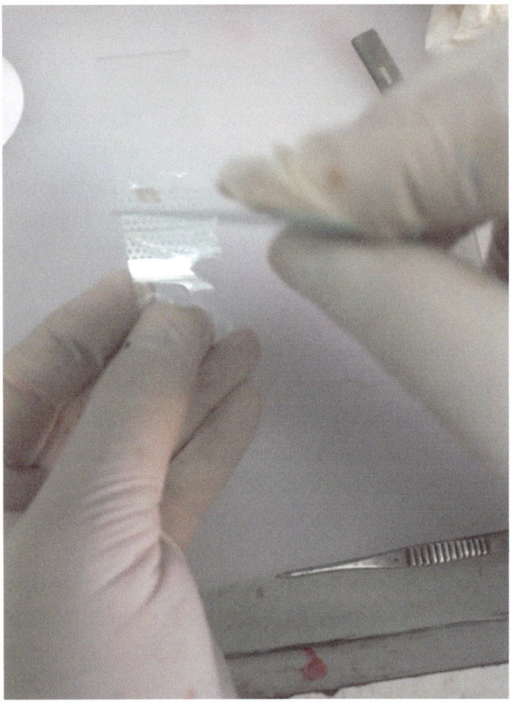

Fig. 9.14 Picture shows the technique of doing imprint cytology wherein a small bit of fresh tissue is kept on the center of a glass slide and then with the help of another glass slide placed perpendicular to it, the tissue is firmly spread across the glass slide

9.7 Method

Fresh unfixed tissue obtained at the time of diagnostic or excision biopsy can be used for making squash preparation and impressions on glass slides. The procedure for making squash or imprint smears is usually based on the size, shape, consistency, and crushable properties of the tissue submitted. For soft, easy-to-spread tissues, tiny bit of the fresh tissue is placed between two clean glass slides and gently drawn apart (Fig. 9.13). For large firm specimens, the imprint smears are prepared by touching the freshly cut surface of the lesion with clean slides, avoiding smearing to retain cell morphology (Fig. 9.14). If the surface was covered with blood or exudates, more number of smears are made, after gently wiping the surface clean. It is preferable to make a minimum of three slides for each case. It is advisable to preserve extra unstained smears for further tests like immunocytochemistry or for any molecular studies in future.

These smears are either alcohol-fixed for rapid hematoxylin and eosin staining, or fixed by air-drying for Diff-quick staining. A provisional cytologic diagnosis can be made by the pathologist based on the cellular and architectural features seen on smears prepared from either or both techniques. After reporting on the cytology slides, the remaining tissue should be fixed in 10% buffered formalin and processed for permanent sections, and stained by hematoxylin and eosin, and periodic acid Schiff's stain. Special and immunohistochemical stains can be done. Though the accuracy of combined frozen section and cytology is the ideal method of intraoperative diagnosis, imprint and squash cytology alone gives 96% accuracy [56].

9.8 Fluid (Vitreous, Aqueous, or Other Fluids) Cytology

The most common fluid sample from ophthalmic surgeries is vitreous fluid. The vitreous sample is obtained as a vitreous biopsy (undiluted) or from vitrectomy procedures (diluted). The fluid obtained is therefore unfixed and therefore requires urgent attention in the laboratory. The samples can be processed in different ways: celloidin bag techniques, cytocentrifugation, direct smears, and by Millipore filtration devices [57, 58]. Most commonly used technique is cytospin, which gives good cellular recovery and excellent cytologic details. Here the sample is fed into the plastic tube, and arranged in a holder, which contains a filter paper, glass slide, and the plastic tube. The cytospin is usually set for 10 minutes at 1000 revolutions per minute, which concentrates the cells into a focal area on the glass slide. The slides are then fixed either in alcohol or by rapid air-drying. Depending on the indication of the vitreous biopsy, the sample is then submitted for routine cytology, electron microscopy, immunocytochemistry, special stains, and flow cytometry.

9.8.1 Conjunctival Impression Cytology

One of the tests that is frequently done in diagnosing squamous metaplasia of the ocular surface is Impression cytology of the ocular surface using a nitrocellulose paper [59–62]. This is based on the principle that by capillary action, the superficial cells of ocular surface are transferred to the filter paper, which can be stained and interpreted for the type of cells lining the ocular surface. This was initially frequently used for diagnosing squamous metaplasia for Vitamin A deficiency wherein there was a loss of goblet cells with gradual change of columnar cells to squamous cells with keratinization [61, 62]. The other indications include identification of goblet cells over the corneal region to confirm conjunctivalization of cornea, which is one of the features characterizing the limbal stem cell deficiency [63, 64]. The other indication could be to diagnose ocular surface squamous neoplasia, to evaluate the extent of involvement of ocular surface by the tumor, and to confirm or rule out the recurrence in a diagnosed case of squamous cell carcinoma of ocular surface [65, 66]. The goblet cells and the cellular morphology is well identified by PAS–hematoxylin and Eosin staining. In this technique, a 5 × 5 mm of sterile nitrocellulose paper is gently placed in the conjunctival and corneal surface of the diseased eye for 5 seconds. Then the filter paper is gently peeled off from the surface and dipped in alcohol-filled petri dishes. The membrane is stained by modified periodic acid–Schiff stain.

Method

1. Fix the filter paper in 70% ethanol for 2 minutes.
2. Wash in tap water × 10 dips.
3. Apply Periodic acid Schiff reagent 0.5% for 2 minutes.
4. Wash in tap water × 10 dips.
5. Immerse in 5% Sodium metabisufite for 2 minutes.
6. Stain with Hematoxylin for 2 minutes.
7. Dehydrate in 95% ethyl alcohol × 10 dips.
8. Stain with Eosin for 2 minutes.
9. Dehydrate in absolute alcohol for 2 minutes.
10. Transfer into Xylene.
11. Mount with glycerin mount or Paramount.

The filter paper becomes transparent in the organic solvents. Under the microscope, observe for the presence of goblet cells, which appear as magenta pink cells (Fig. 9.15).

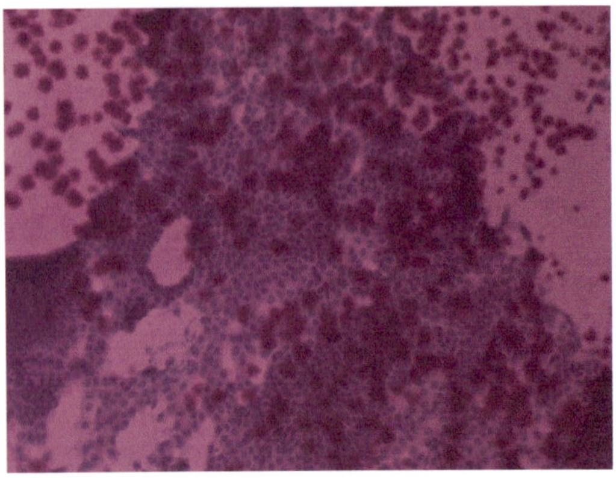

Fig. 9.15 The picture of the conjunctival impression cytology using nitrocellulose paper shows sheets of epithelial cells on the filter paper along with large PAS-positive goblet cells (PAS-hematoxylin stain, 400)

9.9 Ophthalmic Photography

Documentation of the cases is not only important for academic interest or teaching purposes but also is considered as a legal document. Hence, gross and microphotography is extensively used in this specialty. It could be done with the help of a digital camera or a well-equipped photographic system [67]. Ideally, the photograph of the specimen is taken when it is submerged in 60% of ethanol, which restores the color of the specimen even after initial fixation in 10% formaldehyde. Use of appropriate lighting, good-quality camera roll, appropriate use of close-up and zoom lenses, and clean background free of artifacts, all these can surely give good-quality pictures. Similar care should be taken for microphotographs [67, 68]. The pictures can be taken with a digital camera in built or external or with traditional film. The pictures should be taken at appropriate magnification so as to highlight the relevant features of the case. Even though the new photoshopping software can manipulate the picture, it is ideal to take good pictures in the first instance, which requires minimal modification.

9.10 Summary: Ophthalmologists and the Pathology Laboratory

To maintain a good relationship between the ophthalmologist and the pathologist, there should be an effective, timely, and accurate communication between the two. This is generally done by the ophthalmologist who fills up the pathology lab requisition form, thus providing information on the age, sex, race, laterality, location of the lesion, and other clinical details, including the provisional clinical diagnosis. This will allow the pathologist to prepare for special fixation, or preparation of the sample as may be indicated by the clinician's provisional diagnosis of the lesion. Care should be taken to fix the tissues in an appropriate manner, in consultation with the pathologist. For all interesting and unusual cases, request for photography should be made at the time of submitting the sample so that the pathologist can take pictures before grossing the sample. The ophthalmologists are advised to visit the laboratory to look at the slides of all the specimens that they had referred to the pathologist. In case of any discrepancy in clinico-pathological correlation, it is in the interest of the patient and the clinician to discuss the case in person referring to the complete records of the patient.

Acknowledgments I am grateful to my technicians Mr. Chenchu Naidu and Mr. G Sridhar Rao for providing high-quality sections, with special stains and immunohistochemistry slides. I sincerely thank Mr. SNL Chary and Mr. Jangaiah for the excellent digital photographs and for developing the microphotographs. We thank Secretary Ms. Uma Maheshwari for her secretarial assistance.

Financial Disclosures None

Conflict of Interest None

References

1. Pearse AGE. Histochemistry theoretical and applied, vol. 1. 4th ed. Edinburgh: Churchill Livingstone; 1975.
2. Hopwood D. Fixation and fixatives. In: Bancroft JD, Stevens A, editors. Theory and practise of histological techniques. 3rd ed. Churchill Livingstone; 1990. p. 21–34.
3. Hopwood D. Theoretical and practical aspects of glutaraldehyde fixation. Histochem J. 1972;4:267–303.
4. Prophet EB, Mills B, Arrinton JB, Sobin LH. AFIP laboratory methods in histotechnology. Washington, DC: American Registry of Pathology; 1992. p. 25–8.
5. Margo CE, Saxe S, Grossniklaus HE. Microwave-stimulated chemical fixation of whole eyes. Ophthalmology. 1992;99:1117–22.
6. Torczynski E. Preparation of ocular specimens for histopathologic examination. Ophthalmology. 1981;88:1367–71.
7. Folberg R, Verdick R, Weingeist TA, Montague PR. The gross examination of eyes removed for choroidal and ciliary body melanomas. Ophthalmology. 1986;93(12):1643–7.
8. Rosai J. Gross techniques in surgical pathology. Ackerman's surgical pathology. 7th ed. St Loius: CV Mosby Co; 1989. p. 13–29.
9. Gravanis MB, Rietz CW. The problem-oriented postmortem examination and record: an educational challenge. Am J Clin Pathol. 1973;60:522–35.
10. Hall J. Embedding. In: Prophet EB, Mills B, editors. Laboratory methods in histochemistry. Washington DC: Armed Forces Institute of Pathology, American Registry of Pathology; 1992. p. 39–44.
11. Emanuele PV. Ocular histotechnology. In: Prophet EB, Mills B, editors. Laboratory methods in histochemistry. Washington DC: Armed Forces Institute of Pathology, American Registry of Pathology; 1992. p. 109–15.
12. Bancroft JD. Frozen and related section. In: Theory and practise of histological techniques. Edinburg, London: Churchill Livingstone; 1990. p. 81–92.
13. Horobin RW. An overview of the theory of staining. In: Theory and practise of histological techniques. Edinburg, London: Churchill Livingstone; 1990. p. 81–92.
14. White VA. Advanced diagnostic techniques-diagnostic immunohistochemistry. In: Albert DM, Jokobiec FA, editors. Principles and practise of ophthalmology. Philadelphia: WB Saunders; 1994. p. 2372–86.
15. Erfandson RA, Erlandson RA. Application of transmission electron microscopy to human tumor diagnosis: an historical perspective. Cancer Investig. 1987;5:487–505.
16. Fine BS, Ts'o MO, Font RL, Zimmerman LE. Electron microscopy of pathologic ocular tissue. Int Ophthalmol Clin. 1971;11:57–86.
17. Mukai K, Rosai J. Immunocytochemistry in diagnostic histopathology: its contributions and limitations. Basic Appl Histochem. 1981;25:153–8.
18. Eagle RC Jr. Immunohistochemistry in ophthalmic pathology. In: Liabson PR, editor. The year book of ophthalmology. St Louis: Mosby Year Book; 1990. p. 133–6.
19. Eagle RC Jr. Specimen handling in the ophthalmic pathology laboratory. Ophthalmol Clin North Am. 1995;8:1–15.
20. Mullis K, Faloona F, Scharf S, Saiki R, Hom G, Erlich H. Specific enzymatic amplification of DNA *in vitro*: the polymerase chain reaction. Cold Spring Harb Symo Quant Biol. 1986;51:263–73.
21. Erlich HA. Basic methodology in PCR technology. Principles and application for DNA amplification. New York: W H Freeman and Co; 1992.
22. Madhavan HN, Therese KL, Gunisha P, Jayanthi U, Biswas J. Polymerase chain reaction for detection of Mycobacterium tuberculosis in epiretinal membrane in Eales' disease. Invest Ophthalmol Vis Sci. 2000;41:822–5.
23. Chichili GR, Athmanathan S, Farhatullah S, Gangopadhyay N, Jalali S, Pasricha G, Sharma S. Multiplex polymerase chain reaction for the detection of herpes simplex virus, varicella-zoster virus and cytomegalovirus in ocular specimens. Curr Eye Res. 2003;27:85–90.
24. Grody WW, Cheng L, Lewin KJ. Application of in-situ DNA hybridization in diagnostic surgical pathology. Pathol Annu. 1987:151–75.
25. Sklar J. DNA hybridization in diagnostic pathology. Hum Pathol. 1985;16:654–8.
26. Nakamura Y, Mashima Y, Kameyama K, Mukai M, Oguchi Y. Detection of human papillomavirus infection in squamous tumours of the conjunctiva and lacrimal sac by immunohistochemistry, in situ hybridisation, and polymerase chain reaction. Br J Ophthalmol. 1997;81:308–13.
27. Saegusa M, Takano Y, Hashimura M, Okayasu I, Shiga J. HPV type 16 in conjunctival and junctional papilloma, dysplasia, and squamous cell carcinoma. J Clin Pathol. 1995;48:1106–10.
28. De Gaetani C, Ferrari G, Righi E, Bettelli S, Migaldi M, Ferrari P, Trentini GP. Detection of human papillomavirus DNA in urinary bladder carcinoma by in situ hybridisation. J Clin Pathol. 1999;52:103–6.
29. Braylum RC. Flow cytometry. Arch Pathol Lab Med. 1983;107:1–6.

30. Coon JS, Landay AL, Weinstein RS. Biology of disease. Advances in flow cytometry for diagnostic pathology. Lab Investig. 1987;57:453–79.
31. Frierson HF Jr. Flow cytometric analysis of ploidy in solid neoplasm. Comparison of fresh tissue with formalin-fixed paraffin-embedded specimen. Hum Pathol. 1988;19:290–4.
32. Wolska-Szmidt E, Masiuk M, Krzystolik K, Chosia M. Flow cytometry in the diagnosis of lymphoproliferative lesions of the orbit and eye adnexa in fine needle aspiration biopsy. Pol J Pathol. 2003;54:253–9.
33. Laucirica R, Font RL. Cytologic evaluation of lymphoproliferative lesions of the orbit/ocular adnexa: an analysis of 46 cases. Diagn Cytopathol. 1996;15:241–5.
34. Murray MR, Stout AP. The classification and diagnosis of human tumors by tissue culture methods. Tex Rep Biol Med. 1954;12:898–915.
35. Char DH, Wood IS, Huhta K, Rand N, Morita CT, Howes EL Jr. Retinoblastoma: tissue culture lines and monoclonal antibody studies. Invest Ophthalmol Vis Sci. 1984;25:30–40.
36. Albert DM, Rabson AS, Dalton AJ. Tissue culture study of human retinoblastoma. Investig Ophthalmol. 1970;9:64–72.
37. Lauer SA, Levin RJ, Bradley MK, Rosenbaum PS, Rameau R. An immortalized cell culture from a malignant mixed tumor of the lacrimal gland. Ophthalmic Plast Reconstr Surg. 1997;13:168–73.
38. McNamara M, Clynes M, Dunne B, NicAmhlaoibh R, Lee WR, Barnes C, Kennedy SM. Multidrug resistance in ocular melanoma. Br J Ophthalmol. 1996;80.1009–12.
39. Dillman RO, Nayak SK, Barth NM, DeLeon C, Schwartzberg LS, Spitler LE, Church C, O'Connor AA, Beutel LD. Clinical experience with autologous tumor cell lines for patient-specific vaccine therapy in metastatic melanoma. Cancer Biother Radiopharm. 1998;13:165–76.
40. Koss LG. Aspiration biopsy. A tool in surgical pathology. Am J Surg Pathol. 1988;12:43.
41. Schyberg E. Fine needle biopsy of orbital tumors. Acta Ophthalmol. 1975;125:11–2.
42. Kennerdell JS, Slamovits TL, Dekker A, Johnson BL. Orbital fine-needle aspiration biopsy. Am J Ophthalmol. 1985;99:547–51.
43. Czerniak B, Woyke S, Danieal B, Krzysztolik Z, Koss LG. Diagnosis of orbital tumors by aspiration biopsy guided by computerized tomography. Cancer. 1984;54:2385–9.
44. Santos JE, Leiman G. Nonaspiration fine needle cytology. Application of a new technique to nodular thyroid disease. Acta Cytol. 1988;32:353–6.
45. Zajdela A, de Maublanc MA, Schlienger P, Haye C. Cytologic diagnosis of orbital and periorbital palpable tumors using fine needle sampling without aspiration. Diagn Cytopathol. 1986;2:17–20.
46. Krohel GB, Tobin D, Chavis RM. Inaccuracy of orbital fine needle aspiration biopsy. Ophthalmology. 1984;91:83.
47. Liu D. Complications of fine needle aspiration biopsy of the orbit. Ophthalmology. 1985;92:1768–71.
48. Tijl JW, Koornneef L. Fine needle aspiration biopsy in orbital tumours. Br J Ophthalmol. 1991;75:491–2.
49. Ackerman LV, Ramirez GA. Indication for and limitation of frozen section diagnosis. A review of 1269 consecutive frozen section diagnosis. Br J Surg. 1959;46:336.
50. Dallow RL, Pratt SG. Approach to orbital disorders and frequency of disease occurrence. In: Albert DM, Jokobiec FA, editors. Principles and practise of ophthalmology. Philadelphia: WB Saunders; 1994. p. 1881–9.
51. Young I. Use of the cryostat. An aid to frozen section diagnosis in surgical pathology. J Albert Einstein Med Cent (Phila). 1963;11:82–5.
52. Older JJ, Quickert MH, Beard C. Surgical removal of basal cell carcinoma of the eyelids utilizing frozen section control. Trans Am Acad Ophthalmol Otolaryngol. 1975;79:658–63.
53. Fuchs U. Smear and imprint technique in malignant lesions of the eye. Acta Ophthalmol (Copenh). 1988;66:445–9.
54. Font RL, Laucirica R, Ramzy I. Cytologic evaluation of tumors of the orbit and ocular adnexa: an analysis of 84 cases studied by the "squash technique". Diagn Cytopathol. 1994;10:135–42.
55. Vemuganti GK, Naik M, Honavar SG, Shekar GC. Rapid intraoperative diagnosis of tumors of the eye and orbit by squash and imprint cytology. Ophthalmology. 2004;111(5):1009–15.
56. Mair S, Lash RH, Suskin D, Mendelsohn G. Intraoperative surgical specimen evaluation: frozen section analysis, cytological examination, or both ? A comparative study of 206 cases. Am J Clin Pathol. 1991;96:8–14.
57. Engel H, de la Cruz ZC, Jimenez-Abalahin LD, Green WR, et al. Cytopreparatory techniques for eye fluid specimens obtained by vitrectomy. Acta Cytol. 1982;26:551–60.
58. Chess J, Sebeg J, Tolentino FI, Schepens L, Calderone JP, et al. Pathologic processing of vitrectomy specimensl; a comparison of pathologic findings with celloidin bag and cytocentrifugation preparation of 102 vitrecomy specimens. Ophthalmology. 1983;90:1560–4.
59. Egbert PR, Lauber S, Maurice DM. A simple conjunctival biopsy. Am J Ophthalmol. 1977;84:798–801.

60. Tseng SC. Staging of conjunctival squamous metaplasia by impression cytology. Ophthalmology. 1985;92:728–33.
61. Nelson JD. Impression cytology. Cornea. 1988;7:71–81.
62. Nolan GR, Hirst LW, Bancroft BJ. Impression cytology for detection of vitamin A deficiency. Arch Ophthalmol. 1987;105:1224–8.
63. Puangsricharern V, Tseng SC. Cytologic evidence of corneal diseases with limbal stem cell deficiency. Ophthalmology. 1995;102:1476–85.
64. Sridhar MS, Vemuganti GK, Bansal AK, Rao GN. Impression cytology-proven corneal stem cell deficiency in patients after surgeries involving the limbus. Cornea. 2001;20:145–8.
65. Spinak M, Friedman AH. Squamous cell carcinoma of the conjunctiva. Value of exfoliative cytology in diagnosis. Surv Ophthalmol. 1977;21:351–5.
66. Nolan GR, Hirst LW, Bancroft BJ. Efficacy of a training programme designed to teach cervical smear screeners to identify ocular surface squamous neoplasia using conjunctival impression cytology. Cytopathology. 1997;8:388–96.
67. Eagle RC. Photographic tips for the ophthalmic pathology laboratory. In: Wilson R, editor. The year book of ophthalmology. St Louis: Mosby; 1997. p. 341–54.
68. Biswas J, Babu K, Krishnakumar S, Vanitha K, Vaijayanthi P. Gross photography of ophthalmic pathology specimens. Indian J Ophthalmol. 2001;49:273–6.

Corneal Pathology

10

Neha Jain, Somasheila Murthy, Varsha M. Rathi, Sujata Das, Saumya Jakati, Dilip K. Mishra, Geeta K. Vemuganti, and Muralidhar Ramappa

Contents

N. Jain · M. Ramappa
Cornea Service, Shantilal Shangvi Cornea Institute, L V Prasad Eye Institute, Hyderabad, Telangana, India
e-mail: muralidhar@lvpei.org

S. Murthy (✉)
Specialist in Corneal Diseases, Uveitis, Cataract and Refractive Surgery
Shantilal Shanghvi Eye Institute, Mumbai, Maharashtra, India
e-mail: smurthy@lvpei.org

V. M. Rathi
Allen Foster Community Eye Health Research Centre, Gullapalli Pratibha Rao International Centre for Advancement of Rural Eye care, LV Prasad Eye Institute, Hyderabad, Telangana, India
e-mail: varsharathi@lvpei.org

S. Das
Shantilal Shangvi Cornea Institute, L V Prasad Eye Institute, Bhubaneswar, Odisha, India
e-mail: sujatadas@lvpei.org

S. Jakati · D. K. Mishra
Ophthalmic Pathology Laboratory, L V Prasad Eye Institute, Hyderabad, Telangana, India
e-mail: saumyajakati@lvpei.org; dilipkumarmishra@lvpei.org

G. K. Vemuganti
School of Medical Sciences, University of Hyderabad, Hyderabad, Telangana, India
e-mail: gkvemuganti@gmail.com

G. K. Vemuganti et al. (eds.), *Ocular Pathology*, https://doi.org/10.1007/978-981-96-8614-8_10

10.1 Introduction

Cornea is the transparent avascular anatomical structure with a stereotyped pathological response. Its stratified architecture allows a systematic approach to diagnose pathological states affecting all the 5 layers, namely, the external epithelium, Bowman's layer, stroma, and the Descemet's membrane with the endothelial cell layer. Being the most exposed part with a specific visual function, any pathology such as infection, inflammation, dystrophy, edema, or scarring that compromises its transparency is of concern. Hence, understanding the pathobiology of different diseases is crucial. This chapter is divided into five sections: developmental conditions; corneal infections and inflammation; dystrophies; ectasias; and degenerations.

10.2 Embryology and Developmental Anomalies of the Cornea [1, 2]

10.2.1 Embryology

10.2.1.1 Epithelium

It is derived from the surface ectoderm and consists of a superficial squamous cell layer and basal cuboidal epithelial cell layer at 40 days of gestation (embryo is 17–18 mm in length). It attains the normal adult appearance by 5–6 months of pregnancy when the eyelids open in utero.

10.2.1.2 Stroma and Bowman's Layer

The development of the remaining layers of cornea takes place from the mesenchymal cells, which differentiate to form a superficial fibrous layer that later forms the anterior part of corneal stroma among other structures. Primary corneal stroma is secreted by the basal layer of epithelium and is replaced by the migrating mesenchymal cells at the 7th week (22–24 mm). This mesenchyme present between the surface ectoderm and developing lens forms the stroma thereafter. Initially, the stroma consists of filaments, amorphous material, and only a few collagen fibrils. After the mesenchymal cells form the stroma, they differentiate into stromal fibroblasts or keratocytes that secrete type I collagen fibrils and matrix of mature (secondary) corneal stroma. At 4-months of gestation, the most superficial acellular part of the corneal stroma condenses to form the bowman's layer. By the 5th month, the corneal nerves are formed.

10.2.1.3 Endothelium and Descemet's Membrane

The mesenchymal cells present at the rim of the optic cup's rim migrate beneath the corneal epithelium's basal lamina of the corneal epithelium to form the primordial corneal endothelium. At 40 days of gestation, the endothelium consists of two layers of flattened cells. By the 3rd month, the central endothelium becomes a single layer of flattened cells overlying an interrupted basal lamina forming the Descemet's layer later. By the 6th gestation month, the Descemet's layer is clearly demarcated.

10.2.1.4 Limbus

Formation of the limbal anlage occurs in the 7th–10th gestational week. It is derived from the mesenchymal cells of neural crest cells and allows the differentiation into sclera or cornea and allows the corneal curvature to exceed the scleral curvature.

10.2.2 Developmental Anomalies of the Cornea

10.2.2.1 Normal Parameters at Birth

The newborn cornea is steep at birth and gets flattered as the limbal ring expands in the first 2–3 years. Normal newborn cornea measures 10 mm in horizontal diameter and acquires a standard adult diameter of 12 mm by the age of 2 years [3].

Developmental anomalies are structural and functional anomalies that develop in utero or during early childhood. They could be abnormalities in size, location, organization, or amount of tissue. The etiology could be multifactorial, that is, genetic, infectious, toxic, traumatic, inflammatory, metabolic, or mechanical processes affecting the development of the anterior segment of the eye during tissue induction, differentiation, or maturation. Most the etiologies affect the eye during organogenesis (4th–6th gestational week) or during the period of anterior segment differentiation (6th–16th gestational week). The earlier the insult occurs, the more severe is the effect. These can occur as isolated defects or can be associated with other ocular or systemic anomalies due to the close embryologic relationship between the affected structures and the cornea and can often be associated with glaucoma [4]. The abnormalities characterizing anterior segment dysgenesis (ASDs) are complex and involve multiple structures, which have made their clinical classification and description difficult.

10.2.2.2 Dermoid

An epibulbar dermoid is a benign choristoma consisting of histologically mature tissue that presents in an abnormal location. Ocular surface dermoid can occur in isolation or manifestation of oculo-neurocutaneous or Goldenhar Syndrome, organoid naevus syndrome. Limbal dermoids are pinkish, solitary, or multiple well-defined elevated lesions that are often straddling the limbus (Fig. 10.1a) with a presence of skin appendages on the surface [4]. While dermolipomas are encased within the conjunctiva and Tenon's capsule that are located at the lateral or medial canthus. Histologically, they are classified as simple when lined by either squamous epithelium or keratinized epidermal lining with dermal appendages like pilosebaceous units, sweat glands, and fat (Fig. 10.1b). The term complex choristoma is used when the underlying collagenous tissue contains mesenchymal elements like cartilage, bone, smooth muscle bundles, or ectopic lacrimal gland [5, 6].

10.2.2.3 Peters Anomaly

- This is a part of the anterior segment dysgenesis syndromes. The mesenchyme, which is predominantly involved in the formation of the cornea, is derived from the neural crest. Lack of migration or differentiation of the neural crest cells during embryological development affects the anterior segment. A localized centrally or para-central defect of the endothelium and Descemet's membrane develops, known as internal or posterior ulcer of von Hippel. Iris strands adhere at the edges of this defect in the posterior corneal surface. The lens placode separates from the surface ectoderm during embryogenesis, and if this cleavage of lens-corneal endothelium is incomplete, it leads to severe forms of Peter's anomaly (Fig. 10.1c). The anterior chamber angle may also be malformed, leading to an increased risk of secondary developmental glaucoma [7]. Clinically, this presents as cor-

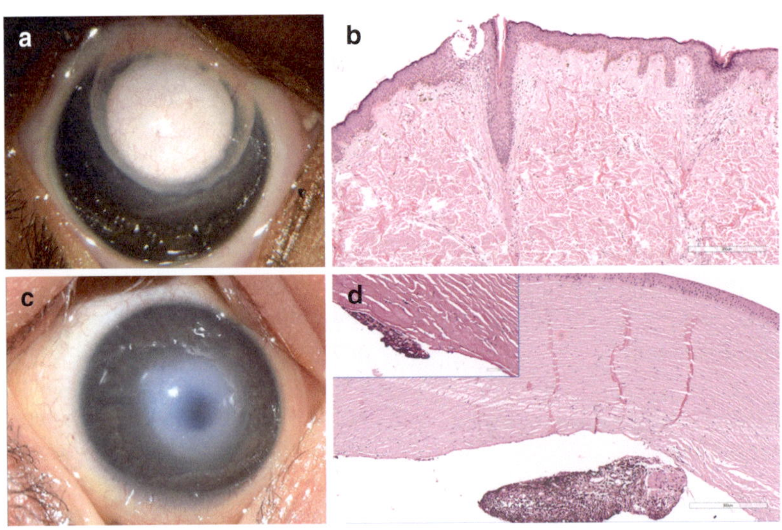

Fig. 10.1 (**a**) Clinical photograph of the right eye shows a large limbal dermoid obscuring the visual axis. (**b**) Scanner view of the excised dermoid showing stratified squamous epithelial lining with pilosebaceous units and collagenous tissue in the stroma resembling smooth muscle bundles. (Hematoxylin and eosin (H&E); 4× original magnification). (**c**) Clinical photograph of the right eye of an infant shows corneal opacification involving the visual axis. (**d**) The corneal button shows corneal scarring with iridocorneal adhesions, noted on the Hematoxylin and eosin (H&E); 10× original magnification and in the insert: Periodic acid Schiff (PAS) stain, 40× original magnification

neal opacification usually involving the central visual axis and based on the severity can be noted to be in contact with the iris and lens. The cornea may show central corneal scaring with disruptions in Bowman's layer, iridocorneal and keratolenticular adhesions (Fig. 10.1d), breaks in the Descemet's membrane, and at times adherent anterior polar cataract. They may be associated with PAX 6 mutations, and can occur with fetal-alcohol syndrome.

10.2.2.4 Sclerocornea and Cornea Plana

- Sclerocornea is characterized by peripheral corneal stromal opacification and vascularization (Fig. 10.2a). Histologically, the cornea shows thickened epithelium, irregular basement membrane, and absent Bowman's layer. The stroma consists of irregular stromal arrangement similar to scleral tissue with vascularization. Descemet's membrane may be very thin or disrupted (Fig. 10.2b, c).
- In cornea plana, progressive scleralization of the cornea occurs from periphery to center and is associated with a flat cornea (Fig. 10.2d). The absence of limbal anlage is noted, which is the structure responsible for limbal differentiation and corneal curvature, leading to disruption of the normal interface between the sclera and cornea and the surface curvature is flattened. Initially considered as the same entity by some [8], this was later characterized as two different entities [7, 9]. Bilateral cornea plana is a familial trait (autosomal dominant or recessive) characterized by corneal flattening and peripheral opacification [10] (Fig. 10.2b).

10.2.2.5 Megalocornea

The horizontal diameter of more than or equal to 12 mm in children or 13 mm at any age is categorized as megalocornea (Fig. 10.2e). It is nonprogressive, usually bilateral and symmetrical. It is hypothesized to occur due to a defect in the growth of the optic cup, wherein the anterior tips

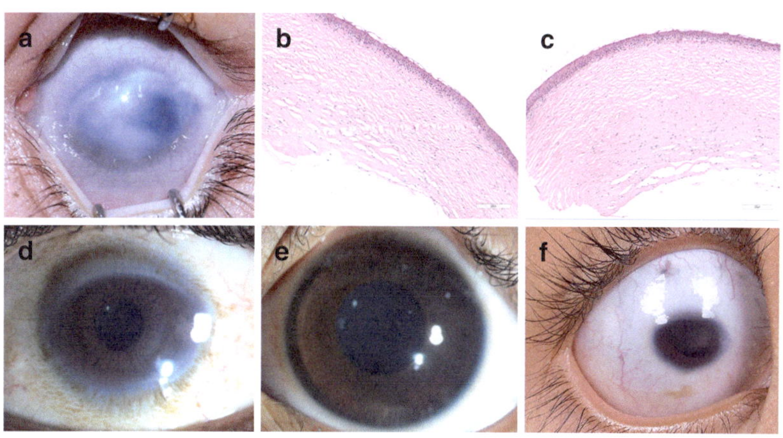

Fig. 10.2 (**a**) Clinical photograph obtained during examination under anesthesia in an infant showing corneal stromal opacification and vascularization typical for sclerocornea. Histologically, the cornea shows thickened epithelium, irregular basement membrane, and absent Bowman's layer. The stroma consists of irregular stromal arrangement similar to scleral tissue with vascularization. Descemet's membrane may be very thin or disrupted (Hematoxylin and eosin (H&E). (**b**) 6× original magnification. (**c**) 4× original magnification. (**d**) Slit-lamp photograph shows peripheral corneal opacification with flattened corneal curvature in cornea plana. (**e**) Slit-lamp photograph of megalocornea shows an otherwise normal appearing cornea; however, the white-to-white measurement is 14.5 mm horizontally. (**f**) Slit-lamp photograph shows an abnormally small cornea measuring 5 mm horizontally, with reduced anterior and posterior segment, confirming the diagnosis of microcornea with micro-ophthalmos

of the optic cup fail to close, thereby leaving a larger space to be taken up by the cornea [11, 12]. Another possible explanation includes exaggerated growth of the cornea relative to the rest of the eye and abnormal collagen production as it can be associated with systemic collagen synthesis disorders.

10.2.2.6 Microcornea

The horizontal corneal diameter is less than or equal to 10 mm in an otherwise standard-sized globe is defined as microcornea (Fig. 10.2f). It possibly occurs due to arrest in the growth of the cornea, which occurs after 5th gestational month when the differentiation is complete. Another postulated explanation is that the anterior tips of the optic cup overgrow, thereby leaving less space for the cornea opposed to the mechanism of development of megalocornea. It can occur either in isolation or associated with microophthalmos and lens-irido-choridal colobomas, cataract, myopia, and posterior staphylomas [13].

10.2.2.7 Absence of the Cornea

It is an extremely rare condition. Agenesis of various other anterior segment structures is seen as well due to close relation in the embryological development of other ocular structures. Anophthalmos, that is, complete absence of the eye, is the most extreme manifestation of this spectrum.

10.3 Corneal Infection

Microbial keratitis is an important cause of corneal blindness. Prompt diagnosis and appropriate therapy reduce the morbidity. While microbiology aids in early identification, tissue diagnosis may confirm and provide additional information in some cases [14]. The specimens included are corneal biopsy, corneal tissue after keratoplasty [15].

Routine Hematoxylin and Eosin (H&E) staining along with Periodic Acid Schiff (PAS) stain is routinely done on all sections. Special stains such as Grocott-Gomori Methenamine Silver stain (GMS) and Acid-Fast (AF) stain, etc., are used as per the suspected diagnosis on clinical or histologic findings [16].

10.3.1 Bacterial Keratitis

10.3.1.1 Clinical Features

Bacterial keratitis is a leading cause of visual morbidity and blindness worldwide [13]. *Staphylococci, Streptococci,* and *Pseudomonas* species were identified as common etiological agents [17, 18]. Common risk factors associated with bacterial keratitis include trauma, contact lens, and ocular surface disorders.

The rate of disease progression depends on the virulence of the organism and host factors. Highly virulent organisms such as *Pseudomonas* cause rapid tissue destruction, whereas organisms like *Streptococcus* viridians are associated with indolent course. Clinical features suggestive of bacterial keratitis are suppurative stromal defect associated with overlying epithelial defect with indistinct edge, edema, and white cell infiltration of surrounding stroma. There may be hypopyon in some cases [19].

10.3.1.2 Histopathology Features

Bacterial colonization occurs due to alteration of the corneal surface due to ulceration due to trauma or due to decreased tear film formation. Dense infiltration of polymorpho-nuclear leukocytes from the adjacent limbal vessels is seen. These infiltrate the stromal lamellae forming abscess. The karyorrhectic debris released from the inflammatory cells gives a basophilic hue to the background stroma. Stromal necrosis is caused by the collagenolytic enzymes released by the microbes and inflammatory cells. Stromal edema can also be seen in few cases. Special stains for bacteria such as Gram's stain aid in the detection of the bacteria: Gram positive stain blue and Gram negative stain red. Histology of the corneal button reveals completely ulcerated epithelium and Bowman's layer. Ulcer is often sealed by cyanoacrylate glue, which appears as refractile substance at area of ulceration. Stroma shows dense collection of polymorphonuclear leukocytes and necrotic stroma. Descemetocele formation can be seen.

In cases of infectious crystalline keratopathy, multiple large colonies of bacteria are noted with little or no stromal inflammation. The local immune-compromised state in cornea facilitates the bacteria to flourish in colonies and develop a protective biofilm. In advanced cases, severe inflammation of the stroma can be seen. *Nocardia* infection has also been reported after laser refractive surgery and trauma. Histopathologically, clusters of thin branching filament-like organisms are noted in Gram-stained specimens. These organisms are acid-fast in 1% modified Ziehl-Neelson stained preparation and seen at 1000× magnification (oil immersion) [20]. The *Bacilli* are noted as bright red staining bodies. Nontuberculous mycobacteria (NTM) are noted as dense colonies within the corneal stromal pockets, or within amputated LASIK flaps in cases of Atypical mycobacterial keratitis.

Salient Points

1. Bacteria can often be confused with the uveal pigment, which are round, larger, brown colored than bacteria.
2. Bacteria must often be searched in the center of abscess and areas of injury.

Case Illustration—1

A 55-year-old female presented with gradual decreased vision in OD eye for 1 month. There was past history of phacoemulsification with intraocular lens implantation. On examination, there was a corneal epithelial defect of 3 × 2 mm with deep stromal infiltrates and circum-ciliary congestion (Fig. 10.3a). Patient was treated with ciprofloxacin 0.3% and prednisolone 1%. Therapeutic penetrating keratoplasty was done. Histopathology revealed the stromal infiltrates and (Fig. 10.3b, c) the presence of Gram-negative *Bacilli* (Fig. 10.3d).

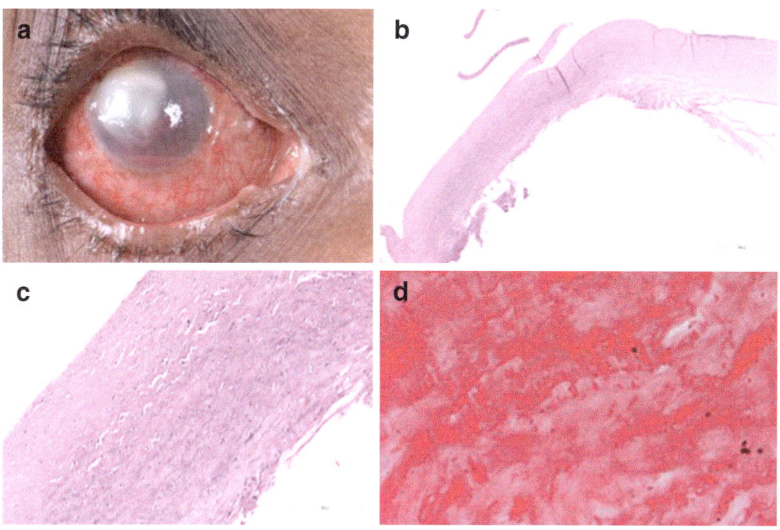

Fig. 10.3 Bacterial keratitis—(**a**) Photograph of the right eye shows corneal ulceration with large epithelial defect and deep stromal infiltrates and circumciliary congestion. (**b**) Scanner view of the excised cornea showing corneal ulceration and stromal infiltrates (Hematoxylin and eosin (H&E); 4× original magnification). (**c**) Higher magnification of the stroma showing scant-to-moderate inflammatory infiltrate with basophilic exudative debris and loss of Descemet's membrane (H&E; 15× original magnification). (**d**) Gram-negative bacteria seen in the stroma (Grams stain; ×1000)

Case Illustration—2

An 82-year-old male presented with watering and redness of OD eye for 5 days. In the past, he had visited multiple hospitals, but there was no relief. On examination, perforated corneal ulcer was seen with no light perception (Fig. 10.4a).

B scan showed diffuse low reflectivity, vitreous opacities, and membranes. Choroidal detachment was seen in all quadrants. Eviscerated contents were sent to histopathology, which should diffuse suppuration with complete stromal necrosis and anterior synechiae (Fig. 10.4b, c). Neutrophilic infiltrates forming abscess were noted in the intraocular structures (Fig. 10.4e). Gram's stain revealed Gram-positive *Bacilli* (Fig. 10.4f).

10.3.2 Fungal Keratitis

10.3.2.1 Clinical Features

The epidemiological features of fungal keratitis vary among different geographic regions and climatic conditions [21]. *Fusarium* spp. and *Aspergillus* spp. are the most common fungi isolated from patients of tropics, while *Candida albicans* is the most common pathogen of mycotic keratitis in temperate region. Trauma with plant materials, indiscriminate use of steroid, and trauma are documented as common risk factors. The onset of fungal infection of cornea is mostly insidious. In cases of keratitis due to dematiaceous fungus, brownish to black pigmentation appearance is seen.

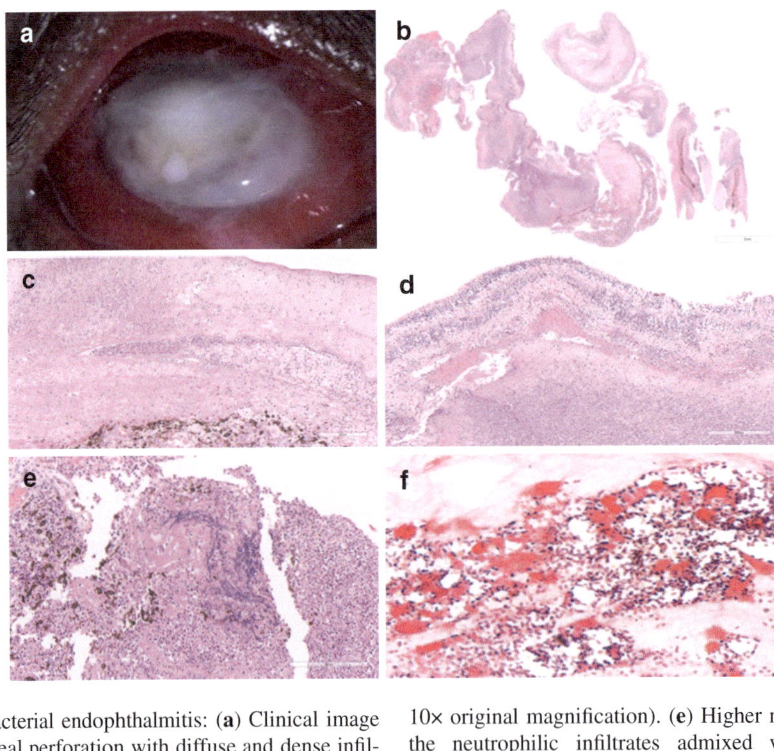

Fig. 10.4 Bacterial endophthalmitis: (**a**) Clinical image showing corneal perforation with diffuse and dense infiltrates with congested sclera. (**b**) Scanner view of the eviscerated contents (H&E; scanner view). (**c**) perforated and necrosed cornea with dense diffuse infiltrates and adherent iris tissue. (H&E; 10× original magnification). (**d**) Necrosed retina with intravitreal pyogenic abscess (H&E; 10× original magnification). (**e**) Higher magnification of the neutrophilic infiltrates admixed with basophilic stained bacterial colonies. (H&E; 20× original magnification). (**f**) Clusters and singly scattered Gram-positive *Bacilli* are noted admixed with infiltrates (Grams stain; ×1000)

10.3.2.2 Histopathology Features

Fungal keratitis mostly present with epithelial ulceration. Destruction of the Bowman's layer with fragmentation could be absent, focal, or total. The stromal inflammation is mostly suppurative with neutrophils. Depending on the duration of infection, treatment received, the extent of stromal thickness, inflammation, and necrosis varies. In the early stages, the inflammation could be in the anterior two-thirds with satellite lesions in the surrounding stroma. The posterior stroma, when affected, may show loss of stromal keratocytes due to apoptosis. Later these abscesses become confluent and lead to destruction of stroma with necrosis and perforation. In a few cases, there could be predominant deep-seated lesions along with anterior chamber exudates and hypopyon. Granulomatous reaction is seen in the posterior stroma and around Descemet's membrane, in few cases [22]. Fungus has been reported in anterior chamber exudates. It has been reported that there is a negative correlation between degree and distribution of inflammatory cells with intensity and distribution of the fungal filaments [23]. Dense carpet-like accumulation of filaments has been reported in cases of dematiaceous fungal keratitis [24]. The underlying stroma showed minimal inflammation and necrosis. Fungal hyphae appear brown colored and are often referred to as "copper penny appearance" on H&E staining.

Salient Points

Fungal hyphae usually are seen away from the infection in the case of necrotic stroma.

Case Illustration—3

A 51-year-old female complained of pain, redness, watering for 25 days in the right eye. On examination, corneal infiltrate of about 8 × 8 mm was noted with temporal limbus involvement (Fig. 10.5a). Hypopyon was about 7 mm and the intraocular pressure was raised. Patient was treated with Natamycin 5%, Ketoconazole 200 mg and taken up for penetrating keratoplasty. Histopathology showed thin, hyaline, basophilic fungal hyphae on H&E staining (Fig. 10.5b). PAS (Fig. 10.5c) and GMS (Fig. 10.5d) highlights the septate branching fungi.

Case Illustration—4

A 60-year-old male complained of pain, watering in the right eye for 1 month. On examination,

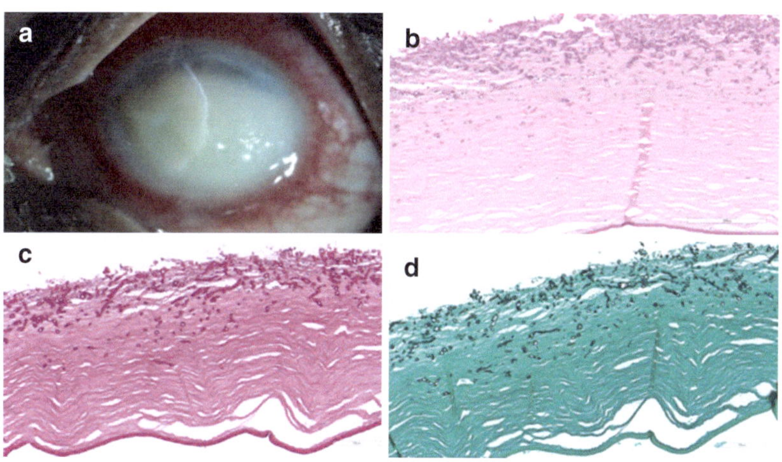

Fig. 10.5 Fungal keratitis: (**a**) Photomicrograph showing diffuse corneal infiltrates with 7 mm hypopyon and circumciliary congestion. (**b**) Histopathology of the corneal button shows ulcerated epithelium and destroyed Bowman's layer with pale acidophilic fungal hyphae in anterior stroma. (H&E; 20× original magnification). (**c**) Anterior stroma shows magenta-colored thin, hyaline, septate, acute angle branched fungal hyphae. Posterior stroma shows loss of keratocytes and mild edema. Descemet's membrane is seen with loss of keratocytes. (PAS; 10× original magnification). (**d**) Fungal hyphae are highlighted on silver stains (GMS; 20× original magnification)

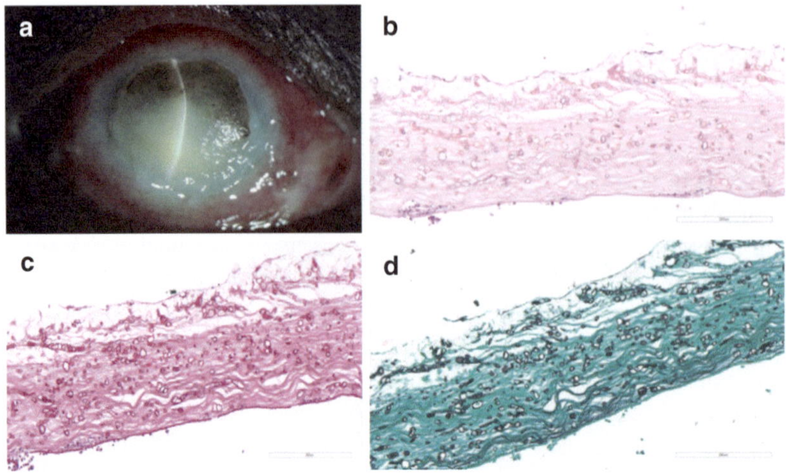

Fig. 10.6 Keratitis by dematiaceous fungi: (**a**) Photograph showing pigmented corneal ulcer. (**b**) Cornea showing ulcerated epithelium with brown pigmented fungal hyphae (PAS; 20× original magnification). (**c**) These hyphae are highlighted on PAS stain (PAS; 20× original magnification). (**d**) GMS stain (GMS; 20× original magnification)

large stromal infiltrates 7.5 × 8 mm with pigmentation were seen (Fig. 10.6a). Corneal scraping revealed fungal filaments. Therapeutic penetrating keratoplasty was performed, which revealed pigmented, septate fungi with copper-penny-like appearance suggestive of dematiaceous fungi (Fig. 10.6 b, c, d).

10.3.3 Pythium Keratitis

10.3.3.1 Clinical Features

Pythium, an oomycete, is a fungus like organism, which causes a highly morbid and infectious form of microbial keratitis. Risk factors for *Pythium* infection are agriculture- or water-related activities. The classical clinical features in *Pythium keratitis* are central deep stromal infiltrates with raised edges with peripheral guttering, which is surrounded by tentacle-like mid-to-deep stromal infiltrates surrounding the central infiltrates [25].

10.3.3.2 Histopathology Features

Histopathology shows ulceration of the epithelium with stromal destruction and varying inflammation. Like fungal keratitis, the load of *Pythium* filaments is maximum in areas where inflammation is scanty. The organisms are noted as wide filaments with admixed narrower structures. The oocyte is stained poorly to well-stained (variable) with PAS and stains well with Potassium Hydroxide-Sulfuric Acid stain [26]. In contrast, fungal filaments stain well with PAS and GMS but not with Potassium Hydroxide-Sulfuric Acid stain. The recommendation is that in a scenario of strong clinical suspicion of *Pythium*, special stains should be performed in the following order: IKI-H_2SO_4, GMS, and PAS [26]. Destaining of H&E-stained slide and restaining it with IKI-H_2SO_4 stain can also be attempted successfully in patients with low microbial load [26].

Salient Features

1. Cellulose, a complex carbohydrate, is the part of the cell wall of *Pythium*. Cellulose is oxidized by strong oxidizing agents such as chromic acid in GMS stain. Periodic acid Schiff's stain is a weak oxidizing agent. Hence, it cannot reduce cellulose.
2. IKI-H2SO4 stain can help in differentiating *Pythium* from Fungus.

Case Illustration—5

A 61-year-old female presented with severe pain, watering, and was unable to open her left eye. She had blurring of vision for distance and vision since past 1 week. There was no history of trauma. On examination, corneal ulcers measuring 6 × 7 mm with stromal infiltrates were seen (Fig. 10.7a). Patient was treated with Linezolid 0.2%, Azithromycin 500 mg and underwent therapeutic penetrating keratoplasty.

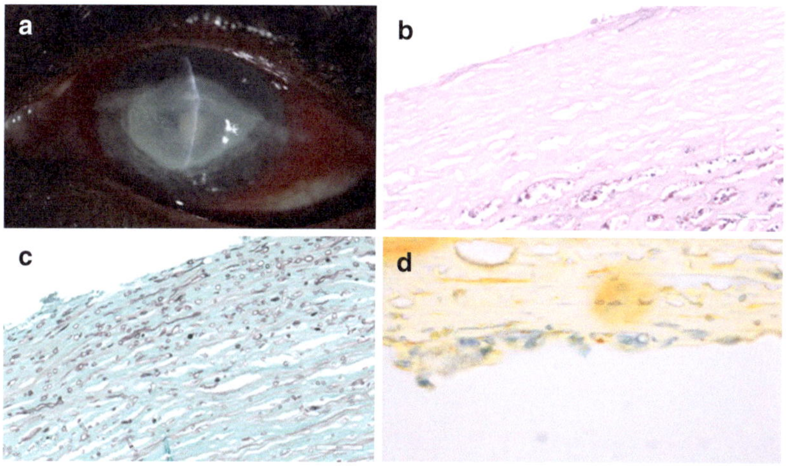

Fig. 10.7 *Pythium keratitis*: (**a**) Photograph showing corneal ulcer in left with stromal infiltrates. (**b**) Histopathology of the cornea showing ulcerated epithelium and destroyed Bowman's. Anterior stroma shows refractile, negative staining structures on per-iodic acid Schiff's stain (PAS; 20× original magnification). (**c**) These filaments are highlighted on GMS (GMS; 20× original magnification). (**d**) on Iodine–Potassium iodate sulfuric acid special stain (IKI-H2SO4; ×1000)

H&E staining showed faint, refractile filaments, which stained negative on PAS stain (Fig. 10.7b) and were highlighted as black filaments on GMS (Fig. 10.7c) and blue on Iodine Potassium iodate–H2SO4 stain (Fig. 10.7d).

10.3.4 Acanthamoeba Keratitis

10.3.4.1 Clinical Features

Although Acanthamoeba keratitis may occur after corneal trauma, particularly in rural environment [27], up to 92% cases have been reported after contact lens use [28]. The earliest signs may be micro-erosion, irregularities, opacities, or micro-cystic edema, often with patchy anterior stromal infiltrate. Radial neuritis is a pathognomonic sign for Acanthamoeba keratitis. Ring infiltrate with an overlying epithelial defect is commonly observed in cases of Acanthamoeba keratitis. Although, the epithelium is intact in early stages, in long-standing cases, a central defect, which is often associated with stromal thinning, is noted. The inflammation may involve sclera [29].

10.3.4.2 Histopathology Features

Ulceration of epithelium and destruction of Bowman's layer is seen like any other microbial keratitis. The hallmark finding in cases of Acanthamoeba keratitis is the presence of cysts as well as trophoziotes. While trophoziotes are oval to elongated basophilic structures larger than keratocytic nuclei and located within collagen lamella, the cysts are more oval, and show classic double-walled staining well with H&E or PAS and GMS. The trophozoites appear smaller than cysts in formalin fixed paraffin embedded tissues. Apart from moderate-to-severe inflammatory infiltration, granulomatous inflammation is seen. New blood vessels and apoptotic loss of keratocytes have also been reported, especially in advanced cases associated with scleritis [30, 31].

Case Illustration—6

A 33-year-old nondiabetic female presented with history of redness, pain, watering, and appearance of white spot in the right eye for 1 month duration. There was no prior history of trauma. On examination, ring infiltrate with guttering along the periphery, endothelial exudates, and

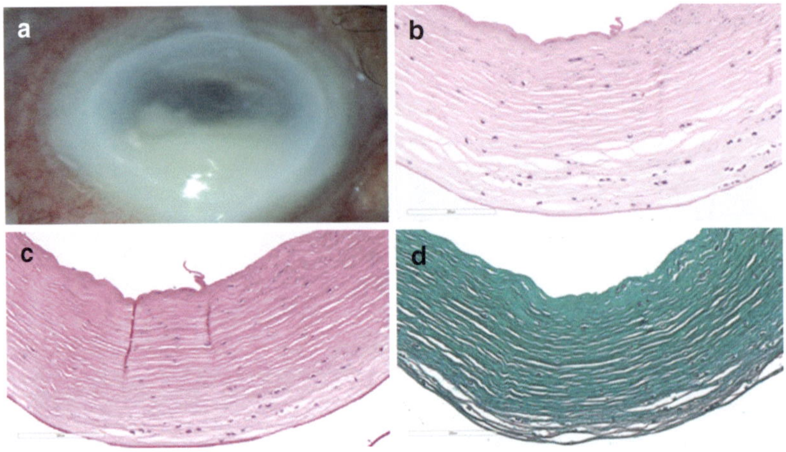

Fig. 10.8 Acanthamoeba keratitis: (**a**) Photograph showing corneal ring infiltrate with hypopyon. (**b**) Corneal stroma showing minimal inflammatory infiltrates with double-walled cysts (H&E; 20× original magnification). (**c**) These cysts are highlighted on PAS stain (PAS; 20× original magnification) and (**d**) on GMS (GMS; 20× original magnification)

4 mm hypopyon were noted (Fig. 10.8a). B scan showed low spikes and few dot echoes. Tissue adhesive and bandage contact lens were applied. Therapeutic penetrating keratoplasty was performed. The corneal button showed trophozoites and cysts in H&E (Fig. 10.8b), PAS (Fig. 10.8c) and GMS preparations (Fig. 10.8d).

10.3.5 Microsporidial Keratitis

10.3.5.1 Clinical Features

Microsporidial keratitis mostly occurs in two forms: (i) superficial keratoconjunctivitis and (ii) deep stromal keratitis. Typical clinical features of superficial keratoconjunctivitis include diffuse, multifocal, coarse, raised, punctate, round-to-oval epithelial lesion in the cornea, with or without anterior chamber reaction. It is usually associated with mild-to-moderate conjunctival congestion. Microsporidial stromal keratitis could mimic suppurative or nonsuppurative inflammation and vascularization of cornea. The durations of symptoms range from few months to years [32].

10.3.5.2 Histopathology Features

Epithelial ulceration, destruction of Bowman's membrane, diffuse stromal necrosis, and neutrophilic infiltrate were seen. Microsporidial spores are described as oval or rounded with a band-like horizontal girdle. Several stains have been used to easily delineate the spores such as Calcofluor White (CFW) with 10% Potassium Hydroxide, GMS, 1% Acid-Fast stain, and Masson's Trichrome stain [33]. Microsporidial spores are inter-lamellar in location and appear as small, oval, refractile, and can be stained with 1% acid-fast stain and stain with Kinyoun stain. Rarely, the spores can be found to traverse the Descemet's membrane and reach the anterior chamber and found in the exudates [34]. Granulomatous reaction has been reported in cases with coexisting HSV infection [35].

Case Illustration—7

A 32-year-old male complained of blurring of vision in right eye associated with redness, pain, and burning sensation since the past one and half years. There was no prior history of injury. On examination, 4.5 × 5.5 mm mid stromal infiltrates were noted with multiple keratic precipitates (Fig. 10.9a). Patient underwent therapeutic penetrating keratoplasty. Histopathology revealed diffuse infiltration in posterior stroma (Fig. 10.9b) and microsporidial spores, which are oval, refractile bodies noted in H&E (Fig. 10.9c), PAS

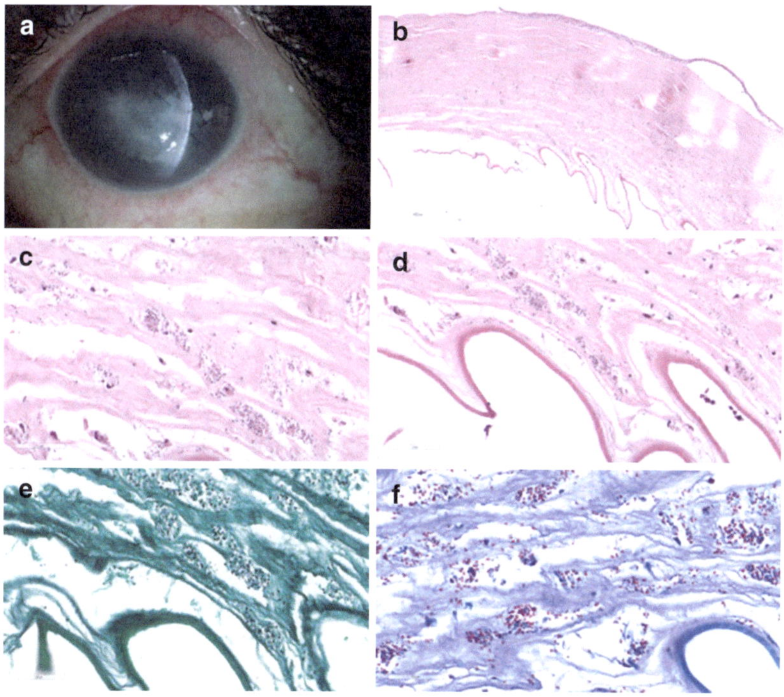

Fig. 10.9 Microsporidial keratitis: (**a**) Photograph shows cornea with stromal infiltrates and sutures placed post corneal scrapping. (**b**) Scanner view of the cornea showing edema and superficial blebs (H&E; scanner view). (**c**) Stromal inter-lamellar clefts show oval, refractile structures in the background of stromal edema (H&E; 30× original magnification). (**d**) refractile organisms are reaching up to Descemet's membrane (H&E; 30× original magnification). (**e**) These structures are highlighted on GMS (GMS; 40× original magnification) and (**f**) are 1% acid-fast (Kinyoun stain; 40× original magnification)

(Fig. 10.9d), GMS (Fig. 10.9e), and Kinyoun stain (Fig. 10.9f).

10.3.6 Viral Keratitis

10.3.6.1 Clinical Features

Herpes simplex virus (HSV) 1, 2 are known to cause keratitis. The clinical spectrum is dendritic ulcer, necrotizing stromal keratitis, immune stromal keratitis, viral endotheliitis, and keratouveitis [36]. Scarring and vascularization are commonly noted clinically. Direct invasion, replicating virus, and severe host inflammatory response lead to destruction of stroma in cases of necrotizing stromal keratitis (NSK). Immune stromal keratitis is predominantly immune mediated.

10.3.6.2 Histopathology Features

Corneal scraping might reveal the characteristic Cowdry "A" type of inclusions in the epithelial cells. On cytopathology, triad of nuclear crowding, nuclear moulding, and intranuclear inclusions is the classic feature for identification of viral infection. The epithelium may show ulceration in cases of NSK. There are neutrophilic infiltrates in stroma and can be either diffuse or focal. Viral etiology includes mononuclear infiltrates, multinucleate giant cells (MNG), and inclusion bodies in the epithelial cells, rarely in deep stroma. In some cases, stromal loss and necrosis with descemetocele formation or perforation with giant cell reaction around Descemet's membrane have been observed. In other cases, especially chronic or recurrent cases, a prominent feature noted is vascularization progressing toward the site of active inflammation. The antigen has been isolated from epithelial cells, keratocytes (less often), and in the MNG and the endothelial cells.

The epithelium is usually intact with minimal inflammation in cases of Immune stromal keratitis. Inflammation is of varying degree, which could be focal, multifocal, or diffuse, associated with stromal edema. Neovascularization with multiple fronds of vessels or ghost vessels with perivascular cuffing is a common feature. Other features suggestive of its chronicity are ingrowth of pannus, fragmented Bowman's layer, lipid keratopathy, stromal scarring, myofibroblast, granulomatous reaction around DM, and duplication of DM.

Case Illustration—8

A 74-year-old male presented with gradual vision loss for distance and near in left eye since 2 months. On examination, dense corneal scarring with vascularization and lipid deposit in mid stromal region (Fig. 10.10a) and dendritic pattern of epithelial defect was seen on fluorescent dye (Fig. 10.10b). Posterior temporal stromal scar was noted. Patient was treated with Aciclovir 3%. Histopathology revealed corneal button with hyperplastic epithelium and solid implantation of epithelium. Stroma showed scarred and vascularization (Fig. 10.10c).

Case Illustration—9

A 72-year-old male diagnosed case of HSV keratitis with endotheliitis presented with complaints of pain, redness, and watering of right eye for 15 days. On examination, perforated ulcer was seen at 7 o clock with iris plugging and surrounding infiltrate with inferior cornea vascularization (Fig. 10.11a, b). Penetrating keratoplasty was done. Histopathology showed para-centrally thinned-out cornea (Fig. 10.11c) with incarceration of Iris and fragmented Descemet's membrane with multinucleate giant cell reaction (Fig. 10.11d).

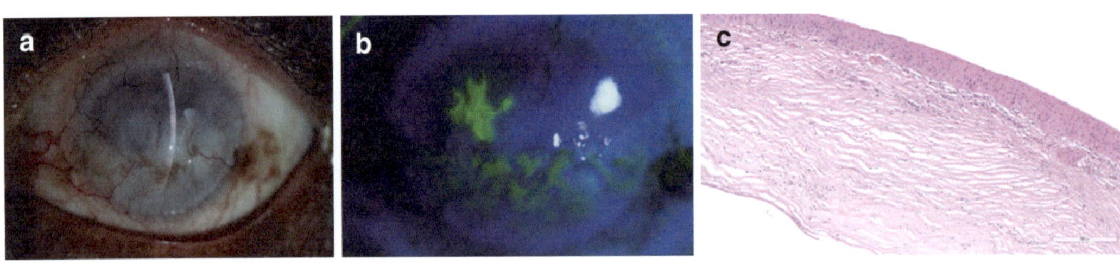

Fig. 10.10 Chronic viral stromal keratitis: (**a**) Photograph shows diffusely scarred and vascularized cornea. (**b**) Dendritic ulcer on fluorescent dye. (**c**) Cornea showing hyperplastic epithelium with scarring and vascularization in the stroma (H&E; 20× original magnification)

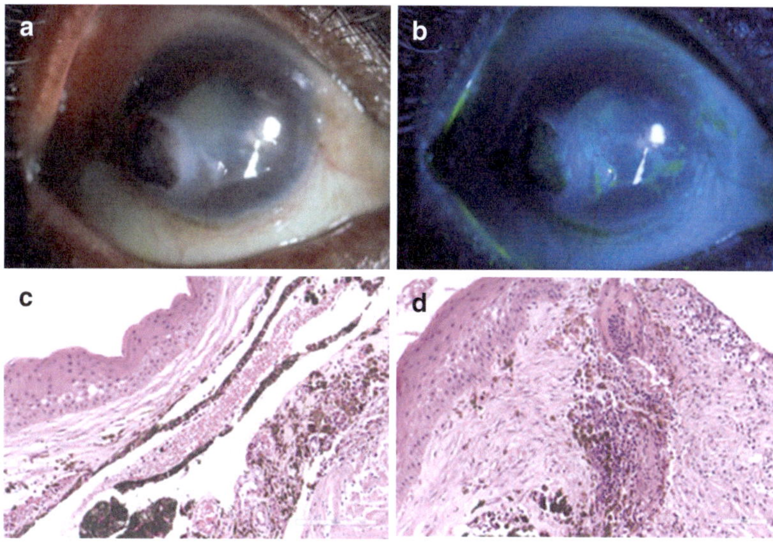

Fig. 10.11 Necrotizing viral stromal keratitis: (**a**) Photomicrograph showing perforated corneal ulcer with Iris plugging. (**b**) Ill-defined margins of the ulcer on the fluorescent dye. (**c**) Corneal thinning with hyperplastic epithelium and anterior synechiae (H&E; 20× original magnification). (**d**) Fragmented Descemet's membrane with adjacent granulomatous inflammation and multinucleated giant cell (H&E; 20× original magnification)

10.4 Corneal Dystrophies

Corneal dystrophies are defined as bilateral, symmetrical, inherited, slowly progressive corneal disorders, usually not associated with systemic diseases and not related to environmental exposure (although secondary changes can be noted in late stages). Table 10.1 shows the differences between dystrophy and degeneration. The first International Classification Committee of corneal Dystrophy IC3D provided a consensus classification in 2008, which was based on the five layers of cornea [37]. Subsequent revision excluded the acellular Bowman's and Descemet's membrane (DM) [38]. Table 10.2 shows the current classification of corneal dystrophies and their categories. The categorization was based on the identification of chromosome and mapping of the gene [39]. Some dystrophies are reported in more than one category as they may have degenerative features, may be unilateral or have systemic associations. Some dystrophies may not progress at all.

Table 10.1 Differences between dystrophy and degeneration

Corneal dystrophy	Corneal degeneration
Bilateral	Unilateral.
Inherited	Not inherited.
Very gradually progressive	Stable.
No vascularization unless other events	Vascularization is often present.
Primary changes not influenced by environment	Occurs due to environmental factors.
No systemic disease (usually)	Systemic disease.

Description of the Dystrophies

The histological, immuno-histological, and ultrastructural changes observed in corneal dystrophies have been described earlier by this group [36]. The findings of confocal microscopy (CM) and spectral domain anterior segment optical coherence tomography (AS-OCT) may help us to understand the corneal dystrophy and diagnose those similar to histopathological studies [40]. In this section, we describe the histopathological findings of dystrophy and correlate them with the diagnostic investigations. The features are described in a tabular form under the following headings: light microscopy (LM), electron microscopy (EM), immunohistochemical (IHC) and other studies, and the findings on anterior segment imaging using the OCT and CM.

Table 10.2 The IC3D Classification of dystrophies based on the anatomy of cornea and evidence-based category

Category 1	Category 2	Category 3	Category 4
Epithelial and subepithelial dystrophies			
Epithelial basement membrane dystrophy (EBMD) majority degenerative, rarely	Lisch epithelial corneal dystrophy (LECD)	Epithelial recurrent erosion dystrophies (EREDs)	Subepithelial mucinous corneal dystrophy (SMCD)
Meesmann corneal dystrophy (MECD)		Franceschetti corneal dystrophy (FRCD)	
Gelatinous drop-like corneal dystrophy (GDLD)		Dystrophia helsinglandica (DH)	
		Dystrophia smolandiensis (DS)	
Epithelial–stromal TGFBI dystrophies			
Reis–Bücklers corneal dystrophy (RBCD)			
Thiel-Behnke corneal dystrophy (TBCD)			
Lattice corneal dystrophy, type 1 (LCD1)—variants (III, IIIA, I/IIIA, IV) of lattice corneal dystrophy			
Granular corneal dystrophy, type 1 (GCD1)			
Granular corneal dystrophy, type 2 (GCD2)			
Stromal dystrophies			
Macular corneal dystrophy (MCD)			Central cloudy dystrophy of François (CCDF)
Schnyder corneal dystrophy (SCD)			
Congenital stromal corneal dystrophy (CSCD)			
Fleck corneal dystrophy (FCD)			
Posterior amorphous corneal dystrophy (PACD)			
Pre-Descemet corneal dystrophy (PDCD)			Pre-Descemet corneal dystrophy (PDCD
Endothelial dystrophies			
Fuchs endothelial corneal dystrophy (FECD)	Fuchs endothelial corneal dystrophy (FECD)	Fuchs endothelial corneal dystrophy (FECD)	
Congenital hereditary endothelial dystrophy (CHED)			
Posterior polymorphous corneal dystrophy (PPCD)	Posterior polymorphous corneal dystrophy (PPCD)		
	X-linked endothelial corneal dystrophy (XECD)		
Removed dystrophies			
			Grayson-Wilbrandt corneal dystrophy (GWCD)

Category 1: the gene is mapped and identified; the specific mutations known
Category 2: the gene is not mapped but chromosome locus known
Category 3: not mapped to chromosome locus
Category 4: no convincing evidence available at present

10.4.1 Epithelial and Subepithelial Dystrophy

Table 10.3 shows the histopathological and investigative findings of the dystrophy

(i) Epithelial basement membrane dystrophy (EBMD) (Map-dot-fingerprint dystrophy, Map, dot, fingerprint, bleb disease): It is the most common corneal dystrophy, with incomplete or affected epithelial-basement membrane complex. Guerry's lines and Cogan's dots in epithelium are visible.

(ii) Meesmann Corneal Dystrophy (MECD) (Juvenile hereditary epithelial dystrophy): This is autosomal-dominant dystrophy and has a known variant (Stocker–Holt dystrophy). The onset is in early childhood with presence of corneal erosions in some cases. Multiple small, clear transparent cysts in the interpalpebral areas are seen on slit-lamp biomicroscopy.

(iii) Gelatinous Drop-Like Corneal Dystrophy (GDLD): (Fig. 10.12a) These present as mulberry-like opacities in the subepithelium and anterior stroma and are known to recur in 100% of cases after surgery. Degenerative changes are also frequently reported with this dystrophy. Histopathological findings include amorphous deposits located in the anterior stroma (Fig. 10.12b), which stain with Congo red (Fig. 10.12c, d)

(iv) Franceschetti corneal dystrophy (FRCD): Recurrent erosions are reported early in life and the severity decreases in adult life [41].

(v) Dystrophia Helsinglandica (DH): Corneal erosions are reported in this autosomal-dominant dystrophy and may last for 1–10 days. Seen early in life, the severity and the frequency of recurrent erosions reduce with age. Subepithelial fibrosis and gelatinous superficial elevations are reported without any/mild visual acuity affectation.

(vi) Subepithelial mucinous corneal dystrophy (SMCD): Recurrent corneal erosions are more common in the first decade of life and gradually subside as the patient ages. Subepithelial haze is more prominent in the central cornea rather than the peripheral cornea and may result in reduced vision [42]. The clinical picture of this dystrophy is similar to the Grayson-Wilbrandt corneal dystrophy (GWCD) (removed from the classification now), but it is different histochemically [42].

10.4.2 Epithelial–Stromal TGFBI Dystrophies [40]

These are all autosomal dominant and usually seen early in life. Recurrent corneal erosions are common in all of these (Table 10.4)

(i) Reis–Bücklers corneal dystrophy (RBCD): Opacities are noted in the superficial stroma and Bowman layer and extend up to the limbus. These opacities have clear areas in between to begin with and then spread up to limbus. The vision is reduced early in childhood, and recurrent corneal erosions are common.

(ii) Thiel-Behnke corneal dystrophy (TBCD): It is characterized by symmetrical, subepithelial honeycomb opacities in the central cornea. Recurrent corneal erosions result in the deterioration of vision.

(iii) Lattice corneal dystrophy, type 1 (LCD1): Variants such as III, IIIA, I/IIIA, IV have been reported. Initially, the superficial stroma shows the presence of fleck-like opacities in the center with dark lines. Later, diffuse subepithelial ground-glass haze and lattice lines are visible in the entire cornea (Fig. 10.13a, b). Vision is reduced because of the involvement of the central cornea. Histopathologically, these deposits are identified better by Congo red stain (Fig. 10.13c, b).

(iv) Granular corneal dystrophy, type 1 (GCD1): Deposition of granules in the superficial layers initially with clear areas in between and sparing the limbus is the hallmark of GCD1. The granules may appear as snowflakes or breadcrumbs (Fig. 10.14a, b, c).

Table 10.3 Histopathological and investigative findings in epithelial and subepithelial dystrophies

Dystrophy	Light microscopy	Transmission electron microscopy	Immunofluorescence Analysis	Immunohistochemical studies	AS OCT	Confocal microscopy
1. Epithelial basement membrane dystrophy (EBMD)	Basement membrane encroaches the epithelium; cysts contain cellular debris and pyknotic nucleus, PAS positive	Fine granular, friable basement membrane			Thickened basement membrane in the epithelium. Hyperreflective dots are seen. The epithelial detachment appears has a stair-step appearance in the epithelium [73].	Highly reflective due to the abnormal basement membrane and also the epithelium.
2. Meesman's dystrophy	Intraepithelial cysts filled with PAS- positive degenerative material—autofluoresces in ultraviolet light. The negatively charged substances such as glycosaminoglycans stain with the Hale colloidal iron technique	Intracytoplasmic "peculiar substance" +				Cysts are hyporeflective and the peculiar substance is reflective [4, 5].
3. Gelatinous drop-like corneal dystrophy	Subepithelial amyloid stains brick red with Congo red stain—seen as nodules or sheet in the anterior stroma		Lactoferrin is expressed in amyloid.	Sub epithelial amyloid stains for anti-apolipoprotein J and antibodies to lactoferrin.		Amyloid is noted in epithelial cells and anterior stroma.
4. Lisch epithelial corneal dystrophy (LECD)	Presence of diffuse cytoplasmic vacuolization, PAS-positive material is noted	Electron-dense whorled inclusions within the entire epithelium			Epithelium is of normal thickness hyperreflective stroma is quite normal, borders sharp [74].	The typical intracytoplasmatic vacuolization of the involved epithelial cells [75]

5. Epithelial recurrent erosion dystrophies (EREDs)—						
6. Franceschetti corneal dystrophy (FRCD)	Irregular enlarged deposits in basal epithelium—both intracellular and intercellular, subepithelial, avascular pannus Negative staining with Congo red [37].	Irregular shape and size of basal epithelial cells, with large intercellular clefts due to presence of Alcian blue-positive deposits.			Hyperreflective and thickened epithelium [4].	Dcorin expression increased and claudin and E-cadherin expression decreased.
7. Subepithelial mucinous corneal dystrophy (SMCD)	PAS positive, Alcian blue positive, material present below epithelium	Subepithelial deposition of glycosaminoglycan		Chondroitin-4-sulfate + dermatan sulfate.		

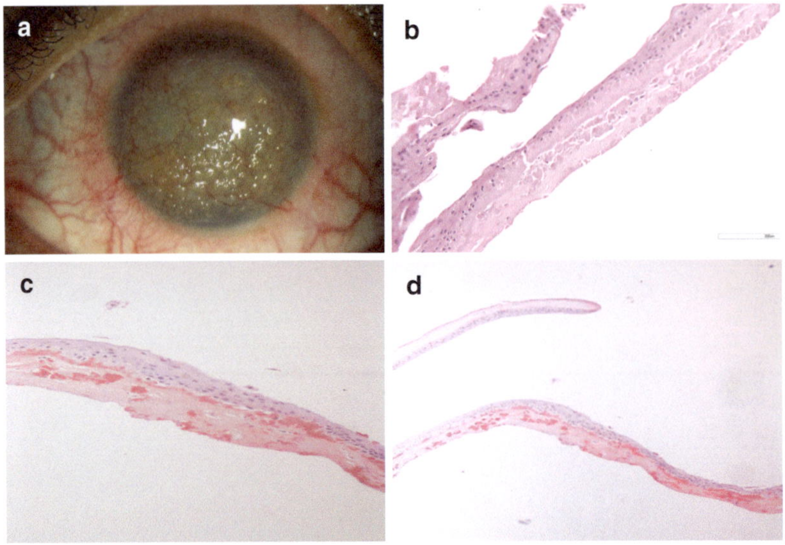

Fig. 10.12 Gelatinous drop-like corneal dystrophy: (**a**) Clinical photograph shows elevated nodular opacities with stromal scarring and vascularization, seen in advanced stages of gelatinous drop-like corneal dystrophy. (**b**) Specimens from lamellar keratectomy show hyperplastic epithelium of variable thickness and deposits of amorphous material in subepithelial and anterior stromal region. (H&E; 10× original magnification). (**c, d**) These deposits stain bright red with Congo stain

Homozygotes have more severe manifestations. The patients present with glare and photophobia, and as the opacities increase, visual acuity decreases. Histopathologically, these deposits stain with Masson's trichrome stain (Fig. 10.14d, e, f).

(v) Granular corneal dystrophy, type 2 (GCD2) Avellino dystrophy: This is considered a combination of GCD1 and lattice lines with presence of dots and lattice-like lines giving it a moth-eaten appearance. The appearance may be translucent on retro-illumination. The lattice lines or dashes are whiter and rarely cross each other as against the refractile lines of lattice dystrophy, which cross each other. With recurrent corneal erosions, and the formation of the scar in visual axis, the vision reduces. It is slowly progressive; however, these dystrophies recur when a patient undergoes procedures such as laser-assisted in situ keratomileusis (LASIK).

10.4.3 Stromal Dystrophies (Table 10.5) [40]

(i) Macular corneal dystrophy (MCD): It is autosomal recessive characterized by the presence of flake-like opacities in the entire cornea with no clear areas (Fig. 10.15a, b) in between and up to the limbus along with the involvement of Descemet's membrane (DM) and endothelium (Fig. 10.15c), picked up on histopathology with Alcian blue stain (Fig. 10.15d). The cornea, despite the presence of deposits, is thinner than normal. Visual acuity is reduced in these patients.

(ii) Schnyder's corneal dystrophy (SCD): It is autosomal dominant and may be seen in childhood, but the diagnosis is usually delayed and more so when patients do not have crystalline deposits, which is in 50% of cases. The clinical features vary according to the age with ring-like or disc-like

Table 10.4 Histopathological and investigative findings of epithelial–stromal TGFBI dystrophies

Dystrophy	Light microscopy	Transmission electron microscopy	Immunofluorescence analysis	Immunohistochemical studies	AS OCT	Confocal microscopy
1. Reis–Bücklers corneal dystrophy (RBCD)	Masson trichrome–red positive deposits in Bowman layer extending into subepithelium up to posterior stroma.	Presence of rod-shaped bodies in subepithelium.		Rod-shaped bodies—positive for kerato-epithelin	Hyperreflective deposits with serrated anterior border at Bowman layer and anterior stroma level. Thicker in the center	High-reflective deposits in supra-basal level, no shadows seen. High-reflective material in Bowman's layer and more deposits in the anterior.
2. Thiel-Behnke corneal dystrophy (TBCD)	Irregular thickening of epithelium to make the surface smooth. Bowman layer has sawtooth appearance.	Presence of curly collagen fibers.		Curly fibers are immune–positive for kerato-epithelin	Prominent hyperreflective sawtooth pattern involving Bowman layer and epithelium	Distinct deposits with shadowing visible.
3. Lattice corneal dystrophy, type 1 (LCD1) — variants (III, IIIA, I/IIIA, IV) of lattice corneal dystrophy	Amyloid deposits in all layers of cornea that stain positive with Congo red	Extracellular amyloid, few keratocytes in the area of amyloid.				Linear branching lines in the stroma.
4. Granular corneal dystrophy, type 1 (GCD1)	Multiple deposits in all layers of cornea, which are positive for Masson trichrome stain.	Dense rod-shaped bodies.		Positive for kerato-epithelin		Abnormal hyperreflective opacities in various shapes.
5. Granular corneal dystrophy, type 2 (GCD2)	Staining is positive with Mason Trichome and/or Congo red stain of deposits—in epithelium and stroma luxol fast blue +	Rod-shaped electron-dense deposits and amyloid fibrils.				Reflective dots and lines are visible.

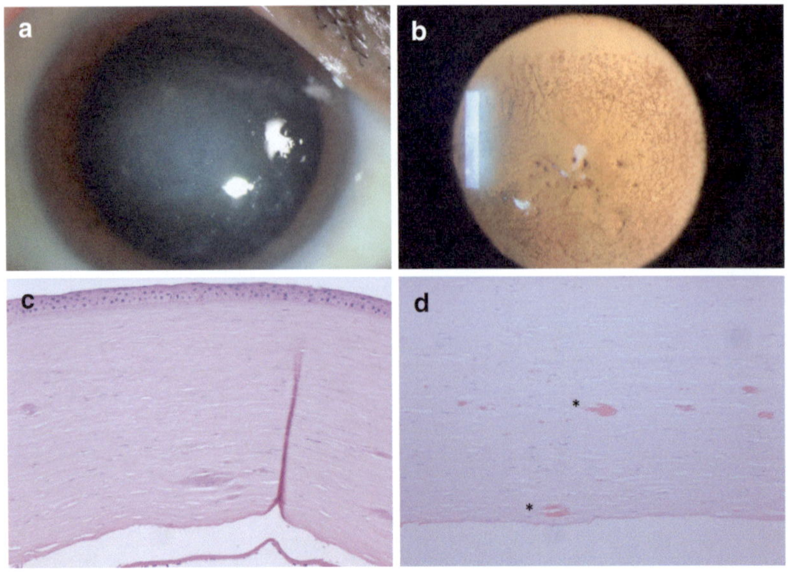

Fig. 10.13 Lattice corneal dystrophy: (**a**) Clinical photograph showing diffuse corneal opacification (ground-glass appearance). (**b**) The lattice lines are prominent on retro-illumination. (**c**) Fusiform deposits are noted in the stroma (H&E; 20× original magnification). (**d**) These deposits are stain pink with Congo red stain (asterisk) (20× original magnification)

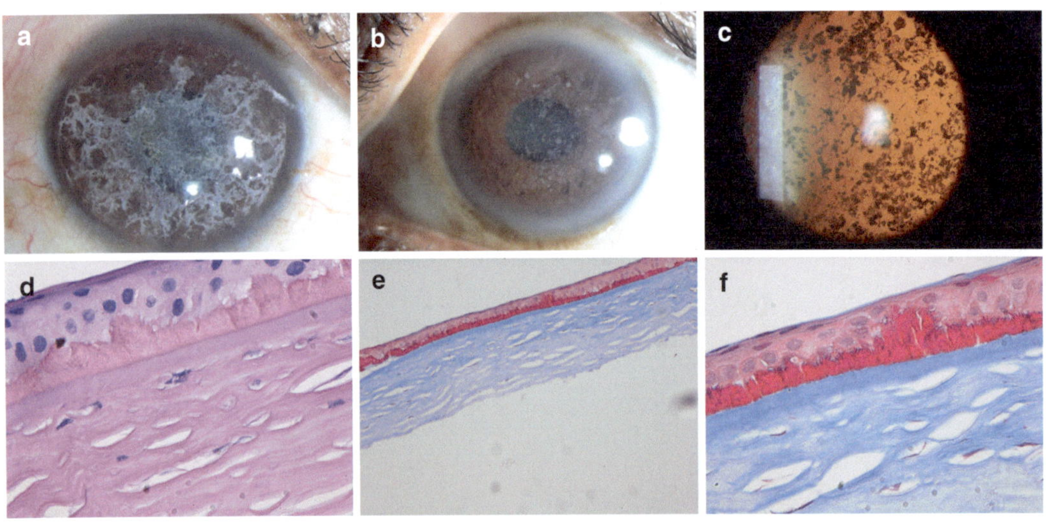

Fig. 10.14 Granular corneal dystrophy: (**a**) Diffuse photograph shows whitish opacities located predominantly in anterior stroma, with clearer intervening areas. (**b**) Snowflake- or bread-crumb-like opacities with clear intervening spaces. (**c**) Retro-illumination captures the opacities located in mid and posterior stroma. (**d**) Histopathologic button of a case of superficial variant of granular dystrophy shows eosinophilic deposits located at the level of the basement membrane (H&E; 20× original magnification), which stain prominently with Masson's trichrome stain (**e**) 10× original magnification and (**f**) 40× original magnification

Table 10.5 Histopathological and investigative findings of stromal dystrophies

Dystrophy	Light microscopy	Transmission electron microscopy	Immunofluorescence analysis	Immunohistochemical studies	AS OCT	Confocal microscopy
1. Macular corneal dystrophy (MCD) C1	All layers of cornea including DM and endothelium involved with glycosaminoglycans (GAGs) stain positive with Hale colloidal iron or Alcian blue.	GAGs are noted throughout cornea.		MCD type I: No keratin sulfate reactivity in the cornea or in the serum. MCD type IA: keratin sulfate reactivity in keratocytes. No activity in serum and extracellular matrix. MCD type II: Serum level normal or low. All deposits show activity.	Hyperreflectivity throughout the entire cornea	Highly reflective deposits in all layers and keratocytes may not be visible.
2. Schnyder corneal dystrophy (SCD) C1	Abnormal deposition of phospholipids and cholesterol in all layers of cornea. Lipids: Positive Congo red staining and Alcian blue.	Deposits in all layers of cornea.				Highly reflective deposits in all layers of cornea
3. Congenital stromal corneal dystrophy (CSCD) C2	The stromal lamellae is thin and stroma contains amorphous material.	Amorphous areas with decorin present. Endothelium is normal.			Increased corneal thickness.	Epithelium is normal with increased reflectivity from stromal surface.
4. Fleck corneal dystrophy (FCD) C2	Keratocytes contain GAGs and are swollen and vacuolated. Positive for Alcian blue and colloidal iron (GAG) and Sudan black and Oil Red O+ (lipid).	Membrane-based inclusion bodies in keratocytes.			Brighter reflections from flecks	Hyperreflective dot-like material in keratocytes with kidney-shaped inclusions in basal nerves

(continued)

Table 10.5 (continued)

Dystrophy	Light microscopy	Transmission electron microscopy	Immunofluorescence analysis	Immunohistochemical studies	AS OCT	Confocal microscopy
5. Posterior amorphous corneal dystrophy (PACD) C2	Colloidal iron staining + in posterior stroma Thin DM and loss of endothelial cells	Abnormal collagen fibrils and keratocytes.				Hyperreflective posterior stroma with microfolds
6. Pre-Descemet corneal dystrophy (PDCD) C1 or C5	Usually, normal cornea; presence of enlarged keratocytes with vacuoles and intracytoplasmic lipid-like inclusions in the posterior stroma.	Lipofuscin-like lipoprotein, no extracellular deposits.				Hyperreflective dots at the level of DM
7. Central cloudy dystrophy of François (CCDF) C5	Positive staining for GAGs; staining for acid mucopolysaccharidosis.	Fibrillogranular electron-dense deposits in extracellular vacuoles, sawtooth lamellar pattern of the endothelium.				Highly refractile deposits with dark striae in between present in the anterior stroma.

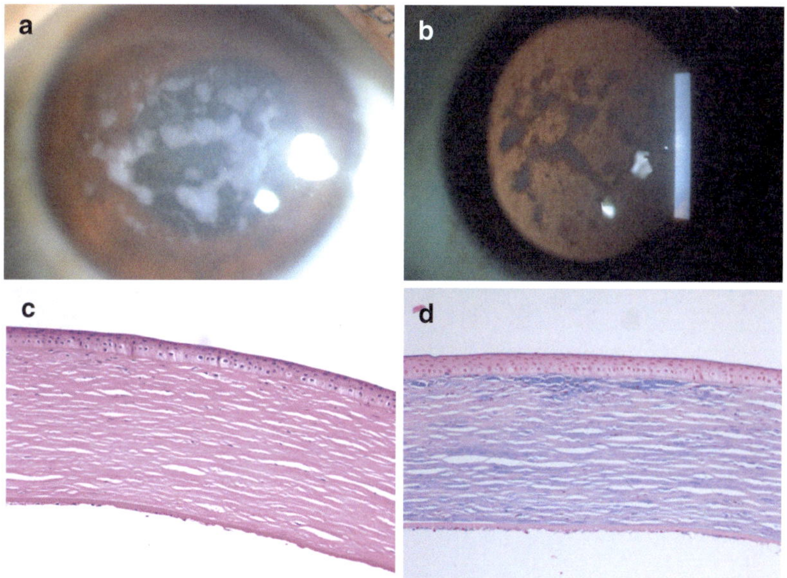

Fig. 10.15 Macular corneal dystrophy: (**a**) Diffuse photograph shows large multiple opacities without clear intervening stroma. (**b**) Retro-illumination captures these dense opacities located in mid and posterior stroma. (**c**) Diffuse deposits are noted throughout the stroma (PAS; 20× original magnification) (**d**) These deposits stain blue with Alcian Blue stain. Note the infiltration of endothelial cells with the deposits (20× original magnification)

opacities to begin with in young adults. Arcus develops later on, and, subsequently, entire cornea becomes hazy. Vision may be reduced during day time, and patient may have photophobia. Hyperlipoproteinemia is reported in these patients

(iii) Congenital Stromal Corneal Dystrophy (CSCD): It is an autosomal-dominant dystrophy present at birth. The opacities are flake-like whitish deposits and the cornea appears thickened but with a smooth corneal surface. There is gradual vision loss in these patients, and the dystrophy usually remains stable.

(iv) Fleck corneal dystrophy (FCD): It is autosomal-dominant, nonprogressive dystrophy with onset in early life. As the name suggests, dandruff-like flecks are seen throughout the stroma up to limbus. The other layers of cornea are not involved. The patients are usually asymptomatic.

(v) Posterior amorphous corneal dystrophy (PACD): It is autosomal dominant and occurs early in life. Diffuse gray-white sheet-like opacities are seen prominently in posterior stroma. Transparent stromal breaks may be noted. Flattening of the cornea, hyperopia, and reduced corneal thickness are characteristic of this dystrophy. Focal endothelial abnormalities may be seen. Presence of other signs such as iris strands, corectopia, and prominent Schwalbe's line indicates it to be a mesodermal dysgenesis.

(vi) Pre-Descemet corneal dystrophy (PDCD): Although familial, there is no defined pattern of inheritance. Many subgroups are described and may represent secondary degenerative changes. There are grayish-white opacities just anterior to the DM as the name suggests and may be focal or diffuse, central, or annular. Usually, these are nonprogressive with stable vision.

(vii) Central cloudy dystrophy of François (CCDF): It is autosomal-dominant, nonprogressive, and mimics posterior crocodile shagreen degeneration of the cornea. The opacities are dense posteriorly and fade anteriorly with a clear cornea around it. Vision is usually not affected.

10.4.4 Endothelial Dystrophies (Table 10.6) [40]

(i) Fuchs endothelial corneal dystrophy (FECD): Usually autosomal dominant; however, cases without a known inheri-

Table 10.6 Histopathological and investigative findings in endothelial dystrophies

Dystrophy	Light microscopy	Transmission electron microscopy	Immunofluorescence Analysis	Immunohistochemical studies	AS OCT	Confocal microscopy
Fuchs endothelial corneal dystrophy (FECD)	Thickened Descemet's membrane, presence of guttae on endothelium, which are reduced in numbers	Thickened anterior banded zone in early onset disease with stromal thickening, Posterior nonbanded zone thickens when occurs late				Polymegethism, pleomorphism, decreased hexagonality, and reduced number of endothelial cells
Congenital hereditary endothelial dystrophy (CHED)	Diffuse epithelial and stromal edema with thickening	Stromal thickening with disrupted lamella. Presence of basement membrane–like material on the Descemet's membrane.		Collagen present within posteriorDescemet's membrane		
Posterior polymorphous corneal dystrophy (PPCD) C1 or C3	Nodular excrescences on Descemet's membrane	Presence of epithelial microstructures on DM		Positive with anti-CK7, CK8, CK18, and CK19 antibodies	Rail-road track sign epithelial-like cells on endothelium with	Polymegethism of endothelial cells

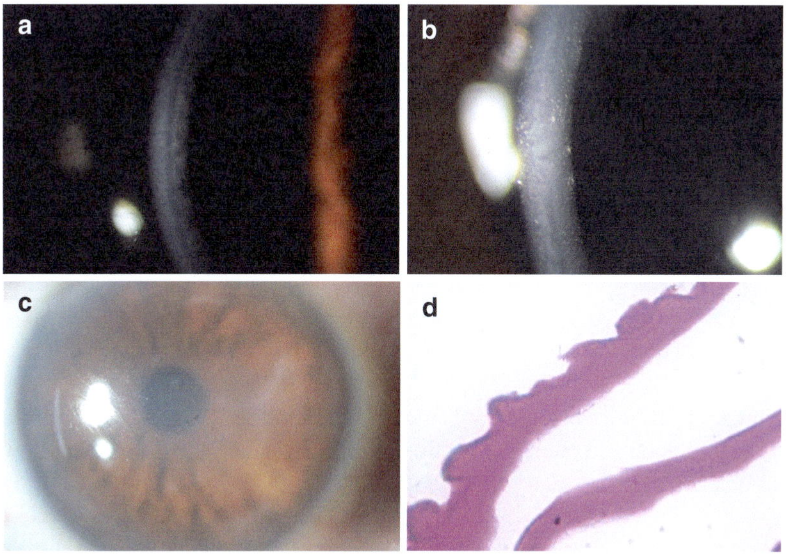

Fig. 10.16 Fuch's endothelial dystrophy: (**a**) Clinical photograph in slit illumination shows guttata. (**b**) These guttata become prominent as the disease progresses and take a "beaten-metal" appearance. (**c**) In later stages, endothelial decompensation leads to presence of stroma edema. (**d**) Specimen from endothelial keratoplasty shows thickened Descemet's membrane with prominent guttata (PAS stain, 40× original magnification)

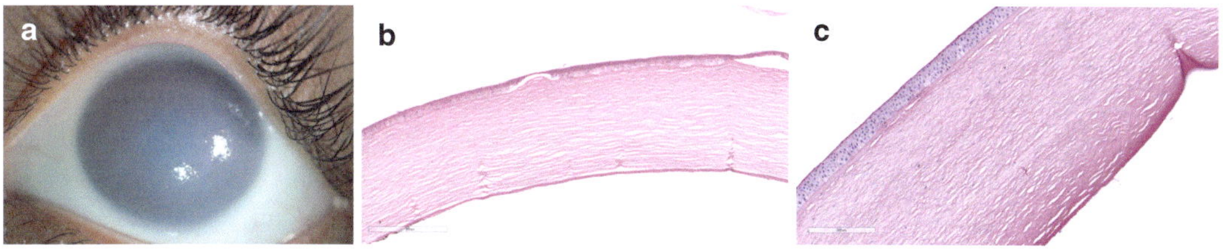

Fig. 10.17 CHED: (**a**) Case of congenital hereditary endothelial dystrophy. Note the corneal clouding due to severe edema. (**b**) Histopathology shows epithelial hypertrophy and edema, dense stromal edema, and thickening (H&E; 10× original magnification), and (**c**) prominently thickened DM, which is seen better on PAS (10× original magnification)

tance are reported too. The condition becomes symptomatic later in life. Presence of cornea guttata (Fig. 10.16a) is the hallmark. Late-onset FECD will have larger guttae (Fig. 10.16b). Guttae may remain stable or progress causing edema. DM is thickened. Stromal edema occurs (Fig. 10.16d), and persistent or worsening of that leads to formation of bullae and bullous keratopathy and subsequently subepithelial fibrosis. Visual acuity is worst in the morning in the early stage, as the cornea swells due to overnight closure of the lids and reduced oxygenation. Formation of bullae may occur, which, on rupture, may cause pain, photophobia, and watering of eyes. As the disease progresses, vision reduces with edema. Histopathological changes show the presence of excrescences and thickening of the Descemet's membrane, more prominent on PAS stain (Fig. 10.16d).

(ii) Congenital hereditary endothelial dystrophy (CHED): It is an autosomal recessive occurring early in life, at birth. There is corneal clouding and thickening of cornea (Fig. 10.17a, b, c), and sometimes, this is confused with congenital glaucoma.

(iii) Posterior polymorphous corneal dystrophy (PPCD): It is autosomal dominant, with opacities at the level of DM and endothelium. Flakes appear on endothelium. Patients may have steepening of cornea with or without keratoconus. Corneal edema, high pressures are known to occur but in later part of life.

10.5 Corneal Ectasias

The noninflammatory ectatic disorders of the cornea include keratoglobus, keratoconus, pellucid marginal degeneration, and posterior keratoconus.

The hallmark of these conditions is corneal thinning [43], but the location of maximal thinning differs, which helps in differentiating the different entities [44].

Distortion in the architecture of the anterior corneal curvature can affect visual acuity variably ranging from mild to severe reduction. Corneal topography and tomography are useful in diagnosing this condition objectively much before they become evident on clinical examination [45]. Usually early in onset (2nd decade) and progressive in nature, these conditions can cause mild-to-severe decrease in vision. In the initial stages, glasses or contact lenses can be useful. The management involves strategies to prevent progression, which includes corneal collagen cross-linking [46] as well as visual improvement by various means, especially contact lenses [47, 48]. Advanced stages need surgical management such as corneal transplantation [49].

The four conditions are discussed below, and the key differentiating features are represented in Table 10.7.

10.5.1 Keratoconus

It is the most common noninflammatory corneal ectatic disorder, which affects both genders [45] and is characterized by localized area of corneal thinning resembling a conical shape [49, 50]. It can occur in all races with a higher incidence in the Middle Eastern countries and Asia [51], and both genetic and environmental factors are implicated in the etiopathogenesis. Systemic associations with atopic diseases, Down syndrome, Ehler-Danlos syndrome, and osteogenesis imperfecta are noted along with ocular conditions such as floppy eyelid vernal keratoconjunctivitis (VKC), retinitis pigmentosa, etc [52]. Eye rubbing causes microtrauma that can predispose the patient to developing keratoconus and may be also the final etiological link that causes its association with the above disorders [44]. The visual distortion can range from mild irregular astigmatism to severe thinning, requiring surgical intervention [44]. Deposition of hemosiderin is manifested as Fleischer's ring at the base of the cone. As the disease progresses, the ring becomes thinner and discrete [44]. Another characteristic feature of the disease is the presence of vertical striae due to Descemet's membrane compression [45].

The patient may present with symptoms of progressive decrease in visual acuity, photophobia, glare, and ocular irritation. Due to progressive ectasia, progressive myopia ensues, requiring frequent change in glass prescription. High, irregular myopic astigmatism with a scissoring reflex is seen on retinoscopy in advanced cases. Munson sign is a V-shaped deformation of the lower lid seen on downward gaze due to angulation caused by corneal protrusion. Slit-lamp examination shows corneal ectasia and thinning corresponding to the area of maximal ectasia (Fig. 10.18a). Corneal hydrops (Fig. 10.18b) occurs due to imbibition of aqueous in the stroma through area of Descemet's rupture. It can occur in advanced cases. On corneal topography, a localized area of corneal steepening eccentrically associated with reduced pachymetry and superior-inferior asymmetry is seen [53]. Histopathological features suggestive of keratoconus include iron deposition in the epithelial basement membrane, stromal thinning, and breaks in bowman's layer Fig. 10.18c, d.

Initially, glasses and contact lens are dispensed to improve visual acuity. In moderate cases, corneal collagen cross-linking (CXL) is done to strengthen the cornea. In advanced cases,

Table 10.7 Differentiating features between various ectatic conditions

Clinical Feature	Keratoconus	Pellucid marginal degeneration	Keratoglobus	Posterior keratoconus
Frequency	Most common	Less common	Rare	Least common
Type of contour abnormality	Anterior	Anterior	Anterior	Posterior
Laterality	Usually bilateral Asymmetrical involvement	Bilateral	Bilateral	Usually unilateral
Age of onset	Puberty	20–40 years	Birth	Birth
Most common site	Central two-third of the cornea, apex just below visual axis	Peripheral	Generalized thinning	Paracentral
Location of thinning	Inferior paracentral	Inferior band 1–2 mm wide, 1–2 mm from the limbus	Generalized, more marked in the periphery	Posterior paracentral excavation
Site of protrusion	Thinnest at the apex	Superior to band of thinning	Generalized	Generally none
Thickness of protruding cornea	Thin	Normal	Thin	Thin
Iron ring	Fleischer ring	Absent	Absent	Occasionally
Vascularization and cellular infiltration	Absent	Absent	Absent	Absent
Scarring	Common	At the level of Descemet's membrane and posterior stroma at superior edge of thinned area if hydrops occurs	Mild	Common
Striae	Vogt striae, common	Uncommon	Occasionally	None
Acute hydrops	Can occur in advanced cases	Can occur	Less frequently	Not seen
Type of astigmatism induced	Irregular astigmatism	Against-the-rule superiorly with-the-rule near point of maximal protrusion	Irregular astigmatism	Mild irregular astigmatism, lesser than keratoconus
Corneal perforation and rupture	Rare	Rarely	Can be seen after trivial trauma also	Not seen
Treatment	Spectacle correction and contact lens fitting CXL to limit progression in mild-to-moderate disease DALK/PK in moderate-to-severe disease	Spectacles, large diameter rigid gas-permeable contact lens, hybrid lenses, PROSE lens, Large diameter or eccentric PK, DALK, crescentric lamellar keratoplasty	Spectacles Customized PROSE lenses Lamellar keratoplasty, partial thickness corneoscleroplasty, large diameter PK	Spectacle PK if corneal scarring occurs

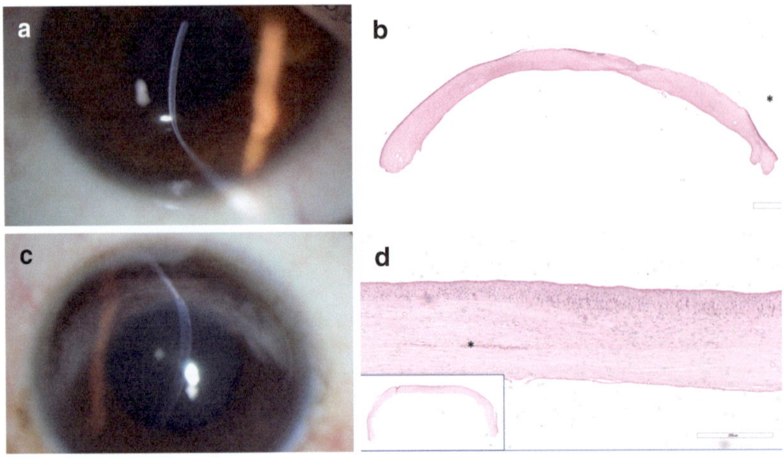

Fig. 10.18 PMD and TMD: (**a**) Pellucid marginal degeneration (PMD): note the area of maximal ectasis is more central, whereas the maximal thinning is inferior, below the area of ectasia. (**b**) Histopathology shows an elongated corneal button with prominent thinning at one end (asterisk) (H&E; 2× original magnification). (**c**) The clinical photograph of a case of Terrien's marginal degeneration (TMD) shows prominent scarring and thinning superiorly, with vascularization. (**d**) Histopathology shows effacement of the corneal button (insert, H&E; 2× original magnification), epithelial irregularity, and hyperplasia, with absence of Bowman's layer, and stroma shows scarring and vascular channels (asterisk) (H&E; 20× original magnification)

where CXL is not possible due to increased risk of endothelial damage, deep anterior lamellar keratoplasty (DALK) or penetrating keratoplasty (PKP) is done depending upon the corneal thickness and the site of corneal scarring.

10.5.2 Pellucid Marginal Degeneration

Peripheral corneal ectatic disorder affecting the cornea inferiorly forms 4–8 o clock in concentrically [54] (Fig. 10.19a, b). Thinning occurs 1–2 mm central to the limbus [49]. It may occur superiorly or if it occurs inferiorly, can be unilateral or may involve more than 4 clock hours. The site of corneal protrusion is superior to the area of thinning. The ectatic cornea is of normal thickness, and the corneal contour resembles the shape of a "beer belly." Crab-claw appearance is seen on power map of corneal topography [55]. The differential diagnosis for peripheral corneal thinning disorders includes Terrien's marginal degeneration (Fig. 10.19c, d), Mooren's ulcer, and furrow degeneration.

The differentiating features in contrast to other ectatic disorders are presented in Table 10.7.

10.5.3 Keratoglobus

Nonprogressive or minimally progressive, bilateral corneal ectatic disorder. Generalized corneal thinning occurs, which is more marked in the periphery, leading to a globular appearance of the cornea [56]. It is usually seen from birth and can be associated with a normal or slightly increased corneal diameter. The differential diagnosis includes congenital glaucoma and megalocornea [12].

It is a congenital disease but can have syndromic association or secondarily acquired as well [56]. It can be seen in patients with inflammatory orbital pseudotumor, chronic eye rubbing, glaucoma after PKP, and chronic marginal blepharitis [57]. It has also been seen in patients with blue sclera and connective tissue disorders like Ehler-Danlos syndrome, and this should be excluded in children presenting with this disorder [58]. Acquired keratoglobus has been seen in patients with hyperthyroidism and vernal kerato-

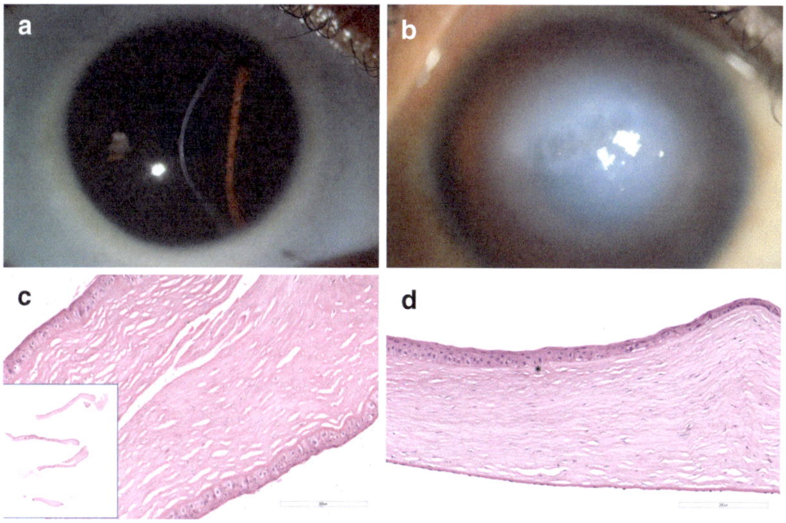

Fig. 10.19 Keratoconus: (**a**) Slit-lamp photograph shows corneal thinning centrally with ectasis coinciding with the area of thinning. (**b**) Corneal hydrops due to break in DM. (**c**) Deep anterior lamellar keratoplasty specimens show linear strips of tissue (insert, H&E; scanner view 2× original magnification), with intact but hypertrophic epithelium and irregular stromal arrangement (H&E; 20× original magnification). (**d**) Bowman's layer breaks and loosely arranged collagen lamella are noted (H&E; 20× original magnification)

conjunctivitis [57]. The initial line of management is spectacle correction. This increases the visual acuity as well as provides protection from trauma as even trivial trauma can cause perforation in such patients. A customized scleral lens improves visual acuity by making the anterior corneal contour regular, but its use should be weighed against the risk of trauma during insertion and removal. Surgical intervention with lamellar graft, epikeratoplasty, partial thickness corneo-scleroplasty, and large diameter PK can be planned when required [57].

10.5.4 Posterior Keratoconus

It is a development disorder, usually unilateral and nonprogressive [43]. Increase in curvature of the posterior cornea causes thinning. It can involve the cornea diffusely where the entire posterior corneal surface has increased curvature, or it can be localized with single or multiple areas of posterior corneal steepening [44]. Mild-to-moderate decrease in visual acuity occurs as only the posterior corneal surface is involved, and the anterior surface maintains its contour [59].

The etiopathogenesis of the disorder is unknown. It is usually congenital or can be seen in association with other abnormalities as well; thus, investigations are required to rule out syndromic associations or ocular associations such as aniridia, ectopia lentis, anterior lens opacities, anterior lenticonus, etc [59, 60]. Trauma can cause acquired posterior keratoconus as well [61]. Early diagnosis is required to decrease the risk of developing amblyopia [62].

Histopathology Epithelial changes are common in keratoconus [62, 63] and show uneven thickness with areas of hyperplasia at the apex to compensate for the thinning or effacement in other areas. Elongation of these cells in the layers of the epithelium is also noted. Iron deposition at the base of the Bowman's layer is noted, which can be picked up by using Perl's Prussian blue stain for iron and can be seen as bluish stippling. Bowman's layer breaks are common [64] and inwardly directed epithelial cells or protrusion of the stromal collagen through these breaks are noted leading to a Z-shaped configuration. Stroma shows thinning more pronounced in the center in keratoconus, whereas the thinning is diffuse in keratoglobus. There are fewer keratocytes in the anterior stroma, and the collagen appears loosely arranged. Areas of focal linear scarring can also be noted. The Descemet's membrane can show breaks and discontinuity, due to previous hydrops and a pseudo-DM can be noted filling in the gap [65, 66].

10.6 Corneal Degeneration

Degeneration is the deterioration in the structure and function of a tissue. These changes can occur primarily due to aging or secondarily due to adverse internal or external influences. Thus, they are classified as involutional (age-related) or noninvolutional (hyaline, amyloid, lipid, calcific based on the type of deposition), and by anatomic location (anterior, posterior, central, peripheral) [67].

Degenerative corneal diseases are associated with delayed onset, peripheral involvement, variable progression, inflammation, and neovascularization. It can be asymmetric and can involve one or both the eyes [67].

The various involutional corneal degenerations, especially those related to increasing age, are discussed in Table 10.8 [68–78]. Certain degenerations can be both involutional and noninvolutional. They have been included in the relevant table with their more common form and the other type has been described at the same place as well for easier understanding.

The various noninvolutional corneal degenerations, especially those due to chronic inflammation or systemic disease, are discussed in Table 10.9. Figure 10.20a–g illustrates the various corneal degenerations.

Table 10.8 Involutional corneal degenerations

	Arcus Senilis	Limbal Girdle of Vogt	Hudson-Stahli line	Crocodile Shagreen	Cornea Farinata	Salzmann's Nodular degeneration	Terrien marginal corneal degeneration
Age	40–60 years If <40: Arcus Juvenilis or anterior embryotoxon	40–60 years	Middle and older age group	–	–	Primary: More common, not associated with any other diseases Secondary: VKC, phlycten, trachoma, measles, interstitial keratitis	Middle age, most commonly in 20–40 years
Gender predilection	Males > Females	–	Males > Females	–	–	Females > Males	Males > Females
Location	Periphery (inferior followed by superior)	Parallel to inter-palpebral limbus (nasal > temporal)	Junction of middle and lower third of cornea	Anterior: due to trauma, hypotony, BSK, megalocornea, keratoconus, central involvement Posterior: age related, peripheral involvement	Central	Midperiphery of the cornea, single or multiple, annular	Starts supero-nasally, fine superficial vascularization present, peripheral thinning disorders, progresses circumferentially
Laterality	Bilateral, symmetric	Symmetric	Bilateral, symmetric	Bilateral, symmetric	Bilateral	Unilateral or bilateral	Bilateral, symmetric; can by asymmetric also
Progression	Slowly over years	–	–	–	–	Slow	Slow
Lucid interval from limbus	Present (lucid interval of Vogt)	Type I: Present Type II: Absent	Present	–	–	–	Present
Deposition	Cholesterol, cholesterol esters, phospholipids, neutral glycerides	Type I: Calcium Type II: Due to chronic exposure to UV rays	Ferritin	–	–	–	Lipid deposition at leading edge, central to thinning
Color of opacity	Gray-white, opaque	Yellowish-white	Faint yellow to dark brown	Gray	Gray brown to white, "flour dust" appearance	Gray-white elevated nodular lesion	–

(continued)

Table 10.8 (continued)

	Arcus Senilis	Limbal Girdle of Vogt	Hudson-Stahli line	Crocodile Shagreen	Cornea Farinata	Salzmann's Nodular degeneration	Terrien marginal corneal degeneration
Location of opacity	Descemet's membrane followed by Bowman's layer	Beneath epithelial layer, adjacent to Bowman's layer	Epithelium	Posterior stroma, just anterior to Descemet's membrane (DM)	Posterior stroma, adjacent to DM	Between epithelium and Bowman's layer	–
Symptoms	Asymptomatic	Asymptomatic	–	Asymptomatic	Asymptomatic	Asymptomatic watering, photophobia, irritation if erosion occurs; decrease in vision if irregular astigmatism in visual axis	Asymptomatic mild irritation occasionally; decrease in vision due to irregular or against-the-rule astigmatism in advanced cases
Histopathology	Extracellular deposition in corneal fibroblasts, absent foam cells, hourglass appearance	Focal areas of hyaline deposition, elastotic degeneration, hypertrophy of overlying epithelium	Ferritin deposition within basal epithelial cells and intercellular spaces	Extracellular stromal vacuoles containing fibrillar-granular material, posterior stroma just anterior to Descemet's membrane	Abnormal posterior keratocytes with membrane-bound intracytoplasmic vacuoles filled with lipid-like inclusions representing lipofuscin	Dense collagen plaques with hyalinization, excessive secretion of basement-membrane-like material, overlying epithelium may be absent or atrophic	Corneal stromal thinning, interstitial vascularization in stromal collagen, disorganized collagen lamella, paucity of inflammatory cells
Treatment	Vo visual significance <40: rule out hyperlipoproteinemia type IIa > type IIb	Not required	Not required	Not required	–	Lubricants superficial keratectomy, phototherapeutic keratectomy, lamellar keratoplasty	Spectacles, rigid gas-permeable lens; scleral contact lenses; peripheral crescentic lamellar graft, penetrating keratoplasty for high astigmatism, for impending or frank perforation

Table 10.9 Secondary corneal degenerations

Characteristics	Calcific band keratopathy	Lipid keratopathy	Spheroidal degeneration/ climatic droplet keratopathy
Precipitating factor	Chronic inflammation, systemic or hereditary diseases associated with abnormalities in calcium metabolism; topical or intraocular medications that cause disturbance in local calcium metabolism. e.g., chronic uveitis in JRA, hypercalcemia in CRF. It can occur primarily as well without any associated inflammation or systemic disease.	Primary: Rare. No inflammation, trauma, infection, or vascularization, normal lipid level. Can occur due to increased vascular permeability of limbal vessels or altered metabolic activity of keratocytes. Secondary: Corneal vascularization due to. e.g. herpetic keratitis, trauma, ulcer, interstitial keratitis	Ultraviolet rays, low humidity, higher winds, microtrauma Type I: Older patients, no associated ocular pathology Type II: Other corneal pathologies present Type III: Conjunctival form, can occur with type I/II, e.g., can be seen with pinguecula
Age	–	–	>40
Gender predilection	–	Secondary: Females>males	Type I, III: Males> Females
Location	Inter-palpebral zone, peripheral involvement along horizontal meridian, progresses centripetally.	Primary: Central or peripheral, localized, or diffuse Secondary: Adjacent to abnormal vessels	Type I: Inter-palpebral limbus Type II: Lower two-thirds of the cornea Type III: Conjunctiva
Laterality	–	Primary: Unilateral or bilateral Secondary: Depends on the precipitating etiology	Type I, III: Bilateral Type II: Unilateral
Progression	Slowly progressive (months to years); Fast progression (weeks to months);can occur rarely, especially in dry eyes.	Slow, can be sudden rarely	Progressive till exposure to precipitating factor persists
Lucid interval from limbus	Present.	–	–
Deposition	Hydroxyapatite, phosphate salt of calcium. Under normal circumstances, the concentration of calcium and phosphate is such that it is soluble. In the presence of low pH or increase in concentration of either ion, precipitation occurs.	Neutral fat, free fatty acids, cholesterol crystals, phospholipids	Hyaline-like material
Color of deposit	Gray to white.	Gray to yellow white	Type I: Clear to yellow gold Type II: Diffuse haze Type III: Light yellow to brownish yellow
Site of deposition	Bowman's layer.	All corneal layers, maximum in mid-stroma	Beneath epithelium, bowman's layer, anterior stroma

(continued)

Table 10.9 (continued)

Characteristics	Calcific band keratopathy	Lipid keratopathy	Spheroidal degeneration/ climatic droplet keratopathy
Symptoms	Initially asymptomatic. Later decrease in vision, foreign body sensation, tearing, photophobia.	Decrease in vision	Decrease in vision when visual axis is involved
Histopathology	Fine basophilic granules in cytoplasm of basal epithelium, extracellular space in Bowman's layer, anterior stroma.	Intracellular and extra cellular lipid deposition, stromal vascularization, necrosis, vacuolization, foam cells	Granular deposition of spherules with hyaline-like material, disruption of Bowman's layer, epithelium elevation and thinning in advanced cases
Treatment	Mechanical debridement, EDTA chelation, phototherapeutic keratectomy.	Argon laser photocoagulation of feeder vessels, administration of VEGF inhibitors, penetrating Keratoplasty if visual axis is involved	Lamellar or penetrating keratoplasty, phototherapeutic keratectomy, excision for conjunctival lesions

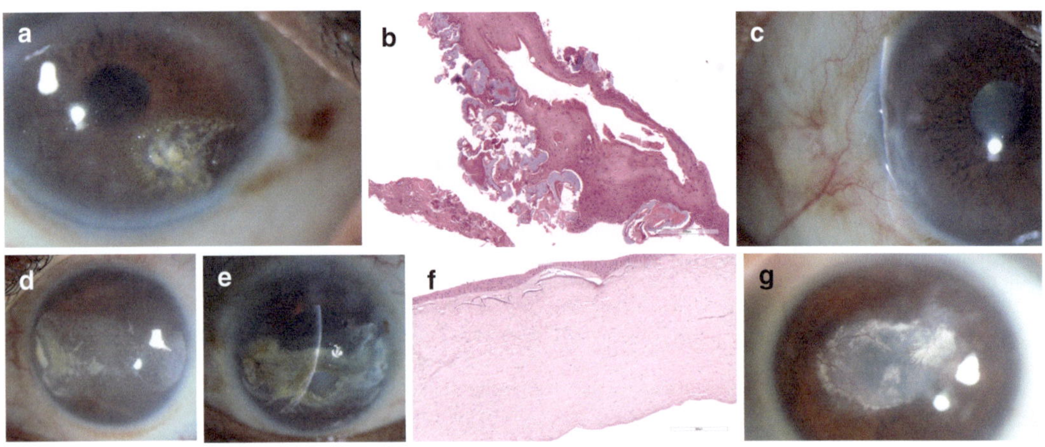

Fig. 10.20 Corneal degenerations: (**a**) A case of spheroidal degeneration. (**b**) Histopathological changes show epithelial hyperplasia and gray amorphous material deposited below the epithelium. (PAS; 10× original magnification). (**c**) Senile furrow degeneration (**d**) Band-shaped keratopathy right eye and (**e**) Left eye. (**f**) Histopathology shows hyperplastic epithelium, disrupted Bowman's layer, and bluish deposits of calcium in the anterior stroma. (H&E; 10× original magnification). (**g**) Slit-lamp photograph of a case of lipid keratopathy in resolved herpes simplex virus keratitis. There is central cornea scarring, and whitish lipid deposition alongside the prominent vascular channels around the scar

Financial disclosures none for all authors

Funding Funding by Hyderabad Eye Research Foundation for Varsha M Rathi, Sujata Das, Soumya Jakati, Dilip K Mishra, Somasheila I Murthy and Muralidhar Ramappa

References

1. Khurana AK, Khurana I. Anatomy and physiology of eye. 3rd ed. CBS Publishers and Distributors; 2019. p. 1–19.
2. Khurana AK. Comprehensive ophthalmology. 7th ed. Jaypee Brothers Medical Publishers; 2019. p. 3–13.

3. Friede R. Surface area of cornea and sclera in embryos and in newborn infants and its relation to megalocornea in adults. Z Augenheilkd. 1933;8:213.
4. Rosa RH, Bloomer MM, Kivelä TT, Milman T, Potter HA, Nasreen AS, et al. Ophthalmic pathology and intraocular tumors. American Academy of Ophthalmology; 2019.
5. Mansour AM, Barber JC, Reinecke RD, et al. Ocular choristomas. Surv Opthalmol. 1989;33(5):339–58.
6. Kausar A, Zafar SN, Altaf S, et al. Opthalmic manifestations of linear nevus sebaceous/organoid nevus syndrome. J Coll Physicians Surg Pak. 2015;25(3):220–2.
7. Nischal KK. Genetics of congenital corneal opacification—impact on diagnosis and treatment. Cornea. 2015;34:S24–34.
8. Idrees F, Vaideanu D, Fraser SG, Sowden JC, Khaw PT. A review of anterior segment dysgeneses. Surv Ophthalmol. 2006;51(3):213–31.
9. Khan AO. Sclerocornea and cornea plana are distinct entities. Surv Ophthalmol. 2007;52(3):325.
10. Waizenegger U, Kohnen T, Weidle E, Schütte E. Congenital familial cornea plana with ptosis, peripheral sclerocornea and conjunctival xerosis. Klinische Monatsblatter fur Augenheilkunde. 1995;207(2):111–6.
11. Roche O, Dureau P, Uteza Y, Dufier J. Congenital megalocornea. J Fr D'ophtalmol. 2002;25(3):312–8.
12. Ong AP, Zhang J, Vincent AL, McGhee CN. Megalocornea, anterior megalophthalmos, keratoglobus and associated anterior segment disorders: a review. Clin Experiment Ophthalmol. 2021;49(5):477–97.
13. Bateman JB, Maumenee IH. Colobomatous macrophthalmia with microcornea. Ophthalmic Paediatr Genet. 1984;4(2):59–66.
14. Das S, Sharma S, Priyadarshini O, Sahu SK, Kar S, Vemuganti GK. Association between culture results of corneal scrapings and culture and histopathology results of corneal tissues in therapeutic keratoplasty. Cornea. 2011;30(9):1003–6.
15. Vemuganti GK, Murthy SI, Mishra DK. Role of histopathology in corneal and conjunctival infection. In: Das S, Jhanji V, editors. Infection of the cornea and conjunctiva. Springer Nature Singapore Pte Ltd; 2021. p. 247–61.
16. Vemuganti GK, Murthy SI, Das S. Update on pathologic diagnosis of corneal infections and inflammations. Middle East Afr J Ophthalmol. 2011;18(4):277.
17. Ung L, Bispo PJ, Shanbhag SS, Gilmore MS, Chodosh J. The persistent dilemma of microbial keratitis: global burden, diagnosis, and antimicrobial resistance. Surv Ophthalmol. 2019;64(3):255–71.
18. Rautaraya B, Sharma S, Ali MH, Kar S, Das S, Sahu SK. A 3½-year study of bacterial Keratitis from Odisha, India. Asia-Pacific J Ophthalmol. 2014;3(3):146–50.
19. Lin A, Rhee MK, Akpek EK, Amescua G, Farid M, Garcia-Ferrer FJ, et al. Bacterial keratitis preferred practice pattern®. Ophthalmology. 2019;126(1):P1–P55.
20. Garg P, Sharma S, Vemuganti GK, Ramamurthy B. A cluster of Nocardia keratitis after LASIK. Thorofare: Slack Incorporated; 2007. p. 309–12.
21. Leck A, Thomas P, Hagan M, Kaliamurthy J, Ackuaku E, John M, et al. Aetiology of suppurative corneal ulcers in Ghana and south India, and epidemiology of fungal keratitis. Br J Ophthalmol. 2002;86(11):1211–5.
22. Panda A, Mohan M, Mukherjee G. Mycotic keratitis in Indian patients. Indian J Ophthalmol. 1984;32(5):311.
23. Vemuganti GK, Garg P, Gopinathan U, Naduvilath TJ, John RK, Buddi R, et al. Evaluation of agent and host factors in progression of mycotic keratitis: a histologic and microbiologic study of 167 corneal buttons. Ophthalmology. 2002;109(8):1538–46.
24. Garg P, Vemuganti GK, Chatarjee S, Gopinathan U, Rao GN. Pigmented plaque presentation of dematiaceous fungal keratitis: a clinicopathologic correlation. Cornea. 2004;23(6):571–6.
25. Vishwakarma P, Mohanty A, Kaur A, Das S, Priyadarshini SR, Mitra S, et al. Pythium keratitis: clinical profile, laboratory diagnosis, treatment, and histopathology features post-treatment at a tertiary eye care center in Eastern India. Indian J Ophthalmol. 2021;69(6):1544.
26. Mittal R, Jena SK, Desai A, Agarwal S. Pythium insidiosum keratitis: histopathology and rapid novel diagnostic staining technique. Cornea. 2017;36(9):1124–32.
27. Sharma S, Garg P, Rao GN. Patient characteristics, diagnosis, and treatment of non-contact lens related Acanthamoeba keratitis. Br J Ophthalmol. 2000;84(10):1103–8.
28. Stehr-Green JK, Bailey TM, Visvesvara GS. The epidemiology of Acanthamoeba keratitis in the United States. Am J Ophthalmol. 1989;107(4):331–6.
29. Jain R, Garg P, Motukupally SR, Geary MB. Clinico-microbiological review of non-contact-lens-associated Acanthamoeba keratitis. Semin Ophthalmol. 2015;30(4):281–8. Taylor & Francis
30. Vemuganti GK, Sharma S, Athmanathan S, Garg P. Keratocyte loss in acanihamoeba keratitis: phagocytosis, necrosis or apoptosis? Indian J Ophthalmol. 2000;48(4):291.
31. Vemuganti G, Pasricha G, Sharma S, Garg P. Granulomatous inflammation in Acanthamoeba keratitis: an immunohistochemical study of five cases and review of literature. Indian J Med Microbiol. 2005;23(4):231–8.
32. Sharma S, Das S, Joseph J, Vemuganti GK, Murthy S. Microsporidial keratitis: need for increased awareness. Surv Ophthalmol. 2011;56(1):1–22.
33. Joseph J, Vemuganti GK, Garg P, Sharma S. Histopathological evaluation of ocular microsporidiosis by different stains. BMC Clin Pathol. 2006;6(1):1 8.
34. Das S, Sharma S, Sahu SK, Vemuganti GK. Intraocular invasion by microsporidial spores in a case of stromal keratitis. Arch Ophthalmol. 2011;129(4):512–26.

35. Mittal R, Balne PK, Sahu S, Das S, Sharma S. Coexistence of herpes simplex virus infection in microsporidial stromal keratitis associated with granulomatous inflammation. Indian J Ophthalmol. 2017;65(4):276.
36. Holland EJ, Schwartz GS. Classification of herpes simplex virus keratitis. Cornea. 1999;18:144–54.
37. Weiss JS, Møller H, Lisch W, Kinoshita S, Aldave AJ, Belin MW, et al. The IC3D classification of the corneal dystrophies. Cornea. 2008;27(Suppl 2):S1.
38. Weiss JS, Moller HU, Aldave AJ, Seitz B, Bredrup C, Kivela T, et al. IC3D classification of corneal dystrophies--edition 2. Cornea. 2015;34(2):117–59.
39. Weiss JS, Moller HU, Lisch W, Kinoshita S, Aldave AJ, Belin MW, et al. The IC3D classification of the corneal dystrophies. Cornea. 2008;27(Suppl 2):S1–83.
40. Vemuganti GK, Rathi VM, Murthy SI. Histological landmarks in corneal dystrophy: pathology of corneal dystrophies. Dev Ophthalmol. 2011;48:24–50.
41. Lisch W, Bron AJ, Munier FL, Schorderet DF, Tiab L, Lange C, et al. Franceschetti hereditary recurrent corneal erosion. Am J Ophthalmol. 2012;153(6):1073–81 e4.
42. Feder RS, Jay M, Yue BY, Stock EL, O'Grady RB, Roth SI. Subepithelial mucinous corneal dystrophy. Clinical and pathological correlations. Arch Ophthalmol. 1993;111(8):1106–14.
43. Krachmer JH, Feder RS, Belin MW. Keratoconus and related noninflammatory corneal thinning disorders. Surv Ophthalmol. 1984;28(4):293–322.
44. Feder RS, Neems LC. Noninflammatory ectatic disorders. In: Mannis MJ, Holland EJ, editors. CORNEA fundamentals, diagnosis and management, vol. 2. 4th ed. Elsevier; 2017. p. 820–43.
45. Naroo SA. Contact lens & anterior eye. The journal of the British Contact Lens Association. Editorial. Cont Lens Anterior Eye. 2008;31(4):173–5.
46. Perez-Straziota C, Gaster RN, Rabinowitz YS. Corneal cross-linking for pediatric keratcoconus review. Cornea. 2018;37(6):802.
47. Kumar M, Shetty R, Lalgudi VG, Khamar P, Vincent SJ, Atchison DA. The effect of scleral lenses on vision, refraction and aberrations in post-LASIK ectasia, keratoconus and pellucid marginal degeneration. Ophthalmic Physiol Opt. 2021;41(4):664–72.
48. Lim L, Lim EWL. Current perspectives in the management of keratoconus with contact lenses. Eye. 2020;34(12):2175–96.
49. Gomes JA, Tan D, Rapuano CJ, Belin MW, Ambrósio R Jr, Guell JL, et al. Global consensus on keratoconus and ectatic diseases. Cornea. 2015;34(4):359–69.
50. Millodot M, Shneor E, Albou S, Atlani E, Gordon-Shaag A. Prevalence and associated factors of keratoconus in Jerusalem: a cross-sectional study. Ophthalmic Epidemiol. 2011;18(2):91–7.
51. Georgiou T, Funnell C, Cassels-Brown A, O'Conor R. Influence of ethnic origin on the incidence of keratoconus and associated atopic disease in Asians and white patients. Eye. 2004;18(4):379–83.
52. Vazirani J, Basu S. Keratoconus: current perspectives. Clin Ophthalmol (Auckland, NZ). 2013;7:2019.
53. Rabinowitz YS. Keratoconus. Surv Ophthalmol. 1998;42(4):297–319.
54. Martínez-Abad A, Piñero DP. Pellucid marginal degeneration: detection, discrimination from other corneal ectatic disorders and progression. Cont Lens Anterior Eye. 2019;42(4):341–9.
55. Karabatsas C, Cook S. Topographic analysis in pellucid marginal corneal degeneration and keratoglobus. Eye. 1996;10(4):451–5.
56. Wallang B, Das S. Keratoglobus. Eye. 2013;27(9):1004–12.
57. Cameron JA. Keratoglobus. Cornea. 1993;12(2):124–30.
58. Brooks JK. A review of syndromes associated with blue sclera, with inclusion of malformations of the head and neck. Oral Surg Oral Med Oral Pathol Oral Radiol. 2018;126(3):252–63.
59. Silas MR, Hilkert SM, Reidy JJ, Farooq AV. Posterior keratoconus. Br J Ophthalmol. 2018;102(7):863–7.
60. Ganesan N, Narayana S, Kasturi N, Kaliaperumal S, Srinivasan R, Vallinayagam M. Varied presentations of posterior keratoconus: a clinical case series. Cornea. 2020;39(11):1348–53.
61. Williams R. Acquired posterior keratoconus. Br J Ophthalmol. 1987;71(1):16–7.
62. Sykakis E, Carley F, Irion L, Denton J, Hillarby M. An in depth analysis of histopathological characteristics found in keratoconus. Pathology. 2012;44(3):234–9.
63. Tsubota K, Mashima Y, Murata H, Sato N, Ogata T. Corneal epithelium in keratoconus. Cornea. 1995;14(1):77–83.
64. Naderan M, Jahanrad A, Balali S. Histopathologic findings of keratoconus corneas underwent penetrating keratoplasty according to topographic measurements and keratoconus severity. Int J Ophthalmol. 2017;10(11):1640.
65. Bergeron S, Fernandes BF, Logan P, Burnier MN. Histopathological findings in keratoconus. In: New frontiers for the treatment of keratoconus. Cham: Springer; 2021. p. 49–53.
66. Santodomingo-Rubido J, Carracedo G, Suzaki A, Villa-Collar C, Vincent SJ, Wolffsohn JS. Keratoconus: an updated review. Cont Lens Anterior Eye. 2022;45:101559.
67. Reidy JJ. Corneal and conjunctival degenerations. In: Mannis MJ, Holland EJ, editors. CORNEA fundamentals, diagnosis and management, vol. 2. 4th ed. Elsevier; 2017. p. 856–74.
68. Sugar HS, Kobernick S. The white limbus girdle of Vogt. Am J Ophthalmol. 1960;50(1):101–7.
69. Rose GE, Lavin MJ. The Hudson-Stahli line III: observations on morphology, a critical review of aetiology and a unified theory for the forma-

tion of iron lines of the corneal epithelium. Eye. 1987;1(4):475–9.
70. Paranjpe V, Galor A, Monsalve P, Dubovy SR, Karp CL. Salzmann nodular degeneration: prevalence, impact, and management strategies. Clin Ophthalmol (Auckland, NZ). 2019;13:1305.
71. Chan AT, Ulate R, Goldich Y, Rootman DS, Chan CC. Terrien marginal degeneration: clinical characteristics and outcomes. Am J Ophthalmol. 2015;160(5):867–72. e1
72. Ding Y, Murri MS, Birdsong OC, Ronquillo Y, Moshirfar M. Terrien marginal degeneration. Surv Ophthalmol. 2019;64(2):162–74.
73. Crispin S. Ocular lipid deposition and hyperlipoproteinaemia. Prog Retin Eye Res. 2002;21(2):169–224.
74. Belliveau MJ, Brownstein S, Agapitos P, Font RL. Ultrastructural features of posterior crocodile shagreen of the cornea. Surv Ophthalmol. 2009;54(5):569–75.
75. Mahadevan R, Fathima A, Rajan R, Arumugam AO. An ocular surface prosthesis for keratoglobus and Terrien's marginal degeneration. Optom Vis Sci. 2014;91(4):S34–S9.
76. Jhanji V, Rapuano CJ, Vajpayee RB. Corneal calcific band keratopathy. Curr Opin Ophthalmol. 2011;22(4):283–9.
77. Hall MN, Moshirfar M, Amin-Javaheri A, Ouano DP, Ronquillo Y, Hoopes PC. Lipid keratopathy: a review of pathophysiology, differential diagnosis, and management. Ophthalmol Therapy. 2020;9(4):833–52.
78. Stevenson W, Cheng S-F, Dastjerdi MH, Ferrari G, Dana R. Corneal neovascularization and the utility of topical VEGF inhibition: ranibizumab (Lucentis) vs bevacizumab (Avastin). Ocul Surf. 2012;10(2):67–83.

Pathology of the Sclera

11

Isha Chaudhari, Manisha Acharya, Arpan Gandhi, and Somasheila Murthy

Contents

I. Chaudhari (✉) · M. Acharya
Department of Cornea and Refractive Services, Dr. Shroff's Charity Eye Hospital, New Delhi, India

A. Gandhi
Chairperson Laboratory Services, Dr Shroff's Charity Eye Hospital, Secondary Centres, New Delhi, India

S. Murthy
Specialist in Corneal Diseases, Uveitis, Cataract and Refractive Surgery, Shantilal Shanghvi Eye Institute, Mumbai, Maharashtra, India

G. K. Vemuganti et al. (eds.), *Ocular Pathology*, https://doi.org/10.1007/978-981-96-8614-8_11

11.1 Introduction

The sclera is the tough, white, collagenous, outer coat of the eye that gives protection and contour to the eye and also attachment to the extraocular muscles. Diseases of the sclera can be congenital, metabolic, degenerative, acquired inflammatory, or acquired noninflammatory. It is infrequent to find a scleral disease in isolation. Infective scleritis may be due to the spread of infection from a contiguous structure like the cornea; noninfectious scleritis is usually due to an underlying connective tissue disease. Noninflammatory diseases of the sclera may be early signs of metabolic, hematological, and connective tissue abnormalities. Nearly 50% of patients with scleritis have evidence of underlying systemic disease. Hence, the importance of knowing about scleral diseases with their systemic association as a scleral manifestation may be the first sign of a more sinister pathology. In this chapter, we shall be discussing some common diseases of the sclera in brief starting with the embryological derivation of the sclera, the congenital conditions of the sclera, which mainly includes blue sclera and its associations, commonly encountered metabolic diseases of the sclera, scleritis—infectious and noninfectious, and degenerative conditions like plaque and phthisis bulbi.

11.2 Embryology and Congenital Conditions of the Sclera

11.2.1 Embryology

The sclera, along with other structures such as corneal endothelium and stroma, are formed by the extracellular mesenchyme [1, 2]. This extracellular mesenchyme consists of the mesoderm and the neural crest cells, both of which contribute to the formation of the sclera. From the first sign of optic primordia on day 22 of gestation, to the formation of aqueous humor by the seventh week, a protective shell is required to cover the complex structure that has now evolved. Under the influence of the inductive forces of the pigmented outer layer of the optic cup, the mesenchyme surrounding the optic cup forms a vascularized pigmented layer, the choroid and the collagenous layer, the sclera, which is continuous with the dura mater of the brain [3]. The sclera also contributes to the stroma of the cornea. The limbus receives a massive contribution of the neural crest cells, which are responsible for the linkage between the sclera and the irido-corneal angle [4]. The neural crest cells migration takes place in three waves. The first wave occurs in the fourth week, forming the corneal endothelium and an acellular stroma. The second wave takes place in the seventh week, where these cells invade the corneal stroma and condense to form the sclera. The third wave occurs at the eighth week and forms the iris stroma. The formation of the choroid and the sclera marks the onset of the mature form of the eye in embryogenesis.

11.2.2 Congenital Conditions of the Sclera

11.2.2.1 Nevus of Ota

Nevus of Ota, also known as ocular dermal melanocytosis, is a dermal melanocytic hamartoma, with an incidence of 0.4% [5]. There is a female preponderance, with the most common age of presentation being either at birth or between 11 and 20 years of age. It is thought to occur due to an abnormality of neural crest cell migration.

It typically presents as a unilateral blue-black or slate gray hyperpigmented macules of the eye, adnexa, and face, rarely palate, which are located along the distribution of the first or second branches of the trigeminal nerve. The hyperpigmentation occurs due to entrapped melanocytes of the conjunctiva and sclera. There is an increased risk of uveal melanoma and glaucoma in these cases [6].

About 22–77% of patients have ocular involvement. It can be associated with increased intraocular pressure, asymmetric cupping, uveitis, cataract, and melanoma [7–9].

11.2.2.2 Blue Sclera

Bluish color of the sclera occurs in conditions of scleral thinning. The color is imparted by the increased visibility of the underlying uvea through the area of scleral thinning. Various causes of scleral thinning are enumerated in Table 11.1.

Marfan Syndrome

This is a congenital mesodermal dystrophy. Its classical triad includes a triad of subluxated lens, cardiovascular disease, and skeletal anomalies. As the basic connective tissue is anomalous, the sclera lacks the rigidity to resist deformation due to raised intraocular pressure and allows the intraocular contents of the globe to bulge, resulting in a staphyloma. Homocystinuria is a common differential of Marfan syndrome; however, in this disease, the scleral connective tissue is thicker [10].

Osteogenesis Imperfecta

This syndrome is characterized by a blue sclera, brittle bones, and deafness. It is due to an inherent defect in the synthesis of extracellular matrix leading to abnormalities in connective tissue. Blue sclera is seen in all types of osteogenesis imperfecta and is the most characteristic ocular finding. These patients have significantly less ocular rigidity [11].

Ehlers–Danlos Syndrome

It is characterized by hyperelasticity and fragility of the skin, atrophic scars, and hemangiomatous pseudotumors. Nine types have been described, of which type VI has prominent ocular involvement. The sclera is thin and may lead to spontaneous perforation [12].

Degenerative Myopia

This is another condition associated with thin sclera, especially posteriorly, and may cause staphylomas as a result of stretching of fibers or due to increased scleral growth.

Iron Deficiency Anemia

This is the most frequent metabolic cause of acquired blue sclera.

Table 11.1 Causes of scleral thinning

Inherited/congenital diseases		Acquired diseases	
Systemic	Ocular	Systemic	Ocular
Marfan syndrome	Keratoconus	Iron deficiency anemia	Paralimbic scleromalacia
Osteogenesis imperfecta	Buphthalomos	Myasthenia gravis	
Pseudoxanthoma elasticum	Colobomas		
Ehlers–Danlos syndrome	Myopia		

Histology of Bluish Sclera In conditions of bluish appearing sclera, the sclera is usually thinner than normal, but may be thicker and more cellular than normal. Its collagen fibers are abnormal, being reduced by about 25–30% in the cornea and more than 50% in the sclera.

11.3 Metabolic Diseases of the Sclera

11.3.1 Porphyria

Porphyria is caused by an excessive excretion of one or more fluorescent pigments called porphyrins due to the absence of one or more enzymes responsible for their metabolism. Porphyrias can be divided into erythropoietic and hepatic types based on the site of accumulation of porphyrins. Scleral involvement is generally rare and is present only in the congenital variety, porphyria cutanea tarda, and porphyria variegate. Deposition of porphyrins leads to severe photosensitization. Scleral thinning is present, which is bilateral, painless, and symmetrical. These areas are usually localized to sun-exposed interpalpebral fissures. Active scleral inflammation may also occur [13, 14]. Features such as low hairline, long eyelashes, facial hypertrichosis, flat nasal bridge, pink discoloration of teeth, and pseudoscleroderma changes on the face, hands, and feet are noted [15]. These features, along with simple biochemical tests on urine and blood, can clinch the diagnosis.

11.3.2 Cystinosis

Cystinosis is a defect of amino acid metabolism that leads to intracellular crystalline cysteine deposition. The three forms of cystinosis, the infantile form, the benign adult form, and the adolescent form, may have ocular involvement. Ocular findings are noninflammatory deposition of polychromatic, needle-like, glistening cystine crystals in the cornea, conjunctiva, episclera, superficial sclera, and iris [16].

11.3.3 Alkaptonuria

Alkaptonuria is another disorder of metabolism, which leads to deposition of homogentisate due to the absence of an enzyme responsible for phenylalanine and tyrosine metabolism. It is characterized by urine that turns black on standing. Ocular findings include scleral pigmentation of the interpalpebral area, seen as triangular patches, especially at the insertion of horizontal rectus muscles. It is a gray or bluish black pigmentation that increases with age [17]. Histologically, amorphous strands and curlicues are seen within the sclera and overlying substantia propria of the conjunctiva

11.3.4 Amyloid

Amyloid is an eosinophilic hyaline extracellular material that may be deposited in various tissues of the body. Scleral amyloidosis is mostly asymptomatic and does not show any specific lesion but rarely may be associated with glaucoma [18]

11.3.5 Miscellaneous Conditions

Other metabolic diseases that can affect the sclera are gout, hypercholesterolemia, Hand–Schuller–Christian disease, Letterer–Siwe Disease, Hyperparathyroidism, and Hypervitaminosis D.

11.4 Scleritis

11.4.1 Introduction and Classification

Scleritis is defined as the inflammation of the sclera. Typically, it is a very painful condition and may involve the cornea, the episclera, or the underlying uvea. Many classifications of scleral disease have been proposed, based on both clinical and pathological observations. A simple yet commonly used classification, proposed by Watson and Hayreh, based on the location and extent of involvement of the sclera, is as follows [19].

1. Anterior scleritis
   (a) Diffuse scleritis
   (b) Nodular Scleritis
   (c) Necrotizing scleritis
      (i) With inflammation
      (ii) Without inflammation (scleromalacia perforans)
2. Posterior scleritis

Anterior scleritis is the most common pattern and may be diffuse (Fig. 11.1), nodular (Fig. 11.1b), or necrotizing (Fig. 11.1c) type. When scleritis occurs without clinical inflammation and in the absence of pain, such as in long-standing rheumatoid arthritis (RA), it is termed as scleromalacia perforans (Fig. 11.1d). It of the sclera posterior to the insertion of rectus muscle is termed posterior scleritis. Based on the etiology, scleritis can be caused by infectious and noninfectious or immune-mediated causes (Table 11.2). The importance of differentiating infectious from noninfectious causes lies in the fact that antimicrobials are the mainstay for infectious causes, immunosuppressives are the treatment of choice for immune-mediated causes. The use of immunosuppressives in infectious scleritis, due to lack of knowledge of etiology, can lead to clinical worsening [20].

It is often difficult to differentiate solely between the two entities on the basis of initial presentation alone, and therefore relevant laboratory investigations are required. A thorough knowledge of the subtle differences can help make a timely diagnosis.

In this chapter, we have divided scleritis into infectious and noninfectious causes and discussed the common causes with their clinic-pathological correlation.

Table 11.2 Causes of noninfectious and infectious scleritis

Noninfectious scleritis	Infectious (direct invasion or immune response) scleritis
Associated with connective tissue diseases and other inflammatory conditions in which vasculitis may occur, e.g., rheumatoid arthritis	Bacterial
Associated with vasculitic diseases, e.g., Wegener's granulomatosis	Tubercular
Surgically induced necrotizing scleritis (SINS)	Fungal
Medication induced	Viral
Miscellaneous	Parasitic

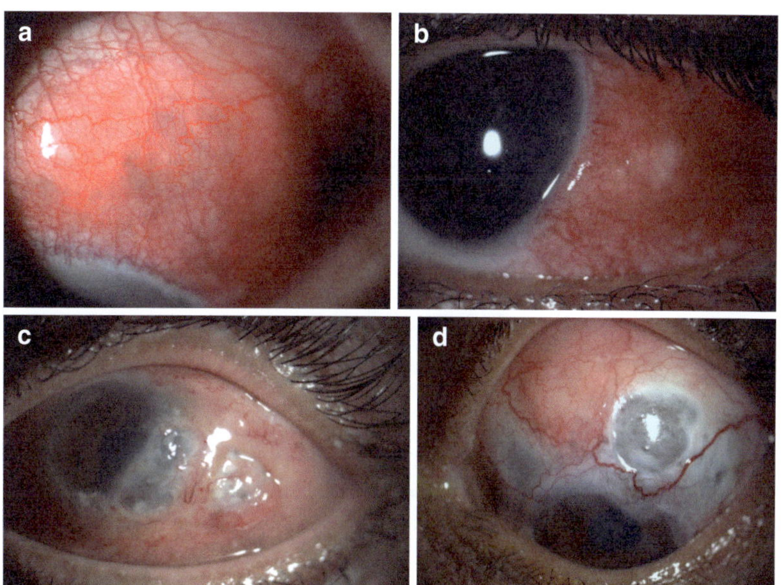

Fig. 11.1 (**a**) Diffuse scleritis, (**b**) Nodular scleritis, (**c**) Necrotizing scleritis, more common in patients with systemic vasculitis, (**d**) scleritis associated with rheumatoid arthritis (scleromalacia perforans or low-grade chronic scleritis)

11.4.2 Noninfectious Scleritis

Underlying autoimmune diseases are responsible for 30–50% of non-infectious scleritis [20, 21]. Another importance of identifying the underlying cause is the fact that around 15–59% patients present with scleritis as the first manifestation of a possible life-threatening disease. Rheumatoid arthritis (RA) and granulomatosis with polyangiitis (GPA) (Fig. 11.2a, b) are two most common diseases associated with scleritis. Clinical features of noninfectious scleritis depend on the degree and site of inflammation. The most characteristic symptom is pain, severe enough to awaken the patient at night, often radiating to involve forehead, brow, ear, jaw, or face. Firm, immobile, and tender nodules are a feature of nodular scleritis

11.4.2.1 Rheumatoid Arthritis (RA)-Associated Scleritis

Rheumatoid arthritis is a systemic disease, which principally affects the joints. Its most common ocular association is Sjogren's syndrome, followed by episcleritis, scleritis and peripheral ulcerative keratitis (PUK). Scleritis affects 0.2–6.3% patients with RA [22, 23]. It has been reported that scleritis associated with RA is more severe than idiopathic scleritis but as severe as scleritis associated with other immune-mediated diseases [24].

11.4.2.2 Granulomatosis with Polyangiitis

It is a multisystem granulomatous inflammatory disorder. In the eye, it is known to cause diseases ranging from conjunctivitis and episcleritis to the more severe uveitis, scleritis, keratitis and retinal vasculitis. Scleritis of the necrotizing type is the most common type seen in WG and can lead to permanent visual loss [25, 26]. Scleritis in GPA tends to progress rapidly, whereas it is insidious in RA (Fig. 11.2b).

11.4.2.3 Surgically Induced Necrotizing Scleritis (SINS)

Surgically induced necrotizing scleritis has been described following cataract, glaucoma, strabismus and retinal detachment surgery and has been noted that scleritis develops more frequently following multiple surgical events, rather than after a single operation. The predisposing factor for SINS is usually excessive conjunctival manipulation and episcleral vessel cautery such as after extracapsular cataract surgery with a limbal incision, or a pterygium surgery [19, 21, 27]. For example, the cataract incision may be central to the inflammatory process, however, minor procedures such as suture removal, YAG-laser capsulotomy or wound leak repair could be a provocative factor. Increased likelihood of scleritis after multiple surgeries suggests that the condition may be the result of a hypersensitivity reaction directed against an antigen revealed or altered by tissue injury [27]. Scleritis after a surgical procedure is most likely to be of the necrotizing type (Fig. 11.3). About 63% of patients with SINS have an underlying systemic disorder, most commonly a connective tissue disorder [27], either due to a primary event like vasculitis in the deep episcleral venous plexus or due to the tendency for organ-specific autoreactivity due to another autoimmune disease. The time to presentation has been reported to range from

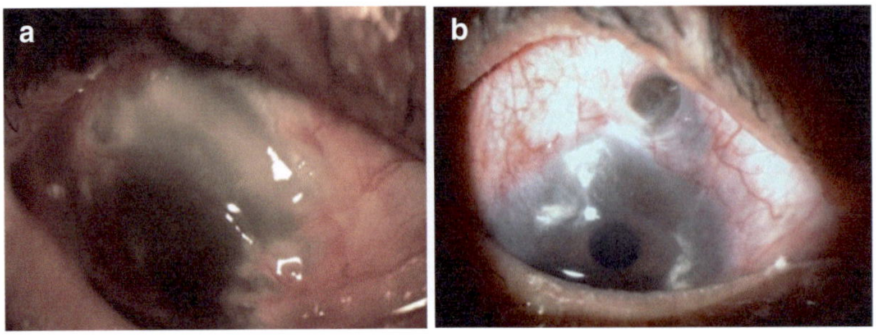

Fig. 11.2 (**a**, **b**) Scleritis associated with Granulomatosis polyangiitis (GPA); (**a**) shows necrotizing scleritis before, and (**b**) shows resolution after treatment with systemic immunosuppressives

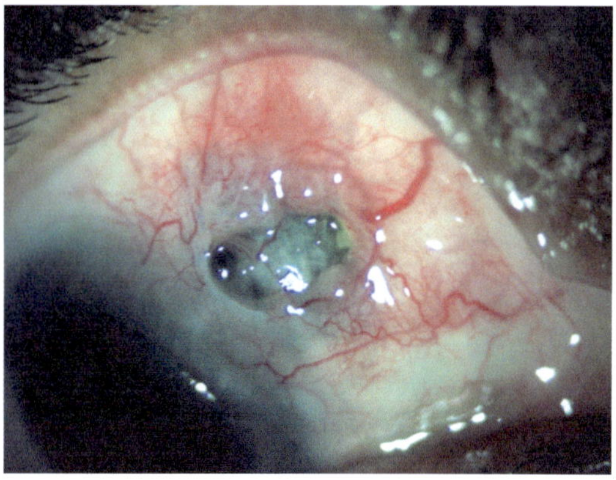

Fig. 11.3 Surgically induced necrotising scleritis (SINS)

2 weeks to 6 months [28]. Surgically induced diffuse scleritis (SIDS) has also been reported [29].

11.4.3 Infectious Scleritis

Infectious scleritis can be bacterial, fungal, viral, or parasitic and can also occur with concomitant keratitis. In a study from India, of the enrolled scleritis patients, 17.87% were diagnosed to have an infection [30]. The two main pathogenic mechanisms involved in the development of infectious scleritis are, firstly, direct invasion of replicating organisms due to breach in the overlying barriers and causing tissue destruction, and secondly, due to immune reactions triggered by the infective organism [31]. Infectious scleritis can be classified into two types [2]:

1. Exogenous scleritis: caused due to either post-traumatic or postsurgical infections, or an extension of keratitis.
2. Endogenous scleritis: associated with systemic infections like syphilis and tuberculosis. This entity is less frequent and can mimic noninfectious scleritis.

Common predisposing factors include ocular trauma, contiguous spread of infection from microbial keratitis, recent ocular surgery, most commonly pterygium surgery, use of antimetabolite like Mitomycin C, use of local radiotherapy, systemic immunosuppressed condition, debilitating ocular disease such as varicella zoster recurrent keratitis, herpes simplex keratitis, dry eye, or ocular immunosuppression by the use of topical steroids [32]. In a series of 97 patients, the most common infection was found to be Herpes Zoster ophthalmicus [33].

Points to differentiate infectious from noninfectious scleritis are:

1. The precipitating cause, like concurrent keratitis, history of recent surgery, or past pterygium surgery, is obvious. SINS can be differentiated by its longer latent period.
2. Immune-mediated scleritis waxes and wanes with the underlying systemic disease. The time for resolution if associated with infectious keratitis is longer.
3. Immune-mediated scleritis: the sclera appears deep red to purplish with overlying conjunctival congestion, whereas infective scleritis is identified with conjunctival ulceration and slough, purulent exudates, abscesses or pus points, or in association with hypopyon and keratitis precipitates (Fig. 11.4).

11.4.3.1 Bacterial Scleritis

The most commonly incriminated organisms are Pseudomonas aeruginosa, Streptococcus pneumonia, and in cases of scleral buckle, Staphylococcus may also be involved.

Nontuberculous mycobacterial (NTM) scleritis is more commonly seen in immune-compromised individuals. The most commonly associated NTM is *Mycobacteroides chelonae*. There should be a high suspicion of NTM infection if the scleritis is following minor office ophthalmic procedures or in cases of injuries associated with soil or contaminated water.

11.4.3.2 Tuberculous Scleritis

Tuberculous scleritis though rare in the west, is still a fairly common entity in a developing country like India. A study suggested that presumed ocular tuberculosis was responsible for 75% of infectious cases in India [34]. Immune mediated process in tuberculosis infection is more common than direct invasion. Immune mediated tuberculous scleritis is a type 4 hypersensitivity reaction, and is often associated with

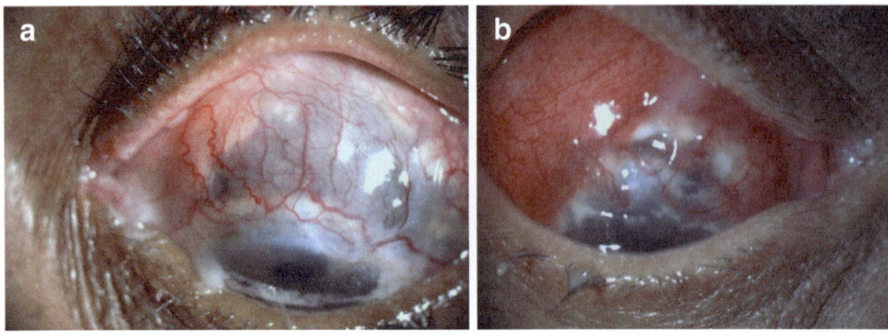

Fig. 11.4 (**a**) Bacterial scleritis: note the multiple areas of thinning and areas of healing, (**b**) Fungal scleritis: showing multinodular appearance with purulent cheesy material at the base of nodules

an active inflammatory component of the scleritis rather than an active infection of the scleral tissue.

11.4.3.3 Fungal Scleritis

Fungal scleritis is the most devastating type of infectious scleritis due to difficulty in controlling the infection, potential of worsening in case of inadvertent steroid treatment and globe destruction leading to visual loss (Fig. 11.4b).

Studies have shown a prevalence of scleritis due to fungal origin to range from 5–38% [35–37]. The most commonly involved fungi are filamentous of which Aspergillus flavus is the most frequent.

11.4.3.4 Viral Scleritis

The most commonly implicated viruses belong to the herpes family, including Varicella Zoster virus (VZV) and Herpes simplex virus type 1(HSV-1). Herpes Zoster scleritis is the most common cause of infectious scleritis, and scleritis may occur months or years after the onset of infection. It is a viral-induced immune mediated manifestation of the infection.

11.4.3.5 Cases

Case 1

Aa 25-year old lady was diagnosed as acanthamoeba keratitis (Fig. 11.6a) based on the presence of nonmotile cysts on KOH mount from corneal scrapings. Patient was started on topical chlorhexidine and topical PHMB treatment. Patient showed response over the next week and complete resolution of infection in two months. A few days after resolution of corneal infection, a nodule involving the conjunctiva and sclera was noted, two millimeters temporal to the limbus (Fig. 11.5b). Clinical suspicion was suggestive of conjunctival tuberculosis. No evidence of acid-fast bacilli was seen on scraping of the lesion. As the conjunctival mass was increasing in size (Fig. 11.5c, d), an excision biopsy with amniotic membrane grafting was performed. Histopathology showed suppurative necrotizing lesion with histiocytic proliferation (Fig. 11.5f–h). TB-PCR of the lesion came out negative. A systemic evaluation of collagen vascular diseases was performed. Apart from ANA, which was mildly raised, the rest was within normal limits. Culture of the lesion didn't grow any organism. Patient was continued on topical anti-amoebic therapy and steroids along with oral and topical antibiotics and the patient responded to it (Fig. 11.5e).

Case 2

A 50 years old male presented with a punched out defect in sclera, temporal to the limbus, 15 days after an uneventful temporal phacoemulsification cataract surgery (Fig. 11.6a). There was a past history of pulmonary Koch's ten years back with completed treatment. Patient was also HbsAg positive. A diagnosis of SINS was made; and the patient was started on oral steroids and planned for a scleral patch graft. The steroids were gradually tapered and the lesion healed on treatment (Fig. 11.6b).

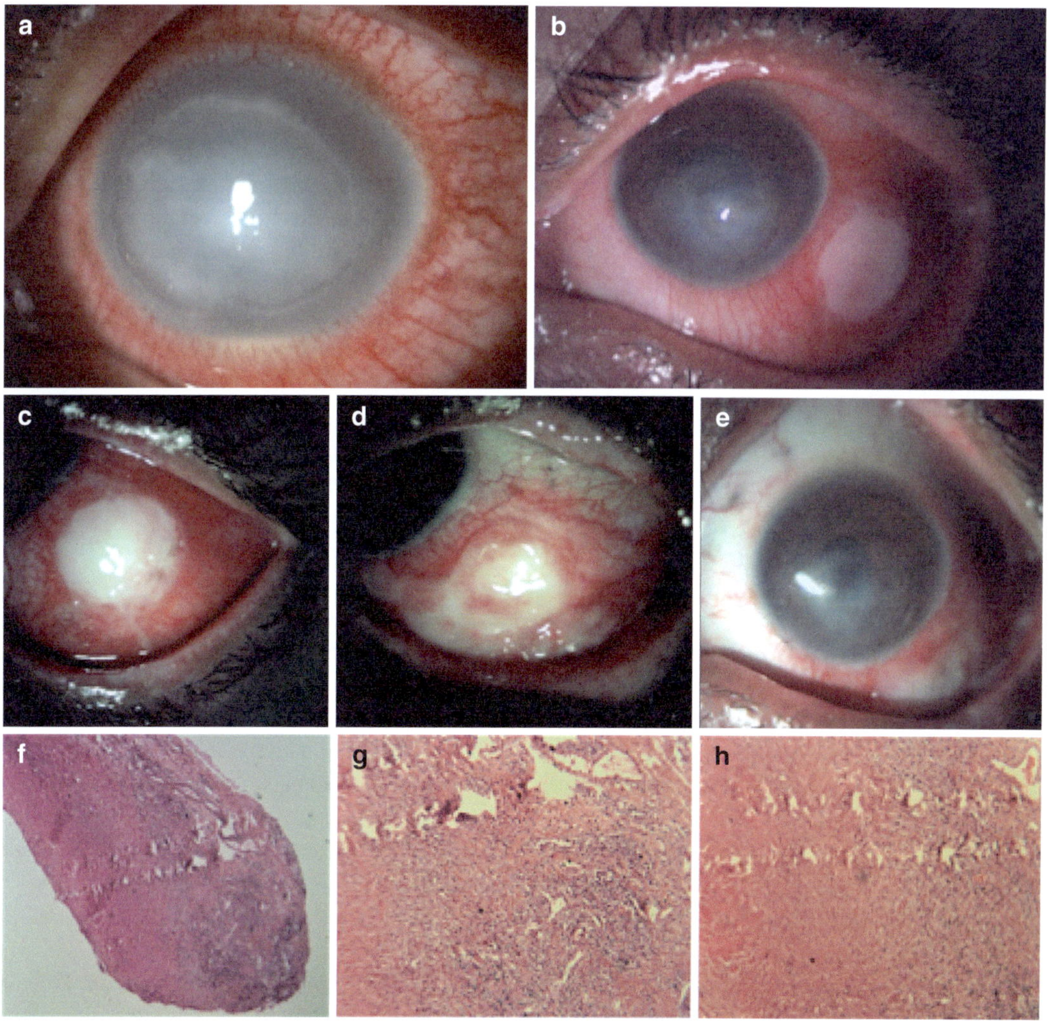

Fig. 11.5 (**a**) Acanthamoeba keratitis in a 25-year-old lady, (**b**) Scleral nodule developed a few days after resolution of corneal infection, (**c**, **d**) Increase in the size of the lesion, (**e**) Resolution on anti-amebic and steroid therapy. (**f**–**h**) Histopathology

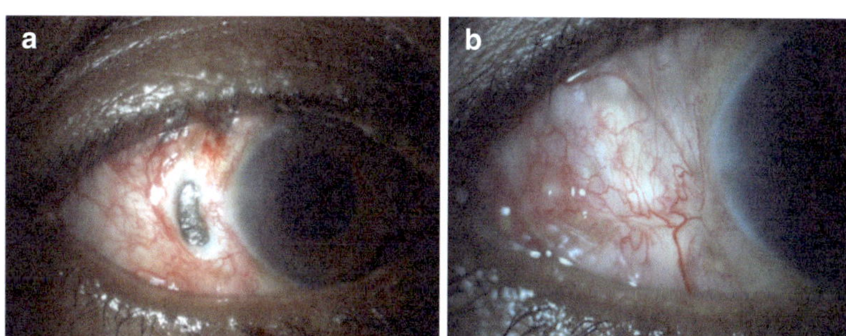

Fig. 11.6 (**a**) Punched out defect in the sclera, in a 50-year-old male, after an uneventful phacoemulsification surgery, (**b**) condition post patch-graft

11.5 Degenerative Diseases of the Sclera

11.5.1 Senile Scleral Hyaline Plaques

Occur in individuals over 60 years of age and appear as dark, nonprogressive, oval patch surrounded by a dense calcareous yellowish ring. The center of the ring is translucent and the underlying uvea is seen through it. These are usually bilateral, symmetrical and present in the interpalpebral area [38].

11.5.2 Phthisis bulbi

Phthisis bulbi is an end-stage eye disease with functional loss, characterized by shrinkage and disorganization of the eye. The sclera in phthisis bulbi is thickened, upto 40% in the anterior part and 60% in the posterior part. The phthisical eye shows a squared-off shape due to folding in of the thickened sclera behind the Spiral of Tillaux. This folding is responsible for the smaller size of the globe [39].

11.6 Histopathological Findings of Scleritis

11.6.1 Histopathology of Scleritis

It is an inflammatory-based process that is seen in the extracellular matrix (ECM) in the sclera. Histopathological studies on sclera alone in immune-mediated scleritis are lacking, as scleral tissue is rarely biopsied in the case of noninfectious scleritis. The sclera that an ocular pathologist sees is part of eviscerated specimens in cases of phthisis bulbi and panophthalmitis, or as part of tumor histopathology specimens [40].

Rao et al. [41] reported histopathological changes from eyeballs received at autopsy scleritis: sections from different scleral specimens showed mainly three types of inflammatory processes. The first showed suppurative inflammatory cell changes with areas of necrosis, and these biopsies are also sent to the ocular microbiology laboratory to prove the causative microorganism. The other type was of an autoimmune etiology, and under the microscope this showed necrotic areas involving the collagen with surrounding suppurative debris and neutrophils along with palisading histiocytes, but no evidence of infection. There were no disease-specific changes noted in the biopsies. Some of the histological findings also included a few loci of vasculitis and scattered giant cells.

In the third type of findings, often referred to as idiopathic scleritis, they noted an absence of necrosis with features of chronic inflammation mainly lymphocytes and scattered plasma cells and histiocytes. The microscopic sections also showed granulation tissue and occasional fibrosis. Also, a detailed serum and immunohistochemistry workup to rule out associated IgG4-positive diseases was indicated in some cases.

Therefore, the histopathological examination under the microscope can offer some histomorphological evidence toward the etiology, at least to help differentiate infectious from noninfectious etiologies when classical and definite clinical features are not seen.

11.6.2 Histopathology of Scleral Biopsy Specimens from Infectious Scleritis

Scleral or sclerocorneal biopsy is advised in suspected infectious scleritis: a part of the deeper tissue obtained at the time of scleral biopsy in suspected infectious scleritis should be sent in 20% formalin. This tissue can further be processed and apart from routine Hematoxylin–Eosin (H&E) and Periodic acid schiff (PAS) stain, Gram's, Acid-fast, and Gomori Methenamine Silver (GMS) stain should also be performed.

11.6.3 Sclera in Ocular Tumors

Enucleation specimens in retinoblastoma: the sclera can be involved microscopically, and vascular invasion too should be looked for. Sclera can be normal in the case of an intraocular tumor. Other tumors such as melanoma can also undergo enucleation and any scleral involvement should be looked for.

In the case of ocular surface squamous neoplasia, scleral involvement may be present and should be looked for in all map biopsy fragments sent for histopathological evaluation.

11.6.4 Specimens Obtained as Evisceration Samples

11.6.4.1 End-Stage Infection

End-stage infection such as panophthalmitis or severe endophthalmitis with microbial keratitis are often received in the pathology laboratory. Special stains should be performed to identify the infectious organisms, such as Gram's stain, Acid-fast, and GMS stain. In H& E stain, the tissue fragments would show edema, red blood cells—areas of hemorrhage and inflammatory infiltrates with extensive neutrophilic infiltrates invading the scleral tissue and clusters of infectious organisms may be noted.

11.6.4.2 Evisceration Specimens in Cases of Phthisis Bulbi (Done for Cosmetic Implants)

Sclera in phthisis bulbi would show thinning or sometimes thickening due to edema, with disorganization of normal scleral architecture.

Figure 11.7 shows sections of scleral tissue with inflammatory cell infiltrate and fibrosis (10× and 20×)in a case of infection with features of necrosis and chronic inflammation; mainly consisting of lymphocytes and scattered plasma cells and histiocytes—10×, 20×, 40× and 100×—H and E stain. The various histopathological features of the sclera are depicted in Fig. 11.7a–i.

Financial Disclosures NFigone

Funding For Somasheila Murthy: Hyderabad Eye Research Foundation, Hyderabad

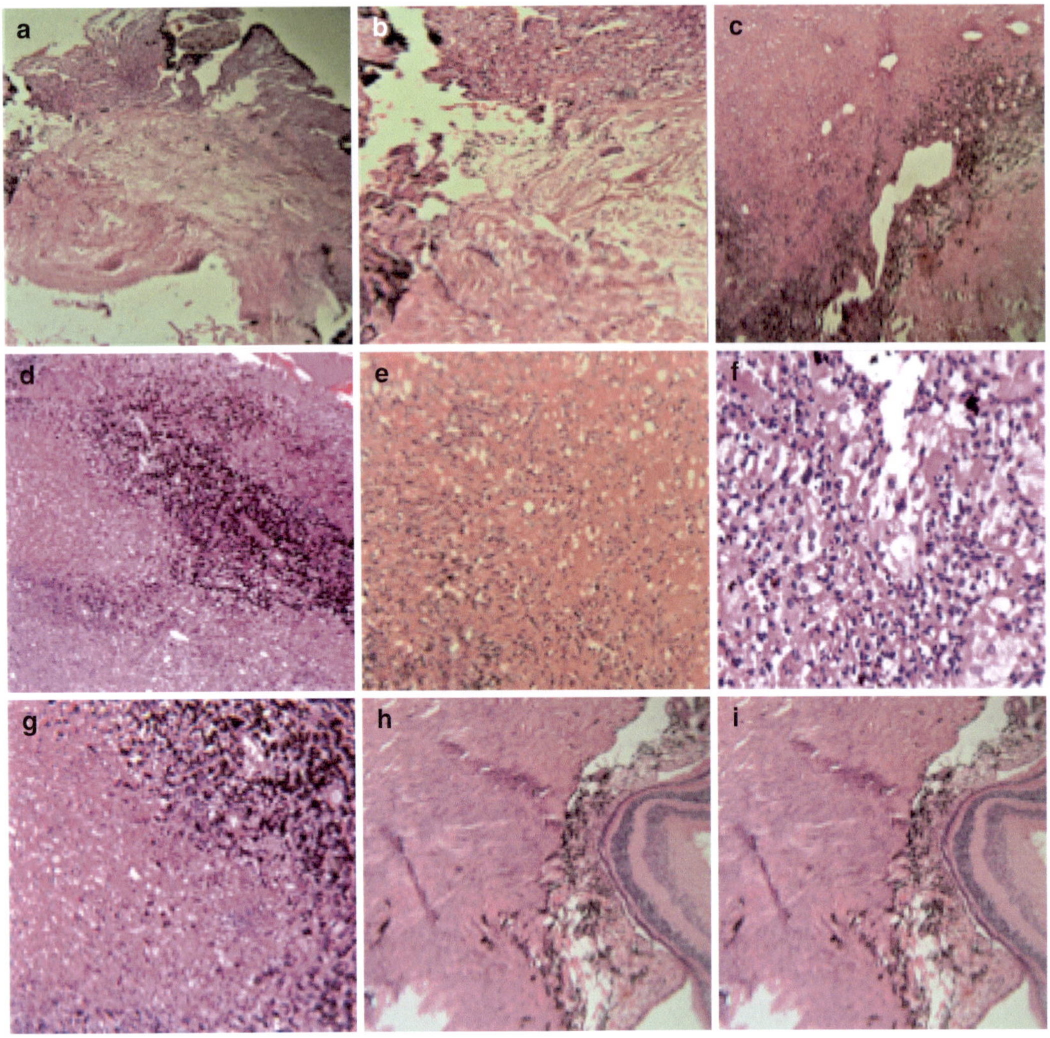

Fig. 11.7 (:**a**) Disorganized scleral tissue with adhered uveal tissue; hematoxylin and eosin (H& E) stained sections under low magnification. (**b**) Scleral tissue of a case of phthisis bulbi; H& E stained section 20× magnification. (**c**) Scleral tissue of a case of phthisis bulbi; H& E stained section 10× magnification. (**d**–**g**) Suppurative panophthalmitis 40× magnification sections show sheets of suppurative inflammation with neutrophils, nuclear debris, and few areas of necrosis: (**d**, **f**, **g**) PAS-stained section, (**e**) H&E stained, (**h**) PAS stained, 100× magnification. (**i**) Scleral tissue from eviscerated contents of a globe with anterior staphyloma: PAS-stained section,20× magnification. The section shows scleral tissue and retinal tissue in the eviscerated specimen

References

1. Hosseini, HS, Beebe, DC, Taber LA. Mechanical effects of the surface ectoderm on optic vesicle morphogenesis in the chick embryo. J Biomech. 47(16): 3837–46.
2. Hosseini HS, Taber LA. How mechanical forces shape the developing eye. Progr Biophys Mol Biol. 137(16): 25–36.
3. Hoar RM. Embryology of the eye. Environ Health Perspect. 1982;44:31–4.
4. Creuzet S, Vincent C, Couly G. Neural crest derivatives in ocular and periocular structures. Int J Dev Biol. 2005;49(2–3):161–71.
5. Yoshida K. Naevus fuscocaeruleus opthalmomaxillaris Ota. Tohoku J Exp Med. 1952;55(S1):34–43.

6. Hori Y, Takayama O. Circumscribed dermal melanoses. Classification and histologic features. Dermatol Clin. 1988;6(2):315–26.
7. Teekhasaenee C, Ritch R, Rutnin U, et al. Ocular findings in oculodermal melanocytosis. Arch Ophthalmol. 1990;108:1114–20.
8. Kumar A, Singh J. Naevus of Ota with primary retinitis pigmentosa: a syndrome. Can J Ophthalmol. 1985;20:261–3.
9. Chan HH, Kono T. Nevus of Ota: clinical aspects and management. Skinmed. 2003;2(2):89–96.
10. Cross HE, Jensen AD. Ocular manifestations in the Marfan syndrome and homocystinuria. A m J Ophthalmol. 1973;75:405.
11. Kaiser-Kupfer MI, McCain L, Shapiro JR, Podgor MJ, Kupfer C, Rowe D. Low ocular rigidity in patients with osteogenesis imperfecta. Invest Ophthalmol Vis Sci. 1981;20:807.
12. McKusick VA. Multiple forms of the Ehlers- Danlos syndrome. Arch Surg. 1974;109:475.
13. Salmon JF, Strauss PC, Todd G, Murray ADN. Acute scleritis in porphyria cutanea tarda. Am J Ophthalmol. 1990;109:400.
14. Chumbley LC. Scleral involvement in symptomatic porphyria. A m J Ophthalmol. 1977;84:729.
15. Veenashree MP, Sangwan VS, Vemuganti GK, Parthasaradhi A. Acute scleritis as a manifestation of congenital erythropoietic porphyria. Cornea. 2002;21(5):530–1.
16. Sanderson PO, Kuwabara T, Stark WJ, Wong VG, Collins E. Cystinosis: a clinical, histopathologic, and ultrastructural study. Arch Ophthalmol. 1974;91:270.
17. Wirtschafter JD. The eye in alkaptonuria. Birth Defects. 1976;12(3):279.
18. Nelson GA, Edward DP, Wilnesky WT. Ocular amyloidosis and secondary glaucoma. Ophthalmology. 1999;106(7):1363–6.
19. Watson PG, Hayreh SS. Scleritis and episcleritis. Br J Ophthalmol. 1976;60(3):163–91.
20. Murthy SI, Sabhapandit S, Balamurugan S, Subramaniam P, Sainz-de-la-Maza M, Agarwal M, Parvesio C. Scleritis: differentiating infectious from non-infectious entities. Indian J Ophthalmol. 2020;68(9):1818–28.
21. Okhravi N, Odufuwa B, McCluskey P, Lightman S. Scleritis. Surv Ophthalmol 2005;50(4):351–63.
22. Smith JR, Mackensen F, Rosenbaum JT. Therapy insight: scleritis and its relationship to systemic autoimmune disease. Nat Clin Pract Rheumatol. 2007;3:219–26.
23. Jayson MI, Jones DE. Scleritis and rheumatoid arthritis. Ann Rheum Dis. 1971;30(4):343–7.
24. Sainz de la Maza M, Foster CS, Jabbur NS. Scleritis associated with rheumatoid arthritis and with other systemic immune-mediated diseases. Ophthalmology. 1994;101(7):1281–6; discussion 1287–8.
25. Harper SL, Letko E, Samson CM, Zafirakis P, Sangwan V, Nguyen Q, et al. Wegener's granulomatosis: the relationship between ocular and systemic disease. J Rheumatol 2001;28:1025–1032
26. Pakrou N, Selva D, Leibovitch I. Wegener's granulomatosis: ophthalmic manifestations and management. Semin Arthritis Rheum. 2006 Apr;35(5):284–92.
27. O'Donoghue E, Lightman S, Tuft S, et al. Surgically induced necrotising sclerokeratitis (SINS)—precipitating factors and response to treatment. Br J Ophthalmol. 1992;76:17–21.
28. Sainz de la Maza M, Foster CS, Jabbur NS. Scleritis-associated uveitis. Ophthalmology. 1997;104:58–63.
29. Scott JA, Clearkin LG. Surgically induced diffuse scleritis following cataract surgery. Eye. 1994;8(Pt 3):292–7.
30. Reddy JC, Murthy SI, Reddy AK, Garg P. Risk factors and clinical outcomes of bacterial and fungal scleritis at a tertiary eye care hospital. Middle East Afr J Ophthalmol. 2015;22:203–11.
31. Ramenaden ER, Raiji VR. Clinical characteristics and visual outcomes in infectious scleritis: a review. Clin Ophthalmol. 2013;7:2113–22.
32. Pavesio C, editor. Scleritis. Cham: Springer International Publishing; 2017.
33. McCluskey PJ, Watson PG, Lightman S, et al. Posterior scleritis: clinical features, systemic associations, and outcome in a large series of patients. Ophthalmology. 1999;106:2380–6.
34. Lane J, Nyugen E, Lim L, Stawell R, Hodgson L, Ismail MAB, et al. Clinical features of scleritis across the Asia-Pacific region. Ocular Immunol In Amm. 2019;27:920–6.
35. Ho YF, Yeh LK, Tan HY, Chen HC, Yeong-Fong Chen YF, Lin HC, et al. Infectious scleritis in Taiwan—a 10-year review in a tertiary-care hospital. Cornea. 2014;33:838–43.
36. Murthy SI, Reddy JC, Sharma S, Sangwan VS. Infectious scleritis. Curr Ophthalmol Rep. 2015;3:147–57.
37. Pradhan Z, Jacob P. Infectious scleritis: clinical spectrum and management outcomes in India. Indian J Ophthalmol. 2013;61:590–3.
38. Roper KL. Senile hyaline scleral plaques. Arch Ophthalmol. 1945;34:283.
39. Tripathy K, Chawla R, Temkar S, Sagar P, Kashyap S, Pushker N, Sharma YR. Phthisis Bulbi-a clinicopathological perspective. Semin Ophthalmol. 2018;33(6):788–803.
40. Hankins M, Margo CE. Histopathological evaluation of scleritis. J Clin Pathol. 2019;72:386–90.
41. Rao NA, Marak GE, Hidayat AA. Necrotizing scleritis. A clinico-pathologic study of 41 cases. Ophthalmology. 1985;92:1542–8.

Eyelids: Benign and Malignant Lesions

12

Seema Sen and Milind Naik

Contents

S. Sen (✉)
Ocular Pathology, Dr. R.P Centre for Ophthalmic Sciences, AIIMS, New Delhi, India

M. Naik
Ophthalmic Plastic Surgery Service, LV Prasad Eye Institute, Hyderabad, India
e-mail: milind@drmilindnaik.com

12.1 Introduction

Eyelids protect the eye from excessive light and injury by forming a mechanical barrier and maintaining lubrication. Eyelid lesions are very com-

G. K. Vemuganti et al. (eds.), *Ocular Pathology*, https://doi.org/10.1007/978-981-96-8614-8_12

mon in ophthalmic practice. Benign lesions predominate (84%). However, frequency varies with geographical location, genetic background, and socioeconomic status [1].

12.2 Anatomy/Histology of the Eyelid

Eyelid skin is one of the thinnest in the whole body and is loosely bound to the dermis. Clinically, the eyelid is a bilamellar tissue. The anterior lamella(a) consists of the skin and orbicularis muscle, whereas the posterior lamella (p) consists of the tarsal plate, levator muscle, and palpebral conjunctiva (Fig. 12.1a). Histologically, these layers are clearly identified (Fig. 12.1b, c). The dermis has fibrous tissue, blood vessels, lymphatics, and nerves. There is no fat in subcutaneous layer. Various glands including eccrine sweat glands of the skin, apocrine Moll's glands and accessory lacrimal glands of Krause and Wolfring are located in the forniceal conjunctiva and upper margin of tarsal conjunctiva, respectively.

12.2.1 Skin–Epidermal Layer

The epidermal layer of the skin is composed of stratified squamous epithelium with mild keratinization. Appendages include hair follicles, sebaceous glands (glands of Zeiss), and sweat glands (Fig. 12.1d). Melanocytes are present in the basal layer.

Lid margin: Most anterior aspect of lid margin is round and post margin is right angled—epidermis is more finally attached to dermis. At the mucocutaneous junction the keratinized epithelium of lid transforms to nonkeratinized conjunctival epithelium. Glands of Moll are apocrine sweat glands located near lid margin in association with the cilia.

12.2.2 Muscular Layer

Muscular layer consists of orbicularis oculi (skeletal muscle) and tendon of levator palpebrae superioris muscle (LPS) inserts into the lid (pretarsal connective tissue) and surface tarsus. The muscular part of LPS lies in the orbital roof and is innervated by oculomotor nerve. Smooth

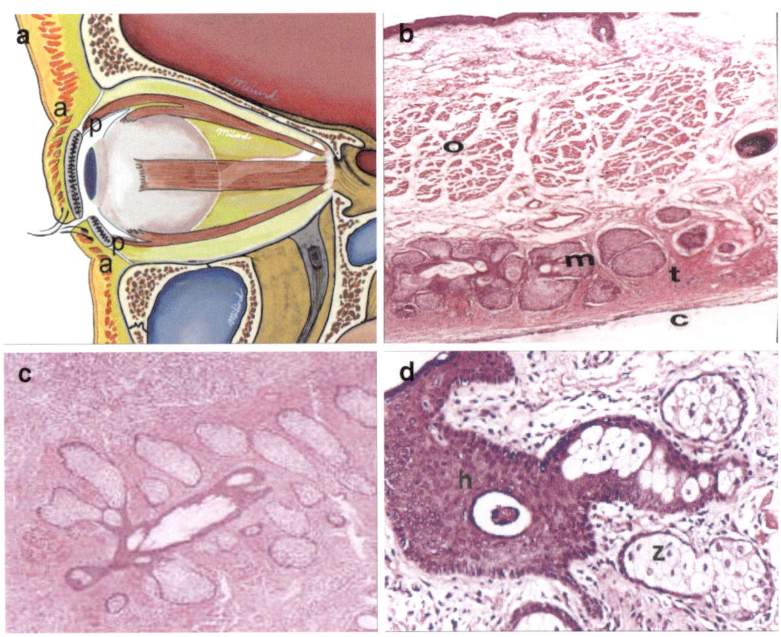

Fig. 12.1 (**a**) Diagrammatic representation of the layers of the eyelid. The anterior lamella (a) consists of skin and orbicularis, and posterior lamella (p) constitutes the tarsus, levator, and conjunctiva. (**b**) Low power view to show conjunctival surface(c), meibomian gland(m) orbicularis muscle (o). (**c**) Higher magnification to show the meibomian glands in the tarsal plate. (**d**) The pilosebaceous unit comprising the hair follicle(h) with Zeiss gland(z)

muscle of Muller is posterior to the levator and is sympathetically innervated.

12.2.3 Tarsal Layer

Dense fibrous tissue provides structural support and stiffness to the eyelid. The meibomian glands are branching tubule alveolar sebaceous glands (40–50 in the upper and 20 in the lower eyelid) and have no association with hair follicles. Eccrine glands are present in preseptal (preorbital skin) skin in the thin reticular dermis [2].

12.2.4 Palpebral Conjunctiva

The posterior eyelid surface is lined by a thin mucous membrane (palpebral conjunctiva) comprising cuboidal epithelium with goblet cells and fibrovascular stroma.

Eyelid lesions and tumors can be classified in several ways. Popularly, they are classified either based on the histologic origin of the tumor, or the pathophysiologic mechanism (Table 12.1). Here, we shall follow the pathophysiologic classification, as that is more practical in the clinical setting.

Table 12.1 Classification of eyelid lesions based on pathophysiologic mechanism

Inflammatory lesions
Chalazion:
Molluscum contagiosum
Neoplastic conditions: Benign
Squamous papillomas
Epidermal Inclusion cysts
Melanocytic nevi
Seborrheic keratosis
Hidrocystoma: Eccrine and apocrine
Xanthelasma
Actinic keratosis
Keratoacanthoma
Neoplastic lesions: Malignant
Basal cell carcinoma
Squamous cell carcinoma
Sebaceous carcinoma
Metastatic carcinoma
Lymphomas
Melanomas

12.3 Inflammatory Lesions

12.3.1 Chalazion

Chalazion is a frequently observed chronic granulomatous inflammatory lesion involving the glands of Zeis or the meibomian glands of the eyelid.

Etiopathogenesis: They are caused by obstruction of the meibomian or glands of Zeis.

Clinical Picture: A chalazion presents as a long-standing, painless nodule on the eyelid. Patients are usually bothered by the unsightly appearance, but rarely may complain about impaired vision (due to astigmatism) or discomfort when it becomes inflamed, or infected. It can either present as an inflamed tender nodule (Fig. 12.2a) or as a painless bump (Fig. 12.2b). Often, there is a history of previous chalazia, or even rosacea.

Histopathology: Microscopically, there is an epithelioid and giant cell reaction to the liberated fat from the sebaceous glands (Fig. 12.2c, d). Fat appears as non-stainable lipid vacuoles (empty spaces produced by lipid dissolved by organic solvents during tissue processing) within the tissue is a reliable indicator. Usually mixed inflammatory infiltrate is rich in plasma cells, varying degree of fibrosis may be seen in older lesions. Differential diagnosis includes sarcoidosis, fungal disease, leprosy, tuberculosis, foreign body giant cell reaction, and syphilis.

Differential Diagnosis The two most common differentials include epidermoid cyst (in young) and sebaceous gland carcinoma (SGC, in elderly). Cysts are usually well defined, with a sharp, abrupt distinction between the lesion and the surrounding normal tissue. Sebaceous gland carcinoma can mimic a chalazion in early stages but is identified by the distorted microanatomy of the posterior lamella and loss of lashes.

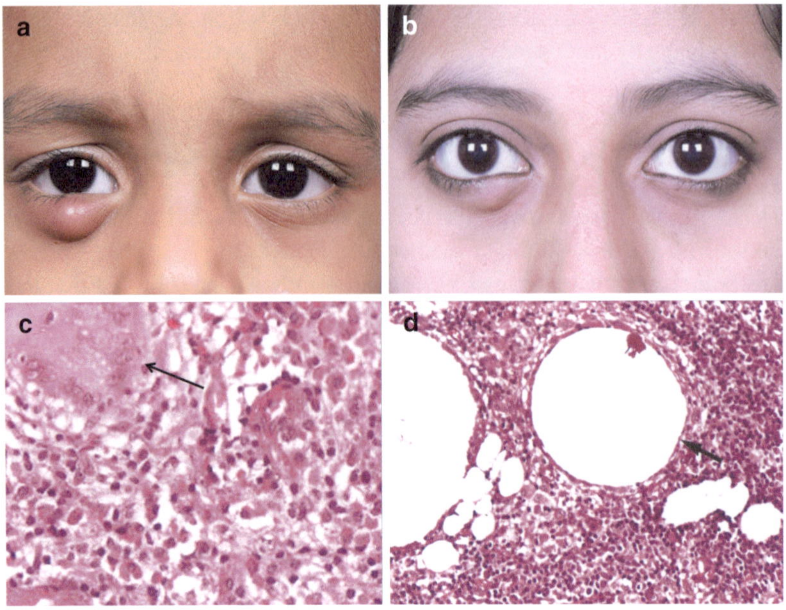

Fig. 12.2 (**a**) An active, inflamed chalazion in a 8-year-old child, amenable to conservative medical therapy. (**b**) A chronic, long-standing chalazion in a 22-year-old lady, which may require surgical curettage. (**c**) Lipogranulomatous inflammation with giant cell (arrow), histiocytes, and chronic inflammatory cells. (**d**) Clear areas in the center (arrow) represent lipid dissolved during processing

Clinicopathologic Correlation Any age can be affected, the lesion may be red or white based on duration. Inflamed lesions are amenable to topical antibiotics or steroid injections, whereas long-standing ones require surgical curettage. Multiple, medial, or marginal ones are best treated with steroid injections rather than surgery (3 M rule) [4]. Multiple or recurrent lesions should always be subjected to histopathology to rule out underlying sebaceous gland carcinoma.

12.4 Molluscum Contagiosum

Etiopathogenesis Molluscum Contagiosum is caused by molluscum virus, a DNA Pox virus.

Clinical picture: It affects young children and immunocompromised adults. Clinically, it appears as skin nodules over the eyelid skin or eyelid margin. The nodules are 2–5 mm in size, pearl-like, raised with an umbilicated center (Fig. 12.3a, b). Since the clinical picture is classic, usually a biopsy is unnecessary.

Histopathology On microscopy, the lobulated lesion shows inverted acanthosis of epithelium, and the cells contain characteristic cytoplasmic eosinophilic inclusions, termed molluscum or Henderson–Paterson bodies (Fig. 12.3c, d). Infection begins in the deeper layers of epidermis, and as the involved cells move toward the surface, the molluscum bodies become more basophilic and eventually replace the cells [5].

Differential Diagnosis The common differentials for molluscum include warts (verruca vulgaris which has a rough, hard texture), chicken pox (varicella have fluid-filled blisters), and eyelid papilloma (usually occurs in the middle-aged or elderly with finger-like fronds).

Clinicopathologic Correlation Molluscum lesions are self-limiting and resolve in a few weeks or months. Watchful observation is usually enough, and treatment is not mandatory. In cases with extensive lesions, treatment options include surgical removal or cryotherapy. In immunosuppressed individuals, antiviral medications may be required. Recurrence is possible in predisposed patients.

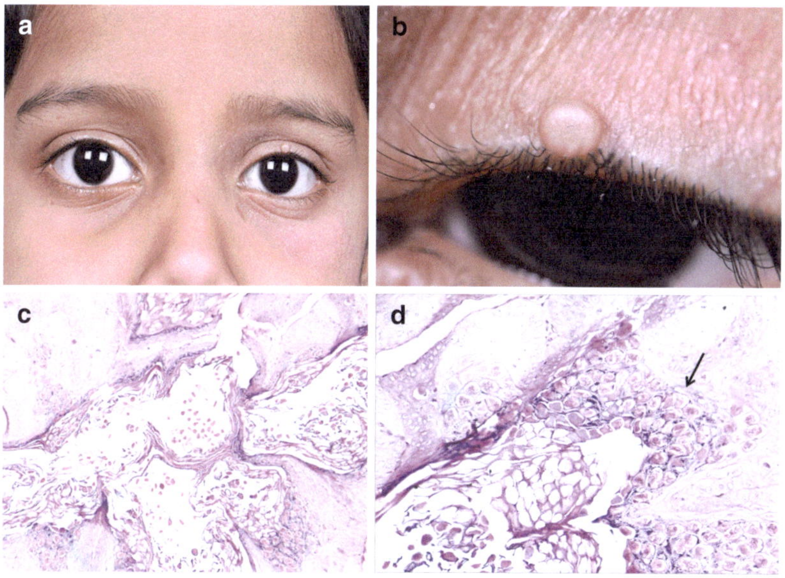

Fig. 12.3 (**a**, **b**) An 11-year-old child with a single 3-mm nodule over the left upper lid with an umbilicated center, suggestive of molluscum contagiosum. (**c**) Invagination of epidermis containing numerous eosinophilic molluscum bodies. (**d**) Higher magnification shows intracytoplasmic molluscum bodies (arrow)

12.5 Neoplastic Lesions: Benign

12.5.1 Squamous Papilloma

Etiopathogenesis Squamous papilloma is an idiopathic benign cellular proliferation. Solar irritation is the most likely cause, and they are often not associated with papillomavirus.

Clinical features Squamous papilloma, also referred to as a skin tag or a wart, represents a soft, pedunculated or sessile flesh-colored lesion with finger-like processes (Fig. 12.4a, b). They may be multiple.

Histopathology On microscopy, papillary appearance was observed with hyperplasia of epithelium. There was acanthosis (thickening) of the surface epithelium and hyperkeratosis with parakeratosis. Fibrovascular core is characteristic (Fig. 12.4c, d).

Clinicopathologic correlation Small lesions can be observed. If cosmetically unacceptable, it can be excised by shave biopsy.

12.5.2 Seborrheic Keratosis

Etiopathogenesis Seborrheic Keratosis is an idiopathic benign cellular proliferation. It could be due to genetic predisposition or sun exposure.

Clinical features Epithelial-derived benign neoplasm of the skin cells, often with a well-circumscribed, elevated stuck-on appearance (Fig. 12.5a). It is usually seen in older individuals, and often has a variable degree of pigmentation.

Histopathology Microscopically, there is a hyperplasia of basaloid cells associated with variable hyperkeratosis and keratin-filled cysts (pseudohorn cysts). Hyperkeratosis causes papillomatosis (Fig. 12.5b, c).

Differential diagnosis Normally, seborrheic keratosis is benign, but the sudden appearance of multiple seborrheic keratoses could raise the suspicion of a paraneoplastic process. The inverted variant can clinically mimic SCC or actinic

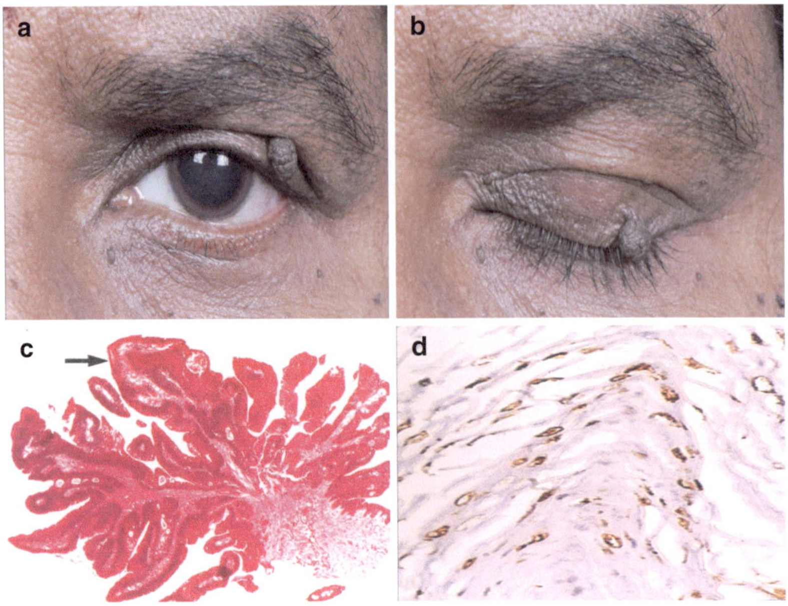

Fig. 12.4 (**a**, **b**) Pedunculated, papillary growth arising from the upper eyelid skin, suggestive of a benign papilloma. (**c**) Light microscopy shows the finger-like projections (arrow) lined by squamous epithelium enclosing a fibrovascular core. (**d**) Cytoplasmic positivity for HPV virus is seen on immunohistochemistry

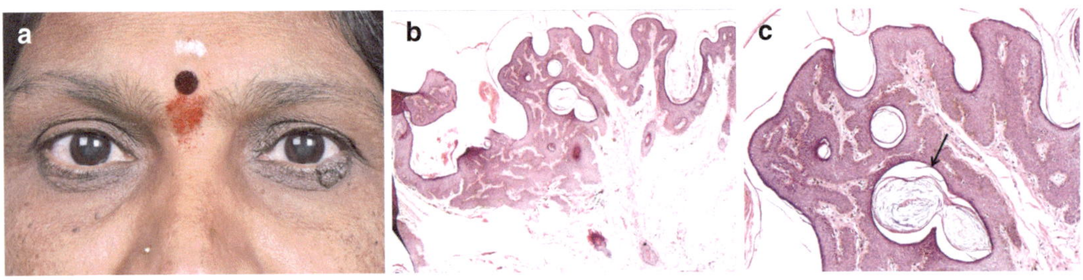

Fig. 12.5 (**a**) 45-year-old lady with a flat pigmented growth over the left lower lid, extending over the eyelid margin. The lesion is asymptomatic, long-standing and does not disrupt the normal architecture of the eyelid margin. (**b**) Histopathology shows a papillomatous lesion above the skin surface. (**c**) Higher magnification to show cystic accumulation of keratin (arrow)

keratosis. Other pigmented differential lesions include melanoma, pigmented BCC, and nevus.

Clinicopathologic correlation Shave excision biopsy is usually curative and provides histopathologic confirmation. Large lesions may require primary closure with undermining, or a skin graft to cover the defect.

12.5.3 Keratoacanthoma

Etiopathogenesis Possible etiologies including ultraviolet (UV) radiation, chemical carcinogens, immunocompromised state, use of BRAF inhibitors, genetic mutations of p53 or H-Ras, human papillomavirus (HPV), and recent trauma or surgery. It arises from the pilosebaceous unit. It is sunlight-related, viral, or genetic. About 25% may be premalignant [6].

Clinical Features

Dome-shaped skin tumor with central keratinous plug and rolled margins (Fig. 12.6a, b). It is characterized by initial rapid growth followed by a period of tumor stability and spontaneous regression.

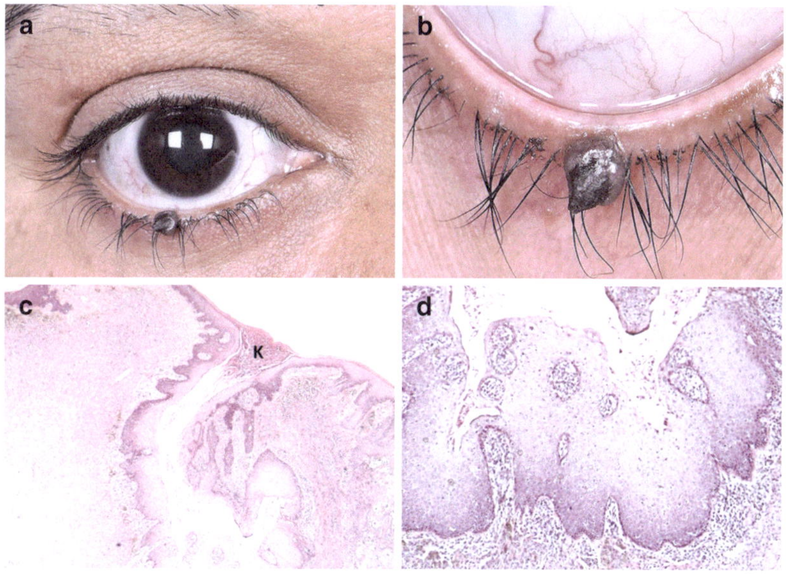

Fig. 12.6 (**a**, **b**) Keratoacanthoma of the right lower eyelid, showing a dome-shaped mass with a central keratinous plug. (**c**) Cup-shaped configuration with central keratin (k). (**d**) Higher magnification shows acanthotic epithelium

Histopathology Histopathologically, there is a cup-shaped lesion with thickened epidermis composed of proliferating well-differentiated squamous epithelium surrounding a central mass of keratin (Fig. 12.6c, d).

Clinicopathologic correlation Best diagnostic test is an excision biopsy with 4-mm margin.

12.5.4 Xanthelasma

Etiopathogenesis Patients with Xanthelasma may have normal or high cholesterol levels (50%). It is seen more commonly in Asian females who are overweight. Patients should be investigated for underlying inherited dyslipidemia. *Clinical Features*: Xanthelasma appear insidiously as yellowish flat or slightly raised plaques in the upper and lower eyelid, usually around the inner canthus. They represent dermal deposition of lipids (Fig. 12.7a, b).

Histopathology The dermis contains nests of xanthoma cells or foam cells in the superficial dermis. These cells are lipid-laden histiocytes in which the cytoplasm appears empty in hematoxylin and eosin sections. Xanthoma cells are located in the periadnexal or perivascular location (Fig. 12.7c, d).

Clinicopathologic correlation Correction is usually surgical and for cosmetic reasons. New lesions may appear, especially if dyslipidemia continues.

12.5.5 Epidermoid Cyst and Epidermal Inclusion Cyst

Etiopathogenesis Proliferation of benign cells within a confined space results in formation of a cyst. Mechanisms of formation include sequestration of epidermal cells along fusion planes during embryonic development, epidermal proliferation from the pilosebaceous unit, or implantation of epidermal elements as a result of trauma or surgery [7].

Clinical features Epidermoid cysts are slow-growing benign cysts that can commonly affect the eyelid [8]. They differ from dermoid cysts only in that dermal appendages are lacking. They present as solitary elevated, oval, and mobile

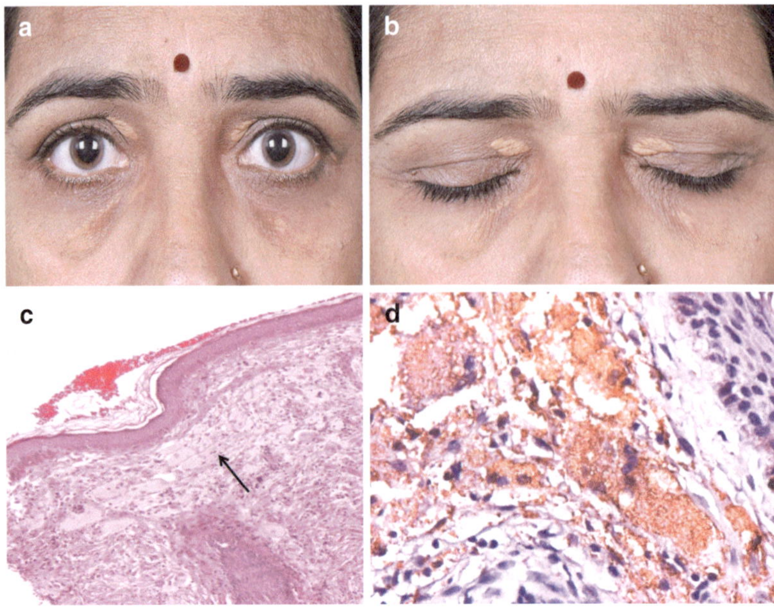

Fig. 12.7 (**a**, **b**) An asymptomatic, flat, yellowish plaque along the medial aspect of upper and lower eyelids in a 35-year-old lady is suggestive of Xanthelasma (**c**) Clusters of lipid-laden foam cells in superficial dermis, mostly perivascular. (**d**). CD-68 positivity is seen in cytoplasm of the macrophages

subcutaneous masses (Fig. 12.8a–d). A central pore may firmly connect the tumor to the overlying skin. Rupture of an epidermoid cyst may incite a foreign body granulomatous reaction in the surrounding tissues.

Histopathology Cysts are named based on the type of epithelium lining the cysts. Epidermoid or sebaceous cysts are lined by laminated keratinizing squamous epithelium. Most are derived from plugged hair follicles.

Contents are cheesy material derived from hyperkeratotic squamous epithelium with the granular layer seen on microscopy. Most are derived from plugged hair follicles. Dermal appendages including hair follicles and sebaceous glands are not seen (Fig. 12.8e–g).

The term epidermal inclusion cysts is used for traumatic cases in which epithelial cells are implanted in the dermis following injury.

Clinicopathologic correlation When these cysts are tarsus-based, they are often misdiagnosed as chalazion, and a mere incision and curettage is likely to lead to a recurrence. Tarsus-based epidermoid cysts require an eyelid crease incision and complete removal of its wall.

12.5.6 Dermoid Cyst

Etiopathogenesis Dermoid cysts are choristomas, which are caused by sequestration of embryonic epithelium.

Clinical features Periocular dermoids can take several forms, which include angular dermoids, orbital dermoids, and rarely, tarsal dermoid [9, 10]. Angular dermoids are usually seen in children and adolescents, as smooth, fixed, firm masses superomedial or superolateral in the anterior orbit (Fig. 12.9a). They may create a bump over the eyelid, but truly are orbital in location along the bony suture lines. Tarsal dermoid is rare and can mimic a chalazion.

Histopathology Dermoid cysts are squamous epithelium-lined keratin-filled cysts identical to epidermoid cysts but are characterized by the presence of skin appendages as hair, sweat

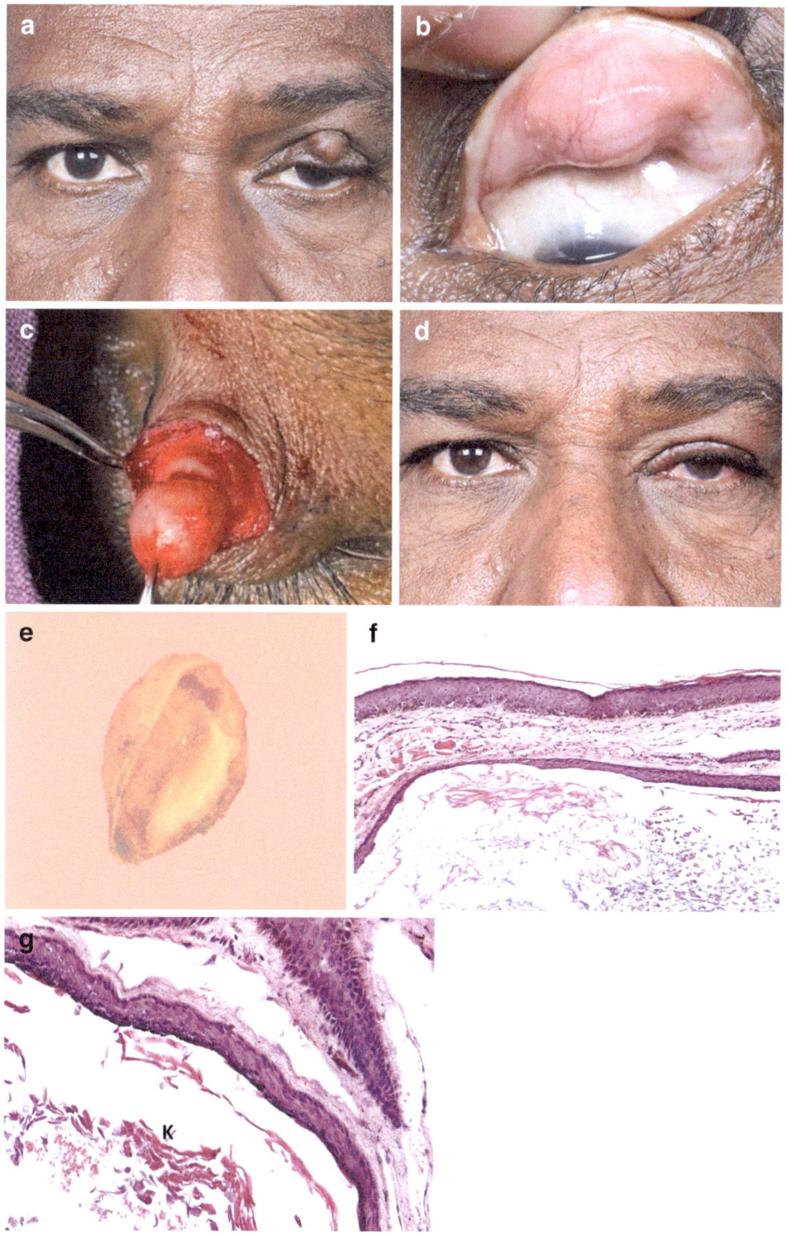

Fig. 12.8 A 50-year-old male with a well-defined tarsus-based nodule over the left upper lid (**a**). Upon eversion of the eyelid, the tarsus appeared normal (**b**), suggestive of an epidermoid cyst. A common misdiagnosis in such a case is chalazion, and classic curettage procedure may lead to recurrence. Treatment involves complete removal of the cyst wall via an eyelid crease incision (**c**), followed by normalization of eyelid contour (**d**). (**e**) Gross appearance of epidermoid cyst. Lumen contains yellowish material (**f**) Low power view shows a cyst in the dermis, and cyst wall lacks appendages. (**g**) Higher magnification shows the cyst to be lined by stratified squamous epithelium. Lumen contains desquamated keratin (k)

glands, or sebaceous glands, derived from the lining epithelium of the cyst (Fig. 12.9b, c).

Clinicopathologic correlation Dermolipoma of the conjunctiva is an epibulbar choristoma, and is quite distinct from eyelid or orbital dermoids. Dermoids often require dissection up to the bone, as they are firmly adherent to the suture lines. Surgical removal and sclerotherapy are the treatment options.

12.5.7 Sweat Gland Cysts (Hidrocystomas)

Etiopathogenesis Hidrocystomas may be single or multiple cysts, lined by a double layer of

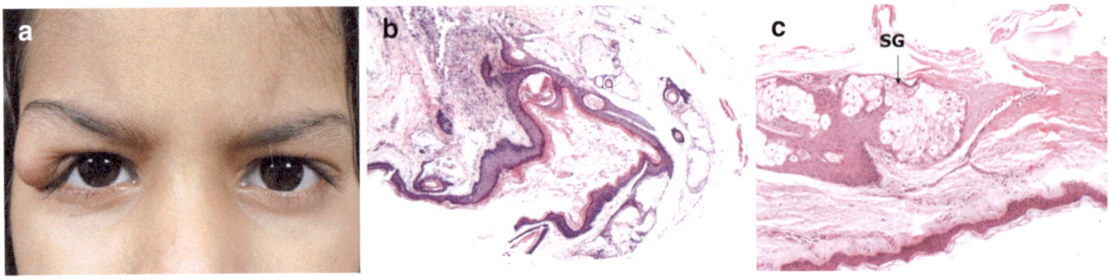

Fig. 12.9 (**a**) An external angular dermoid cyst protruding through the right upper eyelid in a 14-year-old child. It is a slow-growing oval, fixed cystic mass with bony attachment along the fronto-zygomatic suture. (**b**) Low power view of cyst in dermis with numerous appendages in its wall. (**c**) Higher magnification to show the squamous lining epithelium and adnexal structures like hair follicle and sebaceous gland (SG) in the cyst wall

Fig. 12.10 (**a**) An apocrine hidrocystoma along the lateral canthus in a 47-year-old man, showing a well-defined cystic mass filled with clear fluid, and preserved eyelid architecture. (**b**) The cyst in the dermis is lined by cuboidal epithelium with eosinophilic cytoplasm. (**c**) Higher magnification shows apical bulbous protrusions (arrow). (**d**) Eccrine hidrocystoma is lined by flattened cuboidal epithelium (arrow)

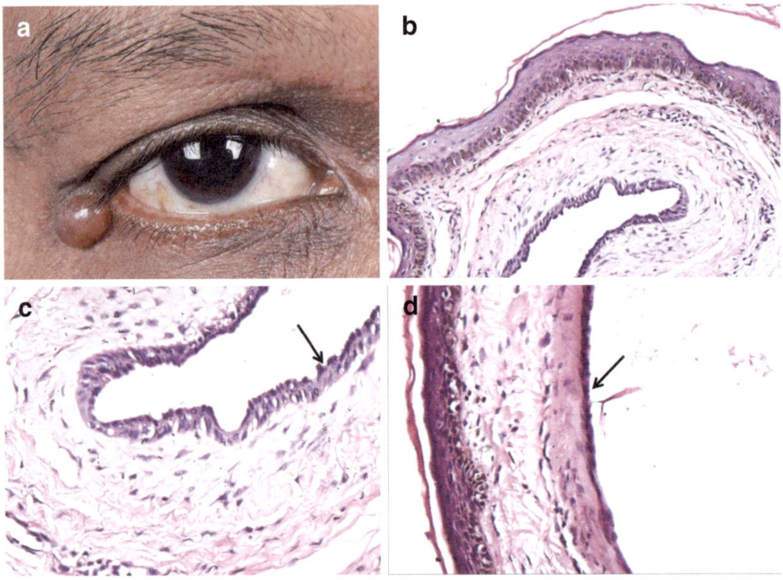

epithelium and result from the blocked duct of Moll's gland. They were first described by Dutch ophthalmologist Jacob Moll.

Clinical features Sweat gland cysts, also known as sudoriferous cysts, are derived from the eccrine glands and usually contain a watery fluid. They are small 2–3 mm in size, located at the lateral canthal region (Fig. 12.10a). Apocrine hidrocystomas are seen at the eyelid margin and are more common than eccrine hidrocystomas.

Histopathology Eccrine hidrocystomas have a low cuboidal to flattened epithelium, paler cytoplasm. No goblet cells are seen. Microscopically, these are lined by single or double cuboidal epithelium mimicking the gland or duct. No myoepithelial cells are seen (Fig. 12.10d). In apocrine hidrocystomas, the inner layer is columnar with deeply eosinophilic cytoplasm, oval to round basal nuclei and apical decapitation secretions. Outer myoepithelial cells are seen [11] (Fig. 12.10b–c).

Clinicopathologic correlation They can be often confused with epidermal inclusion cysts, due to their translucent wall with clear fluid.

12.5.8 Pilomatrixoma (Calcifying Epithelioma of Malherbe)

Etiopathogenesis Pilomatrixoma arises from hair matrix cells. It results from disruption of normal hair anagen progression. 75% of pilomatrixomas harbor mutations to beta catenin gene CTNNB1 [12].

Clinical features It is seen in children and young adults, in the upper eyelid or brow region as a solid or cystic swelling in the subcutaneous tissue.

Histopathology In pilomatrixoma, two populations of cells including large masses of shadow (ghost-like cells) in the center and basophilic basaloid cells at periphery are seen. These have deeply basophilic round to oval nuclei and scant cytoplasm. As the cells transform from peripheral basophilic to central shadow cells, pyknotic nuclei may be seen. Calcification and ossification may occur, which elicits a foreign body giant cell reaction (Fig. 12.11a, b).

Clinicopathologic Correlation

It may recur if incompletely excised. Malignant transformation is rare.

12.5.9 Sebaceous Gland Adenomas

Etiopathogenesis Germline mutations in one allele of the mismatch DNA MMR genes (mismatch repair) are seen in most of the sebaceous neoplasms.

Clinical features Sebaceous adenomas have a predilection for the eyelids due to the abundance of meibomian and other sebaceous glands in this location. It is rare and seen in younger patients. Up to 50% may be associated with Muir–Torre syndrome, an autosomal dominant condition in which at least one sebaceous tumor is associated with a visceral malignancy—GIT, breast [13].

Histopathology Sebaceous adenomas are lobulated lesions with dark and light areas corresponding to germinative and sebaceous cells. The mature sebaceous cells with clear cytoplasm contain lipid and are seen toward center. The peripheral cells are basaloid darker cells, and these layers are >2 (Fig. 12.12a, b).

Clinicopathologic correlation Clinical diagnosis is often confused with other possibilities like chalazion and basal cell carcinoma (BCC).

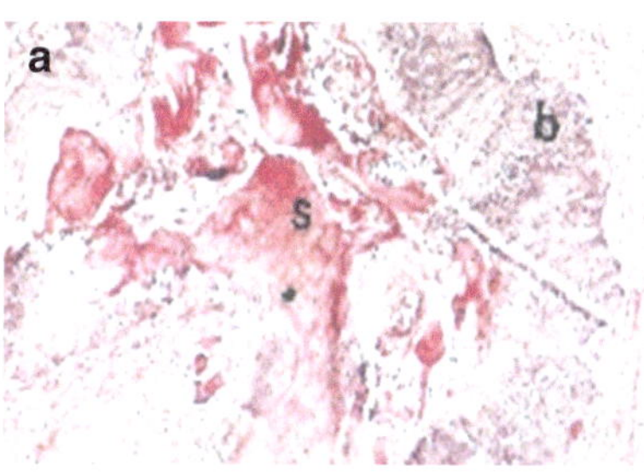

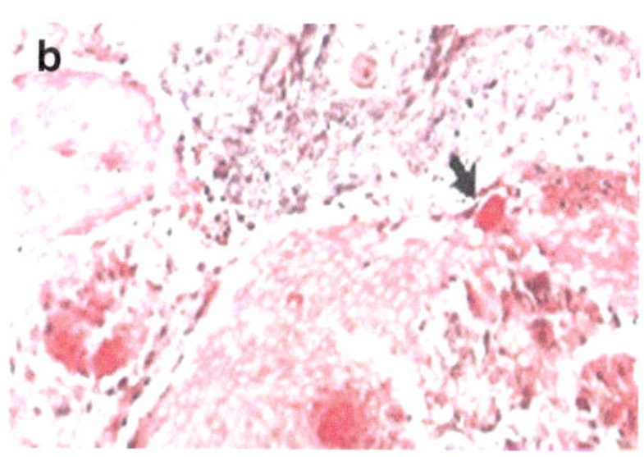

Fig. 12.11 Calcifying epithelioma of Malherbe. (**a**) Irregular islands of tumor embedded in a cellular stroma. Peripheral basophilic cells (b) and central shadow cells(s). (**b**) High power to show eosinophilic shadow cells with a central unstained area. Arrow points to the keratinization. The basophilic cells resemble hair follicular cells

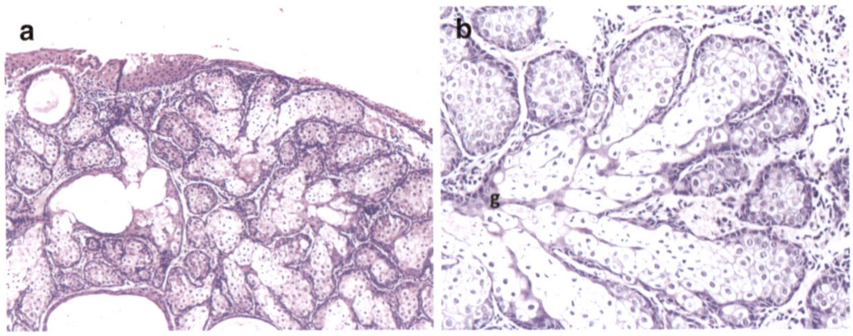

Fig. 12.12 Sebaceous gland adenoma. (**a**) The tumor is located in the dermis, composed of lobules of sebaceous glands. (**b**) Higher magnification to show varying proportion of germinative (g) and mature sebaceous cells

12.6 Neoplastic Lesions: Malignant

Introduction

Skin cancers are the most common malignancies in the human body, and the eyelids are a common site of involvement [14, 15]. The incidence varies based on geographic variability, skin type, and sun exposure. In the white population, basal cell carcinoma (BCC) and squamous cell carcinoma (SCC) are the most common, whereas in more pigmented populations, UV-related epidermal tumors is less common than appendageal tumors such as sebaceous gland carcinoma (SGC) [1–3].

Here, we shall describe the most common malignant eyelid tumors.

12.6.1 Sebaceous Gland Carcinoma

Clinical features A highly malignant eyelid tumor, common in Asians. It has a wide range of presentations (Fig. 12.13a–d) and can masquerade as benign conditions (like chalazion), leading to delayed diagnosis. It is twice as common in the upper eyelid as in the lower eyelid. Classic presentation is an uninflamed tarsus-based nodule or mass with a yellowish lipid tinge. It often leads to distortion of the normal eyelid margin architecture, and loss of lashes. A less common presentation is a diffuse pseudo-inflammatory form where the eyelid margin is thickened, and conjunctiva is diffusely congested, mimicking a chronic blepharo-conjunctivitis. The tumor is aggressive with a strong propensity for intraepithelial (pagetoid) spread, local spread to orbital soft tissues, regional lymph nodes, and even distant metastases to lung, liver, bone, and brain. Tumor-related mortality may be as high as 35% [16].

Etiopathogenesis Sebaceous gland Carcinoma is derived from adnexal sebaceous glands: Meibomian, Glands of Zeis, and sebaceous glands in the caruncle or the brow.

Risk factors Old age (seventh decade), female gender, and south-east Asian ethnicity are known risk factors. Muir–Torre syndrome is an autosomal dominant condition characterized by sebaceous neoplasms and visceral malignancy. Previous irradiation, such as past treatment of retinoblastoma, may pose a slightly higher risk.

Histopathology The tumor may be well, moderately, or poorly differentiated. Patterns include lobular, papillary, infiltrative, and trabecular. Well-differentiated sebaceous gland carcinoma (SGC) shows the tumor cells with vacuolated cytoplasm toward the center of lobule, whereas in the poorly differentiated type the cells show marked pleomorphism, hyperchromatic nuclei, mitotic figures, and prominent nucleoli. The cells in the poorly differentiated tumors were basaloid, basosquamous, or epidermoid type. In the comedo pattern type, there is central necrosis. Oil red "O" for lipids helps in establishing the diagnosis. Pagetoid spread is characterized by tumor cells infiltrating the overlying epidermis or conjunctiva. It is seen in 30% of cases with tumor cells spreading to overlying epidermis or conjunctiva (Fig. 12.13e–g). Adipolipin membranous stain-

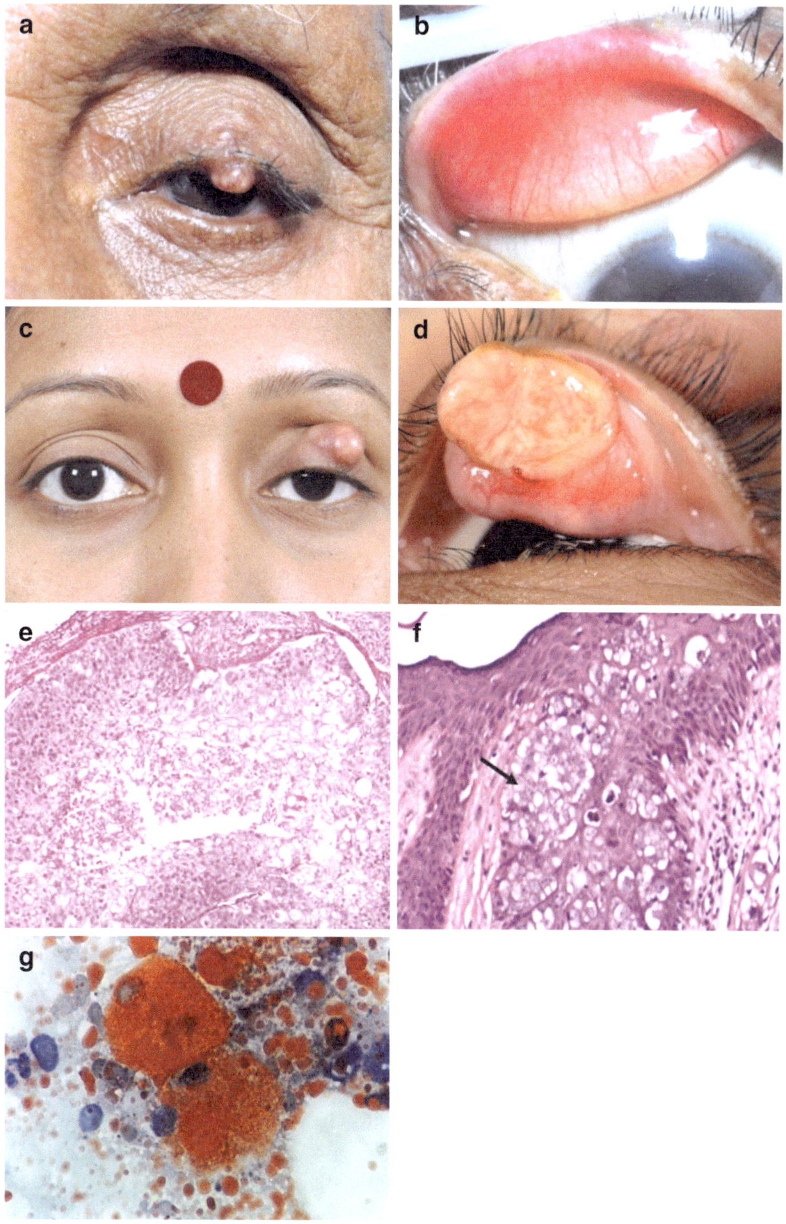

Fig. 12.13 Various clinical presentations of sebaceous gland carcinoma. (**a**) A 70-year-old lady with a painless marginal nodule in the left upper lid, mimicking a chalazion. The lipid deposits and telangiectasia should raise the suspicion of SGC. (**b**) Chronic upper lid blepharoconjunctivitis not responding to conservative measures could be a pagetoid variant of SGC. (**c**, **d**) A 45-year-old lady with a tarsus-based left upper lid lesion with a lipid-rich exophytic component on the tarsal side, suggestive of SGC. Well-differentiated sebaceous gland carcinoma. (**e**) Tumor in dermis shows cells with vacuolated cytoplasm and central necrosis. (**f**) Pagetoid invasion (arrow) of the overlying epidermis by sebaceous carcinoma tumor cells. (**g**) Intracytoplasmic lipid appears orange as demonstrated by oil red "O" stain

ing is useful in the differential diagnosis of poorly differentiated tumors [17].

Clinicopathologic correlation This condition may masquerade as a chalazion, pyogenic granuloma, and chronic blepharoconjunctivitis. Poor prognostic factors include metastasis, multicentricity, pagetoid spread, perineural vascular, and lymphatic invasion.

12.6.2 Basal Cell Carcinoma

Clinical features Basal cell carcinoma (BCC) is the most common tumor in non-Asian countries, where it accounts for 85–95% of malignant eyelid tumors. Mean age reported is 62.4 years [18]. A pearly or pigmented papule with raised edges, central crater, and telangiectasis is the classic presentation (Fig. 12.14a). Other rare presentations include morpheic, linear, pigmented, and

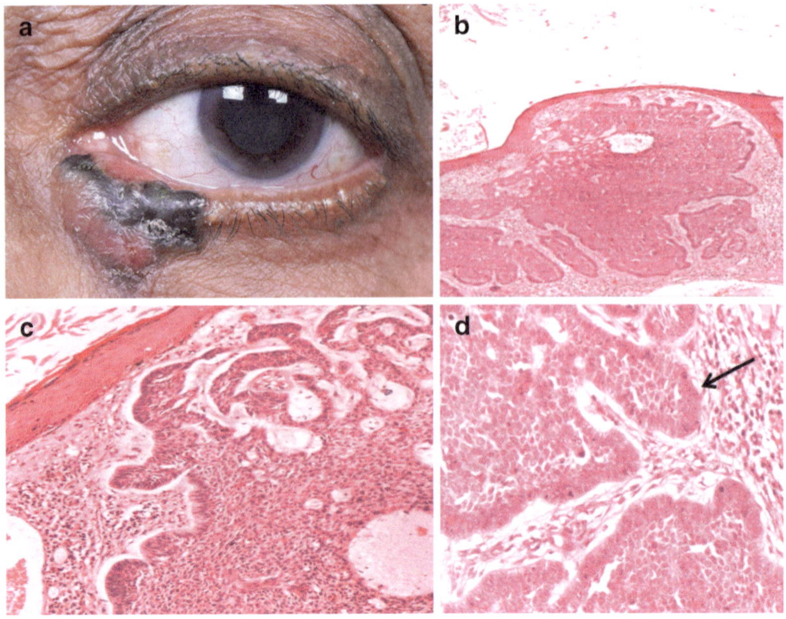

Fig. 12.14 Basal cell carcinoma. (**a**) 60-year-old lady with left lower lid pigmented papule with raised edges, and telangiectasis suggestive of basal cell carcinoma. (**b**) Tumor cells are arranged as basophilic geographical lobules of varying sizes in the dermis and originate from the epidermis. (**c**, **d**) Higher magnification to show peripheral palisading in the lobule (arrow)

cystic. The lower eyelid and inner canthus in adults are commonly affected. Locally aggressive, when multiple may be associated with xeroderma pigmentosa and Nevoid basal cell carcinoma.

Etiopathogenesis BCC is associated with an inherited or acquired mutation in the sonic hedgehog pathway.

Risk factors Ultraviolet exposure, fair complexion, immunosuppression, cutaneous scars, ionizing radiation, and ultraviolet A are known risk factors. Basal cell nevus syndrome is an autosomal dominant multisystem disease characterized by multiple BCCs, odontogenic cysts, skeletal anomalies, and keratinizing palmar pits. Albinism, Bazex syndrome, Rombo syndrome, and Xeroderma pigmentosum are other known risk factors.

Histopathology Histopathologically two main types include the solid (clinically nodular) and morphea/sclerosing (clinically infiltrating). The solid type is composed of various-sized lobules of basaloid cells consisting of oval nuclei and scanty cytoplasm and peripheral palisading of nuclei in a fibromyxoid stroma (Fig. 12.14b–d). Clefting artefact is also characteristic. Due to the high nucleocytoplasmic ratio, they appear blue. BCC with differentiation may be keratotic, adenoid or cystic [18, 19]. The morphea type is characterized by infiltrating basaloid tumor cells in fibrous stroma. This is the most aggressive type which may involve the orbit, sinuses, or rarely intraocular. Basosquamous variant has features of basal and squamous cell carcinoma and has a worse prognosis [3].

Clinicopathologic Correlation Pigmented tumors may be mistaken for melanoma. Recurrence rate reported is 11%.Tumor-related mortality is very low, but it can spread locally leading to functional and structural deficits.

12.6.3 Squamous cell carcinoma

Clinical features Eyelid squamous cell carcinoma accounts for 5–10% of eyelid malignancies, with mean age of 65 years and male preponderance. It commonly involves lower eyelid and medial canthus. Classic presentation is a

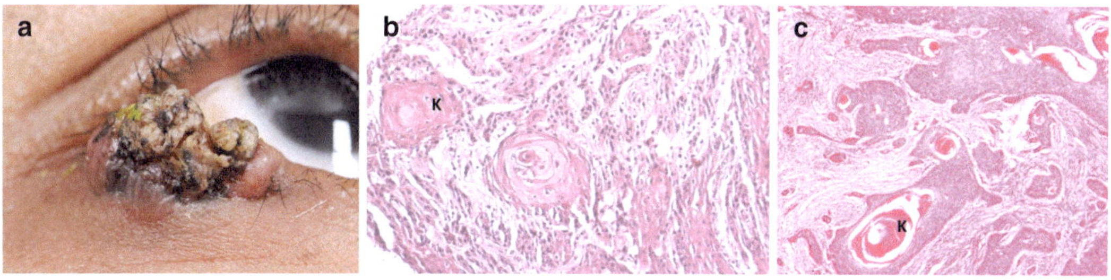

Fig. 12.15 Squamous cell carcinoma. (**a**) Right lower eyelid ulcerative lesion with keratin and loss of normal eyelid architecture, suggestive of squamous cell carcinoma. (**b**, **c**) Tumor cells with eosinophilic cytoplasm invading the underlying stroma and producing keratin pearls (k)

painless scaling nodule or plaque, with ulceration and keratin (Fig. 12.15a). Rarely, it may present as a cutaneous horn, or large fungating mass. Keratoacanthoma is a form of well-differentiated SCC with a propensity for spontaneous regression. Perineural and orbital invasion is seen, along with regional lymph node and distant metastases. A varied clinical presentation can make diagnosis difficult.

Etiopathogenesis Ultraviolet light is the most common extrinsic risk factor, and it may arise de novo or from preexisting lesions as actinic keratosis, xeroderma pigmentosa, and posttransplantation. UVB exposure causes mutations in the DNA of keratinocytes. SCC develops through a pathway involving proto-oncogenes and tumor suppressor genes.

Risk factors: Some of the risk factors include UVB radiation. Pre-existing skin trauma, immunosuppression, precancerous condition (actinic keratosis), xeroderma pigmentosum, and HPV infection.

Histopathology Histopathologically, they may be well or poorly differentiated based on the keratinization. Well-differentiated tumors have large tumor cells with abundant eosinophilic cytoplasm, dyskeratotic cells, keratin pearls, and intercellular junctions. Poorly differentiated tumors are pleomorphic with no evidence of keratinization and high mitotic rate (Fig. 12.15b–d). Variants include the spindle cell and rarely adenoid (pseudoglandular) SCC. Orbital and perineural invasion are poor prognostic features [3]. Aggressive neoplasm with several histologic subtypes, including adenoid, mucin-producing, and acantholytic [19, 20].

Clinicopathologic correlation Prognosis depends on location, depth, AJCC staging, and perineural invasion. Radiotherapy for perineural invasion is recommended. Metastasis including lymph node varies between 1 and 21%.

References

1. Deprez M, Uffer S. Clinicopathological features of eyelid skin tumors. A retrospective study of 5504 cases and review of literature. Am J Dermatopathol. 2009;31:256–62. https://doi.org/10.1097/DAD.0b013e3181961861.
2. Apple DJ, Rabb MF. Ocular pathology: clinical applications and self-assessment. 5th ed. 1998 Mosby Year Book; 1991. p. 565–8.
3. Pe'er J. Pathology of eyelid tumors. Indian J Ophthalmol. 2016;64(3):177–90. https://doi.org/10.4103/0301-4738.181752.
4. Bothra N, Ali MJ, Naik MN. To know when to prick!! Saudi J Ophthalmol. 2017;31(3):203–5.
5. Bipasha M, Harshit V, Shahid AM. Clinical profile and management outcomes of periocular molluscum contagiosum. TNOA J Ophthal Sci Res. 2020;58:5–8.
6. Chow T, Chacko E, Cleary C, et al. Keratoacanthoma of the lower eyelid. Eye. 2005;19:689–90. https://doi.org/10.1038/sj.eye.6701549.
7. Kronish JW, Sneed SR, Tse DT. Epidermal cysts of the eyelid. Arch Ophthalmol. 1988;106:270.
8. Vagefi MR, Lin CC, McCann JD, Anderson RL. Epidermoid cyst of the upper eyelid tarsal plate,

Ophthal Plast Reconstruct Surg. 2008;24(4):323–4. Naik MN, Batra J, Nair AG, Ali MJ, Kaliki S, Mishra DK. Foam sclerotherapy for periorbital dermoid cysts. Ophthalmic PlastReconstr Surg. 2014;30(3):267–70.

9. Koreen IV, Kahana A, Gausas RE, Potter HD, Lemke BN, Elner VM. Tarsal dermoid cyst: clinical presentation and treatment. Ophthal Plast Reconst Surg. 2009;25(2):146–7.
10. Pushker N, Meel R, Kumar A, Kashyap S, Sen S, Bajaj MS. Orbital and periorbital dermoid/epidermoid cyst: a series of 280 cases and a brief review. Can J Ophthalmol. 2020;55(2):167–71.
11. Jakobiec FA, Zakka FR. A reappraisal of eyelid eccrine and apocrine Hidrocystomas: microanatomic and immunohistochemical studies of 40 lesions. Am J Ophthalmol. 2011;151(2):358.
12. Levy J, Ilsar M, Deckel Y, Maly A, Anteby I, Pe'er J. Eyelid pilomatrixoma: a description of 16 cases and a review of the literature. Surv Ophthalmol. 2008;53(5):526–35. https://doi.org/10.1016/j.survophthal.2008.06.007. PMID: 18929763.
13. Dias MBB, Morales MC, Fernandes AG, et al. Sebaceous adenoma of the conjunctiva and caruncle: a clinicopathological report of three cases and literature review. Arquivos Brasileiros de Oftalmologia. https://doi.org/10.5935/0004-2749.20220023.
14. Miller DL, Weinstock MA. Nonmelanoma skin cancer in the United States: incidence. I Am Acad Dermatol. 1994;30(5 Pt 1):774–8.
15. Staples MP, Elwood M, Burton RC, et al. Nonmelanoma skincancer in Australia: the 2002 national survey and trends since1985. Med Aust. 2006;184(1):6–10.
16. Gupta R, Bhaduri A, Desai S, Das S, Menon V. Malignant tumors of the eyelid in India: a multicenter, multizone study on clinicopathologic features and outcomes. Indian J Ophthalmol. 2020;68(11):2466–70.
17. Jakobiec FA, Mendoza PR. Eyelid sebaceous carcinoma: clinicopathologic and multiparametric immunohistochemical analysis that includes adipophilin. Am J Ophthalmol. 2014;157(1):186–208.
18. Wang CJ, Zhang HN, Wu H, et al. Clinicopathologic features and prognostic factors of malignant eyelid tumors. Int J Ophthalmol. 2013;6(4):442–7.
19. Donaldson MJ, Sullivan TJ, Whitehead KJ, Williamson RM. Squamous cell carcinoma of the eyelids. Br J Ophthalmol. 2002;86(10):1161–5.
20. Olver JM, Muhtaseb M, Chauhan D, Mannion E. Well-differentiated squamous cell carcinoma of the eyelid arising during a 20-year period. Arch Ophthalmol. 2000;118(3):422–4. https://doi.org/10.1001/archopht.118.3.422.

Biopsy Pathology of the Uveal Tract

13

Arkaprava Pradhan and Jyotirmay Biswas

Contents

A. Pradhan
Vitreo Retina Consultant, Medical Research Foundation, Sankara Nethralaya, Chennai, India
e-mail: drkap@snmail.org

J. Biswas (✉)
Uveitis and Ocular Pathology Department, Medical Research Foundation, Sankara Nethralaya, Chennai, India
e-mail: drjb@snmail.org

G. K. Vemuganti et al. (eds.), *Ocular Pathology*, https://doi.org/10.1007/978-981-96-8614-8_13

13.1 Introduction

The iris and ciliary body, which together comprise the anterior part of uvea, contain melanocytes, smooth muscles, pigmented epithelium, vascular channels, stromal fibroblasts and nerves. The choroid, which comprises the posterior part of the uvea, is predominantly composed of blood vessels, melanocytes, nerves, fibrocytes, collagen, and interstitial fluid. As uveitis is frequently associated with systemic diseases, a patient's examination must be extremely specific. Clinical features alone are often used to diagnose uveitis, as in the cases of Fuchs' heterochromic iridocyclitis and serpiginous choroiditis. Other ancillary tests, such as fundus fluorescein angiography, indocyanine green angiography, and optical coherence tomography, may also be used, or laboratory tests may be used to diagnose sarcoid, tuberculous, and syphilitic uveitis. However, biopsy plays a big part in masquerade syndromes.

13.2 Anatomy

Histologically, the iris can be divided into four layers: (1) anterior border layer, (2) stroma and sphincter muscles, (3) anterior epithelium and dilator muscles, and (4) posterior pigment epithelium. The anterior border layer consists of condensed connective tissue stroma. This layer has a paucity of collagen but dense accumulation of melanocytes which contain variable amounts of uveal pigments. The sphincter muscle is present in the pupillary portion of the stroma as a ribbon-like band. Comprising smooth muscle cells, it is arranged parallel to the pupillary margin. The dilator muscle is a thin sheet that extends from the sphincter muscles to the peripheral iris. A small aggregation of dilator muscle cells, known as Fuchs' spur, sometimes passes obliquely between the posterior surfaces of the sphincter. Similar smooth muscle bundles which connect the dilator and peripheral border of the sphincter are known as Miclel's spur. The sphincter muscle is supplied by parasympathetic nerves. The anterior epithelium and dilator muscle layer is composed of myoepithelial cells with a cellular part and a muscular basal portion. The muscular extension from one or both poles of the cells (dilator muscle) is oriented in a radial direction from the iris root toward the pupil. The posterior pigment epithelium layer consists of heavily pigmented, low columnar cells. These cells from the pigmented ruff are seen at the pupillary margin. The dilator muscle of the iris lies just anterior to the anterior epithelial layers [1].

The ciliary body forms a 6-mm girdle extending from the ora serrata posteriorly to the scleral spur anteriorly. The anterior 2 mm of the ciliary body, the pars plicata, contains 60–70 radiating folds known as ciliary processes. The posterior 4 mm of ciliary body, pars plana, is continuous with the choroid posteriorly at the ora serrata. Histologically, ciliary body has four parts. From inside to outside they are: nonpigmented ciliary epithelium, pigmented ciliary epithelium, stroma, and ciliary muscles. The nonpigmented ciliary epithelium is a continuous layer, extending from the base of the iris over the surface of pars plicata and the pars plana to the junction with the sensory retina at the ora serrata. This portion, containing a large number of mitochondria and other specialized cell organelles, is the possible site of active secretion of aqueous. Zonules arise from the non-pigmented epithelial cells in the posterior pars plana region and in the valleys between the ciliary processes. The pigmented ciliary epithelium is a single layer pigmented, low columnar cells, continuous with the retinal pigment epithelium at the ora serrata. The ciliary muscles have three parts: the meridional or longitudinal muscles, the radial muscles, and the circular muscles. The bulk of ciliary muscles consists of the longitudinal fibers seen in the outermost part of the ciliary body. These muscles are formed by the anterior part of the longitudinal muscle and pass obliquely to merge with the circular fibers underneath. The circular muscles lie in the innermost part of the ciliary body, originating from the scleral spur region and inserting into the iris, the ciliary processes, and the choroid. The major arterial circle lies anterior to the circular muscle fibers. The space between the muscle bundles contains connective tissue, nerves, blood vessels, melanocytes, and fibroblasts. The ciliary muscles are supplied by both parasympathetic and sympathetic fibers. Parasympathetic fibers are derived from the oculomotor nerve, sympathetic fibers enter with arteries and arterioles, and innervate the ciliary muscle [2].

The choroid is predominantly composed of blood vessels, melanocytes, nerves, fibrocytes, collagen, and interstitial fluid. It is bound internally by Bruch's membrane and externally by suprachoroidal lamellae; between these are the middle vascular layers. Bruch's membrane is composed of a middle elastic layer surrounded by inner and outer collagenous layers. The collagenous layers are bound by inner and outer layers of the basement membrane. The vascular layer of the choroid is composed of an external layer of large vessels (Haller's layer), a middle layer of medium-sized vessels (Sattler layer), and an innermost capillary layer (choriocapillaris). The choriocapillaris is arranged in lobules with precapillary arterioles in the centers of the lobules. Middle choroidal layer vessels form anastomoses posteriorly and are parallel to each other from the equator to the periphery. Outer choroidal vessels are tortuous, interlace posteriorly and run parallel from under the macula to the equator. Melanocytes are most prominent in the outer choroid and around blood vessels. The interface between the middle layer of the choroid and the sclera is the suprachoroid. The suprachoroid is composed of thin interconnected lamellar fibers that bind the choroid and sclera together. Melanocytes, fibrocytes, nerve fibers, and ganglion cells are present in the suprachoroid [3].

It should be noted that choroidal biopsies often contain retinal pigment epithelium and a fragment of neurosensory retina adherent to the inner surface of the specimen. Hence, choroidal biopsies are often chorioretinal biopsies.

13.3 Inflammatory Pathology

Inflammation of the uveal tract—the iris, the ciliary body, and the choroid in general—is called uveitis. When the inflammation involves only the iris, it is called iritis; inflammation of the ciliary body alone is known as cyclitis. However, inflammation involving both structures occurs quite frequently and is known as anterior uveitis. In contrast, when the inflammation involves predominantly the pars plana region, it is called intermediate uveitis. The term posterior uveitis is applied to inflammation involving the choroid; pan uveitis is the term used if both anterior and posterior uveitis are present.

Anterior uveitis is classified as either non-granulomatous or granulomatous, depending upon the pathological basis of the cellular reaction. Non-granulomatous anterior uveitis is characterized by a predominant infiltration of lymphocytes and plasma cells. Granulomatous anterior uveitis, on the other hand, exhibits epithelioid cells, mixed with lymphocytes and giant cells. Non-granulomatous anterior uveitis may have infectious or noninfectious (autoimmune or idiopathic) etiology; infections can be bacterial, viral, fungal, protozoal, or parasitic.

13.4 Infectious Non-granulomatous

Bacterial infections rarely cause an isolated anterior uveitis. The iris and ciliary body may be secondarily inflamed, particularly in acute systemic bacterial infection, leading to endogenous endophthalmitis. It can be caused by bacteria, viruses, and fungi.

Bacterial Individuals with HLAB-27 are known to develop an acute non-granulomatous anterior uveitis, which is believed to be due to an autoimmune process. It is usually triggered by enteric infections caused by Gram-negative bacteria such as *klebsiella* and *Yersinia*. The infiltrating cells may be polymorphonuclear leukocytes mixed with lymphocytes [4].

Viral Several viruses, for example, herpes simplex, herpes zoster, cytomegalovirus, and rubella, can cause anterior uveitis. Herpes zoster causes a non-granulomatous inflammation in early or mild cases, but a granulomatous inflammation is usually observed in the advanced or late stages. Usually, necrosis of the iris stroma or other structures is noted with this viral infection. Rubella can produce a non-granulomatous iridocyclitis with a mild lymphocytic infiltration. Iris hypoplasia also can occur [4].

Fungal Fungi such as *Candida albicans* or *Coccidiodes imitis* can involve the anterior uvea. Candida infection usually occurs in the choroid, but a chronic non-granulomatous inflammation can occur in the iris and the cilliary body also. Fungal anterior uveitis may be a part of the systemic infection. Rarely, however, isolated iridocyclitis is observed with purulent inflammation mixed with granulomas. However, in early stages, the inflammation is generally non-granulomatous [5].

Protozoal Protozoal infections, such as toxoplasmosis or Acanthamoeba keratouveitis, show marked infiltration of chronic inflammatory cells with few epithelioid cells and giant cells. Necrosis and intense inflammation of the ciliary body are seen in toxoplasmosis. Although *Toxoplasma gondii* may be found in the retina of immunocompetent individuals, it is not seen in the iris and the ciliary body of these patients. In the patients with AIDS, the protozoans are observed in the iris as cystic structures, surrounded by a mild non-granulomatous inflammatory reaction. Several nematodes, microfilaria, *Angiostrongylosis*, *Gnathostomaspinegarum*, can produce uveitis, although such cases are very rare. *Gnathostoma* can present as iris holes and severe inflammatory reaction including hypopyon. Parasites should be removed in these cases by anterior chamber tap and identified microscopically [6].

13.5 Infectious Granulomatous Anterior Uveitis

Tuberculosis A patient with tuberculous iridocyclitis often presents with chronic granulomatous uveitis with or without iris nodules. Ciliary body tuberculosis may also present with chronic symptoms and is sometimes associated with involvement of adjacent structures such as choroid, retina, and sclera [7].

Leprosy Lesions occur during the early stage of the tuberculoid type of leprosy; where as in the leapromatous type they occur at a later stage. Anterior uveal involvement is more common in lepromatous leprosy than in the tuberculoid type and may include chronic granulomatous iridocyclitis, inflammatory exudative reactions, or solitary leproma. Histopathology of the lesion reveals infiltration of chronic inflammatory cells with large pale staining histiocytes with abundant cytoplasm, called lepra cells. Acid-fast bacilli can be demonstrated in the lepra cells by a modified acid-fast stain [8].

Syphilis Both the congenital and the acquired forms of syphilis can affect the eye, commonly involving the cornea. Iridocyclitis commonly develops in acquired syphilis and generally occurs during the secondary stage of the disease. Granulomatous as well as non-granulomatous anterior uveitis are seen. Sometimes the iris develops a nectrotizing granuloma, which can clinically simulate melanocytic tumors [9].

Fungal infections *Coccidiodes immitis* and *Blastomyces* can cause granulomatous uveitis. The iridocyclitis in coccidioidomycosis [5] is initially non-granulomatous; however, granulomatous inflammation can occur, particularly in chronic stage. Histopathologically, *C. immitis* evokes a pyogenic reaction around the conidia of this organism, with a granulomatous response around the developing spherules. Iritis or iridocyclitis is rare in blastomycosis. Histologically, the specimen exhibits a granulomatous inflammatory process, with several yeast forms seen within the granuloma. The organisms can be demonstrated vividly by PAS and GMS.

13.6 Noninfectious Non-granulomatous

Behcet's Disease This is a multisystem vasculitis occurring most commonly in Mediterranean countries and Japan and is less common in other parts of the world. Ocular lesions include panuveitis, recurrent iritis associated with hypopyon, necrotizing retinitis and retinal vasculitis. In the early stage, retinal vasculitis and inflammation around the pars plana are observed. In the late stage, along with the neovascularization and the formation of neovascular membranes on the anterior surface of the iris, there is granulation tissue formation resulting in cyclitic membrane and tractional retinal detachment. Occlusive vasculitis and organization of inflammation at the pars plana region are typical in such cases [10].

Intraocular Lens-Related Anterior Uveitis Inflammation induced by an intraocular lens (IOL) has become much rare due to improvements in lens design and to the change from anterior chamber placement of the IOL to positioning in the posterior chamber and the haptics are inserted in the capsular bag. Insertion of haptics in the anterior chamber is associated with frequent complications due to recurrent trauma to the iris and ciliary body. Even a posterior chamber IOL can induce persistent, low-grade, non-granulomatous anterior uveitis due to mechanical irritation, particularly on the posterior surface of iris and ciliary body. The IOL-related ocular inflammation, which is believed to be secondary to mechanical injury to the iris and or the anterior chamber angle, sometimes necessitates the removal of the IOL. The explanted IOL is often coated by a thick membrane containing acute and chronic inflammatory cells, multinucleated foreign body type giant cells, and red blood cells. Propionibacterium acne can cause delayed-onset endophthalmitis after intraocular surgery [11].

Phacogenic Non-granulomatous Uveitis The anterior uveitis, which occurs following disruption of the lens capsule, is thought to be a variant of phaco-anaphylactic endophthalmitis. Histopathologically, this phacogenic uveitis shows non-granulomatous inflammation around the disrupted lens involving the iris and the ciliary body. The cellular infiltrate consists of lymphocytes, histiocytes, and an occasional polymorphonuclear leukocyte.

Fuchs' Heterochromatic Iridocyclitis This non-granulomatous anterior uveitis is typically seen in young adults. Clinically, it is characterized by heterochromia of the iris and small white keratic precipitates, often stellate, scattered throughout the endothelium of the cornea. The anterior chamber cellular reaction is usually minimal. Histopathological features include cellular infiltration by lymphocytes and plasma cells with few eosinophils and mast cells. Occasional Russell bodies (plasma cells loaded with immunoglobulin) are observed. Depigmentation of iris, iris stromal atrophy, and hyalinization of blood vessels walls are also seen [12].

Juvenile Idiopathic Arthritis It is the most common systemic disorder associated with anterior uveitis in children, particularly those with pauci-articular involvement, and is associated with positive serology for antinuclear antibody and negative rheumatoid factor. During the late stage of the disease, histologic examination of the iris tissue shows predominant infiltration of lymphocytes mixed with plasma cells, plasmacytoid cells, and Russell bodies [13].

Neoplastic Lesions It can be divided into melanotic or non-melanotic.

Melanotic It can be benign and malignant.

13.7 Benign

Iris melanocytosis Histologically, these lesions are composed of collections of densely pigmented fusiform melanocytes. They often resemble stromal melanocytes of the iris. This benign condition can be distinguished from melanoma by the presence of orthochromatic nuclei devoid of nucleoli and by the absence of mitotic figures [14].

Melanocytoma of Iris This heavily pigmented tumor is most commonly seen over the optic nerve head but can also occur in the iris and ciliary body. Histologically, the tumor cells are heavily loaded with melanin granules, which often obscure the cellular details. These tumors are benign and rarely undergo malignant transformation [15].

Iris Nevus This common melanotic lesion of the iris is usually flat and pigmented. It can involve the iris from the pupillary margin to the iris root. Lesions are primarily located in the inferior quadrant. The histology of the iris nevus shows an aggregation of melanotic spindle-shaped cells containing small nuclei and generally without nucleoli. Diffuse nevus of the iris, containing nodules, ectropion uvea, and descemetization of the anterior chamber angle and the anterior surface of the iris, is observed in a distinct clinical entity called iridocorneal endothelial (ICE) syndrome [16].

13.8 Malignant

Melanoma of the Iris It comprises 3–10% of all malignant melanomas of the uveal tract. In younger people, iris melanomas are seen more

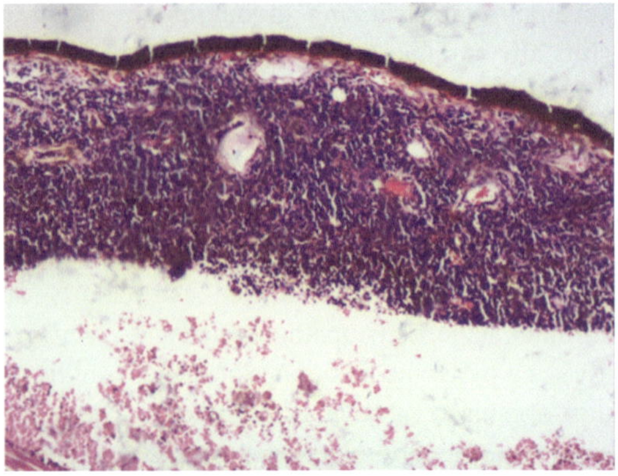

Fig. 13.1 Iris melanoma: Spindle-shaped cells with large oval nuclei and distinct nucleoli

often than choroidal melanomas. Unlike malignant melanoma of the choroid, the iris melanoma can also occur in children. Iris melanoma may present as a localized or diffuse mass, arising most often in the inferior quadrant. In a rare variant of iris melanoma, lightly pigmented, often pedunculated nodules resembling tapioca are present. Histopathologically, iris melanomas are made up of predominantly cohesive spindle cells with prominently cohesive spindle-shaped cells with prominent nuclei and nucleoli (Fig. 13.1). Spindle cell melanoma of the iris is made up of spindle A and spindle B cells. Mixed-cell melanoma of the iris primarily includes spindle B cells mixed with varying proportions of epithelioid cells. Epitheloid cell melanomas of the iris consist of large and small epitheloid cells with plump nuclei and large eosinophilic nucleoli, abundant cytoplasm and high nuclear to cytoplasm ratio. Most frequently, the excised tumors are the spindle cell variety. Iris melanomas have a better prognosis than melanomas of the ciliary body or choroid [17].

13.9 Non-melanotic Lesions

13.9.1 Benign

Leiomyoma It can arise from the iris, the ciliary body, or the choroid. It often causes a diagnostic dilemma. Tumor of the iris or ciliary body occurs in young patients and is more common in females than in males. It clinically presents as a slowly growing, grayish white, vascularized, flat, or elevated lesion. The tumor is characteristically nonpigmented. Clinically, iris leiomyoma is often difficult to differentiate from amelanotic melanoma [18]. It is composed of interlacing compact bundles of spindle cells (Fig. 13.1). The spindle cells were arranged in fascicles running in various directions. Sclero-uvectomy has been found to be beneficial in the management of iris and ciliary body leiomyoma [19].Cytoplasmic filaments of the tumor can be stained positive by Smooth Muscle Actin (SMA) and Muscle Specific Actin (MSA).

Leiomyoepithelioma This tumor occurs in children, presenting as a nodular lesion in the iris pigment epithelium. Histologically, two types of tumor cells (polygonal and spindle) of benign cytology are noted. Polygonal cells exhibit epithelial characteristics, and spindle cells show leiomyomatous differentiation.

Hemangioma Intraocular hemangiomas are seen primarily in the choroid, but they are also observed in the iris and the ciliary body. Hemangiomas which are usually noted at or shortly after birth tend to enlarge, although some hemangiomas are known to regress spontaneously during childhood. Histologically, iris hemangioma is of either capillary or cavernous type and can be associated with diffuse hemangiomas involving choroid and other sites. The cavernous hemangioma shows large, thin-walled vascular structures, lined by endothelial cells and traversed by connective tissue septa. A capillary type shows a multi-lobular pattern containing multiple small vascular spaces, lined by thin walls and endothelium [20].

Neurofibroma This is rarely seen in the iris. They may, however, occur in association with neurofibromatosis. Clinically, these lesions may resemble Lisch nodules, schwannoma, or leiomyoma. Light microscopy demonstrates long, narrow, spindle-shaped cells, with some areas of palisade arrangement as seen in neurofibromas arising from other sites.

13.10 Malignant

Leiomyosarcoma It is a rare tumor that exhibits histologic features of invasiveness, in contrast to leiomyoma. Cytologically, the tumor may show prominent nuclei and the presence of nucleoli and abnormal mitotic figures [21].

Rhabdomyosarcoma This rare iris tumor arises from primitive mesenchymal cells and is seen mostly in children. Histopathologically, the tumor consists of sheets of malignant oval or round cells with prominent nucleoli and scant cytoplasm. Clusters of large polyhedral cells containing eosinophilic cytoplasm may be present [22].

Juvenile Xanthogranuloma JXG is the most common form of non-Langerhans' cell histiocytoses. It is characterized by the presence of Touton giant cells.[23]Iris lesions are the most common intraocular manifestation of the disease (68%) [23] and are virtually always unilateral. Iris lesions may be localized, yellowish, vascularized elevated masses or may appear as a diffuse thin layer on the iris surface, causing heterochromia (Figure) [24].Spontaneous hyphema can occur from these lesions and may lead to secondary glaucoma.

Metastatic tumors Metastases usually involve the choroid, less frequently the iris, and the ciliary body. The most common primary sites in males are the prostate and lungs; in females the breast is the most common primary sites. Another frequent primary site is gastrointestinal tract [25].

13.11 Tumors of Ciliary Body

13.11.1 Melanocytic Tumors

13.11.1.1 Benign

Nevus It is very rare. Histologic features of these tumors are similar to those observed in iris nevi [26].

Melanocytoma These tumors are often associated with transscleral and extrascleral pigmentation. Clinically, they mimic melanoma, but histologically they are quite characteristic, consisting of deeply pigmented large cells when stained with hematoxylin and eosin [14].

13.11.1.2 Malignant

Malignant Melanoma Melanoma of the ciliary body is less common than melanoma of the choroid but more common than melanoma of the iris and Is seen in the fourth or fifth decade of life. Ciliary body melanomas are usually pigmented but can be amelanotic. A smaller ciliary body melanoma may be removed surgically by iridocyclotomy. Microscopically, ciliary body melanomas show features similar to those observed in choroidal melanomas [16].

13.11.2 Neuroepithelial Tumors

Glioneuroma These are very rare congenital tumors of the ciliary body that originate from the medullary epithelium at the anterior margin of the primitive optic cup and are seen primarily in young children, presenting as a slowly growing white fleshy mass in the anterior chamber angle. Histologic analysis reveals a well-differentiated neural tissue, similar to that of the brain. The tumor is benign with an excellent prognosis for life, although the vision usually remains poor [27].

Meduloepithelioma It originates from ciliary epithelium. It may arise from optic nerve and retina on rare occasions. It was earlier known as Diktyoma. Histologically, the tumor consists of multilayered sheets and cords of poorly differentiated neuroepithelial cells similar to those of embryonic retina and ciliary epithelium. The tumor can be either benign or malignant.

In benign non-teratoid medulloepithelioma, a major part of the tumor contains multilayered sheets and cords of neuroepithelial cells. In the malignant variant, these components consist of poorly differentiated neuroepithelial cells.

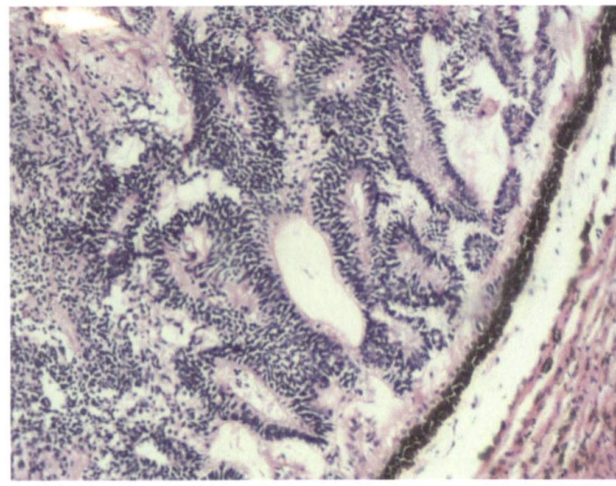

Fig. 13.2 Medulloepithelioma of ciliary body: Tumor comprises neuroepithelial cords and tubules that contain cytoplasmic pigments along with the presence of multilayered tumor cells and central lumen

Benign teratoid medulloepitheliomas usually contain heteroplastic tissues such as hyaline cartilage. In contrast, malignant teratoid medulloepithelioma may show areas of undifferentiated cartilaginous tissue as well as rhabdomyoblasts [28]. (Fig. 13.2).

Immunohistochemistry shows positive neuron-specific enolase, vimentin, and S-100 protein. Medulloepitheliomas appear to be radioresistant. Surgical excision by cyclectomy according to the extent of tumor invasion into the ocular or orbital tissue, is the best modality of treatment.

Adenoma of the Nonpigmented Epithelium Adenoma can be solid, papillary, tubuloacinar, or pleomorphic. Multiple acini and lobules are seen in loose fibrillary and mucoid material in the tubuloacinar type, whereas in the pleomorphic type there are also sheets and cords of neoplastic epithelium. The fibrillary material within the tumor stains positive with PAS, mucicarmine, and Alcian blue; the Alcian blue-positive material is found to be hyaluronidase-sensitive. Some of the tumors mimic malignant melanoma [29]. There can be extensive iris atrophy with focal infiltration of mononuclear cells [30].

Nonpigmented Adenocarcinoma It is a rare tumor that presents as an epibulbar tumor in a phthisical eye. Histopathologic analysis reveals tubules and gland-like formations of pleomorphic epithelial cells surrounded by hyalinized stroma. Immunohistochemistry reveals strong positivity for vimentin, focal positivity for epithelial membrane antigen and S-100 protein, and weak positivity for neuron-specific enolase.

Adenoma of Pigment Epithelium Histologically, these adenomas are composed of large pigmented cells, arranged in lobules, nodules, and sheets.

Adenocarcinoma of the Pigment Epithelium This rare tumors exhibit cytologic features of adenocarcinoma with local invasion and may contain both pigmented and nonpigmented pleomorphic epithelium of the ciliary body.

13.11.2.1 Myogenic

Leiomyoma It appears as a dome-shaped mass with dilated episcleral vessels overlying the quadrant of the tumor. Histopathologically, they are of two types: mesectodermal and mesodermal.

Mesectodermal leiomyomas show amelanotic, spindle-shaped cells with eosinophilic cytoplasm and long oval nuclei.

Mesodermal leiomyomas show interlacing bundles of spindle cells on histologic analysis. These neoplastic cells contain fibrillary eosinophilic cytoplasm and oval nuclei. Mesectodermal and mesodermal leiomyomas can be successfully removed by lamellar sclerocyclectomy.

13.11.3 Vascular

Hemangioma It is extremely rare. Histologically, they contain multiple capillary channels surrounded by densely packed cells with foamy cytoplasm.

Neural Tumors Schwannoma and neurofibroma are the most common neural tumours.

Schwannoma This encapsulated tumor arises from the Schwann cells of the peripheral nerves and is composed of spindle-shaped cells. Schwannomas are composed of cellular Antoni A areas alternating with hypocellular Antoni B areas. Antoni A areas are composed of interlacing bundles of spindle cells (Schwanncells) with wavy or oval nuclei, eosinophilic cytoplasm, and indistinct cytoplasmic borders. Intranuclear vacuoles may be present. Antoni B areas are hypocellular and less compact than Antoni A areas. They consist of haphazardly arranged spindle cells in a loose myxoid or hyalinized stroma containing a few inflammatory cells and delicate collagen fibers [31].

Neurofibroma This neurogenic tumor of the ciliary body is seen in association with iris and choroidal neurofibromatosis.

13.12 Choroidal Lesions

13.12.1 Inflammatory Lesions

Sympathetic ophthalmia (SO) shows diffuse uveal infiltrate of lymphocytes with overlying noncaseating granulomas. The choriocapillaris and retina are usually spared from the inflammatory infiltrate. Dalen Fuchs' nodules composed of T cells, macrophages, and retinal pigment epithelium may be present on the inner surface of Bruch's membrane.

Vogt Koyanagi Harada (VKH) disease has a similar histologic appearance to SO, with the exception of involvement of the choriocapillaris and the retina with the inflammatory process in the chronic stage.

Several other ocular inflammatory diseases, including Multiple Evanescent White Dot Syndrome, Acute Posterior Multifocal Placoid Pigment Epitheliopathy, Punctate Inner Choroiditis, Birdshot chorioretinopathy, and serpiginous choroiditis may manifest with inflammatory infiltrates in the choroid.

Behcet's disease is associated with acute inflammation, whereas uveitis associated with juvenile rheumatoid arthritis is associated with chronic inflammation. It is unlikely that patients with these diseases will undergo choroidal biopsy.

13.12.2 Neoplasia

Melanoma is the most common primary intraocular malignancy in adults. Choroidal melanoma cells may be elongated with fusiform nuclei and prominent nucleoli(spindle melanoma cells); they may have large round nuclei with prominent eosinophilic nucleoli and abundant cytoplasm, or most frequently, they may have a mixture of spindle and epithelioid cells. The tumor composed of benign nevus cells and melanoma cells led to the diagnosis of choroidal melanoma, probably arising in bilateral diffuse uveal melanocytic proliferation [32].

Another primary uveal tumor that has been diagnosed by choroidal biopsy is primary intraocular lymphoma. Although most intraocular lymphomas that involve the uvea are secondary and occur after the diagnosis has been established. The B-cell lymphoma may infiltrate the retina, subretinal pigment epithelium, and choroid. Nodular subretinal pigment epithelium infiltrates are characteristic of primary intraocular large cell lymphoma that may be diagnosed by examination of a vitreous cytology specimen. Subretinal pigment epithelium infiltrates of large cell lymphoma were found.

Metastatic tumors to the choroid are more common than primary intraocular tumors in autopsy material. The diagnosis of a metastatic neoplasm to the choroid is carcinomas, in particular lung and breast. The diagnosis of a metastatic neoplasm to the eye is usually clinically apparent, because patients often present with a known primary malignancy and multiple uveal tumors. The different neoplasia may be encountered in the choroid, that is, nevi, melanocytosis, hemangioma, neurofibroma, schwannoma, osteoma, leiomyoma, leiomyosarcoma, fibrosarcoma, Hodgkin's disease, mycosis fungoides, etc. But choroidal biopsy and fine needle aspiration biopsy can be done to diagnose these cases (Figs. 13.3 and 13.4).

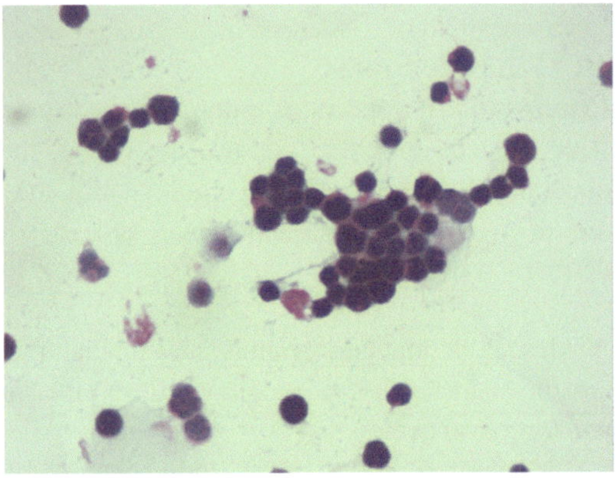

Fig. 13.4 AC tap sample of a 7 year old child of Acute lymphoblastic leukaemia shows lymphoblasts

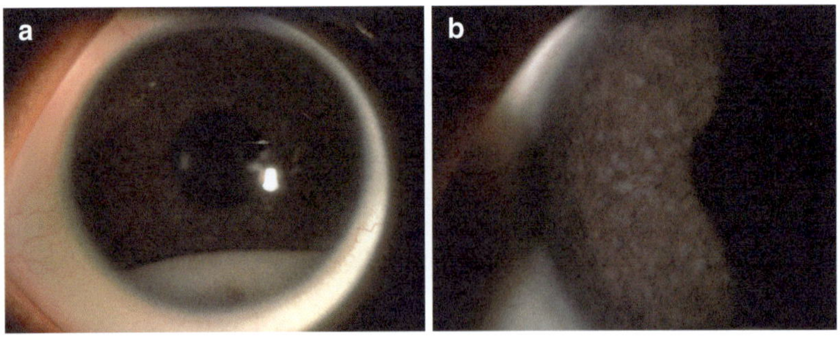

Fig. 13.3 Leucocytic infiltration in a 7 year old child of Acute lymphoblastic leukaemia (ALL) (**a**) Pseudo-hypopyon (**b**) Leukemic infiltrates over the iris

References

1. Yanoff M, Fine BS, Berkow JW. Diabetic lacy vacuolation of iris pigment epithelium; a histopathologic report. Am J Ophthalmol. 1970;69(2):201–10.
2. Anatomy of ciliary body. Basic and clinical science course (BCSC): Section 2 - Fundamentals and Principles of Ophthalmology. 2020.
3. Palestine AG, Nussenblatt RB, Chan C-C, Hooks JJ, Friedman L, Kuwabara T. Histopathology of the subretinal fibrosis and uveitis syndrome. Ophthalmology. 1985;92(6):838–44.
4. Agrawal RV, et al. Current approach in diagnosis and management of anterior uveitis. Indian J Ophthalmol. 2010;58(1):11–9. https://doi.org/10.4103/0301-4738.58468.
5. Moorthy RS, Rao NA, Sidikaro Y, Foos RY. Coccidioidomycosisiridocyclitis. Ophthalmology. 1994;101(12):1923–8.
6. Biswas J, Gopal L, Sharma T, Badrinath SS. Intraocular Gnathostomaspinigerum. Clinicopathologic study of two cases with review of literature. Retina. 1994;14(5):438–44.
7. Biswas J, Badrinath SS. Ocular morbidity in patients with active systemic tuberculosis. Int Ophthalmol. 1995;19:293–8.
8. Rathinam SR. Leprosy uveitis in the developing world. Int Ophthalmol Clin. 2010;50(2):99–111.
9. Ryan SJ, Hardy PH, Hardy JM, Oppenheimer EH. Persistence of virulent Treponema pallidum despite penicillin therapy in congenital syphilis. Am J Ophthalmol. 1972;73(2):258–61.
10. Paovic J, et al. Behcet's disease: systemic and ocular manifestations. Biomed Res Int. 2013;2013:247345. https://doi.org/10.1155/2013/247345.
11. Phatak S, Lowder C, Pavesio C. Controversies in intraocular lens implantation in pediatric uveitis. J OphthalInflamm Infect. 2016;6:12.
12. La Hey E, Mooy CM, Baarsma GS, de Vries J, de Jong PT, Kijlstra A. Immune deposits in iris biopsy specimens from patients with Fuchs' heterochromiciridocyclitis. Am J Ophthalmol. 1992;113(1):75–80.
13. Kanski JJ. Juvenile arthritis and uveitis. Surv Ophthalmol. 1990;34(4):253–67.
14. Shammas HJ, Minckler DS, Hulquist R, Sherins RS. Melanocytoma of the ciliary body. Ann Ophthalmol. 1981;13(12):1381–3.
15. Shields JA, Annesley WH Jr, Spaeth GL. Necrotic melanocytoma of iris with secondary glaucoma. Am J Ophthalmol. 1977;84(6):826–9.
16. Naumann G, Yanoff M, Zimmerman LE. Histogenesis of malignant melanomas of the uvea. I. Histopathologic characteristics of nevi of the choroid and ciliary body. Arch Ophthalmol. 1966;76(6):784–96.
17. McLean IW, Foster WD, Zimmerman LE, Gamel JW. Modifications of Callender's classification of uveal melanoma at the Armed Forces Institute of Pathology. Am J Ophthalmol. 1983 Oct;96(4):502–9.
18. Shields JA, Shields CL, Eagle RC Jr, De Potter P. Observations on seven cases of intraocular leiomyoma. The 1993 Byron Demorest Lecture. Arch Ophthalmol. 1994;112(4):521–8.
19. Jyotirmay Biswas S, Kumar K, Gopal L, Bhende MP. Leiomyoma of the ciliary body extending to the anterior chamber: clinicopathologic and ultrasound biomicroscopic correlation. Surv Ophthalmol. 2000;44(4):336–42.
20. Isola VM. Hemangioma of the ciliary body: a case report and review of the literature. Ophthalmologica. 1996;210(4):239–43.
21. Dugmore WN. 11-year follow up of a case of iris leiomyosarcoma. Br J Ophthalmol. 1972;56(4):366–7.
22. Naumann G, Font RL, Zimmerman LE. Electron microscopic verification of primary rhabdomyosarcoma of the iris. Am J ophthal. 1972;74:110–7.
23. Juvenile Xanthogranuloma. In: Basic and clinical science course (BCSC) section 6: pediatric ophthalmology and strabismus. American Academy of Ophthalmology; 2017.
24. Samara WA, Khoo CT, Say EA, et al. Juvenile Xanthogranuloma involving the eye and ocular adnexa: tumor control, visual outcomes, and globe salvage in 30 patients. Ophthalmology. 2015;122(10):2130–8.
25. Ferry AP, Font RL. Carcinoma metastatic to the eye and orbit. I. A clinicopathologic study of 227 cases. Arch Ophthalmol. 1974;92(4):276–86.
26. Nissen E, Armitage J, Thornton S, Coupland SE. Pigmented Limbal nodule consistent with a ciliary body nevus in an organ donor. JAMA Ophthalmol. 2015;133(6):721–3.
27. Addison DJ, Font RL. Glioneuroma of iris and ciliary body. Arch Ophthalmol. 1984;102(3):419–21.
28. Kivelä T, Tarkkanen A. Recurrent medulloepithelioma of the ciliary body. Immunohistochemical characteristics. Ophthalmology. 1988;95(11):1565–75.
29. Chang M, Shields JA, Wachrel DL. Adenoma of the nonpigmented epithelium of the ciliary body simulating a malignant melanoma. Am J Ophthalmol. 1979;88:40–4.
30. Biswas J, Neelakantan A, Rao BS. Adenoma of nonpigmented epithelium of the ciliary body presenting as anterior uveitis and glaucoma: a case report. Indian J Ophthalmol. 1995;43:137–40.
31. You JY, Finger PT, Iacob C, McCormick SA, Milman T. Intraocular schwannoma. SurvOphthalmol. 2013;58(1):77–85.
32. Avery RB, Diener-West M, Reynolds SM, Grossniklaus HE, Green WR, Albert DM. Histopathologic characteristics of choroidal melanoma in eyes enucleated after iodine 125 brachytherapy in the collaborative ocular melanoma study. Arch Ophthalmol. 2008;126(2):207–12.

Pathology of the Lens 14

Aravind Roy, Manjushree Bhate, and Dipankar Das

Contents

A. Roy (✉)
Cornea & Anterior Segment Service, L V Prasad Eye Institute, Vijayawada, Andhra Pradesh, India
e-mail: aravindroy@lvpei.org

M. Bhate
Jasti V Ramanamma Children's Eye Care Center, Kallam Anji Reddy Campus, Hyderabad, Telangana, India
e-mail: manjubhate@lvpei.org

D. Das
Department of Ocular Pathology, Uveitis and Neuro-ophthalmology Services, Sri Sankaradeva Nethralaya, Guwahati, Assam, India

G. K. Vemuganti et al. (eds.), *Ocular Pathology*, https://doi.org/10.1007/978-981-96-8614-8_14

14.1 Introduction

The human crystalline lens focuses light rays from the cornea on the anterior pole of the eye and then to the fovea on the retina located in the posterior pole of the eye. The lens is derived from the surface ectoderm and constitutes the chief focussing structure of the eye. It has the ability to change its shape by its inherent power of accommodation, thereby enabling the focus of light rays from distant as well as near objects. As a part of the normal ageing process the lens continues to harden and progressively resists changes in its shape. This leads to gradual loss of the accommodation and resulting in the inability to visualise near objects. Ultimately, with ageing this mechanism of increased opacification of the lens fibres leads to the formation of cataracts, which usually present with mild to severe decrease in visual acuity. Cataract-related blindness continues to be the leading cause of reversible blindness worldwide despite concerted efforts of cataract surgery in huge numbers due to significant focus of government policies to overcome the cataract burden and significant modifications of the surgical technique directed towards quick recovery. Hence it is important to understand the embryology of the lens and the pathologic processes in development, ageing and local or systemic disease processes that may lead to cataract.

14.2 Embryology

14.2.1 Early Morphogenesis

The appearance of optic grooves (neuroectoderm origin) at the third week of gestation from the developing forebrain marks the first event [1] As the neural folds fuse, the optic grooves evaginate to form the optic vesicle. This protrusion induces changes in the surface ectoderm for lens placode formation. The lens placode invaginates towards the optic vesicle and forms the lens pit. As the pit deepens, it becomes the lens vesicle, and the lens is pinched off from the outer surface ectoderm layer. The lens vesicle eventually lies in the optic cup [2].

At four weeks, the optic vesicle invaginates and creates the optic cup [1]. Grooves form along the ventral surface of the optic cup and stalk, called retinal (or choroid) fissures, to allow the passage of the hyaloid artery and vein [3, 4],which become entrapped in the optic nerve as the optic cup fuses around them. The distal hyaloid vessels, which supplied the developing lens, degenerate in the vitreous body and leave a remnant known as the hyaloid canal [4–6]. Surface ectoderm gives rise to the lens and corneal epithelium [6, 7].

14.2.2 Development of the Lens

With the emergence of optic vesicle, the surface ectoderm differentiates into the lens placode. It then invaginates to become the lens vesicle [4]. The lens vesicle migrates towards the cavity created by the optic cup [1, 8]. With this, the hyaloid artery passes through and supplies the developing lens and the inner layer of the optic cup before later regressing [4]. Primary lens fibres begin to form as the tall columnar cells on the posterior aspect of the lens vesicle lose their nuclei and lengthen [9]. The expression of ordered crystalline proteins lends transparency to the lens fibres [2]. As it proliferates, the cavity of the lens vesicle gets obliterated [4]. The hyaloid artery regresses as the anterior chamber forms, and the lens gets nourished by the aqueous humour. Interestingly, the absence of vitreous haemorrhage during regression is due to the cessation of blood flow before regression begins [10]. Another important aspect of the lens is the lens capsule. The lens vesicle rapidly becomes surrounded by the basement membrane as a result of the invagination from the surface ectoderm and this goes on to form the lens capsule. The lens receives its immune-privilege due to the presence of the lens capsule which offers protection from pathogens while still permitting the passage of solutes and water [11].

14.3 Congenital Lens Anomalies

Congenital anomalies of the crystalline lens include anomalies of development (anatomical or structural), lens shape and position that may be morphological or pathological. They can occur either in isolation or in combination with other ocular anomalies or systemic abnormalities. We have broadly divided and described these in this section.

14.3.1 Absence of Lens: Congenital Aphakia

This is a very rare condition and is commonly reported to occur due to mutations in the FOXE3 gene. One of the largest case series of Congenital Primary Aphakia (CPA) has reported that these eyes show severe panocular dysgenesis, including microphthalmia, retinal dysplasia and corneal opacity. Aphakia was confirmed by B-scan or ultrasound biomicroscopy (UBM). In their series a characteristic silvery appearance of the cornea was noted with peripheral vascularisation [12].

Another series that looked at the histopathological changes in the cornea and anterior segment in cases of CPA has reported a thin corneal stroma and absence of Bowman's membrane. All the eyes were also microphthalmic, as was reported in congenital primary aphakia and other complex anterior segment dysgenesis [13].

Embryologically, the mesodermal and neural crest cell migration and development in the anterior segment are significantly altered in this disorder; thus there is failure of the surface ectoderm to form the lens placode/vesicle. Congenital primary aphakia is due to the failure in forming the lens placode that can also lead to various other ocular defects including microphthalmia, sclerocornea, absence of iris or ciliary body, dysgenesis of trabecular meshwork, cataracts, Peters' anomaly, iris coloboma and optic disc coloboma [13–15].

Although FOXE3 is the most commonly reported associated gene, mutations in PAX6 may also have an association [14].

14.3.2 Anomalies of Lens Shape

This includes lens coloboma, lenticonus, lentiglobus and microspherophakia.

14.3.2.1 Lens Coloboma

This is a flattening of the lens and is associated with antero-posterior thickening of the lens rim in the area attached to the zonular defect [16]. It is characterised by notching of the equator of the lens in any quadrant. The size and shape of the coloboma vary, and the normal curvature of the lens is replaced by a straight line. In majority, the defect is inferiorly placed and can occur as an isolated anomaly in one eye or bilaterally. It could also be associated with colobomas of the uveal system, giant retinal breaks and retinal detachment (Fig. 14.1a). In the region of the coloboma, the zonules may be absent altogether, or represented only by isolated portions which may be attached to a projection on the curve of the coloboma. The pathogenesis of lens coloboma is the failure of the development of the zonule resulting in a deformity of the lens, hence only the more superficial zones of the lens are affected and do not affect the foetal nucleus (which is formed before the zonule fibres exert any pull). Thus, in the true sense it is actually a zonular coloboma rather than a lens coloboma.

14.3.2.2 Lenticonus

Lenticonus is a localised bulging of the lens capsule and the underlying cortex (Fig. 14.1b). It can reach a diameter of 2 to 7 mm and involves the protrusion of the central anterior or posterior part of the lens capsule and is detected on retinoscopy as a distorted reflex.

Posterior lenticonus is a congenital defect that is not associated with systemic disease. It is often unilateral and sporadic. The suggested hypothesis is traction on the posterior lens capsule by remnants of the hyaloid artery system and disturbance of tunica vasculosa lentis. Overgrowth of the posterior lens fibres has also been suggested [17]. The most significant associated visual problem is amblyopia. The indications for lensectomy in these cases include a visual acuity of 20/100 or less, amblyopia not improving on occlusion therapy or a loss of central fixation.

Anterior lenticonus occurs bilaterally in patients with Alport syndrome. The extra-ocular features in Alport syndrome include progressive renal failure and sensorineural hearing loss while the typical ocular associations are posterior polymorphous dystrophy, anterior lenticonus and fleck retinopathy [18]. Alport syndrome occurs due to a mutation in the gene that encodes for one of the chains of collagen type IV. This collagen is common to the basement membranes of the glomerulus, the cochlea, the lens capsule and the cornea. Anterior lenticonus does not manifest in early childhood but develops over time. An initial increase in lens size is observed. Subcapsular and cortical cataracts may subsequently appear at the level of the conus.

14.3.2.3 Lentiglobus

Lentiglobus is the bulging that involves the entire lens surface. Though rare, posterior lentiglobus has been reported and is characterised by unilateral or bilateral conical or hemispherical protrusion of the posterior lens surface. It may occur with or without central posterior subcapsular lens opacity and is usually associated with local thin-

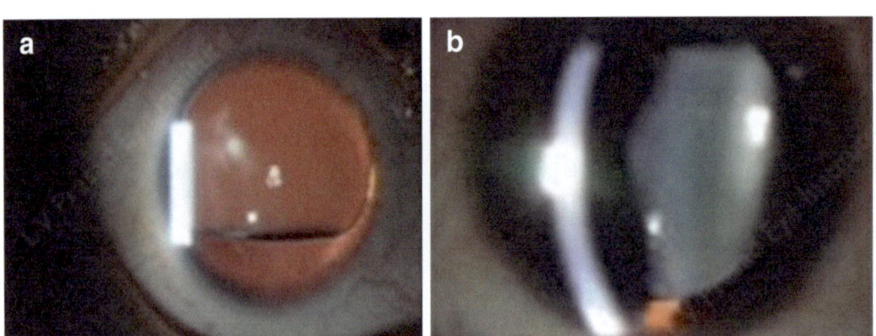

Fig. 14.1 (**a**) Inferior lens coloboma: This diffuse-illumination image is of the right eye of a young girl who presented with nystagmus and poor vision, on examination was detected to have partial aniridia with inferior lens coloboma as depicted in the figure. She was managed conservatively with glasses for refractive error correction and investigated to rule out Wilm's tumour because of the non-familial aniridia (**b**) Anterior lenticonus: Male child presented with reduced vision in both eyes, anterior lenticonus in both eyes detected on slit lamp examination. Corneas were clear, and there was no evidence of fleck retinopathy

ning or absence of the capsule. The pathogenesis in posterior lentiglobus involves subepithelial capsular hyperplasia and subepithelial capsular hyperplasia with inherent weakness of the posterior capsule. While visually significant lentiglobus eyes warrant lensectomy, care in handling of the posterior capsule is important as it tends to be floppy and may flutter intra-operatively [19, 20]. No specific syndromic association has been particularly defined to be associated.

14.3.2.4 Microspherophakia

This is a rare congenitally occurring condition in which the crystalline lens has a spherical shape, increased anteroposterior distance and a reduced equatorial diameter (ED) (Fig. 14.2a, b).

The proposed hypothesis is that there is a lack of nutritional support of the tunica vasculosa lentis which leads to arrest in the development of the secondary lens fibres resulting in weakening and reduced tensile strength of the zonular fibres thus a small spherical crystalline lens without cortico-nuclear demarcation is formed. It is commonly associated with high lenticular myopia, lens dislocation or subluxation and secondary glaucoma [21]. Associated syndromes include Weill–Marchesani syndrome, Marfan syndrome, Alport syndrome and Klinefelter syndrome however most commonly noted in Weill–Marchesani syndrome and is known to be inherited autosomal dominantly, recessively or sporadically [22]. It may present with or without Ectopia lentis, and acute onset of reduced vision, subluxation or dislocation may result in pupillary block and raised intraocular pressure.

14.3.3 Anomalies of Lens Position: Ectopia Lentis

Congenital ectopia lentis is the subluxation of the crystalline lens from its normal position. It is often bilateral. It can result from stretched zonules or absent zonules. A coloboma of the lens and ectopia lentis are a clinical continuum arising from a similar embryonic defect [23, 24].

The most common aetiologies in this condition include Marfan's syndrome (Fig. 14.3a, b), familial or idiopathic ectopia lentis and homocystinuria. In cases of simple ectopia lentis, there is no associated systemic condition [23]. Ectopia lentis et pupillae occurs when the pupil (slit like or oval) is displaced in the direction opposite to that of the crystalline lens. Reduced vision or poor vision due to significant refractive errors commonly myopic astigmatism often lenticular and resultant amblyopia is the commonest presentation. Based on the degree of subluxation and improvement in vision with conservative management like glasses or contact lenses, a decision to perform a lensectomy is usually considered. Visual recovery following lensectomy and rehabilitation for the aphakia or pseudophakia has shown a reasonably significant visual improvement [24]. Systemic work up in each case of ectopia lentis is important for related syndromes such as Marfan's, homocysteinuria, Weill–Marchesani, Ehler Danlos. This is crucial from the perspective of family genetics and life-threatening sequelae such as associated cardiac conditions.

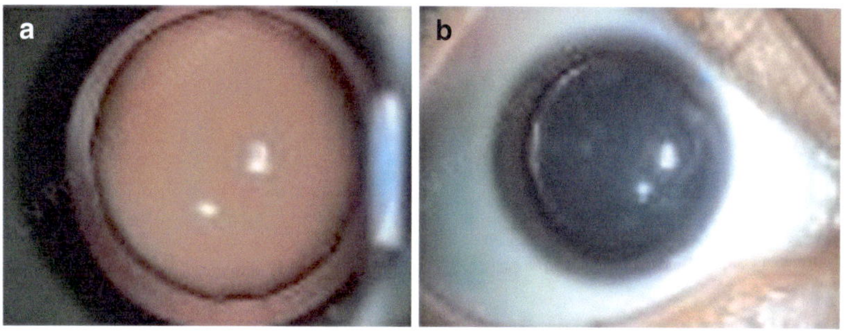

Fig. 14.2 (a, b) Microspherophakia: A patient with suspected Weill–Marchesani was referred for ocular examination by the paediatrician. Bilateral microspherophakia was noted on slit lamp evaluation

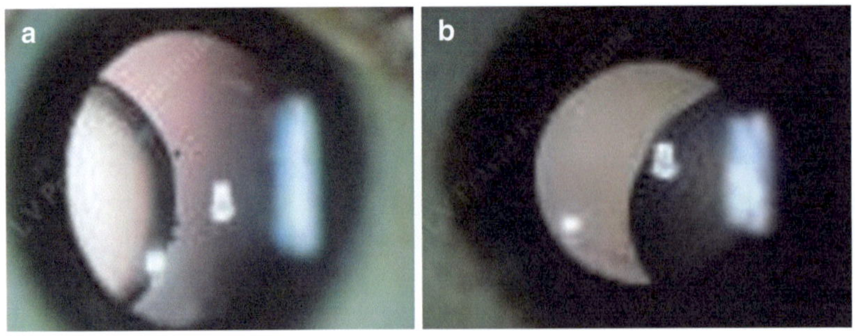

Fig. 14.3 (**a**, **b**) Ectopia lentis in Marfan's (ocular/systemic): Siblings presented with reduced vision, both had a tall stature, increased arm span and suspected Marfan's syndrome. Ocular examination showed an ectopia lentis in both eyes significant to necessitate surgery.

Table 14.1 Morphology of congenital cataracts

Whole lens	Central lens	Anterior	Posterior	Miscellaneous
Total	Lamellar /zonular	Anterior polar–dot	Posterior polar	Oil droplet
Congenital Morgagnian	Nuclear	Anterior polar–Plaque	Posterior subcapsular	Wedge-shaped
Membranous/partially absorbed	Central pulverulent	Anterior pyramidal	Posterior lenticonus	Christmas tree
	Anterior egg	Anterior subcapsular		Blue dot
	Cerulean cataract	Anterior lenticonus		Linear opacities
	Cortical			Crystalline
	Sutural			Nodular

14.3.4 Anomalies of Lens Morphology—Congenital and Developmental Cataracts

Congenital or developmental cataracts may occur either bilaterally or unilaterally and may be sporadic or familial. Typically, congenital cataracts can be classified based on aetiology or morphology (part of the lens that is opaque) [25]. Aetiological classification includes infectious, metabolic and developmental causes, whereas morphological classification includes anterior or posterior subcapsular, polar or involving the nucleus (lamellar), cortical or spoke-wheel like and total cataracts [26]. A number of congenital cataracts, such as blue dot cataracts, are typically visually insignificant, that is, they do not impair vision to a degree that may need surgical intervention. An absent or hazy/obscured view of the retina associated with a central dull glow on retinoscopy and poor vision warrants cataract extraction with habilitation of the resultant aphakia or pseudophakia. Tables 14.1 and 14.2 list the different causes and some of the examples of congenital cataracts with resultant pathology and clinical appearance are in Fig. 14.4a–f.

Table 14.2 Aetiology of congenital cataracts

Bilateral cataracts	Unilateral cataracts
Idiopathic	Idiopathic
Hereditary (autosomal dominant)	Ocular anomalies
Genetic and metabolic diseases	Persistent foetal vasculature
Downs syndrome	Anterior segment dysgenesis
Lowe's syndrome	Posterior lenticonus
Galactosemia	Posterior pole tumours
Marfan's syndrome	Traumatic (rule out birth history/child abuse)
Trisomy 13–15	Rubella (rare)
Hypoglycaemia	
Alport syndrome	
Myotonic dystrophy	
Fabry's disease	
Hypoparathyroidism	
Maternal infection	
Rubella	
Cytomegalovirus	
Varicella	
Syphilis	
Toxoplasmosis	
Ocular anomalies	
Aniridia	
Anterior segment dysgenesis syndrome	
Corticosteroids	

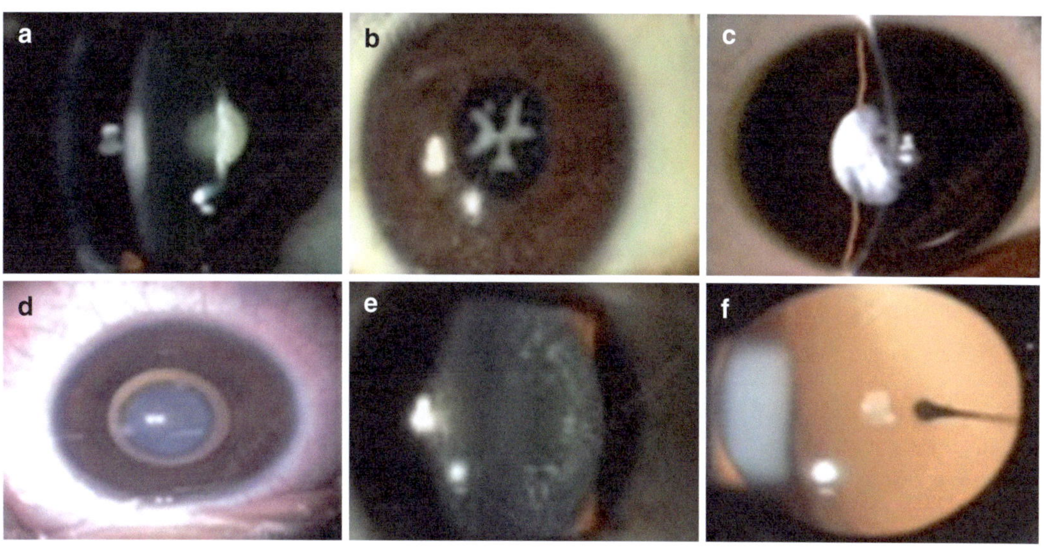

Fig. 14.4 Congenital cataracts: (**a**–**e**) show the varieties of congenital cataract presentations in different patients. All have essentially presented with reduced visual acuity. (**a**) Onion ring -in a patient with posterior lenticonus with cataract (**b**) Sutural Cataract (**c**) PHPV cataract with vessels (**d**) Zonular cataract (**e**) Blue Dot cataract (**f**) PHPV with stalk

14.4 Adult Cataract

The lens is developmentally a part of the ectoderm that invaginates into the mesoderm during development of the optic cup and the capsule of the lens consists of epithelial cells. These are thickest at the equator and thinnest at the posterior capsule. These cells continue to divide and elongate forming the lens capsule. These elongated fibres form Y-shaped intersections and continue to get compacted into the core of the lens forming nucleus, epinucleus, cortex of the lens. The process continues to progress in adults leading to progressive compactness of the nucleus. Along with this process of progressive compactness and metabolic changes the lens continues to harden and become more resistant to deformation, which causes deficiency of near vision or presbyopia due to loss of accommodation and hardening of the nuclear fibres with development of age-related cataracts.

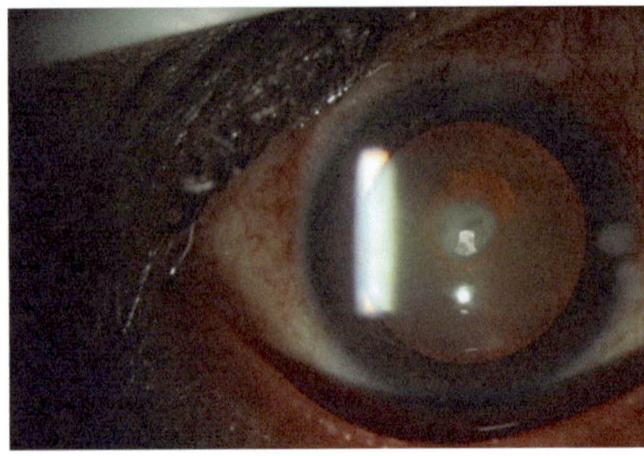

Fig. 14.5 A 66-year-old man with anterior subcapsular cataract

14.4.1 Types of Adult Cataracts Based on Location of the Opacification

Adult cataracts are typically described depending upon their location such as subcapsular, cortical, nuclear, total and Morgagnian cataracts. Based upon their stage of development, they may be immature or mature.

14.4.1.1 Subcapsular Cataract

These cataracts are typically beneath the lens capsule, they may have a plaque or bubble-like appearance. Located at the nodal points of the visual axis, these cataracts usually cause disturbing visual phenomena. Typically they may be posterior or anterior subcapsular cataracts (Fig. 14.5). The patients would complain of difficulty in vision in bright light due to the centrally located cataracts obscuring the visual axis in the constricted pupil. They appear as black or refractive bubbles in retro illumination.

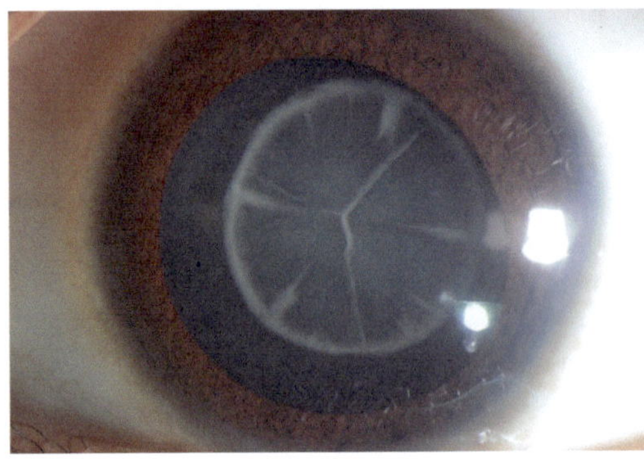

Fig. 14.6 Cortical cataract with opacification of the junctional lens fibres between the nucleus and cortex and sutural junction

14.4.1.2 Cortical Cataracts

Cortical cataracts occur due to opacification of the cortical layers, they occur at variable levels causing wedge-shaped opacities, and this may give a cartwheel appearance to the lens (Fig. 14.6). The variable location of these cataracts causes glare because of scattering of light. Typically the patients may complain of poor vision in dim illumination as these spokes may impede vision in the dilated pupil. These cataracts stand out as radial spokes on retro-illumination.

14.4.1.3 Nuclear Cataracts

Nuclear cataracts occur with progressive condensation and hardening of the central nuclear fibres.

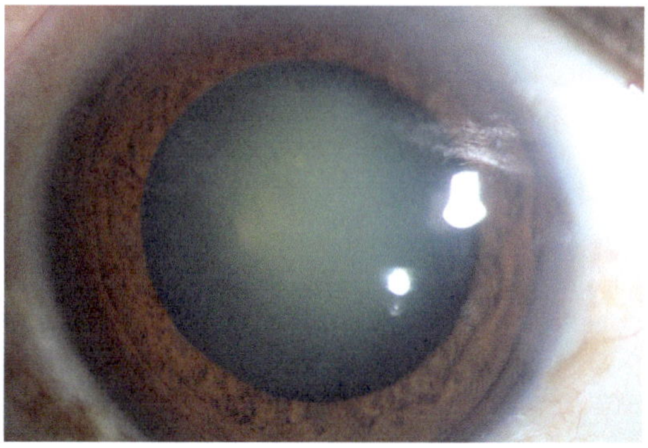

Fig. 14.7 Opacification of the nucleus in an elderly patient

Urochrome deposits in the nucleus impart a yellowish coloration to the central nuclear core. The intensity increases with progressive increase in the hardness of the cataracts (Fig. 14.7). Due to this change the lens becomes progressively myopic and leads to improvement of near vision in elderly: called the 'second sight'. These cataracts are best graded in slit illumination and high beam intensity.

14.4.2 Cataracts Based on Intensity of Opacification

Based on the stage of opacification and morphologic appearance cataracts may be of the following types:

Immature cataract—These are softer cataracts with incomplete loss of transparency.

Mature cataracts—They are completely opaque and do not permit visualisation of the retina and cause gross diminution of vision.

Hypermature cataract—They have a shrunken lens capsule with loss of water from the lens fibres and complete opacification of the lens.

Intumescent cataract—These are totally opacified and swollen cataracts due to hydration of the lens fibres. They are secondary to exposure to heat, trauma, radiation, or drugs such as corticosteroids.

Morgagnian cataracts—This is a variety of hypermature cataract that has a liquified cortex and a dense nucleus that has sunk inferiorly into the substance of the lens.

14.4.3 Traumatic Cataract

Traumatic cataract refers to the loss of clarity of the crystalline lens following a mechanical injury which could be a blunt or a penetrating trauma. There is a loss of transparency, swelling of the lens fibres and opacification of all layers of the lens. In the case of severe blunt or penetrating injury, there can be associated rupture of the lens capsule and fragmentation of the cortical matter. The position may also be disturbed, and the lens may be subluxated or dislocated anteriorly into the anterior chamber or posteriorly into the vitreous cavity. Roseate cataract is a variant of traumatic mechanical cataract that starts as fine feathery posterior subcapsular opacification of the lens fibres. They may remain stable or may progress to involve the entire lens. Other trauma such as electrical shock, radiation or chemical injury may also cause lens opacification.

14.4.4 Cataract in Systemic Diseases

14.4.4.1 Diabetic Cataract

Cataracts in diabetic patients occur due to metabolic imbalance with increased deposition of sorbitol in the lens by altered glucose metabolism which converts glucose to sorbitol. Hyperglycaemia leads to an increase in the glucose levels in the aqueous humour that diffuses into the lens and metabolises to sorbitol causing an increase in the osmotic pressure. This causes accumulation of water in the lens and opacification of the lens fibres. The refractive error and the amplitude of accommodation of the lens are likely to change. There is opacification of the cortex with accumulation of fluid vacuoles and development of snowflake-like opacities. Bread crumb-like or lustrous needle-like opacities may also form in the posterior cortex. The cataractous change may be reversible, or alternatively they may rapidly progress to cause diffuse opacification of the lens [27].

14.4.4.2 Myotonic Dystrophy

Patients with myotonic dystrophy may have fine cortical opacities that may be visually insignificant. Occasionally these cortical opacities may develop into posterior subcapsular cataracts. Ocular complications may be the first clinical sign with nearly all patients having bilateral iridescent cataracts [28].

14.4.4.3 Atopic Dermatitis

Bilateral dense anterior subcapsular shield-like opacities may occur in patients with atopic dermatitis. These typically cause severe visual loss and may progress rapidly. There may be associated posterior subcapsular opacities causing a disabling cataract [29, 30].

14.4.4.4 Neurofibromatosis

Posterior subcapsular and cortical wedge-shaped cataracts may be associated with neurofibromatosis type 2 in 60–90% of patients. These are early-onset and may cause significant visual morbidity [31].

14.4.5 Complicated Cataract

14.4.5.1 Chronic Anterior Uveitis

Anterior chamber inflammation may cause breakdown of the blood–aqueous barrier. There may be concomitant use of corticosteroids for management of this condition. This may lead to development of posterior subcapsular cataract which may progress to involve the entire lens. There may be anterior subcapsular cortical opacities, posterior synechia and associated dense pupillary membranes. The postoperative visual prognosis is related to age of the patient and duration of the disease, clinical course and type of the uveitis and the degree of control of inflammation prior to and after surgery.

14.4.5.2 Acute Angle Closure Glaucoma

Acute angle closure glaucoma may cause small fleck-like greyish white opacities that may be within the pupillary margin (glaucomflecken). Raised intraocular pressure may cause localised infraction of the lens epithelial cells resulting in localised opacification of the anterior and subcapsular areas of the lens.

14.4.5.3 Myopia

Highly myopic eyes are predisposed to nuclear sclerosis or posterior subcapsular cataract.

14.4.5.4 Retinal Dystrophy

Retinal dystrophies may cause variable opacification of the lens fibres. Posterior subcapsular opacities have been described in retinitis pigmentosa, Stickler syndrome, gyrate atrophy, etc.

14.4.5.5 Cataract Following Intraocular Surgery

This kind of cataract commonly occurs following other intraocular surgery such as vitreoretinal surgery, especially with silicone oil injection, following glaucoma filtering surgery and keratoplasty.

14.4.5.6 Steroid-Induced Cataract

Typically noted as a posterior subcapsular cataract, this can be seen in those patients either needing long-term (ocular allergy, uveitis, s/p keratoplasty) steroids or those where indiscriminate use of steroids was noted. Typically presents as a posterior subcapsular cataract.

14.5 Histopathological Findings of Normal Lens and Cataractous Lens

The crystalline lens is a transparent biconvex avascular structure, seen suspended by zonular attachment between the iris and vitreous [32, 33]. The lens consists of three parts—capsule, epithelium and lens fibres (Figs. 14.8 and 14.9) [32, 33]. Lens capsule is transparent and consists of type-IV collagen basement membrane which is resistant to toxic material and facilitates passage of nutrients and by-products in and out of the lens (Fig. 14.10) [32, 33]. The lens capsule is the thickest anteriorly over the lens epithelial cells and appears as pale eosinophilic in haematoxylin and eosin (H&E)-stained section (Figs. 14.11 and 14.12) [32, 33]. The capsule is brightly stained by periodic acid–Schiff (PAS) stain [32–34]. Subcapsular epithelium is composed of a single layer of cuboidal cells, and it is estimated that

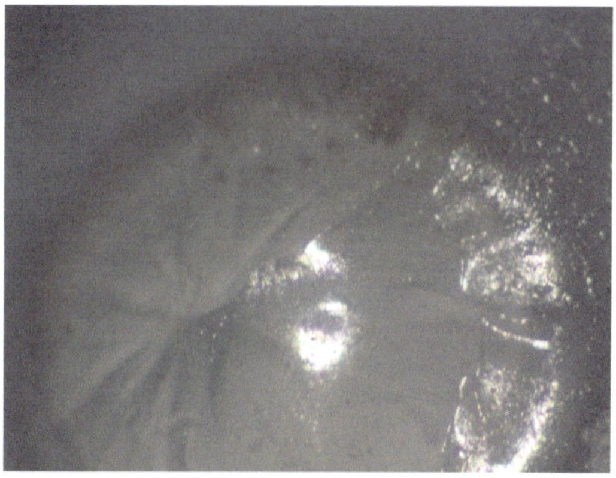

Fig. 14.8 Gross cataractous lens

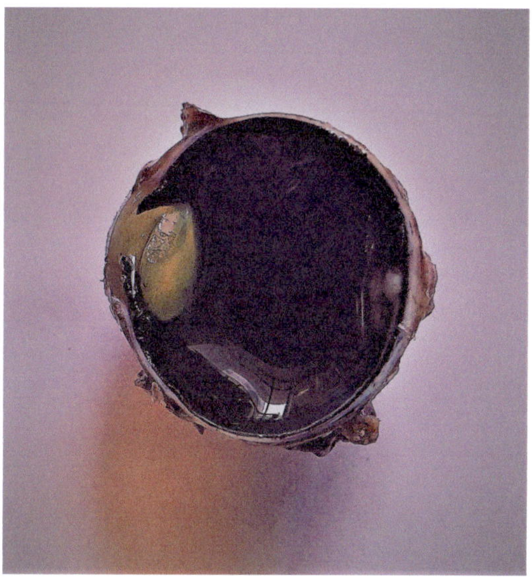

Fig. 14.9 Enucleated eyeball with cataractous lens

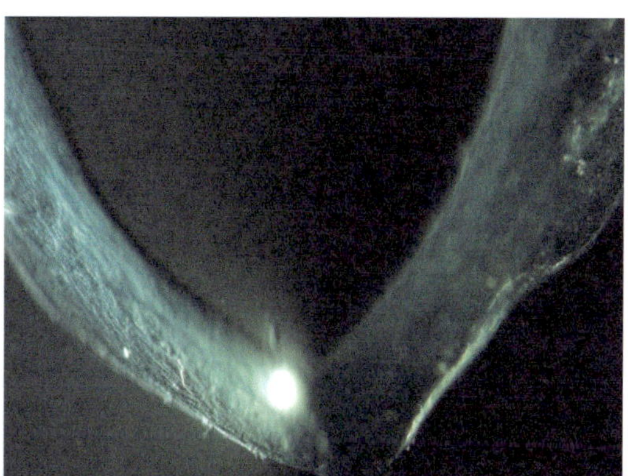

Fig. 14.10 Capsule of crystalline lens in diffraction photography

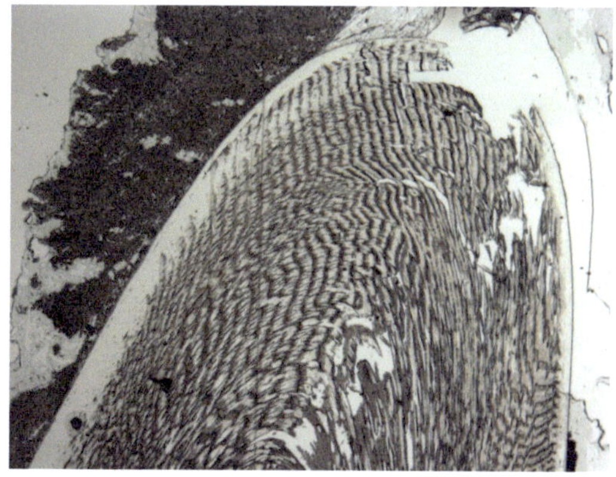

Fig. 14.11 Lens fibre orientation with the capsule in an unstained slide

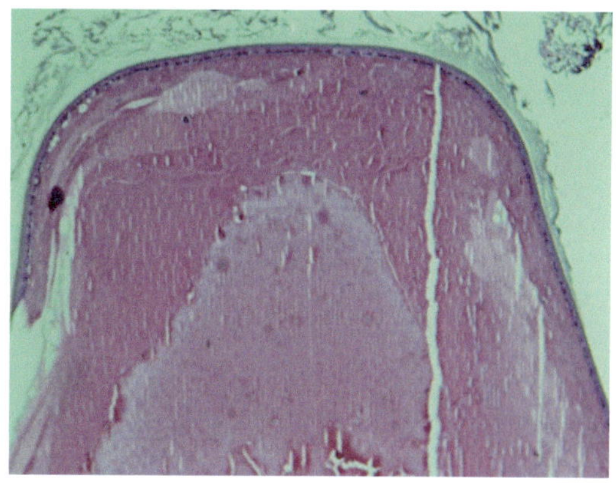

Fig. 14.12 Haematoxylin and eosin stained slide showing capsule and subcapsular epithelium in lens 40×

about 2000 epithelial cells are present in the adult crystalline lens which is attached to the eye via the zomules (Fig. 14.13) [32–34]. Equatorial epithelium consists of differentiating cells which are pyramidal cells [32, 33].

Disease of lens, as explained in the previous sections, includes cataract which is defined as opacity of the lens or its capsule that results in dimness of vision to any extent [32–34]. Pathologically, lens is one of the parts of the body which is incapable of inflammation by itself. As mentioned previously, the degenerative changes in lens are common which result in loss of transparency of lens [32–35].

Congenital anomalies of crystalline lens have been described in the earlier section and include

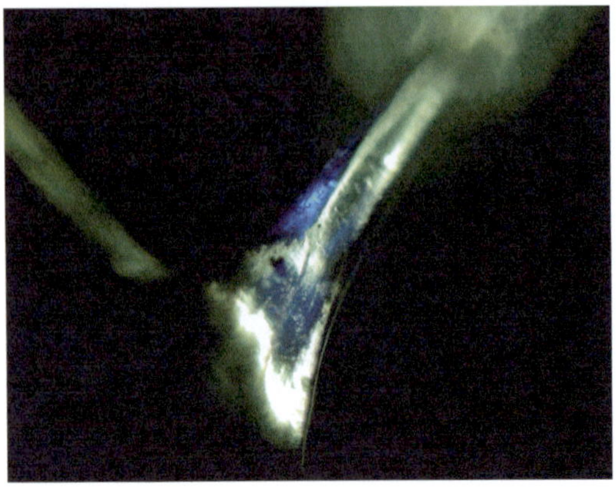

Fig. 14.13 Gross zonular attachment to the lens surface 100×

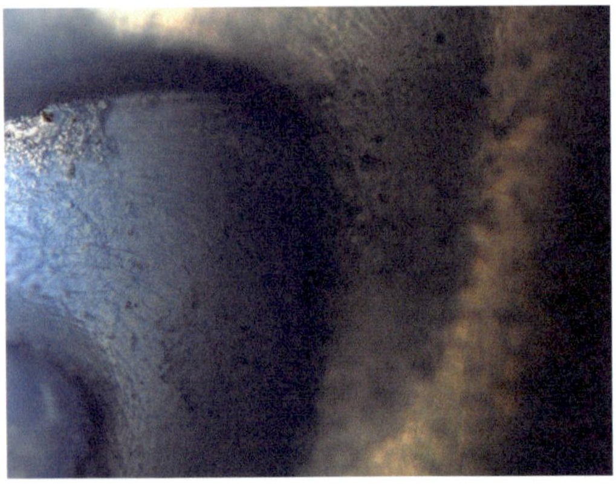

Fig. 14.14 Nucleus and cortex of lens

lens coloboma of lens, spherophakia and dislocation of lens secondary to maldevelopment of zonules [32–35]. Mittendorf's dots are seen on the posterior aspect of the lens as an anterior remnant of persistent hyperplastic primary vitreous [32–36]. Congenital aphakia can exist as primary or secondary. Histopathologically, primary lens aphakia is characterised by absent lens, and there is significant malformation of anterior segment of the eye [32–36].

Morphologically cataract is divided into adult and congenital forms [32–34]. Adult cataract can be cortical or nuclear (Figs. 14.14) and consists of nuclear and peripheral fibres (Figs. 14.15 and 14.16) [32–34]. Age-related senile cataract is due to loss of transparency of lens due to change in the protein content. Environmental and genetic

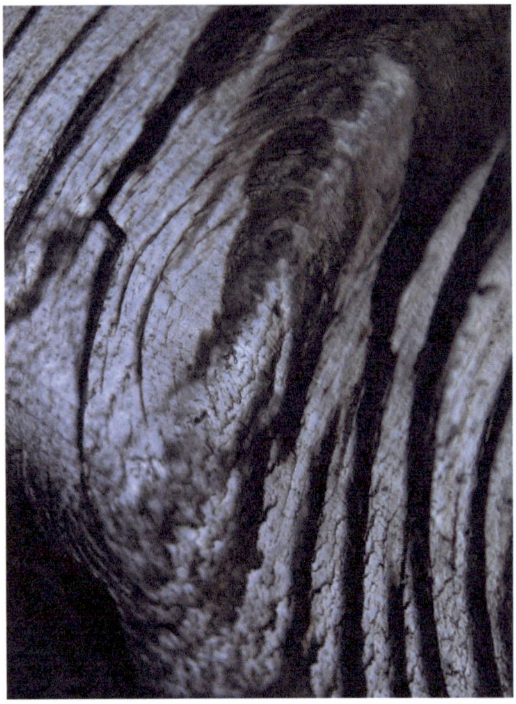

Fig. 14.15 Nuclear fibres

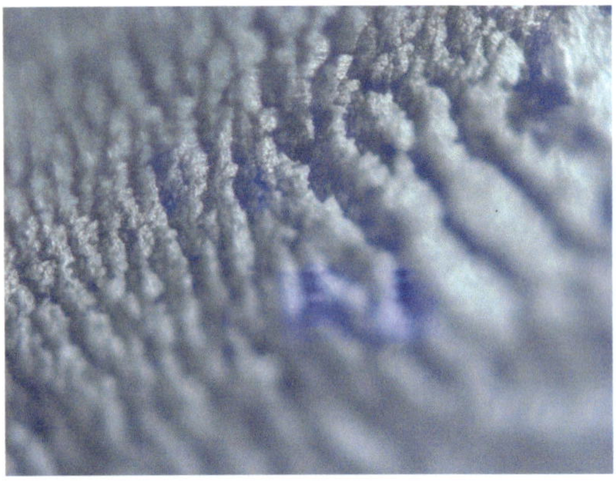

Fig. 14.16 Peripheral fibres orientation

influences affect its occurrence. Cortical cataract affects the cortex of the lens, and nuclear cataract causes the sclerosis of the nuclear segment [32, 37]. In cortical cataract, cortical lens fibre gets separated by fluid imbibition described as lamellar separation. In successive stages, incipient form of cataract is seen where wedge-shaped spokes of opacity with intervening clear areas progress to further hydration of the lens causing

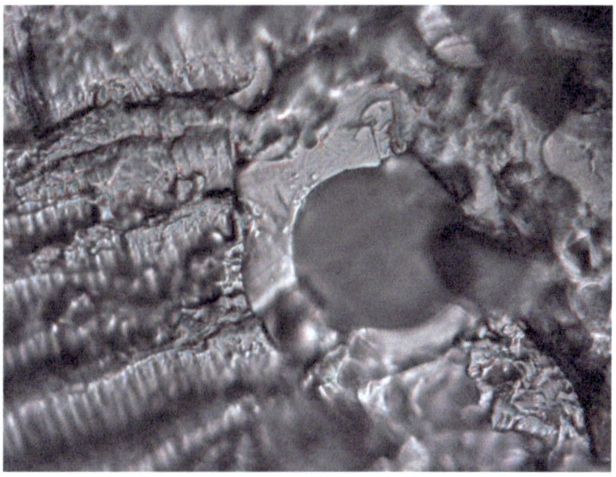

Fig. 14.17 Gross photograph of Morgagnian globules within fractured lens fibres

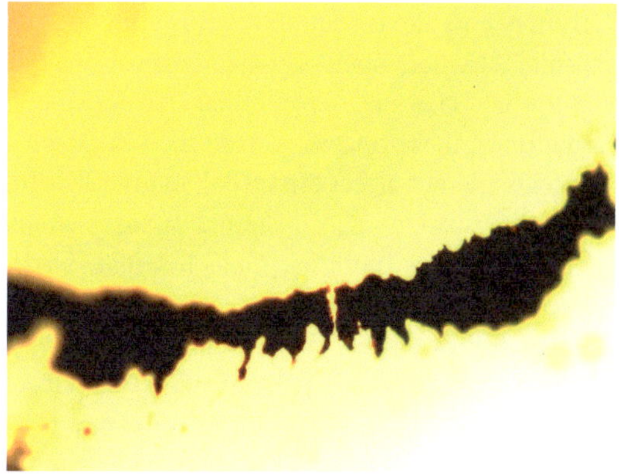

Fig. 14.19 Showing part of Vossius's ring on the anterior surface of the lens

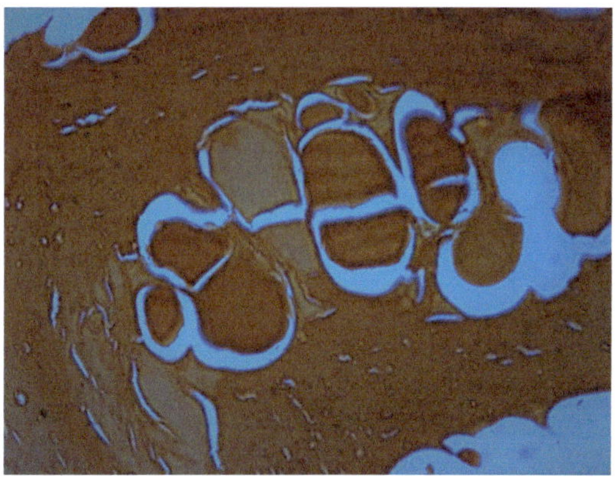

Fig. 14.18 H&E-stained section showing Morgagnian globules

intumescent cataract. Histopathologically, cortical change of the cataractous lens is marked by fluid-filled spaces or clefts within the fractured lens fibres called Morgagnian globules (Figs. 14.17, 14.18, and 14.19). The entire cortex, thereby, gets opaque and leading to 'mature' cataract. If at this stage the cataract is not removed surgically, hypermatured cataract is formed which is usually of two types—shrunken and Morgagnian cataract. Nuclear cataract, on the other hand, is due to intensified sclerosis of nuclear fibres and usually there is deposition of pigmented protein derived from Tryptophan and is known as cataract nigra [32–38]. In certain clinical situation, complicated cataract can develop which is due to alteration of anterior chamber nutrition affecting the lens secondary to inflammation, degeneration, tumours, myopia and conditions like retinitis pigmentosa [38, 39]. This type of cataract starts as opacification in the posterior subcapsular area and they present with polychromatic lustre when observed by slit lamp biomicroscopy [39, 40].

Developmental cataracts can be present at birth or appear during infancy and can be sporadic and familial. This type of cataract is usually seen in both eyes and is symmetric. Developmental opacities are usually small, and often they do not interfere with vision. Some of the cataracts are usually associated with infection such as Rubella [38–40]. Zonular nuclear cataract is seen as a congenital cataract where deposition of a zone of opaque cells is observed surrounded by a clear lens. Some of the opacities are seen in anterior and posterior Y sutures indicating damage in the third to fourth foetal months developing into nuclear cataract. Anterior and posterior polar cataract can be seen in congenital cataract where there is localised loss of central epithelial cells with adjacent cortical degeneration [37–40]. Membranous cataract can be seen in young individuals where developing anterior subcapsular cells at the equator of the lens continue to proliferate forming a Soemmerring's ring cataract.

Coronary cataract is seen in the form of congenital cataract where small dot-like cortical opacification is seen in crown-like arrangement. Sometimes, these opacities were seen in Down's baby who do not affect the visual acuity [38–40]. Cataract is seen in many systemic diseases which include diabetes mellitus, Galactosemia, hyper cupremia, Fabry's disease, myotonic dystrophy, Niemann–Pick disease type A and so on [32–40]. Diabetic cataract can present with snowflake opacities and histological the vacuoles are seen beneath the capsule of the lens and the nucleus is usually free from change [39]. Diabetic cataract is seen in long-standing diabetes and in the patients whose sugar level is uncontrolled. In a few cases, diabetic cataract can be reversible depending on the control of blood sugar. The basic metabolic pathway of diabetes involves the sorbitol pathway thereby affecting glycation in aldose reductase pathways of lens protein [39]. Cataract observed in infant with Galactosemia can be bilateral and in-configurations of 'oil drop' appearance seen in slit lamp examination or direct ophthalmoscopy [32–34]. They are bilateral and appear as a nuclear or zonular opacity. Lenticular appearance induced by copper is seen in Wilson's disease where there is characteristic 'sunflower' appearance where granular deposition of element copper is seen in the anterior and posterior lens capsule in the polar region [32–34]. Feathery or spoke-like deposits of granular material are seen in Fabry's disease which is very rarely seen [32–34]. Cataract in myotonic dystrophy can present as posterior subcapsular star-shaped cataract with cortical vacuoles and clefts in middle-aged patient [32–34].

Cataracts can be seen in various other conditions like steroids usage, anticholinesterases, mercury and due to other medications. Posterior subcapsular cataract can be seen in steroid-induced cases and usually progresses slowly and may be unaltered by stoppage of the medications [33, 34]. Cataract due to trauma can have depositions of iris-pigments on anterior surface of the lens capsules known as Vossius's ring (Fig. 14.19), and the cataract is usually rosette-shaped (Fig. 14.20) [40]. Pathologically they represent irregular separation of intracellular spaces and fragmentation of the cells. First, the opacity appears in the cortical layer and then gets displaced inside the lens.

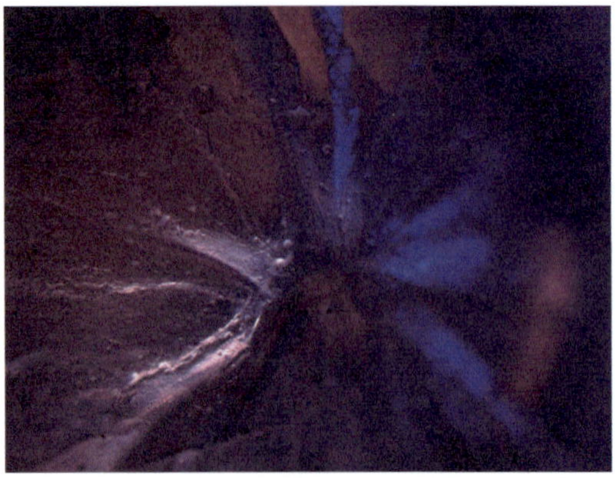

Fig. 14.20 Gross lens fibres orientation in a rosette-shaped traumatic cataract

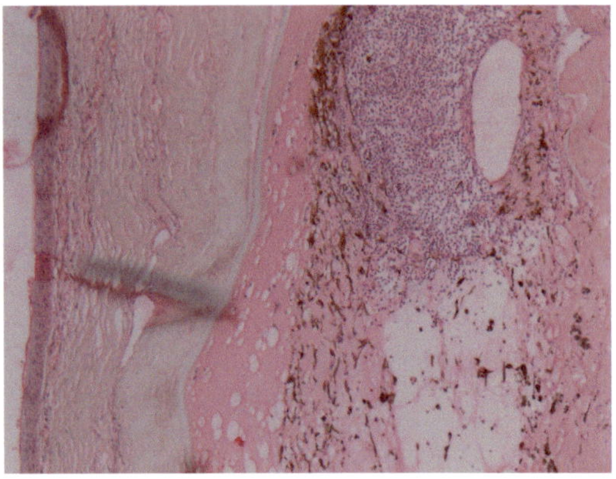

Fig. 14.21 Lens-induced uveitis 20×

Uveitis following a sequela of cataract and its complications is seen in clinical situation and can be complicated by glaucoma [41, 42]. Phacoanaphylactic uveitis has been studied extensively [42, 43]. Hypermature cataract can lead to liquefaction of cortex, and lens protein can extrude into the aqueous causing an inflammatory reaction (Fig. 14.21) [41, 42]. Cytology of aqueous fluid is indicated in this situation where anterior chamber inflammatory cells with macrophages and refractile lens protein can be seen. Rise in intraocular pressure in those eyes is common due to blockage of trabecular meshwork by the lens material and inflammatory by-products in the angle of the anterior chamber. Removal of offending lens material is necessary as soon as the diagnosis is made as this causes significant anterior uveitis [42, 43]. Phacoanaphylactic uveitis is an acute granulomatous inflammation that is seen after extra-capsular cataract surgery with retained lens matter or after lens trauma [41–43]. The inflammation may be so severe and that it sometimes mimics infective endophthalmitis. [41] Anterior synechiae formation and hypopyon uveitis are seen clinically in those situations. In phacoanaphylactic reaction, granulomatous reaction does not affect retina or choroid generally [42, 43]. The occurrence of bilateral granulomatous uveitis after penetrating trauma or surgery should suggest the possibility of sympathetic ophthalmia. In very rare situation, spectrum of sympathetic uveitis and phacoanaphylactic uveitis can occur together [42].

Financial Disclosures None for all authors

Funding Funding by Hyderabad Eye Research Foundation for Aravind Roy and Manjushree Bhate

References

1. Edward DP, Kaufman LM. Anatomy, development, and physiology of the visual system. Pediatr Clin N Am. 2003;50(1):1–23.
2. Wormstone IM, Wride MA. The ocular lens: a classic model for development, physiology and disease. Philos Trans R Soc Lond Ser B Biol Sci. 2011;366(1568):1190–2.
3. Ohuchi H, Sato K, Habuta M, Fujita H, Bando T. Congenital eye anomalies: more mosaic than thought? Congenit Anom (Kyoto). 2019;59(3):56–73.
4. Cvekl A, Tamm ER. Anterior eye development and ocular mesenchyme: new insights from mouse models and human diseases. BioEssays. 2004;26(4):374–86.
5. Barishak RY, Ofri R. Embryogenetics: gene control of the embryogenesis of the eye. Vet Ophthalmol. 2007;10(3):133–6.
6. Creuzet S, Vincent C, Couly G. Neural crest derivatives in ocular and periocular structures. Int J Dev Biol. 2005;49(2–3):161–71.
7. Tawfik HA, Dutton JJ. Embryologic and fetal development of the human orbit. Ophthalmic Plast Reconstr Surg. 2018;34(5):405–21.
8. Fuhrmann S. Eye morphogenesis and patterning of the optic vesicle. Curr Top Dev Biol. 2010;93:61–84.
9. Berthoud VM, Minogue PJ, Osmolak P, Snabb JI, Beyer EC. Roles and regulation of lens epithelial cell connexins. FEBS Lett. 2014;588(8):1297–303.
10. Taniguchi H, Kitaoka T, Gong H, Amemiya T. Apoptosis of the hyaloid artery in the rat eye. Ann Anat. 1999;181(6):555–60.
11. Danysh BP, Duncan MK. The lens capsule. Exp Eye Res. 2009;88(2):151–64.
12. Ernst J, Medsinge A, Scanga HL, Hiasat J, Moore W, Ali A, et al. Congenital primary aphakia. J AAPOS. 2022;S1091-8531(22)00006–4.
13. Chaurasia S, Jakati S, Ramappa M, Mishra DK, Edward DP. Anterior segment alterations in congenital primary aphakia-a clinicopathologic report of five cases. Indian J Ophthalmol. 2020;68(8):1564–8.
14. Sano Y, Matsukane Y, Watanabe A, Sonoda KH, Kondo H. Lack of FOXE3 coding mutation in a case of congenital aphakia. Ophthalmic Genet. 2018;39(1):95–8.
15. Valleix S, Niel F, Nedelec B, Algros MP, Schwartz C, Delbosc B, et al. Homozygous nonsense mutation in the FOXE3 gene as a cause of congenital primary aphakia in humans. Am J Hum Genet. 2006;79(2):358–64.
16. Bavbek T, Ogüt MS, Kazokoglu H. Congenital lens coloboma and associated pathologies. Doc Ophthalmol. 1993;83(4):313–22.
17. Jacobs K, Meire FM. Lenticonus. Bull Soc Belge Ophtalmol. 2000;277:65–70.
18. Savige J, Sheth S, Leys A, Nicholson A, Mack HG, Colville D. Ocular features in Alport syndrome: pathogenesis and clinical significance. Clin J Am Soc Nephrol. 2015;10(4):703–9.
19. Praveen MR, Vasavada AR, Koul A, Ravat FA, Trivedi RH, Shah SK, et al. Intraoperative posterior capsule flutter in posterior lentiglobus. J AAPOS. 2010;14(4):367–8.
20. Murakami Y, Kusaka S, Hayashi N, Soga K, Fujikado T. Wavefront analysis and ultrastructural findings in an eye with posterior lentiglobus. J AAPOS. 2010;14(6):530–1.
21. Yu X, Chen W, Xu W. Diagnosis and treatment of microspherophakia. J Cataract Refract Surg. 2020;46(12):1674–9.
22. Nelson LB, Maumenee IH. Ectopia lentis. Surv Ophthalmol. 1982;27(3):143–60.
23. Neely DE, Plager DA. Management of ectopia lentis in children. Ophthalmol Clin N Am. 2001;14(3):493–9.
24. Simon MA, Origlieri CA, Dinallo AM, Forbes BJ, Wagner RS, Guo S. New management strategies for ectopia lentis. J Pediatr Ophthalmol Strabismus. 2015;52(5):269–81.
25. Amaya L, Taylor D, Russell-Eggitt I, Nischal KK, Lengyel D. The morphology and natural history of childhood cataracts. Surv Ophthalmol. 2003;48(2):125–44.
26. Khokhar SK, Pillay G, Dhull C, Agarwal E, Mahabir M, Aggarwal P. Pediatric cataract. Indian J Ophthalmol. 2017;65(12):1340–9.

27. Kiziltoprak H, Tekin K, Inanc M, Goker YS. Cataract in diabetes mellitus. World J Diabetes. 2019;10(3):140.
28. Kang MJ, Yim HB, Hwang HB. Two cases of myotonic dystrophy manifesting various ophthalmic findings with genetic evaluation. Indian J Ophthalmol. 2016;64(7):535–7.
29. Bair B, Dodd J, Heidelberg K, Krach K. Cataracts in atopic dermatitis: a case presentation and review of the literature. Arch Dermatol. 2011;147(5):585–8.
30. Amemiya T, Matsuda H, Uehara M. Ocular findings in atopic dermatitis with special reference to the clinical features of atopic cataract. Ophthalmologica. 1980;180(3):129–32.
31. Abdolrahimzadeh B, Piraino DC, Albanese G, Cruciani F, Rahimi S. Neurofibromatosis: an update of ophthalmic characteristics and applications of optical coherence tomography. Clin Ophthalmol. 2016;10:851–60.
32. Zigler J. Biology of lens. In: Albert DM, Jakobiec FA, editors. Principles and practice of ophthalmology, basic sciences. Philadelphia: WB Saunders; 1994. p. 97.
33. Eagle R, Spencer W. The lens. In: Spencer W, editor. Ophthalmic pathology: an atlas and textbook, vol. 1. 4th ed. Philadelphia: WB Saunders; 1996. p. 372–437.
34. Yanoff M, Fine BS, Schaffer DB. Histopathology of transient neonatal lens vacuoles. Am J Ophthalmol. 1973;76(3):363–70.
35. Benedek GB. Cataract as a protein condensation disease: the proctor lecture. Invest Ophthalmol Vis Sci. 1997;38(10):1911–21.
36. Font RL, Brownstein S. A light and electron microscopic study of anterior subcapsular cataracts. Am J Ophthalmol. 1974;78(6):972–84.
37. Zimmerman LE, Johnson FB. Calcium oxalate crystals within ocular tissues; a clinicopathologic and histochemical study. AMA Arch Ophthalmol. 1958;60(3):372–83.
38. Apple DJ, Solomon KD, Tetz MR, Assia EI, Holland EY, Legler UF, et al. Posterior capsule opacification. Surv Ophthalmol. 1992;37(2):73–116.
39. Bron AJ, Sparrow J, Brown NA, Harding JJ, Blakytny R. The lens in diabetes. Eye (Lond). 1993;7(Pt 2):260–75.
40. Rafferty NS, Goossens W, March WF. Ultrastructure of human traumatic cataract. Am J Ophthalmol. 1974;78(6):985–95.
41. Nche EN, Amer R. Lens-induced uveitis: an update. Graefes Arch Clin Exp Ophthalmol. 2020;258(7):1359–65.
42. Chu XK, Chan CC. Sympathetic ophthalmia: to the twenty-first century and beyond. J Ophthalmic Inflamm Infect. 2013;3(1):49.
43. Nche EN, Amer R. Lens-induced uveitis: an update. Graefe's Archive for Clinical and Experimental Ophthalmology. 2020;258(7):1359–65.

15 Pathology of Glaucoma

Swathi Vallabh and Geeta K. Vemuganti

Contents

S. Vallabh (✉)
Smt. Jadhavbai Nathamal Singhvee Glaucoma Services, Sankara Nethralaya, Chennai, India
e-mail: drsvh@snmail.org

G. K. Vemuganti
School of Medical Sciences, University of Hyderabad, Hyderabad, India
e-mail: gkvemuganti@gmail.com

G. K. Vemuganti et al. (eds.), *Ocular Pathology*, https://doi.org/10.1007/978-981-96-8614-8_15

15.1 Introduction

Glaucoma is an optic neuropathy associated with characteristic structural damage to the optic nerve and associated visual dysfunction that may be caused by various pathological processes [1].

Earlier, it was described as a triad of high intraocular pressure, optic disc changes, and visual field defects. However, with emerging evidence from various longitudinal studies and imaging modalities, it is now thought of a group of disorders characterized by optic neuropathy due to a multifactorial etiology. To understand the cause and arrive at a diagnosis, it is prudent to be aware of the aqueous humor dynamics and its outflow through the angle, the anatomy of the angle and also the factors affecting the IOP. This chapter gives us an overview about the different types of glaucoma, their mechanisms and their treatment modalities.

In 2020, there were 3.60 million people above the age of 50 years who were blind due to glaucoma, and a further 4.13 million who had moderate to severe visual impairment (MSVI). The age-standardized ratio of women to men was 0.71:1.00 and 0.87:1.00 for glaucoma blindness and MSVI, respectively. Globally, the Sub-Saharan Africa had the highest age-standardized glaucoma blindness rates (blind: 0.66%; 0.52–0.81, MSVI: 0.46%; 0.36–0.57), followed by North African and Middle East (blind: 0.57%; 0.44–0.71, MSVI: 0.38%; 0.29–0.48) [2].

15.2 Anatomy of the Angle of the Anterior Chamber [3]

The aqueous outflow is divided into the conventional or the trabecular outflow and the unconventional or the uveoscleral outflow (Fig. 15.1). The conventional pathway is responsible for 70–95% of the aqueous outflow, while the unconventional pathway is responsible for 5–30% in humans. There is an age-related decline in both the total outflow facility and the trabecular outflow facility. However, there is a relative increase in the contribution of the trabecular pathway and a relative decrease in the uveoscleral pathway with increasing age [4].

15.2.1 Anatomy of the Conventional Aqueous Pathway

15.2.1.1 The Trabecular Meshwork

The trabecular meshwork has a connective tissue core surrounded by endothelium and may be divided into three portions:

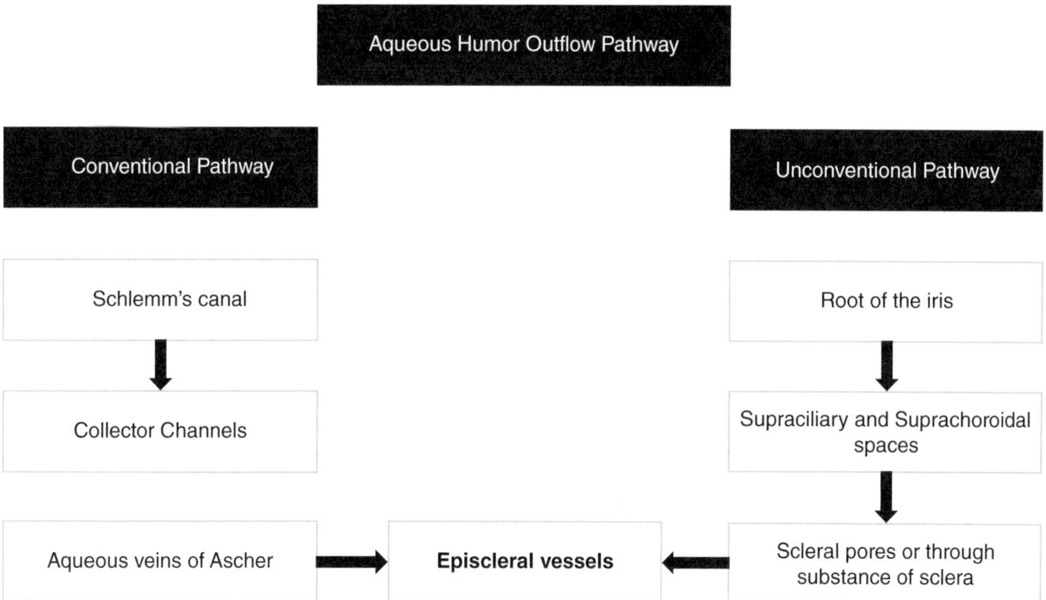

Fig. 15.1 The flowchart depicts the conventional and unconventional pathways of the aqueous humor outflow

(a) The innermost uveal meshwork with irregular openings that vary in size from 25 to 75 μm;
(b) he corneoscleral meshwork extending from the scleral spur to the anterior wall of the scleral sulcus with elliptical openings (diameter range of 5 to 50 μm);
(c) The juxtacanalicular tissue consisting of an inner trabecular endothelial layer, a central connective tissue layer, and an outer layer of Schlemm's canal endothelium [5].

15.2.1.2 Schlemm Canal

The endothelium-lined SC has a diameter of 190 to 370 mm and is present 360 degrees [6]. A complex system of intrascleral channels connects it to the episcleral and conjunctival veins.

15.2.1.3 Episcleral and Conjunctival Veins

The collector channels, previously referred to as the aqueous veins of Ascher [7] originate at the outer wall of the Schlemm canal and terminate in the episcleral and conjunctival veins in a lamination of aqueous humor and blood (the laminated vein of Goldmann).

The inner wall endothelial layer and the adjacent juxtacanalicular tissues are thought to be the site of resistance to the aqueous outflow.

15.2.2 Anatomy of the Unconventional Pathway

In the unconventional pathway, the aqueous humor drains via the root of the iris, passing between the bundles of the ciliary muscle into the supraciliary and suprachoroidal spaces. It then passes, via scleral pores surrounding ciliary blood vessels and nerves, vessels of optic nerve membranes, or directly through the collagen substance of the sclera, into the episcleral veins. The presence of uveal lymphatic channels has been postulated to contribute to the unconventional pathway.

15.2.3 Normal Chamber Angle in an Infant [8]

The angle of healthy infants differs from that of healthy adults.

The differences are:

1. The Schwalbe's line is less distinct.
2. The trabecular meshwork is less pigmented.
3. The junction between the scleral spur and ciliary body is less clear because of a translucent uveal meshwork.

It is important to note that the chamber angle in children continues its development from birth to 2 years of age, when the gonioscopic appearance stabilizes. However, the angle recess appears at 4 or 5 years of age. Normal mesodermal remnants may be present in normal angles which are still evolving into completion.

15.2.4 Age-Related Changes in the Trabecular Meshwork [3]

The morphological changes in the aging angle include:

(a) A change from a long, wedge-shaped form to a shorter, rhomboidal form.
(b) Increase in prominence of the scleral spur.
(c) Increase in compactness of the uveal meshwork.
(d) Localized closures in the Schlemm canal.
(e) Thickening of the trabecular beams.
(f) Denuding of the trabeculae due to a decrease in the endothelial cellularity.
(g) Narrowing of the intertrabecular spaces.
(h) Increase in the extracellular material.

15.3 Classification of Glaucoma

Glaucoma can be classified into primary or idiopathic when there is no known underlying cause, or secondary when there is an underlying cause. It can further be classified based on gonioscopy into open angle or closed angle.

The common finding in all glaucomas is the optic disc damage. This can be seen clinically and leads to corresponding changes in the visual fields and on Optical Coherence Tomography (OCT).

Classification

1. Primary open-angle glaucoma.
2. Primary angle closure glaucoma.
3. Childhood glaucomas—Childhood Glaucoma Research Network Classification.
   (a) Glaucoma in aphakia and pseudophakia.
   (b) Glaucoma associated with non-acquired systemic conditions.
   (c) Glaucoma associated with non-acquired ocular conditions.
   (d) Congenital glaucoma.
4. Secondary open-angle glaucomas.
   (a) Steroid-induced glaucoma.
   (b) Pseudoexfoliation glaucoma.
   (c) Pigment dispersion syndrome and pigmentary glaucoma.
   (d) Glaucoma-associated with elevated episcleral venous pressure.
5. Secondary glaucomas associated with corneal transplantation.
6. Lens-induced glaucoma.
7. Secondary glaucomas associated with retina and vitreoretinal surgery.
   (a) Neovascularization glaucoma.
   (b) Glaucoma associated with vitreoretinal surgery.
   (c) Schwartz syndrome.
8. Malignant glaucoma.
9. Glaucomas associated with ocular tumors.

15.3.1 Primary Open-Angle Glaucoma (POAG) [3, 9]

The prevalence of primary open-angle glaucomas in the <40 years age group is 1–2% in the general population worldwide. Normal tension glaucoma constitutes about a third of all cases of POAG. Most of the cases are asymptomatic and report a slow vision loss.

The risk factors are shown in Table 15.1 [10, 11].

Table 15.1 Risk factors of POAG

Risk factors	Strength of evidence
Elevated IOP	Strong
Increased age	Strong
Race (African American, Hispanic for POAG)	Strong
Optic nerve head alteration	Strong
Thin central corneal thickness	Strong
Confirmed family history in first-degree relatives	Strong
Diabetes mellitus	Moderate
Low blood pressure	Moderate
High myopia	Moderate
Vascular dysregulation (migraine, Raynaud syndrome)	Moderate
Sleep apnea	Moderate
Hypertension	Mild
Hypothyroidism	Mild
Cardiovascular disease	Mild

Table 15.2 The proposed mechanisms of development of POAG

IOP-dependent mechanism	IOP-independent mechanism
TM obstruction by pigments, glycosaminoglycans	Reduced ocular perfusion in diseases like diabetes, hypertension, and peripheral vascular disease
Trabecular endothelial cell loss	Excitotoxic damage from excessive glutamate
Loss of trabecular cell phagocytic activity	Autoimmune-mediated nerve damage
Loss of giant vacuoles from Schlemm's canal endothelium	Loss of neurotrophic factors
Reduced pore size and density in the wall of Schlemm's canal	Failure of cellular repair mechanisms
	Abnormal autoregulation of retinal and choroidal vasculature

15.3.1.1 Proposed Mechanisms of POAG [3, 9]

The main site of aqueous outflow resistance is thought to be in the juxtacanalicular tissue of the trabecular meshwork. There is an age-related decrease in the outflow facility due to the aging changes in the outflow pathway. The resultant IOP is an interplay between the amount of inflow and the age-related decrease in the outflow (Table 15.2).

The characteristic clinical findings include:

(a) Elevated IOP
(b) Open angles of the anterior chamber on gonioscopy
(c) Condition is mostly bilateral but can be asymmetric
(d) Characteristic glaucomatous optic nerve damage—Increase in the cup disc ratio with vertical elongation of the cup, Focal neuroretinal rim thinning or notching, beta zone peripapillary atrophy, disc hemorrhage
(e) Visual field loss on perimetry—nasal step, arcuate scotoma, generalized depression, abnormal glaucoma hemifield test (Fig. 15.2)

Treatment includes medical therapy with IOP lowering agents: Beta blockers (Timolol maleate), Alpha-2 agonists (Brimonidine 0.2%), Carbonic anhydrase inhibitors (Oral—Acetazolamide, Topical—Dorzolamide and Brinzolamide), Miotics (Pilocarpine 2%), Prostaglandin analogs (Latonoporst, bimatoprost, and travoprost).

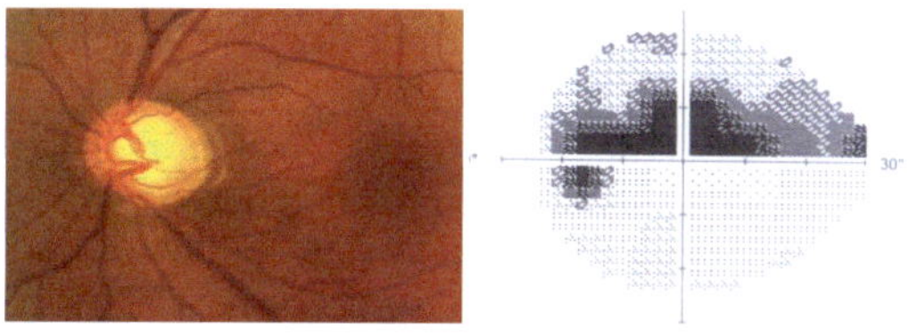

Fig. 15.2 The optic disc of the left eye shows an inferior notch with corresponding superior arcuate defect on the 24–2 test pattern of the Humphrey visual field

Surgical management in cases refractory to medical therapy includes trabeculectomy, angle procedures like goniotomy and laser trabeculoplasty, glaucoma drainage devices, and cyclophotocoagulation.

15.3.2 Primary Angle Closure Glaucoma

This subset of glaucoma is the most common glaucoma in Asians. The prevalence of this subset was 20 million in 2013 and is projected to reach 23 million by 2020 and 32 million by 2040. Seventy-seven percent of the cases are seen in Asia [12].

15.3.2.1 Risk Factors [13]

1. Increasing age
2. Female gender
3. Hyperopia
4. Family history of angle closure
5. Asian or Inuit descent
6. Shallow anterior chamber depth
7. Shorter axial length
8. Thicker lens

15.3.2.2 Mechanism of Primary Angle Closure [13]

The mechanism of angle closure in these eyes is due to relative pupillary block where there is obstruction to aqueous outflow by the apposition of the iris to the lens in the area of the pupil. This results in the accumulation of aqueous in the posterior chamber, leading to anterior bowing of the iris and irido-trabecular contact. The other mechanisms of angle closure described are an anteriorly positioned ciliary body and crowding of the iris caused by a thickened peripheral iris filling the space between the trabecular meshwork and angle recess under dark conditions.

15.3.2.3 Clinical Features [3]

Symptoms The patient can be asymptomatic or present with redness, pain in the eye or over the eyebrows, photophobia, colored haloes, nausea, vomiting.

15.3.2.4 Signs

1. Conjunctiva: circumciliary congestion.
2. Cornea: epithelial and stromal corneal edema in acute cases.
3. Anterior chamber: shallow anterior chamber due to the apposition of the peripheral iris to the trabecular meshwork. This causes the angles also to be occluded.
4. Iris: Iris may be normal or show the following changes:
   (a) Superior segmental iris atrophy: The IOP can cause occlusion of the major arterial circle of iris and subsequent necrosis of the iris. It is usually seen in the superior segment. There can be marked atrophy of the iris stroma and the posterior epithelium.
   (b) Neovascularization of the iris (rubeosis iridis): This usually occurs secondary to an acute attack of elevated IOP leading to retinal vein occlusion. It can also occur due to chronic ischemia in long-standing cases of uncontrolled IOP. NVI can be accompanied by new vessels in the angle termed neovascularization of the angle (NVA).
   (c) Atrophy of the sphincter and dilator pupillae: Ischemia of the muscles can lead to atrophy, resulting in an irregular pupil.
5. Lens: Multiple tiny gray-white lenticular opacities may be seen in the anterior subcapsular region. There are two involved mechanisms: the toxic necrotic products in the aqueous may lead to a metabolic disturbance of the anterior lens cells or an elevated IOP, causing a pressure necrosis.
6. Optic disc changes: An acute attack of rise in IOP can lead to an obstruction of the venous circulation in the optic nerve head, causing the ONH to swell. In chronic cases, characteristic optic nerve changes as described earlier (under POAG) may be seen (Fig. 15.3).

OCT and UBM findings usually aid in the classification of the type of angle closure glaucoma. Salient findings seen in angle closure disease in these eyes include: [3]

(a) A convex iris configuration with an increase in iris thickness causing an anterior bowing of the iris and closure of the angle.
(b) Reduced anterior chamber depth and volume.
(c) Increase in the lens vault: Lens vault is defined as the perpendicular distance between the anterior pole of the crystalline lens and the horizontal line joining the two scleral spurs, on horizontal AS-OCT scans [14].

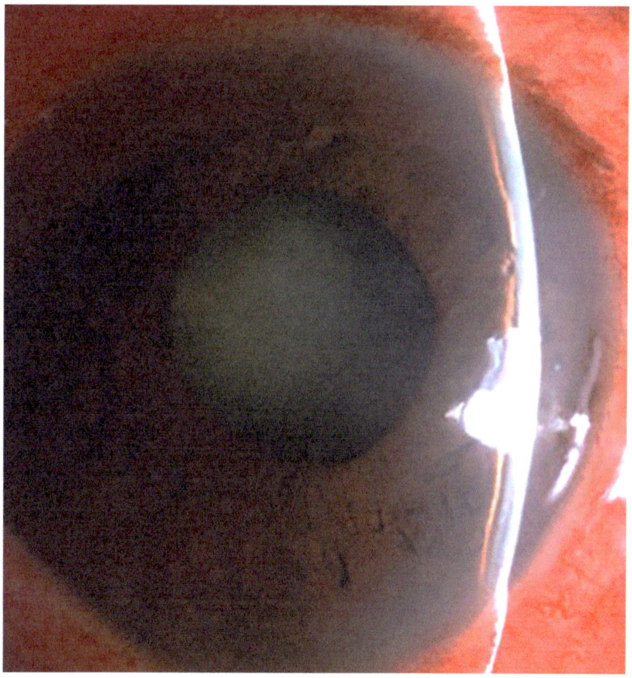

Fig. 15.3 An eye with angle closure glaucoma with conjunctival injection, shallow anterior chamber depth, iris whirling, sphincter atrophy from 12 o' clock to 9 o' clock

(d) Dynamic increase in the iris volume during dilatation.
(e) Choroidal expansion.

15.3.2.5 Management [13]

The treatment goals are to relieve the pupillary block and control the IOP.

The appositional angle closure can be reopened with miotic therapy with Pilocarpine. Pupillary block is relieved by performing a laser or incisional peripheral iridotomy. Once the pupillary block is relieved, routine antiglaucoma medications can be used to control the IOP. Laser trabeculoplasty may also be tried when warranted. Surgical management is reserved for cases refractory to peripheral iridotomy and medical management. The surgical modalities include trabeculectomy, drainage implants, lens extraction, and cyclophotocoagulation.

15.3.3 Childhood Glaucomas

Childhood glaucomas consist of a heterogeneous group of disorders characterized by normal or elevated IOP and characteristic glaucomatous optic nerve damage. The Childhood Glaucoma Research Network [15] has classified childhood glaucomas as shown in Fig. 15.4.

15.3.3.1 Glaucoma Following Cataract Surgery

This group of glaucomas may be described as "glaucomas associated with aphakia and pseudophakia" or "glaucomas in aphakia and pseudophakia".

The prevalence of glaucoma in aphakia is higher than glaucoma in pseudophakia with various studies reporting a prevalence over a 10-year period of 10–33% for the former and 3–13% for the latter.

Mechanisms [16] It can be due to a pupillary block mechanism or open-angle mechanism (Table 15.3).

Age at surgery is the most important risk factor. The earlier the age at surgery, the greater is the risk of developing glaucoma. The highest risk is at less than 1 month of age [17] (Figs. 15.5 and 15.6).

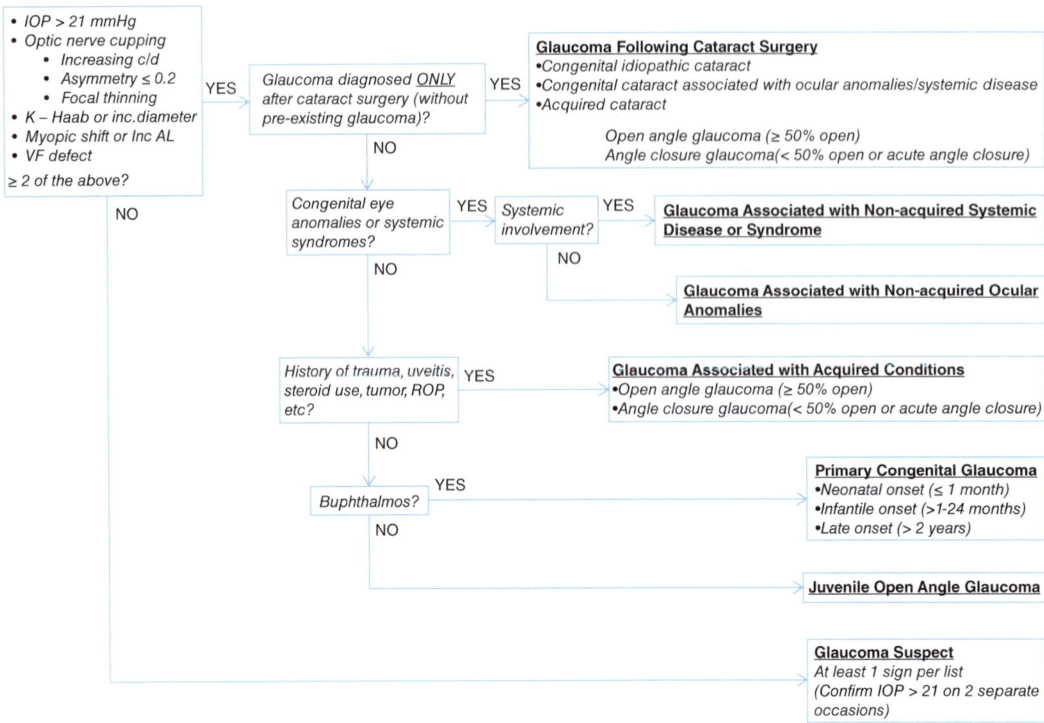

Fig. 15.4 The classification of childhood glaucomas by the Childhood Glaucoma Research Network

Table 15.3 The mechanism of childhood glaucoma following cataract surgery

Pupillary block mechanism	Open-angle mechanism
Inflammation causing membranes with peripheral anterior synechiae formation	Clogging of the angle by inflammatory cells, blood, residual lens particles, or vitreous
Delayed restoration of the anterior chamber due to inadequate vitrectomy or wound leak	Lens removal releases the tension on the zonules and in turn on the trabecular meshwork, leading to collapse of the trabecular spaces and a decrease in outflow
Epithelial ingrowth	Exposed lens epithelial cells can cause undesired changes in the trabecular meshwork structure and function
Inverted insertion of IOL	Steroid-induced mechanism due to postoperative steroids

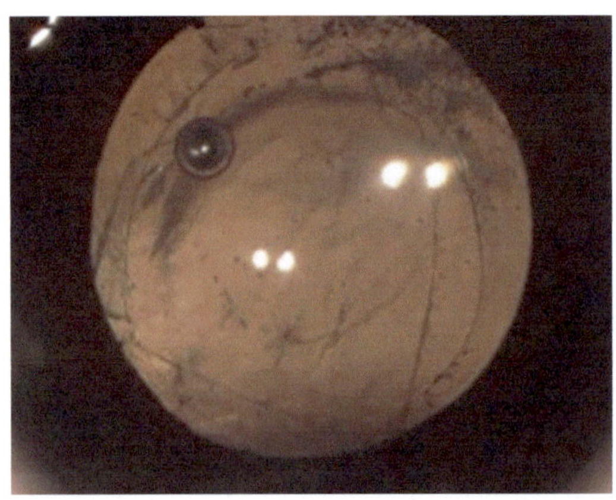

Fig. 15.5 Residual lens epithelial cells following cataract surgery in a child may cause undesired changes in the trabecular meshwork structure and function

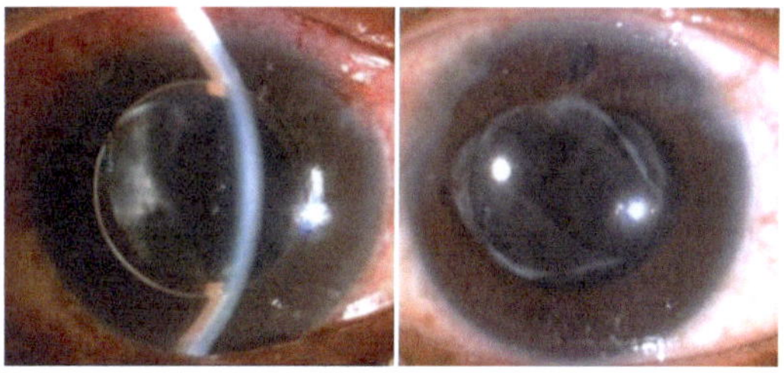

Fig. 15.6 Inverted insertion of 3-piece IOL causing a pupillary block glaucoma with shallow AC (image on the left). The pupillary block is relieved by IOL repositioning in the correct position (image on the right)

Treatment [18] Glaucomas in aphakia and pseudophakia may achieve long-term control of IOP with medical management alone. The surgical management includes goniotomy, trabeculectomy, combined trabeculectomy with trabeculotomy, drainage devices, and cyclophotocoagulation in refractory cases.

Table 15.4 The list of non-acquired systemic diseases or syndromes and ocular anomalies with associated glaucoma [15]

Glaucoma associated with non-acquired systemic disorders	Glaucoma associated with non-acquired ocular anomalies
Congenital rubella	Aniridia
Connective tissue disorders: Marfan syndrome, Weill–Marchesani syndrome	Axenfield–Rieger spectrum
Metabolic disorders: Homocystinuria, Lowe syndrome	Congenital ectropion uvea
Phacomatoses: Neurofibromatosis, Sturge–weber syndrome	Peters anomaly
Chromosomal disorders: Trisomy 21	Microphthalmia
	Ectopia lentis
	Persistent fetal vasculature

15.3.3.2 Glaucomas Associated with Non-acquired Conditions (Table 15.4)

15.3.3.3 Congenital Glaucoma [8]

Primary congenital glaucoma is a rare eye disorder accounting for 0.01–0.04% of total blindness [19]. Incidence in Western countries is 1 in 10,000 births [20]. In the combined states of Andhra Pradesh and Telangana, it is 1 in 3300 births which accounts for 4.2% of all childhood blindness [19].

The involvement is usually bilateral (70%), with a slight preponderance to males (60%) [21].

Most cases of PCG are sporadic in onset. The disease is familial in 10–40% of cases [19]. Patients with a familial pattern usually show an autosomal recessive pattern with incomplete or variable penetrance and possible multifactorial inheritance [22]. An autosomal dominant and pseudo-dominant mode of inheritance has also been reported.

It has been reported that 87% of familial and 27% of sporadic cases are due to mutations in CYP1B1 gene (encoding the cytochrome P450 enzyme) at the locus GLC3A. Another study indicated that a digenic inheritance of CYP1B1 and MYOC mutations results in a phenotype with more pronounced glaucoma, suggesting that CYP1B1 may function as a gene modifier for the MYOC gene [19, 23, 24].

PCG can present with the following symptoms: [8]

- Watering
- Intolerance to light
- Blepharospasm
- Redness
- Sneezing
- Frequent blinking
- Sudden whitish appearance of cornea
- Large eyeball size

The classical triad of PCG includes epiphora, photophobia, and blepharospasm.

The following are the various signs of PCG: [8, 25]

1. The intraocular pressure can be normal or elevated.
2. There can be associated conjunctival congestion.
3. The increase in IOP causes a globe distension, as the scleral and corneal collagens in an

infant are still pliable. This results in Megalocornea and or Buphthalmos [26].

4. When the IOP continues to be elevated, breaks can develop in the already stretched cornea and aqueous gains access into the corneal stroma. This results in acute corneal hydrops [27].
5. Haab's striae [26, 28] (Fig. 15.7).

Haab's striae are tears in the endothelium and Descemet membrane caused by increased intraocular pressure, provided that the cornea has enlarged beyond the elasticity of the membrane. Haab's striae are typically horizontal and linear when they occur centrally in the cornea, but parallel or curvilinear to the limbus when they occur peripherally.

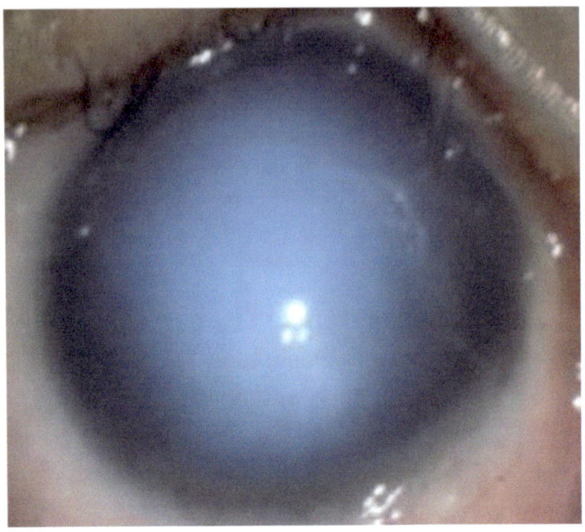

Fig. 15.7 Corneal edema seen in primary congenital glaucoma

- Uncommon in corneas smaller than 12.5 mm in diameter.
- As the edge of the rupture in Descemet's membrane contracts into scrolls and ridges, with aqueous entry into the stroma causing localized corneal edema, compounding any diffuse edema that may also be present simply because of the elevated IOP.

Haab's striae form as a new basement membrane (Descemet's membrane) gets laid down by the Descemet's membrane and hyaline ridges develop.

- Breaks in Descemet's membrane from increased IOP rarely occur after age three (Fig. 15.8).

1. Anomalous iris vessels may also be seen as loops branching from the major arterial circle [29]. The peripheral iris may be covered by fine, fluffy tissue [8].
2. The angle in PCG patients differs from that of healthy infants. There are two types of patho-

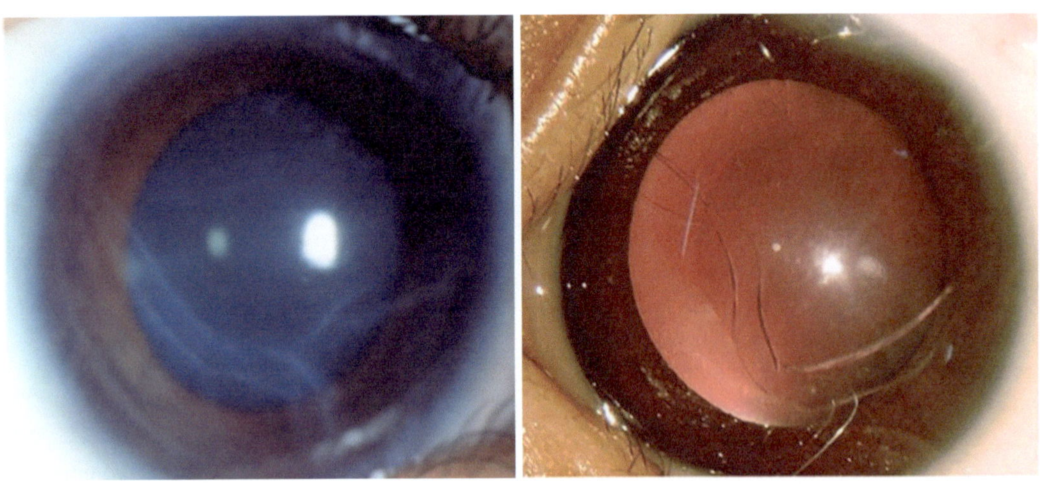

Fig. 15.8 Haab's striae seen in diffuse illumination (image on the left) and retroillumination (image on the right) are tears in the endothelium and the Descemet's membrane and are horizontally oriented in the center of the cornea and curvilinear or parallel to the limbus in the periphery of the cornea

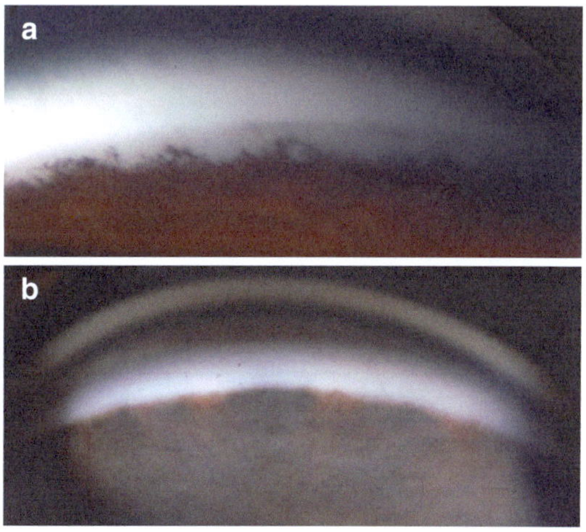

Fig. 15.9 Type I angle with thin pathological mesodermal remnants (**a**) and Type II angle with thick pathological mesodermal remnants and apparent high iris insertion (**b**)

logical chamber angle in children: Type I and Type II [8].

Type 1 angle (Fig. 15.9a) has thin pathological mesodermal remnants that cover the ciliary band and sometimes reach the Schwalbe line. Type II angle (Fig. 15.9b) has thick pathological mesodermal remnants and apparent high iris insertion with black triangles and pillars.

3. There can be limbal ectasia, ciliary, or posterior staphyloma.
4. Late manifestations include fibrosis of the trabecular meshwork and disappearance of the Schlemm's canal.
5. The infant glaucomatous cup usually has a configuration different from adult glaucomas.
   - It is round, steep-walled, and central, surrounded by a uniform pink rim.
   - Circumferential enlargement of the cup due to stretching of the scleral canal.
   - Striking reversal of cupping on IOP reduction with glaucoma surgery [30].

15.3.3.4 Management [19, 25]

The main treatment modality is surgical, with trabeculotomy being the surgery of choice in eyes with hazy corneas and goniotomy in clear corneas. The medical management, if warranted, is with carbonic anhydrase inhibitors as the preferred medication. Alpha agonists are contraindicated in very young children due to the risk of sleep apnea.

Table 15.5 Percentage of steroid responders and the range of IOP elevation

Category of response	IOP elevation in response to glucocorticoids	% of normal population
Nonresponsive	<5 mm hg	61–63%
Moderately responsive	6–15 mm hg	33%
Highly responsive	> 15 mm hg	4–6%

15.3.4 Secondary Glaucomas

15.3.4.1 Steroid-Induced Glaucomas

One of the most common secondary glaucomas occurs secondary to steroid intake in any form. Patients who show an increase in the IOP in the setting of steroid use are labelled as 'steroid responders'.

The prevalence varies widely. Table 15.5 summarizes the percentage of the population who respond to steroid exposure and the range of IOP elevation [31].

The potency, dose, and the route of administration of the glucocorticoid will determine the amount and duration of IOP elevation. Fig. 15.10 depicts the decreasing order of frequency of patients with ocular hypertension with various routes of administration.

Topical administration has the maximum chance of an IOP spike. The elevation in IOP is seen commonly between three to six weeks after initiation of therapy, and typically normalizes within two weeks of the cessation of therapy.

Risk Factors for developing glaucoma with steroid therapy: [3]

- Primary open-angle glaucoma.
- A first-degree relative with POAG.
- A history of previous steroid-induced IOP elevation.
- Type 1 diabetes mellitus.
- Very young age (age less than six years old) or an older age.

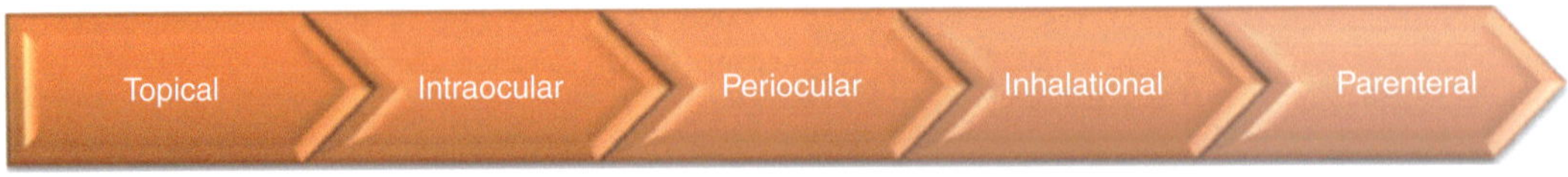

Fig. 15.10 The various routes of administration of steroids in decreasing order of their risk of ocular hypertension

- Connective tissue disease.
- Penetrating keratoplasty, especially in eyes with Fuchs endothelial dystrophy or keratoconus.
- High myopia.

Etiology [31]

Steroids are known to induce physical and physiological changes in the trabecular meshwork and cause an increase in IOP due to decreased outflow of aqueous.

- There is increased accumulation of glycosaminoglycans and extracellular matrix in the trabecular meshwork.
- Corticosteroids induce cytoskeletal changes by the formation of crosslinked actin and increased expression of myocilin, which in turn decreases the outflow.
- Physical obstruction of the trabecular meshwork by glucocorticoids themselves due to steroid-induced suppression of phagocytosis.

Management [31]

All patients on steroid therapy in any form should have IOP monitored regularly.

(a) Discontinue steroids: The first line of therapy includes cessation of steroid therapy in patients for whom it can be stopped.
(b) Steroid-sparing agents: Certain diseases require long-term treatment with steroids. In cases with steroid-induced glaucoma, collaborating with the treating physician and suggesting a steroid-sparing medication can be considered.
(c) Removal of depot steroids; In cases where depot subtenon's or intravitreal steroids have been used, removal of the medication helps in control of IOP.
(d) Management of IOP:
 Antiglaucoma medications: In some patients, even after cessation of steroids, the IOP may remain high. These need to be treated with medications to lower the IOP. In cases where medications fail to correct IOP, surgery in the form of goniotomy, trabeculectomy, or laser trabeculoplasty can be considered.

15.3.4.2 Pseudoexfoliation Glaucoma

Pseudoexfoliation syndrome (PXS) is an age-related systemic disorder caused due to the accumulation of fibrillar extracellular material in the ocular tissues. It was first described by Lindberg in 1917 in Finland [32]. It is the most common cause of open-angle glaucoma globally. Approximately one-fourth of patients with pseudoexfoliation syndrome (PXS) have elevated IOP, and one-third of these have glaucoma [33]. Pseudoexfoliation glaucoma (PXG) comprises as much as 50% of the open-angle glaucoma in Norway, Ireland, Greece, and Saudi Arabia, about 25% in Ethiopia [34].

In a study by Krishnadas et al. [35], the prevalence of glaucoma among subjects with PXF in the South Indian rural population was 7.5%; exfoliation was present in 26.7% of those identified as primary open-angle glaucoma, and increasing age and male gender were significantly associated with PXS.

The precise etiology and pathogenesis are unknown. However, the pathologic process involved is the accumulation of intraocular and extraocular abnormal fibrillar material, either due to its excessive production or inadequate breakdown [36]. Fig. 15.11 explains the various mechanisms of glaucoma in a case of pseudoexfoliation.

It can cause both open-angle and angle closure glaucomas. The factors involved in development of glaucoma are outlined in Table 15.6.

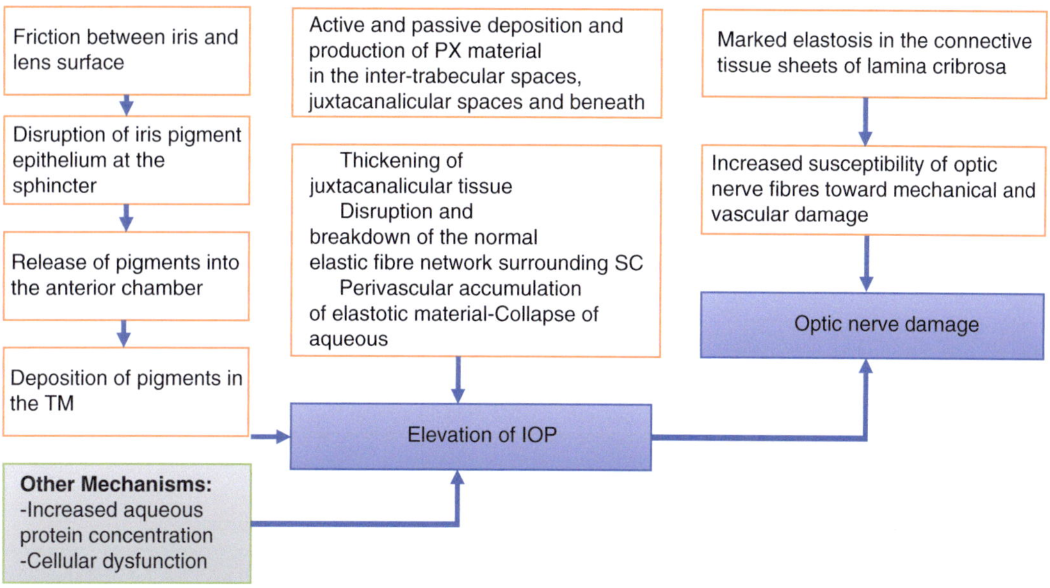

Fig. 15.11 The various possible mechanisms of IOP elevation and optic nerve damage in pseudoexfoliation glaucoma. *TM* Trabecular meshwork, *SC* Schlemm's canal

Table 15.6 The factors involved in the development of pseudoexfoliation glaucoma

Pathogenetic factors of IOP elevation and glaucoma development in PEX syndrome	
1. Ocular hypertension and open-angle glaucoma	Locally produced (endotrabecular) PEX material
	Passively deposited (exotrabecular) PEX material
	Melanin dispersion during mydriasis
	Increased aqueous protein concentrations
	Proliferation/migration of corneal endothelial cells
2. Angle closure glaucomas (pupillary/ciliary block)	Zonular instability and subtle lens subluxation
	Rigid iris and poor mydriasis
	Posterior synechiae
	Protein-rich aqueous humor
	Relative anterior microphthalmos

Reproduced with permission from Schlötzer-Schrehardt et al. [37]

Clinical Features

The clinical signs of PXS have been tabulated in Table 15.7 (Fig. 15.12).

Cataract is often the nuclear type. The causes of cataract development may be linked to: [37]

Ocular ischemia
Aqueous hypoxia
Increased growth factor levels
Reduced protection against ultraviolet radiation by lower levels of ascorbic acid in the aqueous humor

Eyes with pseudoexfoliation have a three- to ten-fold increased risk of zonular rupture and lens dislocation, and cataract surgery in these eyes has an approximately five-fold increased risk of vitreous loss [38].

The first line of management of PXG includes medical management with prostaglandin analogs. PG analogs are known to alter the disease process by affecting the aqueous concentration of TGF-R1, MMP-2, and TIMP-2 [39]. Miotics have a two-fold effect: Increase the aqueous out-

Table 15.7 The clinical manifestations and the surgical challenges in pseudoexfoliation glaucoma based on the tissue involved

Diagnosis of early stages, clinical, and surgical complications of pseudoexfoliation (PEX) syndrome			
Tissue involvement	Early clinical signs	Clinical complications	Surgical complications
Lens, ciliary body, and zonules	Diffuse precapsular layer	Cataract (nuclear)	Zonular rupture/dialysis
	Phacodonesis	Phacodonesis	Vitreous loss
	PEX deposits on zonules (UBM)	Lens subluxation	Posterior capsule rupture
		Angle closure glaucoma due to pupillary and ciliary block	Decentration of lens implant
			Anterior capsule fibrosis
			Secondary cataract
Iris	Peripupillary atrophy and iris sphincter region transillumination	Melanin dispersion	Miosis/poor surgical access
	Melanin dispersion is associated with pupillary dilation	Poor mydriasis	Intra- and postoperative hyphema
	Poor mydriasis, asymmetric pupil sizes	Iris rigidity	Postoperative inflammation
		Capillary hemorrhage	Prolonged blood aqueous barrier breakdown
		Blood-aqueous barrier defects, pseudouveitis	Posterior synechiae and pupillary block
		Anterior chamber hypoxia	
		Posterior synechiae	
Trabecular meshwork	Pigment deposition	Intraocular hypertension	Postoperative IOP rise
	Marked asymmetry of IOP	Open-angle glaucoma	
	Marked IOP rise after pupillary dilation		
Cornea	Atypical corneal guttata	Endothelial decompensation	Endothelial decompensation
		Endothelial migration/ proliferation	
Posterior segment		Retinal vein occlusion	

Reproduced with permission from Schlötzer-Schrehardt et al. [37]

flow, thereby clearing the trabecular meshwork; limit the pupillary movement and slow the progression of the disease. In cases of uncontrolled IOP with medical therapy, cases should be managed with appropriate surgical modalities.

15.3.4.3 Pigmentary Glaucoma and Pigment Dispersion Syndrome

In Pigment dispersion syndrome (PDS), an anomalous Irido-zonular contact leads to melanin dispersion and subsequent deposition on various ocular structures. When this condition leads to an elevated IOP due to aqueous outflow resistance as a result of pigment deposition in the angle, it is termed Pigmentary glaucoma (PG).

About 1–1.5% of glaucoma cases in Caucasian countries are due to PG. The risk of developing PG from PDS is between 35% and 50% [40].

PDS can be an autosomal dominant disease with incomplete penetrance. The risk factors for PG include myopia, male gender, middle age, flat cornea, and a family history of pigmentary glaucoma.

Pathophysiology [3]

Campbell's Mechanical Theory Campbell suggested that the mid-peripheral transillumination defects correspond in number and location to the anterior zonules rubbing against the iris and leading to pigment dispersion. A backward bowing or concavity of the iris was noted in the mid-peripheral region.

The other theories postulated include an inherent weakness of the iris pigment epithelium, elongated anterior zonules which are pigmented (Fig. 15.13).

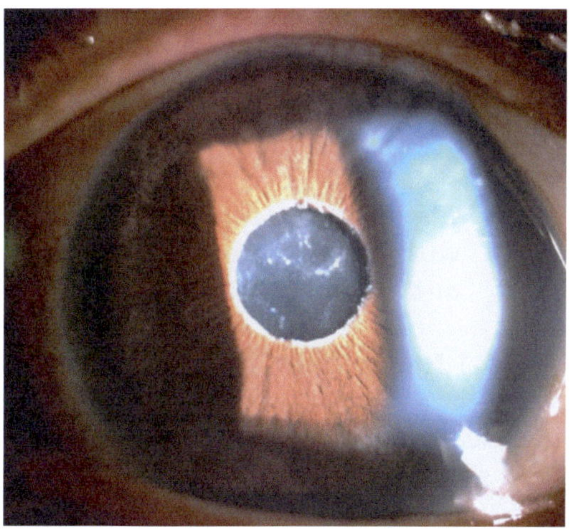

Fig. 15.12 Pseudoexfoliation material seen at the pupillary margin along with cataract in an eye with pseudoexfoliation glaucoma

The mechanism of elevation of IOP is thought to be more than one.

- The pigments physically obstruct the trabecular meshwork and cause resistance to the aqueous outflow.
- The pigments get engulfed by the trabecular cells which cause cell injury and death of these cells. They are then phagocytosed by the macrophages which carry off the melanin pigments through the Schlemm's canal and into the circulation. The loss of trabecular cells causes denudation of collagen beams and obliteration of aqueous channels.

Clinical Features [3, 40]

On slit lamp examination, the following features may be noted:

Cornea: Krukenberg spindles—spindle-shaped pigment deposition in the center of the cornea.

AC: Pigment cells in the anterior chamber may increase after blinking, dilatation, or exercise.

Iris: Iris may show spoke-like mid-peripheral transillumination defects. Heterochromia due to deposition of the pigments on the iris stroma may be seen. Anisocoria with a larger pupil on the side of the PDS may be seen.

Lens: Pigment deposition on the anterior lens capsule and zonules. A pigmented line termed

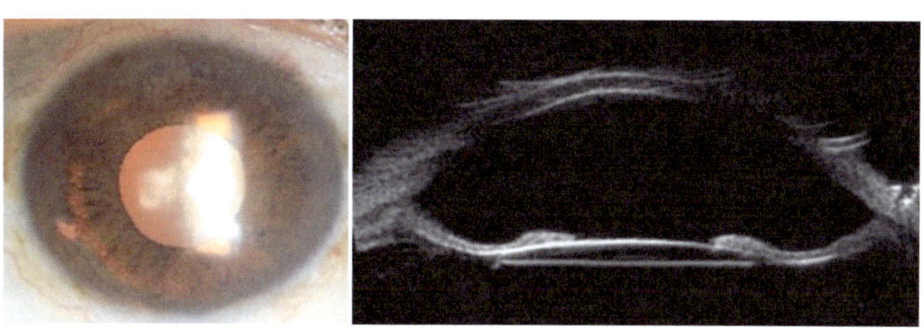

Fig. 15.13 An eye with pigment dispersion syndrome with mid peripheral transillumination defects (image on the left) and UBM of the eye showing posterior bowing of the iris in the corresponding region (image on the right)

the Zentmayer line or Scheie stripe can be seen on the posterior lens capsule.

Gonioscopy: A dense homogenous pigmentation of the trabecular meshwork and occasionally on the Schwalbe's line.

Management [3]

Medical therapy with pilocarpine, apart from lowering the IOP, is theoretically proven to increase the outflow and hence washout of the pigments. It also causes miosis, thereby relieving the mechanism of pigment dispersion. However, young myopes, most affected by this condition, do not tolerate pilocarpine well. All other classes of antiglaucoma medications can be used, but the primary mechanism of pigment dispersion is not treated.

Laser Therapy Some cases show decrease in pigment dispersion and control of IOP with a peripheral iridotomy. This is said to relieve the posterior bowing of the iris and reversal of the 'reverse pupillary block'. Laser trabeculoplasty is one of the treatment modalities when medical therapy fails to control the IOP. Glaucoma filtering surgery is usually indicated when medical and laser treatment have failed to control the IOP.

15.3.5 Glaucoma Following Keratoplasty [41, 42]

Glaucoma occurs commonly following corneal transplantation and is a cause for graft failure. Table 15.8 summarizes the prevalence, the mechanism, and the management of glaucoma in different types of keratoplasty.

15.3.6 Lens-Induced Glaucoma

Lens-induced glaucoma comprises a number of different glaucomatous processes where the mechanism of rise in IOP is due to the crystalline lens.

This can be classified into: [45]

Open-angle mechanism or Lens protein-related: Leakage of lens protein across an intact or a breached lens capsule.

- Phacolytic glaucoma
- Lens-particle induced glaucoma
- Phacoanaphylactic glaucoma

Angle closure mechanism or pupillary block mechanism:

- Phacomorphic glaucoma
- Ectopia lentis

Ectopia Lentis may be associated with Marfan's syndrome, homocystinuria, Weill–Marchesani syndrome, hyperlysinemia, and sulfite oxidase deficiency (Table 15.9; Figs. 15.14 and 15.15).

15.3.7 Glaucoma Associated with Retinal Disorders and Vitreoretinal Surgeries

15.3.7.1 Neovascular Glaucoma (NVG)

Neovascular glaucoma is a secondary glaucoma characterized by rubeosis iridis and raised IOP with retinal ischemia as the underlying mechanism [47]. The proportion of eyes with NVG among the secondary glaucomas is 9–17.4% [48].

The most common causes [48] include:

Ischemic Disorders

- Central retinal vein occlusion
- Diabetic retinopathy
- Carotid insufficiency or ocular ischemic syndrome

Inflammatory Disorders

- Uveitis and retinal vasculitis
- Trauma
- Extraocular inflammatory vascular causes like Giant Cell Arteritis, temporal arteritis

Table 15.8 The prevalence, mechanism, and the management of glaucoma in different types of keratoplasty

Type of keratoplasty	Incidence	Mechanism of glaucoma	Management
Penetrating keratoplasty	9–50% Early post op period: 10–31% Late post op period: 18–35%	*In early post op period:* a. High viscosity viscoelastics or inflammation may impede the aqueous outflow b. Inflammation can also cause pupillary block by the formation of anterior/posterior synechiae c. TM collapse by deep or mid-stromal corneal sutures d. Crowding at TM by same-sized donor button as the recipient's bed, tight sutures, and long bites *The late postoperative period:* a. Corticosteroid-induced IOP elevation b. Inflammation-induced synechial closure leads to the elevation of IOP	Topical management with antiglaucoma medications. YAG laser iridotomy is performed for patients with pupillary block glaucoma. The surgical management includes a. Trabeculectomy or b. Drainage devices (pars plana placement of the tube is preferred due to lesser risk of graft failure) [43, 44] or c. Cyclophotocoagulation in eyes with guarded visual potential
Descemet's membrane endothelial Keratoplasty (DMEK) and Descemet's stripping automated endothelial Keratoplasty (DSAEK)	15.4% in DMEK Post DSAEK: 35%—In eyes with no h/o glaucoma; 45% with prior h/o glaucoma; 43% with prior h/o glaucoma surgery [42]	*Early postoperative period:* a. Angle closure induced by the air bubble introduced at the end of the surgery to hold the DM in place b. Retained viscoelastic can obstruct the aqueous outflow *Late postoperative period:* a. inflammation induced PAS b. Blockage by inflammatory cells c. Steroid-induced ocular hypertension	

Table adapted from: https://eyewiki.aao.org/Cornea_Transplantation-Induced_Glaucoma:_A_Review_of_Glaucoma_Secondary_to_PKP,_DMEK,_and_DSAEK_Procedures
TM Trabeculae Meshwork, *DM* Descemet's membrane

Table 15.9 Classification of lens-induced glaucomas with their clinical features and management [46]

Type of glaucoma	Phacomorphic glaucoma	Ectopia lentis	Phacolytic glaucoma	Lens particle glaucoma	Phacoanaphylactic glaucoma
History of trauma	No	May be present in acquired cases	No	Yes	Yes
Symptoms	Pain, redness	Depends on the state of the lens Diplopia or sudden decrease in vision	Pain, redness	Pain, redness	Pain, redness
Conjunctiva	Congested				
Cornea	May be hazy due to an increase in IOP or long-standing cases due to corneal decompensation				
Anterior chamber depth	Shallow	Variable- deep or shallow	Deep	Deep	Deep
Anterior chamber contents	AC cells and flare	Lens may be in the anterior chamber	Fluffy white particles in the AC, white colored cells in AC	Fluffy white particle in AC	Keratic precipitates and AC reaction with cells and flare
Pupil	Mid-dilated fixed	Normal/ mid-dilated, iridodonesis	Festooned pupil	Festooned pupil	Festooned pupil
Lens	Intumescent cataract	Dislocated or subluxated lens, phacodonesis	Hypermature or mature cataract	Traumatic cataract with breach in the anterior capsule, OR pseudophakia	Traumatic cataract with breach in anterior capsule or pseudophakia s/p cataract surgery
Mechanism of glaucoma	Pupillary block. It can also be seen in eyes with spherophakia	Pupillary block due to dislocation/subluxation of lens	Acute open-angle glaucoma due to TM block by macrophages or lens proteins which have leaked from microdefects of the lens capsule	Open-angle glaucoma due to TM block by lens particles released after cataract surgery or trauma or Nd:YAG capsulotomy	After 1–14 days after the release of lens particles into the aqueous, there is inflammation of TM mediated by IgG and the complement system (type III hypersensitivity—Arthus type reaction)
Laterality	Usually unilateral	Can be bilateral in congenital cases	Usually unilateral	Usually unilateral	Usually unilateral
Management	Immediate management consists of IOP-lowering agents: Mannitol and aqueous suppressants, topical steroids for inflammation, definitive management consists of cataract surgery.	Pupillary block—Laser peripheral iridectomy. Total anterior or posterior dislocation —Removal of the lens. Rise in IOP is treated with antiglaucoma medications	Immediate management consists of IOP-lowering agents: Mannitol and aqueous suppressants. Topical steroids for inflammation. Definitive management consists of cataract surgery.	Immediate management consists of IOP-lowering agents: Mannitol and aqueous suppressants. Topical steroids for inflammation. Persistent inflammation and high IOP warrant removal of lens matter	Immediate management consists of IOP-lowering agents: Mannitol and aqueous suppressants. Topical steroids for inflammation. Persistent inflammation and high IOP warrant removal of lens matter

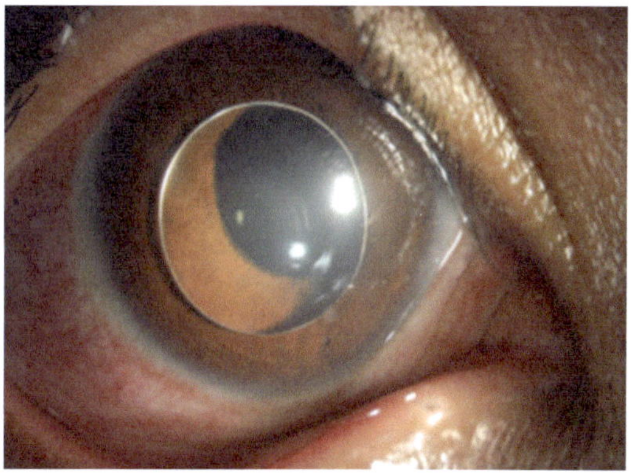

Fig. 15.14 Ectopia lentis in a case of spherophakia resulting in pupillary block glaucoma

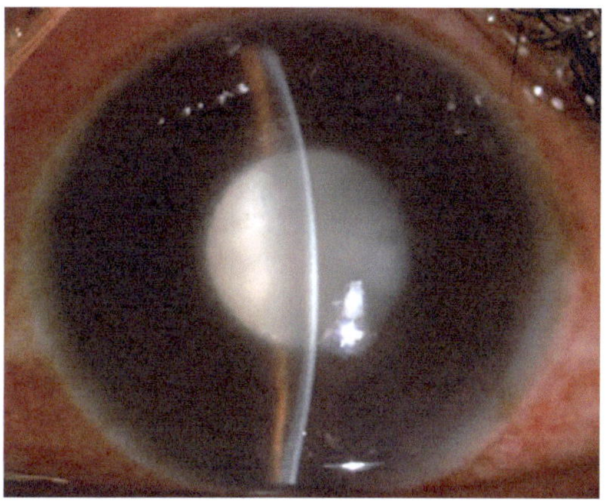

Fig. 15.15 A 60-year-old female with pseudophakia in the right eye presented with sudden pain in the left eye associated with a gradual progressive decrease in vision. On examination, vision in the right eye was 6/6 with glasses, and in the left eye was perception of light. LE showed congested conjunctiva, grade 2 corneal edema, shallow AC, and an intumescent cataract

Retinal Detachment

Tumors

- Ocular melanoma
- Retinoblastoma
- Intraocular metastasis
- Vasoproliferative tumors of the retina

Systemic Diseases

- Systemic lupus erythematosus
- Juvenile xanthogranuloma
- Neurofibromatosis type 1

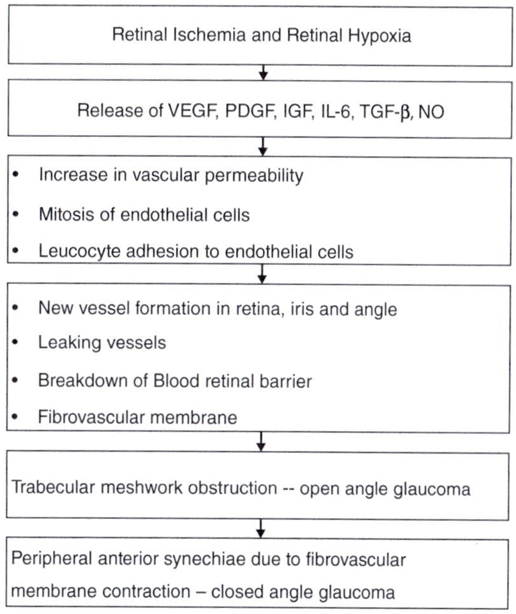

Fig. 15.16 The pathway from the inciting event of retinal hypoxia to the development of angle closure glaucoma. VEGF: Vascular endothelial growth factor; PDGF: Platelet-derived growth factor; IGF: Insulin-like growth factor; IL-6: Interleukin-6; TGF-®: Transforming growth factor-®; NO: Nitric oxide

Pathogenesis of NVG [48]

The primary pathology is a condition which leads to retinal hypoxia and ischemia, thereby disrupting the balance between pro- and antiangiogenic factors. The mechanism is depicted in the flowchart in Fig. 15.16.

Clinical features: NVG could be asymptomatic or could present with a painful red eye. The main signs of NVG include:

Conjunctival congestion

The cornea may be clear or edematous

Elevated IOP (with or without corneal edema)

The iris shows neovascularization, usually seen as thin, tortuous vessels randomly oriented at the pupillary margin. In advanced cases, ectropion uvea may be present.

Gonioscopy shows open or closed angles. Neovascularization of the angles appearing as thin arborizing vessels over the trabecular meshwork may be present.

The fundus reveals the cause of NVG, like diabetic retinopathy, vein occlusion, and ocular ischemic syndrome (Fig. 15.17).

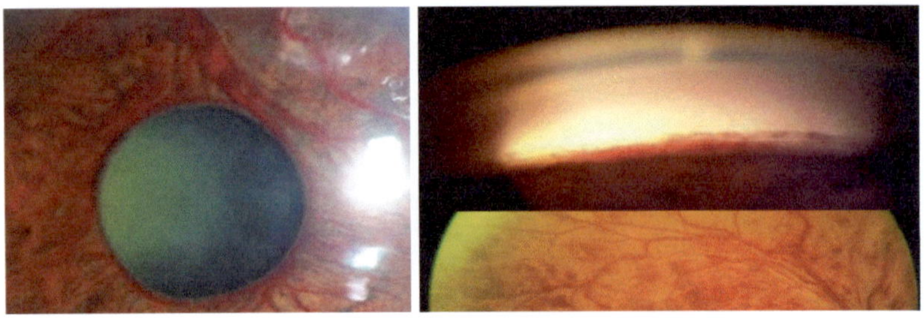

Fig. 15.17 Rubeosis iridis or neovascularization of the iris (image on the left) with blood in the angle (image on the top right) and central retinal vein occlusion (image on the bottom right)

Investigations [48]: Once the diagnosis of NVG is made, the cause needs to be ascertained. Fundus fluorescein angiography is the current gold standard to detect areas of retinal ischemia. Ultrasound B scan may be helpful in conditions where the fundus is not visible to rule out retinal detachment, intraocular tumors. Ultrasound biomicroscopy may be particularly helpful in young patients to rule out ciliary body tumors.

Treatment [48]

The treatment of NVG consists of:

1. Treatment of retinal ischemia with pan-retinal photocoagulation and anti-VEGF (vascular endothelial growth factor)
2. Treatment of any underlying systemic condition like diabetes mellitus, hypertension, and prothrombotic disorders
3. Control of inflammation with topical steroids
4. Control of IOP with antiglaucoma medications or filtering surgery. Trabeculectomy has a high failure rate due to severe inflammation [49].Valved glaucoma drainage devices like the Ahmed valve may be preferred in cases of refractory glaucoma or other filtering surgeries are not feasible. Cyclophotocoagulation can be considered in eyes with guarded potential [50].

15.3.7.2 Glaucoma Following Retinal Surgeries

Glaucoma can occur secondary to vitreoretinal surgeries and can be due to an open-angle mechanism, closed-angle mechanism, or both. Table 15.10 summarizes the incidence, risk factors, pathophysiology, and management of glaucoma secondary to retinal surgeries.

15.3.7.3 Schwatrz Matsuo Syndrome [52]

It is a condition characterized by a rise in IOP associated with rhegmatogenous retinal detachment. The risk factors include rhegmatogenous retinal detachment, retinal tears, or retinal dialysis at the ora serrata. The main mechanism of glaucoma is hypothesized to be the aqueous outflow pathway obstruction by the photoreceptor outer segments which gain access to the aqueous through the retinal detachment. The three main clinical findings include cells in the aqueous with no other signs of uveitis, retinal detachment often involving the macula, and high IOP with marked fluctuations. The angle is usually open or may show angle recession if associated with blunt trauma. The main treatment includes medical management for control of IOP and repair of the retinal detachment. The IOP normalizes after reattachment of the retina.

15.3.8 Glaucoma Associated with Elevated Episcleral Venous Pressure

Elevated IOP secondary to an elevated episcleral venous pressure (EVP) can be acute or chronic. It can be idiopathic or secondary to a pathology. The important disease entities that can lead to this condition are enlisted in Table 15.11.

15.3.8.1 Pathophysiology

The IOP is a balance between the aqueous production and the outflow facility. According to the Goldmann equation IOP = (Rate of aqueous humor production/Facility of aqueous out-

Table 15.10 The incidence, risk factors, pathophysiology, and management of glaucoma secondary to retinal surgeries

Type of retinal intervention	Incidence	Risk factors	Pathophysiology	Management
Glaucoma following PPV	20–60%	Combined surgeries: SB and PPV, PPL and PPV, EL with PPV PPV for PVR	OAG: 80%—Inflammation, corticosteroid response Blood-mediated mechanisms ACG-20%—Silicone oil, fibrin, IOL, Intravitreal gas, ciliary body edema	Most cases have a transient rise in IOP and can be managed medically. Surgical procedures to treat the IOP are chosen based on the mechanism of glaucoma: AC paracentesis, release of oil overfill
Glaucoma following SB	1.4–4.4%—mainly due to angle closure	Preexisting narrow angles, use of an encircling band, high myopia, and older patient age	Impaired venous return to vortex veins or anterior segment ischemia due to SB placement leads to ciliary body swelling, resulting in angle closure	Treatment is with cycloplegics, aqueous suppressants, and topical steroids. Refractory cases respond well to valved implants
Glaucoma following PRP	Transient rise of IOP within 2 hours—Seen in 32–94%	Has not been studied. The higher the amount of laser energy, the greater is the chance of an increase in IOP	Angle closure glaucoma can be seen due to the ciliary body swelling or movement of fluid from choroid into the vitreous Open-angle mechanism is seen due to the impaired uveoscleral outflow following ciliary body congestion; decreased ciliary muscle tone due to short ciliary nerve damage and/or prostaglandin release	Transient IOP rise managed with aqueous suppressants. Pretreatment with an alpha agonist helps to reduce the IOP spike
Glaucoma following intravitreal anti-VEGF	3.45–6%	Injection with bevacizumab, preexisting glaucoma, higher frequency of injections	Immediate increase in IOP due to the volume overload of injection Outflow obstruction by anti-VEGF or its byproducts Repeated injection causes inflammation and chronic trabeculitis, leading to an increase in IOP	Immediate IOP spike usually lasts for three days. Sustained IOP rise can be managed medically or surgically
Glaucoma following IVTA	40% show an IOP > 24 mm hg at 6 months	Preexisting glaucoma or family history of glaucoma, age less than 6 years or older than 60 years, connective tissue disease, type 1 DM, high myopia	Increased accumulation of GAGs; Increased production of TIGR protein; corticosteroid induced cytoskeletal changes; accumulation of ECM in the TM; high levels of TIMP in diabetics	Medical management alone is adequate in the majority of cases. Trabeculectomy alone or combined with vitrectomy for removal of the drug deposit may be needed in some cases

(continued)

Table 15.10 (continued)

Type of retinal intervention	Incidence	Risk factors	Pathophysiology	Management
Glaucoma following the use of silicone oil	2.2–56%	Preexisting glaucoma, diabetes mellitus, aphakia, increased amount of silicone oil in the AC, use of heavy tamponade, emulsified oil, increased duration of oil in the eye	Closure of PI by fibrin, blood or capsule; Pupillary block migration of oil into the angles; Macrophage oil induced endocytosis leading to inflammation and trabeculitis; Synechial angle closure; Overfill of the vitreous cavity with silicone oil; NVI	Along with medical management for IOP, the cause of increase in IOP needs to be treated accordingly. Glaucoma surgery with implants may be considered in refractory glaucomas post-oil removal and in eyes with synechial closure. In a study by Al-Jazzaf et al., the success rate of AGV was 80% at one year after implantation [51]
Glaucoma following intravitreal gas	SF6: 6.1–67% C3F8: 18–59%	Higher concentration of gas, use of C3F8, older age, concurrent PRP, scleral buckle or lensectomy; fibrinous exudate in AC	OAG: When the expansion of the gas exceeds the rate of aqueous outflow, or when the posterior chamber pressure builds up ACG: Expansion of the gas causes an anterior shift in the lens, iris diaphragm, and pupillary block	Elevation in IOP for the first 24 to 72 hours is managed with aqueous suppressants. A severe and persistent rise in IOP may need a partial aspiration of the gas and/or glaucoma surgery with drainage implants

Table adapted from: https://eyewiki.aao.org/Elevated_Intraocular_Pressure_Associated_with_Retinal_Procedures
PPV Pars plana vitrectomy, *SB* Scleral Buckle, *PPL* Pars plana lensectomy, *PVR* Proliferative vitreoretinopathy, *EL* Endolaser, *OAG* Open-angle glaucoma, *ACG* Angle closure glaucoma, *IOP* Intraocular pressure, *AC* Anterior chamber, *VEGF* Vascular endothelial growth factor, *IVTA* Intravitreal triamcinolone, *GAG* Glycosaminoglycans, *TIGR* Trabecular meshwork Inducible Glucocorticoid Response, *ECM* Extracellular matrix, *TM* Trabecular meshwork, *TIMP* Tissue Inhibitor of Matrix Metalloproteinase, *PI* Peripheral iridotomy, *NVI* Neovascularization of iris, *AGV* Ahmed Glaucoma Valve, *SF6* Sulfur hexafluoride, *C3F8* perfluoropropane

Table 15.11 The different disease entities causing glaucoma secondary to raised episcleral venous pressure

Obstruction to the venous return	Arterio-venous anomalies
Retrobulbar tumors	Carotid-cavernous fistula
Thyroid ophthalmopathy	Sturge–weber syndrome
Thrombosis—Cavernous sinus, orbital veins	Orbital varix
Congestive heart failure	Shunts: Orbito-meningeal, carotid-jugular
Orbital amyloidosis	
Episcleral or orbital vein vasculitis	
Mediastinal tumors	

Adapted from: https://eyewiki.org/Elevated_Episcleral_Venous_Pressure_(EVP)

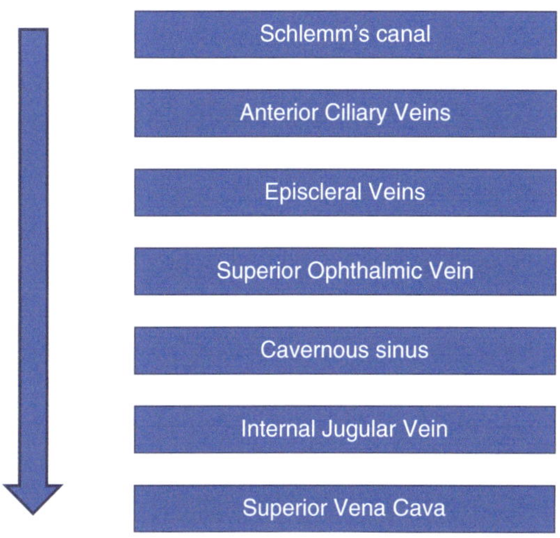

Fig. 15.18 Flowchart showing the drainage of aqueous humor from the Schlemm's canal to the Superior vena cava. (Adapted from https://eyewiki.org/Elevated_Episcleral_Venous_Pressure_(EVP))

flow) + EVP. The normal EVP ranges between 8 and 10 mm Hg [3].

The drainage pathway of the aqueous is as shown in Fig. 15.18:

Any obstruction along this pathway can lead to an increase in EVP and elevated IOP.

15.3.8.2 Clinical Features [3]

A thorough history, including recent history of trauma to the head and history of any systemic illness, needs to be elicited. Patients often present with a chronic red eye. Apart from an elevated IOP, clinical examination shows corkscrew episcleral vessels without inflammation and occasionally chemosis. They may have proptosis, orbital bruit, and in cases of a carotid-cavernous fistula, a pulsatile exophthalmos may be noted. Gonioscopy shows open angles with blood reflux in the Schlemm's canal.

Management: Elevated EVP can be diagnosed by clinical examination. However, the cause of elevated EVP needs to be investigated. Orbital Doppler ultrasound can confirm a dilated superior ophthalmic vein. Cerebral angiography with CT or MRI scan may be considered when an AV fistula is suspected. Treatment of the underlying etiology is the main aim of management. Elevated IOP is best managed by treatment modalities which bypass the conventional outflow pathway. This includes aqueous suppressants medically and trabeculectomy or drainage implants when surgery is warranted.

15.3.9 Malignant Glaucoma (Aqueous Misdirection) [53]

Malignant glaucoma is a type of secondary glaucoma characterized by elevated IOP and shallow anterior chamber, both centrally and peripherally, in the presence of a patent PI.

It is more commonly seen in women and is known to occur more commonly in eyes with angle closure glaucoma after ocular interventions which include cataract surgery, glaucoma surgery, YAG laser capsulotomy, and iridotomy.

15.3.9.1 Mechanism [53, 54]

It is hypothesized that the aqueous humor is misdirected into the vitreous cavity. This is attributed to the anterior rotation of the ciliary body abutting the lens equator, as a consequence of the pressure differential between the anterior and posterior chambers. There are many hypotheses regarding the pathophysiology of malignant glaucoma.

15.3.9.2 Clinical Examination

Slit lamp examination reveals an AC which is shallow peripherally as well as central with a patent PI. The ciliary process is sometimes visible through the PI. Fundus needs to be examined to

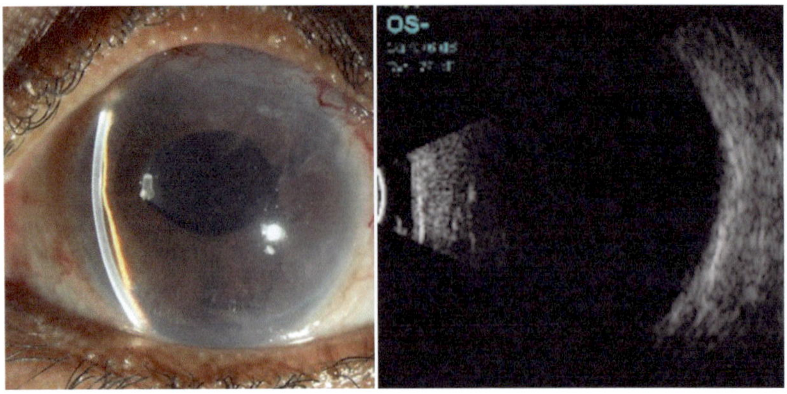

Fig. 15.19 Pseudophakic malignant glaucoma: Shallow anterior chamber depth peripherally and centrally in a pseudophakic eye (image on the left) with a normal B scan (image on the right)

rule out any posterior segment pathology like choroidal hemorrhage or detachment (Fig. 15.19).

15.3.9.3 Investigations

B-scan ultrasonography [53]: In cases where the cornea is not clear, B scan helps to exclude choroidal detachments and suprachoroidal hemorrhage. Ultrasound biomicroscopy (UBM) supplements the physical exam by imaging the anterior chamber angle, iris, and lens configuration.

15.3.9.4 Management [54]

The first line of management consists of controlling the IOP: Osmotic agents like mannitol have a dual role. It dehydrates the vitreous and relieves the primary pathology as well as reduces the IOP. Aqueous suppressants are the drug of choice to control IOP.

Inflammation is controlled by topical steroids. Cycloplegics help in moving the iris–lens diaphragm posteriorly by inhibiting the contraction of the ciliary muscles. Mydriatics help in inhibiting the iris–lens apposition.

In eyes where the above treatment does not relieve an attack of malignant glaucoma, establishing a unicameral chamber by achieving a communication between the anterior and posterior segments is needed. This is done by a YAG hyaloidotomy through a PI, at the optic haptic junction of the IOL, or surgically by irido-zonulo-hyaloido-vitrectomy. Refractory cases need a pars plana vitrectomy. The patients need to be maintained on long-term cycloplegics to prevent recurrences.

15.3.10 Glaucoma Associated with Intraocular Tumors [55, 56]

Rise in IOP is seen in about 5% of eyes with an intraocular tumor. The rise in IOP is dependent on the size of the tumor, its location, and associated signs like hemorrhage, necrosis, and inflammation. Intraocular tumors can lead to secondary elevation in IOP by a variety of mechanisms.

Mechanisms causing an elevation of IOP:

- Direct invasion of the angle, Schlemm's canal, or aqueous channels by the tumor cells
- Seeding of the trabecular meshwork by pigments or macrophages
- Melanomalytic where the pigment-laden macrophages block the aqueous outflow by clogging the angle
- Neovascularization of the iris/angle
- Anterior rotation of the ciliary body
- Anterior chamber angle epithelialization by the tumor
- Elevated episcleral pressure—seen in orbital extension of tumors
- Uveal effusion
- Uveitic—inflammation causes peripheral anterior synechiae and angle closure
- Anterior displacement of the lens-iris diaphragm by the tumor, leading to angle closure

The symptoms and signs depend on the type and location of the malignancy.

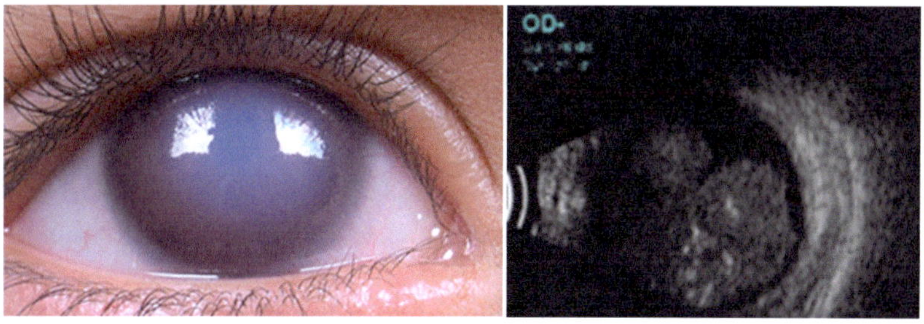

Fig. 15.20 A 2-year-old boy presented with whitish discoloration of the right cornea and an intraocular pressure of 30 mm Hg and deep anterior chamber. B scan of the eye showed hyperechoic lesions with calcifications in the vitreous suggestive of Retinoblastoma

Anterior Segment: Dilated Episcleral vessels, keratic precipitates, anterior chamber cells/pigments, hyphema, Heterochromia, Neovascularization of the iris/angle, transillumination defects of the globe, Mass lesion noted on the uveal tissue.

Posterior Chamber: Vitritis, vitreous hemorrhage, retinal detachment, mass lesions

B scan and UBM may be particularly useful in aiding diagnosis (Fig. 15.20).

The treatment mainly consists of the elimination of the tumor. IOP control is mainly managed medically, as incisional surgeries are contraindicated. Trans scleral cyclophotocoagulation offers a less invasive way of controlling IOP and may be the modality of choice in refractory cases.

Acknowledgements All the clinical pictures used in this chapter are from L V Prasad Eye Institute, Hyderabad.

Conflicts of Interest None.

References

1. Foster PJ, Buhrmann R, Quigley HA, Johnson GJ. The definition and classification of glaucoma in prevalence surveys. Br J Ophthalmol. 2002;86(2):238–42.
2. Bourne RR, Lansingh V, Ehrlich J, et al. Burden of global vision loss due to glaucoma: temporal and regional changes 2000–2020. Invest Ophthalmol Vis Sci. 2021;62(8):1585.
3. Allingham RR. Shields textbook of glaucoma. 6th ed. Wolters Kluwer (India) Pvt Ltd; 2011.
4. Toris CB, Yablonski ME, Wang YL, Camras CB. Aqueous humor dynamics in the aging human eye. Am J Ophthalmol. 1999;127(4):407–12.
5. Tamm ER. The trabecular meshwork outflow pathways: structural and functional aspects. Exp Eye Res. 2009;88(4):648–55.
6. Rohen JW, Rentsch FJ. Morphology of Schlemm's canal and related vessels in the human eye. Albrecht Von Graefes Arch Klin Exp Ophthalmol. 1968;176(4):309–29.
7. Hoffmann F, Dumitrescu L. Schlemm's canal under the scanning electron microscope. Ophthalmic Res. 1971;2(1):37–45.
8. Sampaolesi JZ R, Sampaolesi JR. The Glaucomas-volume 1-pediatric glaucomas, vol. 1. Verlag Berlin Heidelberg: Springer; 2009.
9. Weinreb RN, Khaw PT. Primary open-angle glaucoma. Lancet. 2004;363(9422):1711–20.
10. McMonnies CW. Glaucoma history and risk factors. J Opt. 2017;10(2):71–8.
11. Gordon MO, Beiser JA, Brandt JD, et al. The ocular hypertension treatment study: baseline factors that predict the onset of primary open-angle glaucoma. Arch Ophthalmol. 2002;120(6):714–20. discussion 829–30
12. Tham YC, Li X, Wong TY, et al. Global prevalence of glaucoma and projections of glaucoma burden through 2040: a systematic review and meta-analysis. Ophthalmology. 2014;121(11):2081–90.
13. Sun X, Dai Y, Chen Y, et al. Primary angle closure glaucoma: what we know and what we don't know. Prog Retin Eye Res. 2017;57:26–45.
14. Ozaki M, Nongpiur ME, Aung T, et al. Increased lens vault as a risk factor for angle closure: confirmation in a Japanese population. Graefes Arch Clin Exp Ophthalmol. 2012;250(12):1863–8.
15. Thau A, Lloyd M, Freedman S, et al. New classification system for pediatric glaucoma: implications for clinical care and a research registry. Curr Opin Ophthalmol. 2018;29(5):385–94.
16. Koc F, Kargi S, Biglan AW, et al. The aetiology in paediatric aphakic glaucoma. Eye (Lond). 2006;20(12):1360–5.

17. Mills MD, Robb RM. Glaucoma following childhood cataract surgery. J Pediatr Ophthalmol Strabismus 1994;31(6):355–60; discussion 61.
18. Mandal AK, Netland PA. Glaucoma in aphakia and pseudophakia after congenital cataract surgery. Indian J Ophthalmol. 2004;52(3):185–98.
19. Mandal AK, Chakrabarti D. Update on congenital glaucoma. Indian J Ophthalmol. 2011;59(Suppl1):S148–57.
20. François J. Congenital glaucoma and its inheritance. Ophthalmologica. 1980;181(2):61–73.
21. Dandona L, Williams JD, Williams BC, Rao GN. Population-based assessment of childhood blindness in southern India. Arch Ophthalmol. 1998;116(4):545–6.
22. Genĉík A. Epidemiology and genetics of primary congenital glaucoma in Slovakia. Description of a form of primary congenital glaucoma in gypsies with autosomal-recessive inheritance and complete penetrance. Dev Ophthalmol. 1989;16:76–115.
23. Khan AO. Genetics of primary glaucoma. Curr Opin Ophthalmol. 2011;22(5):347–55.
24. Vincent AL, Billingsley G, Buys Y, et al. Digenic inheritance of early-onset glaucoma: CYP1B1, a potential modifier gene. Am J Hum Genet. 2002;70(2):448–60.
25. Mandal AKNP. The pediatric Glaucomas. Philadelphia: Elsevier Butterworth Heinemann; 2006.
26. deLuise VP, Anderson DR. Primary infantile glaucoma (congenital glaucoma). Surv Ophthalmol. 1983;28(1):1–19.
27. Mandal AK. Acute corneal hydrops in children with primary infantile glaucoma: a report of 31 cases over 23 years at the LVPEI. PLoS One. 2016;11(6):e0156108.
28. WARING GO, GO W Clinical and pathologic alterations of Descemet's membrane: with emphasis on endothelial metaplasia. 1974.
29. Yu Chan JY, Choy BN, Ng AL, Shum JW. Review on the management of primary congenital glaucoma. J Curr Glaucoma Pract. 2015;9(3):92–9.
30. Quigley HA. The pathogenesis of reversible cupping in congenital glaucoma. Am J Ophthalmol. 1977;84(3):358–70.
31. Roberti G, Oddone F, Agnifili L, et al. Steroid-induced glaucoma: epidemiology, pathophysiology, and clinical management. Surv Ophthalmol. 2020;65(4):458–72.
32. Tarkkanen A, Kivelä T, John G. Lindberg and the discovery of exfoliation syndrome. Acta Ophthalmol Scand. 2002;80(2):151–4.
33. Ritch R. Exfoliation syndrome-the most common identifiable cause of open-angle glaucoma. J Glaucoma. 1994;3(2):176–7.
34. Bedri A, Alemu B. Pseudoexfoliation syndrome in Ethiopian glaucoma patients. East Afr Med J. 1999;76(5):278–80.
35. Krishnadas R, Nirmalan PK, Ramakrishnan R, et al. Pseudoexfoliation in a rural population of southern India: the Aravind comprehensive eye survey. Am J Ophthalmol. 2003;135(6):830–7.
36. Ritch R. Ocular and systemic manifestations of exfoliation syndrome. J Glaucoma. 2014;23(8 Suppl 1):S1–8.
37. Schlötzer-Schrehardt U, Naumann GO. Ocular and systemic pseudoexfoliation syndrome. Am J Ophthalmol. 2006;141(5):921–37.
38. Küchle M, Viestenz A, Martus P, et al. Anterior chamber depth and complications during cataract surgery in eyes with pseudoexfoliation syndrome. Am J Ophthalmol. 2000;129(3):281–5.
39. Konstas AG, Koliakos GG, Karabatsas CH, et al. Latanoprost therapy reduces the levels of TGF beta 1 and gelatinases in the aqueous humour of patients with exfoliative glaucoma. Exp Eye Res. 2006;82(2):319–22.
40. Scuderi G, Contestabile MT, Scuderi L, et al. Pigment dispersion syndrome and pigmentary glaucoma: a review and update. Int Ophthalmol. 2019;39(7):1651–62.
41. Al-Mahmood AM, Al-Swailem SA, Edward DP. Glaucoma and corneal transplant procedures. J Ophthalmol. 2012;2012:576394.
42. Banitt MR, Chopra V. Descemet's stripping with automated endothelial keratoplasty and glaucoma. Curr Opin Ophthalmol. 2010;21(2):144–9.
43. Alvarenga LS, Mannis MJ, Brandt JD, et al. The long-term results of keratoplasty in eyes with a glaucoma drainage device. Am J Ophthalmol. 2004;138(2):200–5.
44. Rapuano CJ, Schmidt CM, Cohen EJ, et al. Results of alloplastic tube shunt procedures before, during, or after penetrating keratoplasty. Cornea. 1995;14(1):26–32.
45. Shah SS, Meyer JJ. Lens Induced Glaucoma. StatPearls. Treasure Island: StatPearls Publishing. Copyright © 2022, StatPearls Publishing LLC; 2022.
46. Papaconstantinou D, Georgalas I, Kourtis N, et al. Lens-induced glaucoma in the elderly. Clin Interv Aging. 2009;4:331–6.
47. Hayreh SS. Neovascular glaucoma. Prog Retin Eye Res. 2007;26(5):470–85.
48. Senthil S, Dada T, Das T, et al. Neovascular glaucoma—a review. Indian J Ophthalmol. 2021;69(3):525–34.
49. Takihara Y, Inatani M, Fukushima M, et al. Trabeculectomy with mitomycin C for neovascular glaucoma: prognostic factors for surgical failure. Am J Ophthalmol. 2009;147(5):912–8.
50. Bloom PA, Tsai JC, Sharma K, et al. "Cyclodiode". Trans-scleral diode laser cyclophotocoagulation in the treatment of advanced refractory glaucoma.

Ophthalmology. 1997;104(9):1508–19. discussion 19–20

51. Al-Jazzaf AM, Netland PA, Charles S. Incidence and management of elevated intraocular pressure after silicone oil injection. J Glaucoma. 2005;14(1):40–6.
52. Matsuo T. Photoreceptor outer segments in aqueous humor: key to understanding a new syndrome. Surv Ophthalmol. 1994;39(3):211–33.
53. Chandler PA, Simmons RJ, Grant WM. Malignant glaucoma. Medical and surgical treatment. Am J Ophthalmol. 1968;66(3):495–502.
54. Ruben S, Tsai J, Hitchings RA. Malignant glaucoma and its management. Br J Ophthalmol. 1997;81(2):163–7.
55. Camp DA, Yadav P, Dalvin LA, Shields CL. Glaucoma secondary to intraocular tumors: mechanisms and management. Curr Opin Ophthalmol. 2019;30(2):71–81.
56. Radcliffe NM, Finger PT. Eye cancer related glaucoma: current concepts. Surv Ophthalmol. 2009;54(1):47–73.

16 Retina and Vitreous

Alan Treviño-Herrera, Anamika Patel,
Anirudh Heroor, Avinash Pathengay,
Geeta K. Vemuganti, Shilpa Goyal,
and Somasheila Murthy

Contents

A. Treviño-Herrera · A. Patel (✉) · A. Pathengay
Department of Vitreo-retina and Uveitis, GMRV Campus, L V Prasad Eye Institute, Visakhapatnam, Andhra Pradesh, India
e-mail: avinash@lvpei.org

A. Heroor
Academy of Eye Care Education, L V Prasad Eye Institute, Hyderabad, Telangana, India

G. K. Vemuganti
School of Medical Sciences, University of Hyderabad, Gachibowli, Hyderabad, India
e-mail: gkvemuganti@gmail.com

S. Goyal
Sattvaguna Lab & Healthcare Private Limited, Ambala City, Haryana, India

S. Murthy
Specialist in Corneal Diseases, Uveitis, Cataract and Refractive Surgery
Shantilal Shanghvi Eye Institute, Mumbai, Maharashtra, India

G. K. Vemuganti et al. (eds.), *Ocular Pathology*, https://doi.org/10.1007/978-981-96-8614-8_16

16.1 Introduction

The retina is the innermost layer of the ocular coat and the only light-sensitive layer of the eye, communicating with the brain and central nervous system and thus helping us to see [1, 2]. The vitreous is the acellular material present between the crystalline lens and the retino-choroid complex, with the main function of acting as a refractive medium. The retina comprises ten layers, and each of these layers can be involved in a separate disease process. The retina can also be divided into a central or macular part, which is the most important structure for vision, and the peripheral part. The primary goal of this chapter is to acquaint the readers with the various basic conditions affecting the retina, mainly the congenital conditions, retinal degenerations, macular degenerations, infections and inflammatory conditions, retinal dystrophies, and vascular disorders.

16.2 Embryology

The development of the eye is a complex process and requires extreme coordination among different tissues [2, 3]. The retina is first recognized at day 23 of gestation just before the recognition of the optic vesicles. Optic vesicles are an evagination from the diencephalon, and their position is adjacent to the ectoderm. Neural crest mesenchymal cells interpose between the optic vesicle and the ectoderm, these cells surround the developing cup and will contribute to the formation of the corneal endothelium, the choroid, the ciliary body, and the retinal vasculature. Following this, the optic vesicle folds in on itself, resulting in two tissues: the inner becomes the neural retina, and the outer becomes the retinal pigment epithelium (RPE). The developing cup grows around the optic stalk from the dorsal sides and then fuses in the ventral side at day 33 [1, 4]. The first evidence of vitreous formation is observed in the third to fourth week of gestation when the neural ectoderm separates from the surface ectoderm. In this space, there is evidence of collagen fibrils that become continuous with Müller cells' footplates. At the 10 mm stage, mesodermal cells enter the vitreous space via the fetal fissure. These cells develop into the hyaloid artery that branches throughout the vitreous, known as the *vasa hyaloidea propia*. Fibroblasts in the adventitia of the hyaloid artery are found to synthesize collagen similar to that found in the adult vitreous. By the end of the sixth week, the secondary vitreous begins to appear, consisting primarily of type II collagen. This secondary vitreous displaces the primary vitreous anteriorly and centrally. During the ninth week of gestation, atrophy of vessels starts (*vasa hyaloidea propia* and *tunica vasculosa lentis*). At the seventh month of gestation, hyaloid artery regression begins [2, 4]. The artery completely regresses by birth, and incomplete regressions lead to persistent fetal vasculature (Fig. 16.1a).

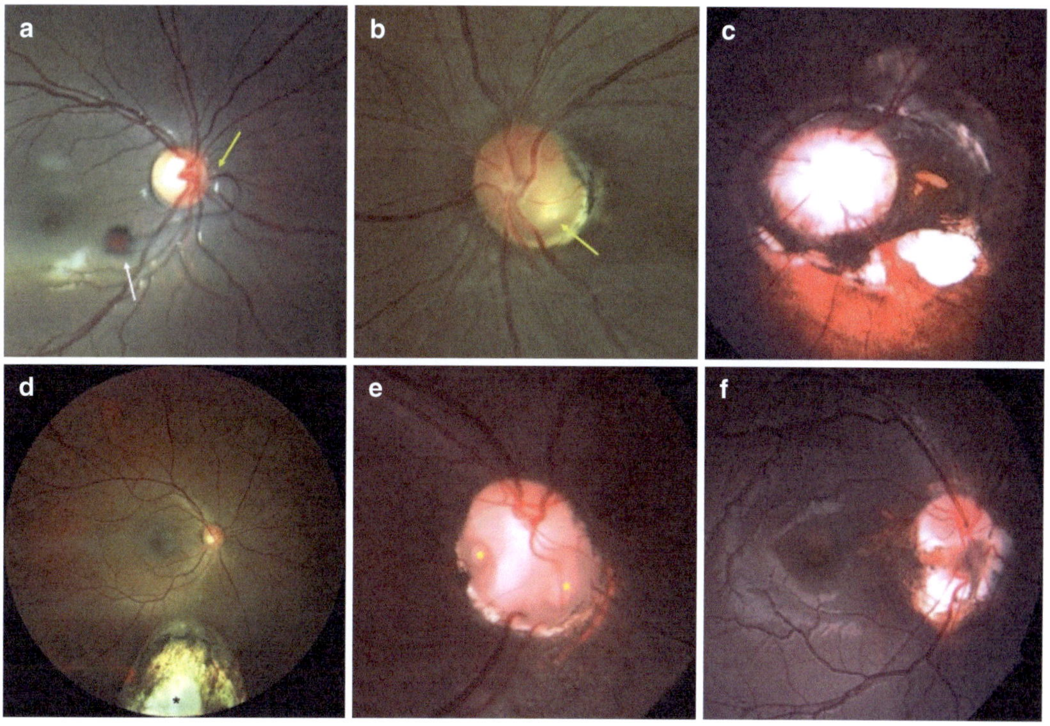

Fig. 16.1 Congenital conditions were found in the Posterior Segment. In (**a**) a persistent hyaloid artery is shown; note the tissue remnants extending from the optic disc (yellow arrow) to the posterior lens capsule (white arrow). In (**b**), a case of congenital optic disc pit is presented; note the depression at the inferotemporal disc (arrow). In (**c**) a morning glory disc anomaly is shown; observe the large and funneled optic nerve appearance, the straight emergence of the retinal vessels from the margin of the disc, and the peripapillary hyperpigmentation. (**d**) shows an inferior choroidal coloboma; observe the absence of choroid and RPE and the bare sclera (asterisk) at the floor of the coloboma. In (**e**) Pedler coloboma is seen; observe the abnormally wide scleral canal; note the optic disc pit at the temporal and nasal aspect of the optic disc (asterisk). (**f**) presents a peripapillary staphyloma; note the atrophic pigmentary changes and the normal vascularity of the disc. In (**g**) solitary congenital hypertrophy of the retinal pigment epithelium (CHRPE) is observed; note the single, flat, round, hyperpigmented retinal lesion at the posterior pole. In (**h**) an ocular albinism fundus is presented; observe the RPE hypopigmentation and the visualization of the choroidal vasculature. The corresponding macular SS-OCT scan of the CHRPE lesion is shown in (**j**); observe the retinal thinning and photoreceptor loss, and RPE absence over the lesion. In (**k**) the corresponding macular SS-OCT is shown; note the absence of foveal depression, compatible with foveal hypoplasia. In (**i**), a myelinated retinal nerve fiber layers (MRNF) case is presented; the white, well-demarcated patch with frayed borders on the anterior surface of the peripapillary neurosensory retina corresponds to the myelin sheath. (**l**) shows the optic disc SS-OCT scan; note that the myelinated retinal nerve fiber layer presents with a hyperreflective appearance

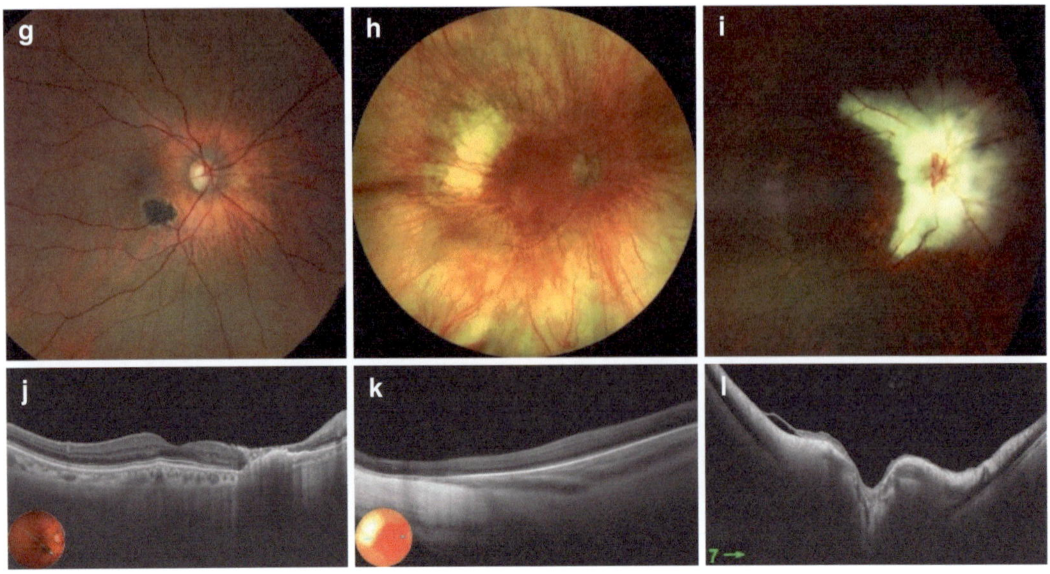

Fig. 16.1 (continued)

16.3 Congenital Conditions

16.3.1 Congenital Conditions of the Vitreous

Congenital conditions affecting the vitreous are mainly persistent primary vitreous and persistent fetal vasculature (Fig. 16.1a) or Persistent Hyperplastic Primary Vitreous [PHPV]. This is a rare congenital anomaly and occurs when the primary vitreous fails to regress [5–7]. Clinically, it is noted as the presence of a vascular membrane behind the lens. It either can be an isolated condition or can have other ocular features like cataract, glaucoma, and a retrolenticular membrane which could mimic retinoblastoma, endophthalmitis (which may occur due to lens-induced uveitis). The management involves surgical removal followed by aggressive amblyopia therapy, however, the results are often suboptimal due to complications such as glaucoma.

Histologically, the hallmark finding is the presence of a dense fibrovascular mass (tunica lentis) along with hyaloid artery arising from the optic nerve, with elongated ciliary processes which represent the primitive hyaloid vascular system [4, 7, 8]. In the case of enucleated globes which may be sent as specimens suspected of retinoblastoma, other developmental anomalies are also noted such as malformed anterior chamber, cataract, and retinal detachment. Some of the cases may also demonstrate inflammatory cells.

16.3.2 Congenital Conditions of the Retina

These can be subclassified into vascular, optic disc such as optic pit (Fig. 16.1b) and morning glory disc (Fig. 16.1c), retinal pigment epithelium abnormalities, and miscellaneous. Further details are tabulated as shown in Table 16.1.

16.3.2.1 Albinism

It presents as ocular (when exclusive eyes are involved) and oculocutaneous (when the skin is also involved). Oculocutaneous albinism is a group of disorders where there is congenital hypopigmentation of skin, hair, and eyes [9, 10]. Presents at birth and has other ocular features like nystagmus, hypopigmented fundus, foveal apla-

Table 16.1 Congenital conditions of the retina

Vascular	Optic disc	RPE abnormalities	Miscellaneous
Prepapillary vascular loops Persistent hyaloid artery Retinal macrovessels Cilioretinal artery Retinal arteriovenous malformation	Congenital optic pits (Fig. 16.1b) Optic nerve hypoplasia and aplasia Morning glory disc anomaly (Fig. 16.1c) Persistent Bergmeister's papilla Coloboma (Fig. 16.1) Inferiorly tilted disc Peripapillary staphyloma (Fig. 16.1f)	Congenital hypertrophy of the retinal pigment epithelium (Fig. 16.1g, j) Grouped hypertrophy of the retinal pigment epithelium Albinism (Fig. 16.1h, k)	Rubella retinopathy Leber's congenital amaurosis Myelinated nerve fibers (Fig. 16.1i, l)

sia, and increased transillumination of light through the iris. These patients tend to have poor visual acuity.

16.3.2.2 Grouped Pigmentation (Bear Tracks)

As the name suggests, there is a resemblance to footprints of bear paws and generally appears mildly pigmented, seen in clusters with the apex at the optic disc in approximately 60% of the patients [11]. It does not have any morbidity, and the patients typically have normal vision.

16.3.2.3 Coloboma

It is a unilateral or bilateral congenital condition that occurs secondary to defective closure of the embryonic fissure. It is one of the causes of severe visual loss in childhood and can be seen in isolation or with other congenital anomalies [4, 12, 13].

There are various manifestations of ocular coloboma, the most common is the retinochoroidal variety (Fig. 16.1d) where the colobomas are noted in the inferior aspect of the retina. Other manifestations include involvement exclusively of the optic nerve alone (Fig. 16.1e) or macular involvement along with the optic disc. These colobomas often include the lens inferonasally as well as the iris. Some of these cases can have microcornea and microphthalmos too [14]. Due to the effaced and abnormal retinal tissue in the colobomatous area, the incidence of atrophy and holes leading to retinal detachment is very high. Less clinically important colobomas include peripapillary staphyloma (Fig. 16.1f).

Histopathologically, colobomas are associated with other malformations such microphthalmos (these eyes are more likely to undergo enucleation for cosmesis and are submitted for histopathology). The retina and choroid over the colobomatous areas are invariably dysplastic and absent in the area of coloboma itself; instead, they are replaced by glial tissue [5, 15].

Morning glory disc can mimic coloboma and pointers such as optic disk lying within the excavation, central glial tuft, severe peripapillary pigmentary disturbance, and anomalous retinal vasculature help to differentiate this condition from the former [5, 16]. Other lesions include hyperpigmented ones such as congenital solitary hypertrophy of the retinal pigment epithelium (Fig. 16.1g, h) and depigmentation such as ocular albinism (Fig. 16.1h). The OCT of the CHRPE lesion is noted in Fig. 16.1j whereas of ocular albinism is noted in Fig. 16.1k. Myelinated nerve fibers are noted as white lesions (Fig. 16.1i) and the corresponding OCT shows hyperreflective appearance (Fig. 16.1l).

16.3.3 Vitreoretinopathies

The affliction of both the vitreous and retina causes vitreoretinopathies. Clinical features include early onset cataract and vitreous abnormalities such as optically empty vitreous and vitreous membranes. Examples of skeletal disorders along with vitreoretinopathies are Sticklers syndrome, Wagner syndrome, and autosomal dominant vitreoretinochoroidopathy (ADVIRC) [17].

Wyburn-Mason syndrome is a rare nonhereditary congenital developmental disorder that affects infants. They demonstrate arteriovenous malformations (AVMs) affecting the blood ves-

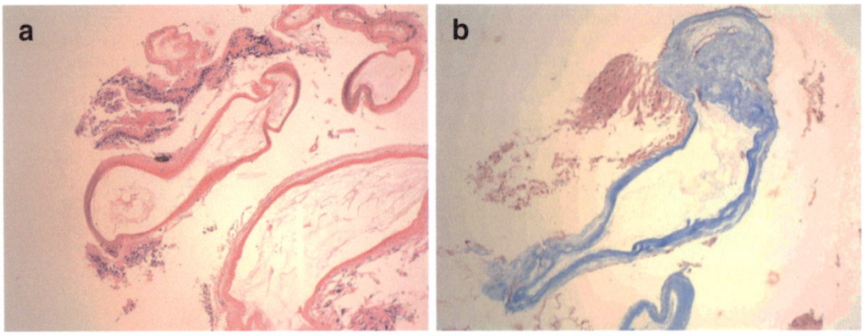

Fig. 16.2 The peeled membrane of Wyburn-Mason syndrome shows a tiny fragment of retinal layer (**a**) with large dilated vessels that are highlighted by blue stain in Masson's trichrome stain (**b**)

sels, specifically the arteries, veins, and capillaries (Fig. 16.2a, b).

16.4 Retinal Degenerations

There have been several proposed classification systems to describe retinal degenerations in previous publications, however, to date, there is no universally accepted classification system for peripheral retinal degenerations. Recently, based on the features detected by imaging with optical coherence tomography (OCT), three subcategories of degeneration have been proposed, namely, vitreoretinal, intraretinal, and chorioretinal (Table 16.2) [17, 18].

Table 16.2 Classification of peripheral retinal degenerations

Structure involved	Conditions
Vitreoretinal degenerations	Snail-track degeneration Lattice degeneration Retinal tufts Peripheral retinal breaks (Fig. 16.2a)
Intraretinal degenerations	Senile retinoschisis (Fig. 16.2b) White-without-pressure Dark-without-pressure Peripheral cystoid degeneration Snowflake degeneration Pearl degeneration
Chorioretinal degenerations	Paving-stone degeneration Hypertrophy of the retinal pigment epithelium Honeycomb degeneration Peripheral retinal drusen

16.4.1 Lattice Degeneration

In this peripheral retinal degeneration, crisscross lines are noted which represent hyalinized retinal blood vessels [18, 19]. They may or may not bear pigmentation (Fig. 16.3a). Approximately 0.5–0.7% of patients with lattice have a long-term increased chance of developing retinal detachment. Also, around 40% of patients with retinal detachment have lattice degeneration as a risk factor [19–23].

16.4.2 Paving Stone Degeneration

This peripheral retinal degeneration is characterized by yellowish, well-defined, flat cobblestone-like lesions with irregular pigmentation [18, 24–26]. Unlike lattice, this is not associated with an increased risk of any complication and is a benign condition. The commonest location is inferior, between the equator and ora serrata.

16.4.3 Snail Track Degeneration

Elongated oval or spindle-shaped white frosty glistening lesions are seen in the temporal quadrant and commonly anterior to the equator [18, 27]. These are bilateral and are seen commonly in myopes.

16.4.4 Pars Plana Cysts

These are 1- to 3-disc diameter clear cystoid spaces between pigmented and nonpigmented

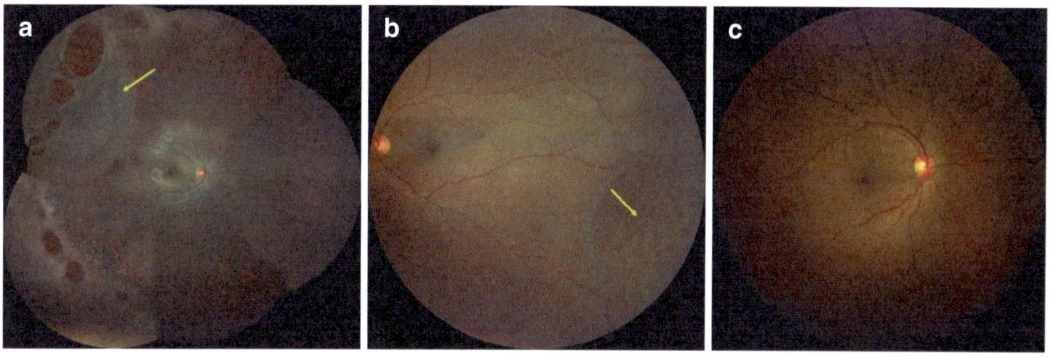

Fig. 16.3 Retinal degenerations and RPE abnormalities. (**a**) presents a case of temporal lattice degeneration with overlying multiple retinal breaks; note the presence of subretinal fluid in the superotemporal quadrant and the presence of laser scars in the inferotemporal quadrant. (**b**) shows an inferotemporal retinoschisis; note the shallow convex elevation of the inner retinal layers and the absence of corrugations. In (**c**) multiple congenital hypertrophy of the retinal pigment epithelium (CHRPE) arranged in clusters is seen in the superior retina; these lesions are called bear tracks

epithelial layers [28]. As the name suggests, they are located at the pars plana, between the ora and the ciliary processes. They can be either solitary or multiple and are generally acquired post-chronic retinal detachments, chronic uveitis and, at times, are seen in post-traumatic uveitis, advanced glaucoma, and multiple myeloma. It should be noted that cysts can be opaque as well in appearance based on their content.

Histologically, they appear as partial detachment of the inner retinal layers, with discontinuity suggestive of retinal breaks and areas of traction, with empty spaces suggestive of fluid. These changes correlate well with those observed on OCT. [29]

Other degenerations include retinoschisis or separation of the retinal layers (Fig. 16.3b) and multiple CHRPE lesions (Fig. 16.3c).

16.4.5 Macular Degeneration

16.4.5.1 Age-Related Macular Degeneration (AMD)

Age-related macular degeneration (AMD) is a complex disease with multifactorial risk factors. It is one of the leading causes of blindness in developed countries. It comprises a series of changes at the macula primarily affecting the outer retina, retinal pigment epithelium (RPE), Bruch's membrane, and choriocapillaris [30–32].

It is classified as non-neovascular (Dry) AMD and vascular (Wet) AMD.

1. Non-neovascular or Dry AMD is essentially identified with the presence of drusen. Other changes include RPE abnormalities such as hyperpigmentation and atrophy.
2. Neovascular or Wet AMD, as the name suggests, has a choroidal neovascular membrane. It is important to note that the disease nearly starts as Dry AMD and gets converted to Wet AMD in a few patients. However, the advanced stage of the disease means either the development of geographical atrophy (GA) in Dry AMD or the development of choroidal neovascular membrane in Wet AMD, or the presence of both.

Salient features of AMD are as follows:

- Age more than 50 years
- Bilateral
- Drusen
- Hyperpigmentation of the retinal pigment epithelium (RPE)
- Hypopigmentation of the RPE
- Geographic atrophy

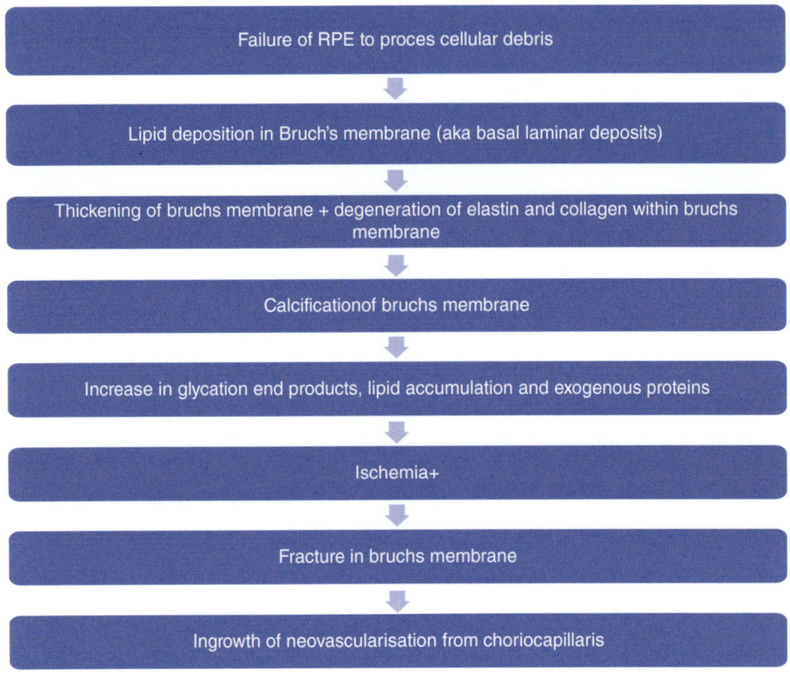

Fig. 16.4 The pathogenesis of age-related macular degeneration is summarized. Note how the alterations at the intracellular level impact the anatomy and physiology of the retina

- Retinal pigment epithelium detachment
- Macular choroidal neovascularization

The pathogenesis of the disease [31, 32] is shown in Fig. 16.4.

16.4.5.2 Drusen

This is the earliest clinical sign of AMD. Clinically, drusen appear as focal, yellow-white lesion commonly seen in the posterior pole, especially the macula [33]. These deposits are located between the RPE and Bruch's membrane. The size of these deposits varies from 20 to 100 μm in diameter and is called small, intermediate, or large based on size.

Histopathologically, hard drusen appear as globular hyaline material, stain red with pico-Mallory stain and periodic acid Schiff stain, whereas soft drusen are powdery and stain blue [34].

16.4.5.3 Geographical Atrophy (GA)

It is seen as a well-defined area of hypopigmentation or depigmentation of the retina due to RPE affliction or damage (Fig. 16.5a–c) [35]. Choroidal vessels can be noted through the hypoplastic area of the GA. The central vision of the patient eventually gets affected secondary to the loss of the outer retina when there is foveal involvement.

16.4.5.4 Wet AMD

It is characterized by the development of a choroidal neovascular membrane (Fig. 16.5d–f). Wet AMD is further classified as occult and classic choroidal neovascular membrane (CNVM) based on the fundus fluorescein angiography pattern and as Types 1, 2, and 3 based on the OCT pattern. Clinically, CNVM is suspected when the following features are noted [36, 37].

1. Presence of yellowish subretinal membrane at fovea/macula
2. Coalescence of drusen
3. Subretinal fluid/hemorrhage
4. Hard exudates
5. Disappearance of drusen

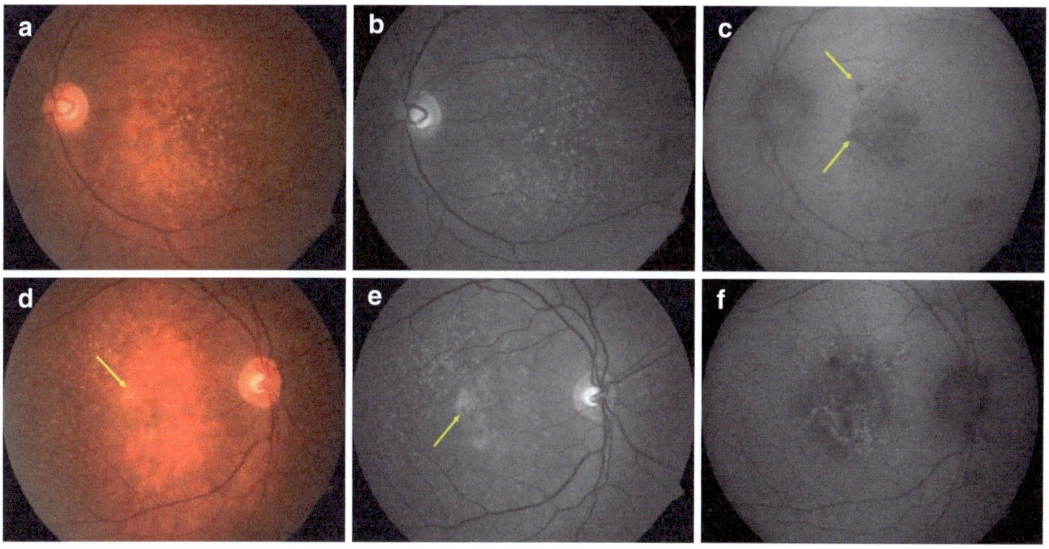

Fig. 16.5 (**a**–**c**) presents a case of dry AMD. Multiple small- and medium-sized hard drusen (**a**) are evidenced in red-free imaging (**b**). Notice the multifocal areas of hypo-autofluorescence suggestive of RPE atrophy (arrow) seen in (**c**). In (**d**–**f**) a case of wet AMD is shown. Multiple small- and medium-sized hard drusen, along with geographic atrophy and with a white to grayish subretinal membrane (arrow) suggestive of a choroidal neovascular membrane (**d**) evidenced in red-free imaging (arrow) shown in (**e**). Notice the multifocal areas of hypoautofluorescence suggestive of RPE geographic atrophy shown in (**f**)

16.5 Infections and Inflammation

Uveitis, as we understand, is an inflammation of the uveal tract where all structures of the uveal tract at once or individually may get affected. The suffix "itis" is added to the name of structures when they get involved. For example, inflammation of the vitreous is called vitritis, retina—retinitis, choroid—choroiditis, and sclera as scleritis. It is important to remember that inflammation is a response secondary to either infectious or noninfectious etiology [38–40].

With this understanding, it is easy to interpret the Standard Uveitis Nomenclature (SUN) classification, which classifies the structural involvement of the uveal tract [41].

Since this chapter deals with only the retina and vitreous, Table 16.3 primarily focuses on the inflammation affecting the uvea secondary to infectious (Fig. 16.6) and noninfectious (Fig. 16.7) etiology [40–42]. Also, it should be noted that the uveal tract is not a tight compartment, and hence one may observe adjacent structural involvement manifesting as either a spillover or multiple structure involvement. For instance, retinitis may involve choroid in retinochoroiditis, and choroiditis may involve partially the retina representing chorioretinitis.

16.5.1 Retinitis

The infectious causes of retinitis [40] are mentioned in Table 16.4.

16.5.2 Endophthalmitis

It is an intraocular inflammation where there is active colonization of microorganisms and accumulation of exudates in the vitreous cavity. The commonest form of presentation of endophthalmitis is post-cataract surgery worldwide [43]. Other exogenous causes include other intraocular surgeries and after penetrating trauma. When the infection of the eye happens

Table 16.3 Infectious conditions affecting the retina and vitreous

Structure	Term	Infectious cause	Noninfectious	Presentation/clinical features
Vitreous	Vitritis	Tuberculosis Syphilis (Fig. 16.5e) Lyme disease Toxocara Chronic endophthalmitis Toxoplasmosis	Sarcoidosis Multiple sclerosis Inflammatory bowel disease	Snowballs, vitreous exudates, pearls of string-like appearance, snowballs, snow banks, Endophthalmitis
Retina	Retinitis	Protozoal, bacterial, fungal, viral, nematode	Sarcoidosis Behcet's (Fig. 16.6c)	Retinitis, retinochoroiditis, chorioretinitis, Endogenous endophthalmitis
Choroid	Choroiditis	Tuberculosis (Fig. 16.5a) Syphilis	Sarcoidosis (Fig. 16.6a) White dots (MEWDS) (Fig. 16.6d) Vogt–Koyanagi–Harada (Panuveitis) (Fig. 16.6b)	Unifocal choroiditis, multifocal choroiditis, SLC, APMPPE, serpiginous choroidopathy, acute syphilitic posterior placoid chorioretinopathy, birdshot chorioretinopathy

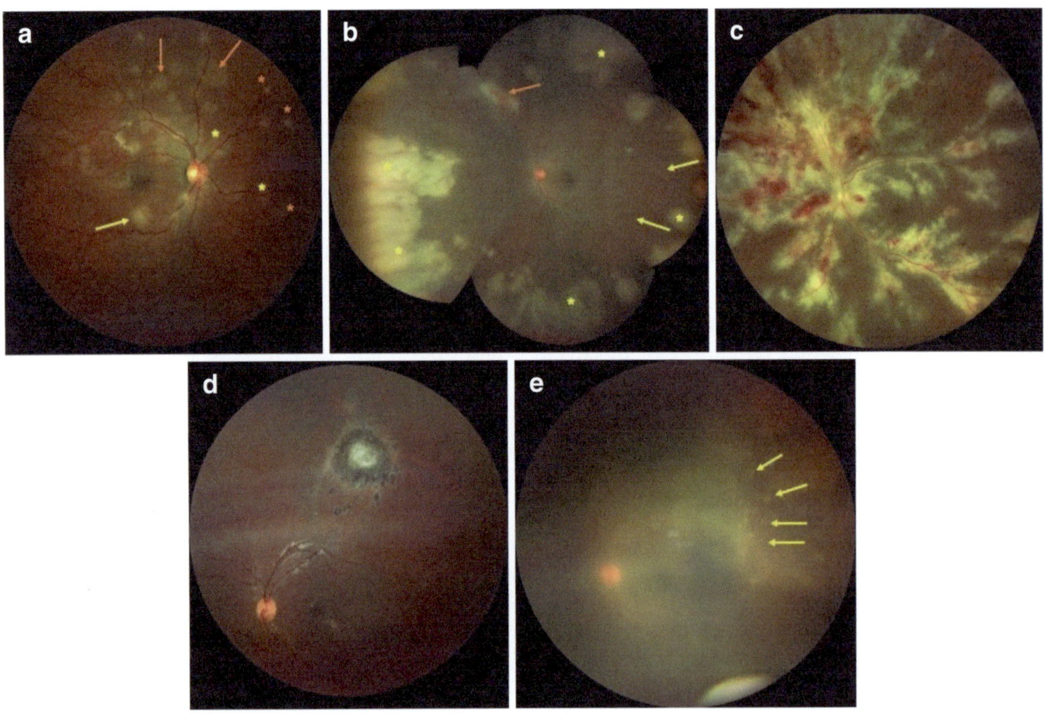

Fig. 16.6 Infections in retina and choroid. In (**a**) a case of ocular tuberculosis (OTB) is shown; note the focal choroiditis (yellow arrow), serpiginous-like choroiditis lesions (white arrows), the sub-vascular lesions (yellow asterisks), and the skip vasculitis (white asterisks). A case of acute retinal necrosis (ARN) syndrome is presented in (**b**) Note the peripheral multifocal areas of retinal whitening (yellow asterisks) and opacification with a tendency to coalesce in the nasal retinal; observe the superior hemorrhage related to vaso-occlusive vasculitis (white arrow) and vasculitis in the temporal retina (yellow arrow). A case of CMV retinitis in a patient with HIV is shown in (**c**). Note the white-yellowish areas which represent active retinitis and the superficial hemorrhages secondary to vaso-occlusive vasculitis. In (**d**) a case of ocular toxoplasmosis is shown; note the superior hyperpigmented chorioretinal scar with central fibrosis and multiple satellite hyperpigmented scars. (**e**) presents a case of ocular syphilis. Note the vitritis, which partially obscures retinal details and the superficial retinal precipitates at the temporal retina (yellow arrow)

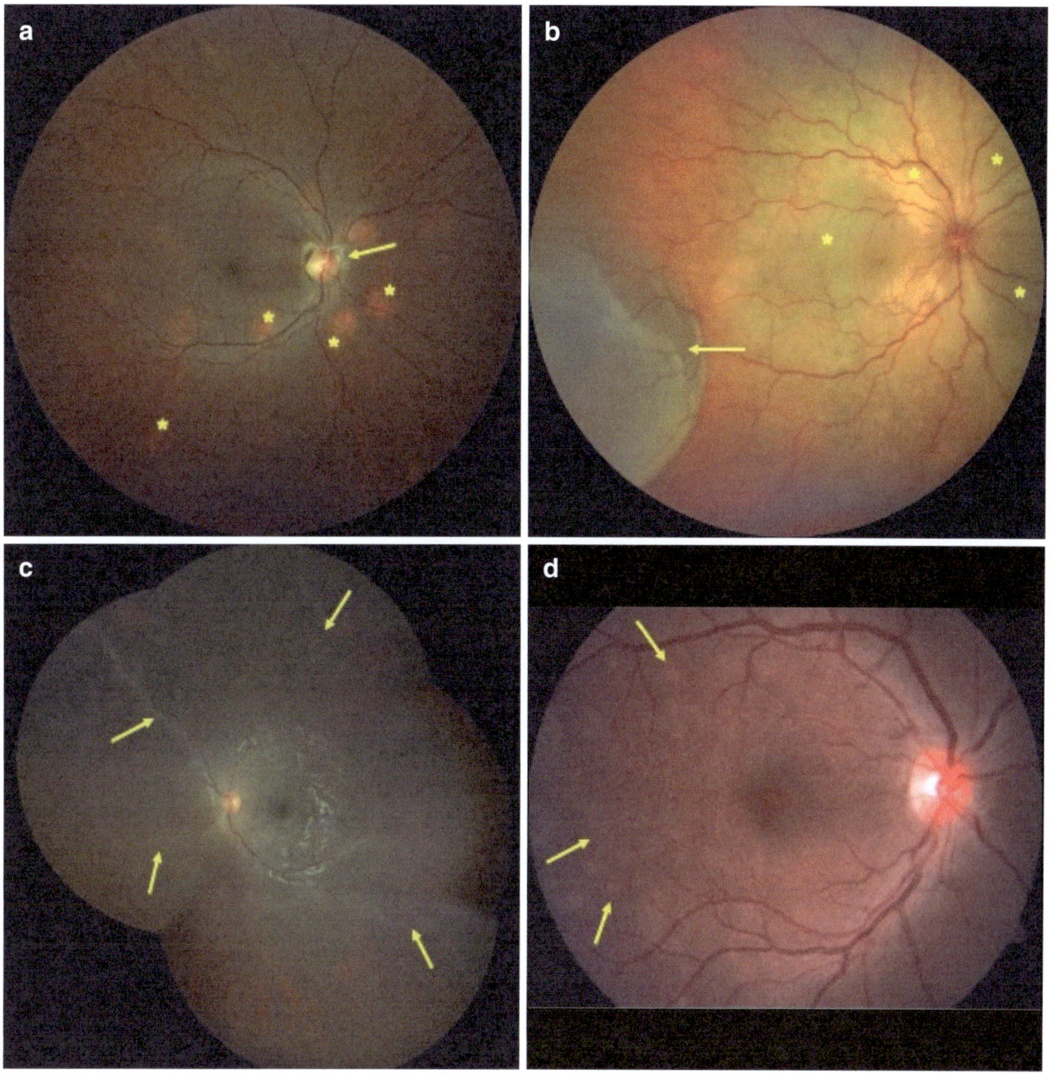

Fig. 16.7 Inflammations in retina and choroid. In (**a**) peripapillary fibrosis (yellow arrow) along with multiple large, round, orangish lesions (yellow asterisks) compatible with multifocal choroiditis in a case of ocular sarcoidosis. (**b**) presents a case of Vogt–Koyanagi–Harada disease. Note the optic disc edema, the vascular tortuosity, the multifocal neurosensory detachments at the posterior pole (yellow asterisk), and the temporal serous bullous retinal detachment (yellow arrow). In (**c**) a case of Behcet's disease is presented; note the grade 1 vitritis, the grayish hue of the retina, and the multifocal skip vasculitis (yellow arrow). (**d**) presents a case of Multiple Evanescent White Dot Syndrome (MEWDS). Note the gray-white lesions appearing to reach the outer retinal layers located temporal to the foveal (yellow arrow). Observe the orange-yellow fovea with granularity, a characteristic finding in MEWDS

Table 16.4 Infectious causes of retinitis

Viral	Cytomegalovirus (Fig. 16.5c) Herpes simplex virus Ebstein Barr virus Varicella zoster virus (Fig. 16.5b) West Nile virus Chikungunya Subacute Sclerosing Panencephalitis (Measles) Zika virus Ebola virus
Bacterial	M. Tuberculosis (Fig. 16.5a) Rickettsiosis (epidemic retinitis) Typhoid Bartonellosis Brucellosis Borreliosis Bacteria causing endogenous endophthalmitis
Spirochetal	*Treponema pallidum* (Fig. 16.5e)
Toxoplasma gondii	*Toxoplasma gondii* (Fig. 16.5d)
Fungal	*Aspergillus*, *candida*
Nematode	Diffuse unilateral subacute necrotizing neuroretinitis (*Toxocara canis*, *Baylisascaris procyonis*, *Ancylostoma caninum*, *Strongyloides* sp., *Alaria mesocercaria*, and filarial worms)

due to the spread of a remote infection elsewhere in the body; this presentation is called endogenous endophthalmitis. Endogenous endophthalmitis can present with focal retinitis along with vitreous involvement, and an upsurge of such presentations was noted in India post-COVID-19 era, where fungal etiology was found to be the most common [42, 43].

The classification of postoperative endophthalmitis is based on the time of onset and the organisms detected.

- Acute-onset endophthalmitis occurs within 6 weeks of intraocular surgery, most frequent pathogens detected are *Staphylococcus* species, *Streptococcus* species, and gram-negative organisms.
- Chronic (delayed-onset) endophthalmitis happens 6 weeks after surgery, and the most frequent pathogens isolated include *Propionibacterium acnes*, coagulase-negative *Staphylococcus* species, and fungi.

The management of postoperative endophthalmitis includes obtaining intraocular cultures and administering intravitreal antibiotics [43, 44]. The vitreous samples are preferred as a biopsy specimen for microbiological cultures as well as histopathology, as the microorganisms can be isolated more frequently from the vitreous, which is the location of the infection, compared to aqueous samples. A vitreous sample can be obtained by either a needle tap (25-gauge on a 3-ml syringe) or by using a vitrectomy instrument (core vitrectomy). Initial therapy includes rapid administration of broad-spectrum antibiotics as intravitreal injections, and later the antibiotic therapy is modified according to the microorganism isolated and cultured. After the infection has been controlled, the introduction of anti-inflammatory drugs such as corticosteroids is necessary to control the severe inflammation which is detrimental to the retina. In acute-onset endophthalmitis, the indication for vitrectomy surgery is guided by the Endophthalmitis Vitrectomy Study (EVS) which concluded that vitrectomy is indicated in patients with acute-onset postoperative endophthalmitis who have very poor (light perception) vision [45]. Patients with hand motions visual acuity or better had equivalent outcomes with or without early surgical intervention. In chronic endophthalmitis, the antibiotic injection usually does not eliminate the infection, and the preferred approach is the surgical route which comprises of pars plana vitrectomy, subtotal or total capsulectomy, and removal of the intraocular lens [44, 46].

Serious complications of endophthalmitis include the development of retinal detachment, choroidal detachment, hypotony, and phthisis bulbi.

Histopathology: pathological specimens that reach the pathology laboratory include vitreous biopsy which may have been sent for microbiological as well as pathological evaluation [44]. The specimen usually consists of fluid. The sample is centrifuged at 3000–4000 g at room temperature for a duration of six to eight minutes, and then using serum, the precipitates are clumped, formalin-fixated (4%), dehydrated, and

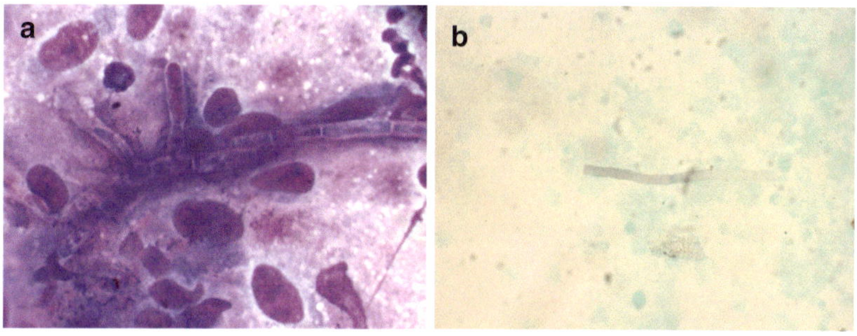

Fig. 16.8 Vitreous smears in a case of fungal endophthalmitis show beaded fungal filaments in PAS (**a**) GMS stain (**b**)

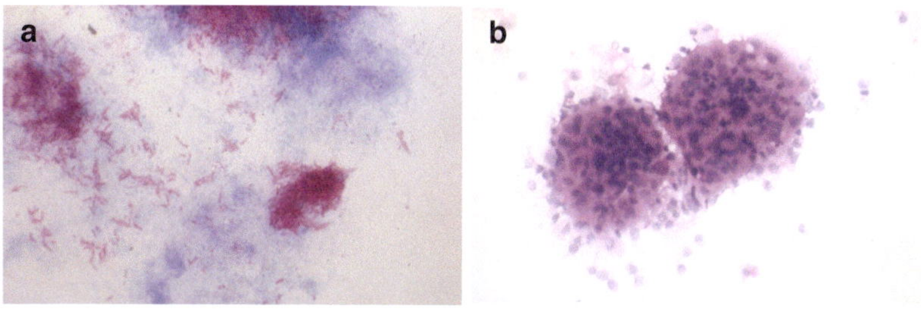

Fig. 16.9 Vitreous smears in a case of mycobacterial endophthalmitis show colonies of bacilli stained pink with 5% acid-fast stain. B also shows granulomatous inflammation

paraffin-embedded to prepare cell blocks. In some cases of infection such as fungal endophthalmitis, fungal filaments can be isolated from the vitreous specimen with the help of special stains such as PAS and GMS (Fig. 16.8) [47]. Chronic endophthalmitis can also be due to mycobacterial etiology, which clinically often resembles noninfectious uveitis and is treated with oral and topical corticosteroids (Fig. 16.9). The nature of the inflammatory cells, whether predominantly neutrophilic or lymphoplasmocytic may also indicate an infection. Rarely, granulomatous inflammation can be noted which can indicate viral infection (Fig. 16.10) [48]. Unusual causes of chronic endophthalmitis include parasites such as microfilaria (Fig. 16.11).

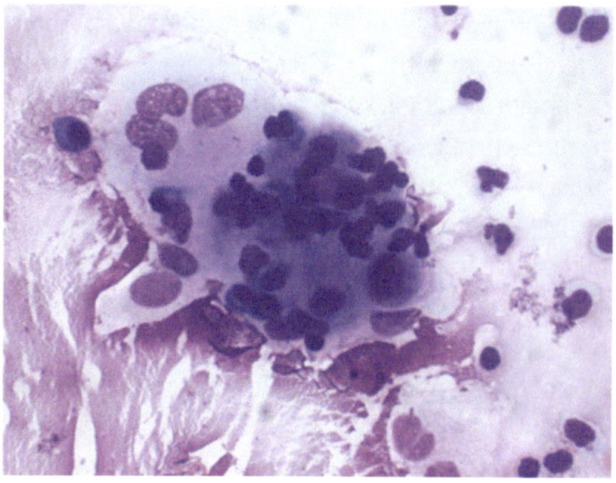

Fig. 16.10 Multinucleated giant cells noted in vitreous fluid specimen, indicative of possible viral etiology

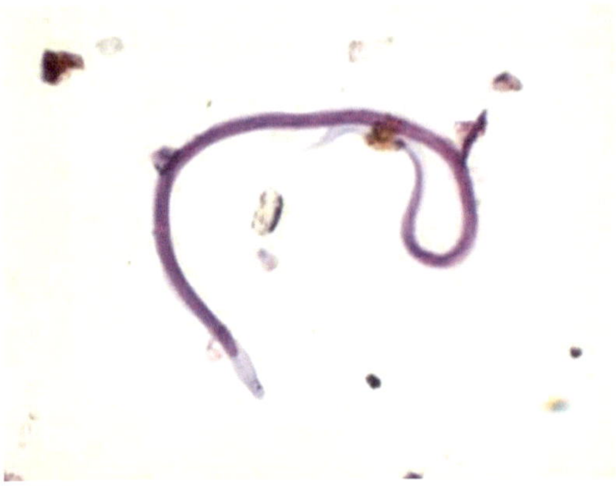

Fig. 16.11 Microfilaria worm is noted in the vitreous specimen in a case of chronic endophthalmitis

16.6 Retinal Dystrophies

These are a heterogeneous group of hereditary degenerative retinal disorders affecting primarily the photoreceptors of the retina resulting in progressive visual impairment. There are two distinct forms of photoreceptors: rods and cones, which differ from each other in both structural and functional capacity [49, 50]. Rods determine the ability to see in the dark (scotopic vision), and cones determine the ability to see in daylight (photopic vision). Hence, patients of retinal dystrophies experience poor night vision or night blindness (nyctalopia), photophobia, reduced central vision, and clinically detectable lesions involving the macula depending upon the type of photoreceptor involvement. They tend to be bilateral and symmetric at presentation and could be stationary or progressive.

The OMIM (Online Mendelian Inheritance in Man) and RetNet (The Retinal Information network online) host more than 750 and 300 genetic disorders with retinal involvement and different retinal degeneration, respectively [51, 52].

For ease of understanding for the readers, we have tabulated the common retinal dystrophies in Table 16.5 to categorize them based on their location.

Table 16.5 Classification of retinal dystrophies

1	Diffuse photoreceptor dystrophies	Rod–cone dystrophies (retinitis pigmentosa) Cone and cone–rod dystrophies Leber congenital amaurosis Enhanced S-cone disease
2	Choroidal dystrophies	Choroideremia Gyrate atrophy Bietti crystalline dystrophy
3	Macular dystrophies	Stargardt disease Best disease or best vitelliform dystrophy Adult-onset vitelliform lesions Early-onset "Drusenoid" macular dystrophies Pattern dystrophies Atypical and "occult" macular dystrophies
4	Inner retinal dystrophies	X-linked retinoschisis

16.7 Vascular Diseases (Fig. 16.12)

Anatomically, the central retinal artery loses its internal elastic lamina and muscular coat when it enters the neural retina. Central retinal vein also is turned into a venule when it loses its thick wall near the first intraneural retinal bifurcation. Therefore, the retinal circulation is predominantly arteriolar and not arterial.

Retinal circulation is divided into two halves: the inner half receives its blood supply from retinal circulation, and the outer half from the choriocapillaris [53].

Retinal ischemia can be secondary to both retinal and choroidal vascular insufficiency due to various causes such as arteriosclerosis, atherosclerosis, dysproteinemias, collagen diseases, malignant hypertension, choroidal nevus, malignant melanoma, choroidal hemangioma, and metastatic carcinoma [54, 55].

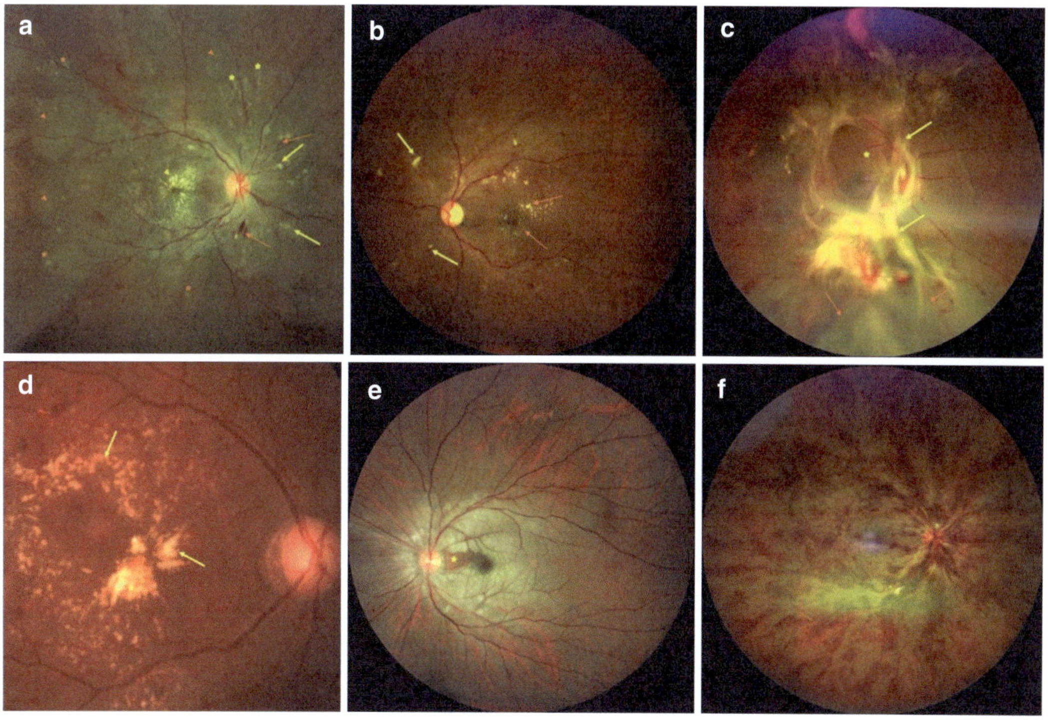

Fig. 16.12 Vascular diseases and retinal circulation. (**a**) shows a case of malignant hypertension is present; note the peripapillary cotton wool spots (CWS) (yellow arrow) and splinter hemorrhages (white arrow), and the hard exudates at the macula forming a macular star (yellow arrowhead). In the mid-periphery multiple neurosensory detachments (white arrowhead) are evident; observe multiple Siegrist streaks (yellow asterisk) and Elschnig spots (white asterisk) indicating hypertensive choroidopathy. (**b**) shows a case of severe nonproliferative diabetic retinopathy with diabetic macular edema (DME), note the CWS (yellow arrow), dot and blot hemorrhages, hard exudates (white arrow), and the DME. (**c**) shows a case of proliferative diabetic retinopathy, observe the fibrovascular proliferation extending from the optic disc to the superior and inferior retina (yellow arrow) with broad adhesion causing inferior focal tractional retinal detachment (white arrow). Note the macular epiretinal membrane with traction (yellow asterisk). (**d**) shows a case of diabetic macular edema, observe the circinate pattern of hard exudates (yellow arrow) at the macula with a plaque of hard exudates (yellow asterisk). Note the multiple microaneurysms and dot blot hemorrhages temporal to the macula. (**e**) shows a case of acute central retinal artery occlusion with a patent cilioretinal artery and nasal foveal sparing. Note the retinal whitening indicating retinal edema and the cilioretinal artery patency (asterisk). (**f**) is a case of acute ischemic central retinal vein occlusion; note the peripapillary splinter hemorrhages and the dot and blot hemorrhages in the mid-periphery. Observe the dilatation and tortuosity of veins, and along the inferotemporal arcade, a CWS is present. In (**g**) a case of acute nonischemic central retinal vein occlusion is presented; note the splinter hemorrhages (yellow arrow) at the peripapillary area, the dot and blot hemorrhages (white arrow), and the Roth spots (yellow asterisk) at the mid-periphery. At the posterior pole, retinal whitening is observed, indicating patchy ischemic retinal whitening (PIRW) (white asterisk), and at the macula, a cystoid macular edema is noted. In (**h**) a case of acute inferior hemiretinal vein occlusion is presented; observe the dilatation and tortuosity of veins. Note the dot and blot hemorrhages and the subhyaloid hemorrhage (white asterisk) at the inferior macula, indicating a breakthrough hemorrhage. In (**i**) a case of acute macular branch retinal vein occlusion is presented. Note the splinter hemorrhages and CWS (yellow asterisk) along the inferior macula. Observe the inferior cystoid macular edema

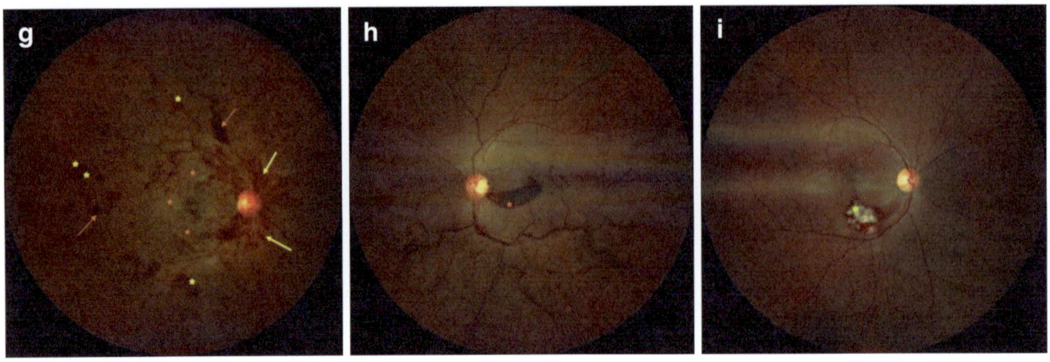

Fig. 16.12 (continued)

Table 16.6 Retinal vascular diseases and the etiology

Ocular manifestation	Causes
Retinal hemorrhage	Diabetes mellitus (DM), hypertension, (HTN), vascular occlusion, arterial embolism, blood dyscrasias, ocular ischemic syndrome, Purtscher retinopathy
Cotton wool spots	DM, HTN, HIV, SLE, septic embolism, radiation retinopathy, Purtscher retinopathy
Hard exudates	DM, HTN, coats disease, resolving CME
Microaneurysm	DM, Takayasu arteritis
Neovascularization	DM, BRVO, CRVO, Takayasu arteritis, sickling hemoglobinopathies

The commonest ocular manifestations of retinal vascular disease are tabulated in Table 16.6 along with their causes.

16.7.1 Hypertensive Retinopathy

Systemic hypertension affects the retina, optic nerve, and choroid which manifests as hypertensive retinopathy, optic neuropathy, and choroidopathy. The ocular manifestations depend upon the onset which could be acute or chronic [56].

In the acute stage which is also called malignant hypertension retina, the optic nerve and choroid can get affected. On ophthalmoscopy, retinal nerve fiber layer (RNFL) hemorrhages, cotton wool spots, hard exudates, disc edema, chorioretinal infarcts (Elschnig's spots), and lineal hyperpigmented streaks over choroidal arteries (Siegrist streaks) are noted [56, 57] (Fig. 16.12a). In a chronic setting, change in the retinal vasculature is noted in the form of arteriovenous crossing, retinal arteriolar sclerosis with associated cotton wool spots, disc edema, flame-shaped hemorrhages, etc.

16.7.2 Diabetes Mellitus

Diabetes affects many ocular tissues, including the cornea, lens, optic nerve, and retina.

It is postulated that prolonged exposure to hyperglycemia leads to biochemical and molecular pathway changes, which cause loss of pericytes and endothelial damage. Also, with the advent of various imaging techniques, the vascular abnormalities at both superficial and deep plexuses are understood better [58].

Diabetic retinopathy is classified (Table 16.7) as mild, moderate, and severe nonproliferative diabetic retinopathy (NPDR) based on the extent and severity level of the findings depicted in standard photographs of Early Treatment Diabetic Retinopathy Study (ETDRS) [59, 60]. The main features of diabetic retinopathy are intraretinal hemorrhages, microaneurysms, cotton-wool spots, intraretinal microvascular abnormalities (IRMAs), and dilation and beading of retinal veins. The severe NPDR follows the "4-2-1 rule" which means severe intraretinal hemorrhages and microaneurysms in 4 quadrants

Table 16.7 Classification and treatment of diabetic retinopathy

Classification	Features	Treatment
Mild	Few microaneurysms	Metabolic control Treatment in case of DME
Moderate	Increased number of microaneurysms and dot-blot hemorrhages. Cotton wool spots and hard exudates may be present	Metabolic control Treatment in case of DME
Severe: "4-2-1 rule"	Four quadrants of diffuse retinal hemorrhages and microaneurysms, 2 or more quadrants of venous beading, or 1 or more quadrants of IRMA	Metabolic control Treatment in case of DME PRP in selected cases[a]
Proliferative	The presence of NVI, NVD, NVE, vitreous hemorrhage, and/or fibrovascular proliferation—TRD	Metabolic control PRP Anti-VEGF selected cases Vitreoretinal surgery

DME diabetic macular edema, *IRMA* Intraretinal microvascular abnormality, *NVD* neovascularization of the disc, *NVE* neovascularization elsewhere, *NVI* neovascularization of the iris, *PRP* pan-retinal photocoagulation, *TRD* tractional retinal detachment

[a] In patients at high risk of progression and noncompliance with follow-up

or definite venous beading in 2 or more quadrants or moderate IRMA in 1 or more quadrants (Fig. 16.12b).

Progression from nonproliferative to proliferative diabetic retinopathy manifests as retinal neovascularization or neovascular proliferation either involving the disc or one disc diameter from the optic disc, or retinal neovascularization elsewhere (Fig. 16.12c).

Diabetic macular edema: It is the result of fluid extravasation from retinal vessels into the surrounding neural retina due to the hyperglycemia-induced breakdown of the blood–retinal barrier. It can be either a central subfield or a non-center.

In the management of diabetic retinopathy (DR) and diabetic macular edema (DME), metabolic control by the patient is essential for a proper and sustained response to treatment. Different treatment modalities are available in the treatment of DR including pan-retinal photocoagulation, anti-VEGF injections, and vitreoretinal surgery. The treatment is defined according to the stage of the disease, refer to Table 16.7 for further details on the treatment of DR and DME.

Epiretinal Membranes

With the advances in vitreoretinal microsurgical technique, epiretinal membranes are now made available to the pathologists and cell biologists which have significantly improved our understanding of the pathobiology. Especially with the expanding armamentarium of molecular tools like immunohistochemistry (IHC), PCR, in situ hybridization, autoradiography etc. available molecular. The epiretinal membrane arises on the inner retinal surface, while the subretinal membranes arise beneath the neurosensory retina [61, 62]. The formation of epiretinal membranes is believed to be a wound-healing process. It arises in response to ischemia of the inner retina and is a serious complication of proliferative diabetic retinopathy. The membrane consists of glial cells, prominent blood vessels, fibroblasts, and inflammatory cells with or without the retinal pigment epithelial cells. Gandorfer et al. [63] reported the ultrastructural changes of the vitreomacular interface of 55 consecutive patients of diabetic macular edema, wherein the internal limiting membrane consisted of isolated cells embedded in vitreous collagen attached to the membrane in nonproliferative diabetic retinopathy (NPDR). Fibrous astrocytes, fibroblasts and myofibroblasts, and macrophages were present in both NPDR and proliferative diabetic retinopathy (PDR). Ultrastructural analysis demonstrated both monolayer and multilayer cells (up to 6 layers) situated on the native vitreous collagen. Fibroblasts and fibrous astrocytes were predominant in PDR, with the formation of new vessels. Nicoletti et al. [64] proposed that the vascular endothelial growth factor (VEGF) is produced locally and plays a fundamental, but not specific, role in diabetic retinal neovascularization and proliferation. Ishida et al. [65] added that coexpression of VEGF-R2 and neuropilin-1 is indicative of fibrovascular proliferation in diabetic retinopathy. New insights are obtained related to cell proliferation and cell death within these membranes; this could pave the way for newer treatment modalities [66, 67]. It is not only the cells and the growth factors but also the extracellular matrix proteases are crucial in the remodeling and penetration of the capillary basement membrane by the migrating endothelial cells [68]. Das et al. [69, 70] studied the role of proteolysis of basement membrane components by a variety of proteinases. They determined the expression of proteinases in human retinal tissues with active neovascularization and demonstrated the increased activity of proteinases in the final common pathway of retinal neovascularization. Many drug combinations including corticosteroids, antiproliferative, and antineoplastic drugs like 5-fluorouracil and daunorubicin have been tried with variable efficacy in the prevention or treatment of proliferative vitreoretinal disease [71–74]. Clinical trials are already underway with other drugs like retinoic acid and idelalisib (phosphoinositide 3-kinase inhibitor) as an adjunct to membrane peeling with the objective of preventing membrane recurrences following rhegmatogenous retinal detachment [75–77]. It would be a challenge to see which molecules- the proteinases, inhibitors of growth factors, factors controlling the cell kinetics, would finally help large-scale treatment of this blinding retinal disease.

16.7.3 Retinal Vascular Occlusion

Based on the type of artery occlusion, retinal arteriolar occlusion can manifest either as central retinal artery (CRAO) (Fig. 16.12e, f), branch retinal artery (BRAO), or cilioretinal artery occlusion (CLRAO) [78]. The causative factor is the presence of either a thrombus or an embolus causing the interruption in blood supply to the retina. It is very important to assess the cardiovascular risk factors and to treat them, due to the high probability of cardiovascular death [78, 79].

CRAO Patients will present with acute and painless loss of vision, which in some cases may be preceded by amaurosis fugax [78, 80]. Vision will be just counting fingers or light perception in 90% of the cases. In 25% of the population, a permeable cilio-retinal artery (CLRA) will be present. In 10% of the cases, the CLRA will respect the fovea, and vision will improve to 20/50 in up to 80% of these patients. In the acute phase, a relative afferent pupillary defect (RPAD) will be found, and whitening of the retina will be present, which resolves in 4–6 weeks leaving a pale optic disc, attenuated retinal vessels, and thinned retinal nerve fiber layer (RNFL). In the fovea, a cherry red spot will be present [78, 81, 82].

The objectives of the ocular treatment include the increase of the perfusion pressure of the retinal circulation and the dislocation of the thrombus or embolus. This could be achieved with ocular massage (fluctuation of the IOP and intraocular vascular dilatation), antiglaucoma medication (lower IOP), and AC paracentesis (lower IOP) [83]. Clinical trials are going on for the use of intravenous fibrinolytics in treatment of acute CRAO and have shown promising results [83–85]. Visual prognosis is poor; in cases of patent CLRA, vision may be functional.

BRAO Patients will present with partial, painless, unilateral, and acute diminution of vision. The visual field defect may be central or sectorial, and in some patients may present asymptomatic and be found incidentally. The visual prognosis is good and, in most cases, vision is equal to or better than 20/40 [86].

Based on the type of vein occlusion, retinal vein occlusion can manifest either as central retinal vein (CRVO) (Fig. 16.12f, g), branch retinal vein (BRVO), or hemiretinal vein occlusion (HRVO) (Fig. 16.12h). It is very important to assess the cardiovascular risk factors and to treat them, due to persistent or recurrent retinal vein occlusions and cardiovascular risk [86, 87].

CRVO The different clinical features in the acute phase of CRVO include intraretinal hemorrhages, and the presence of dilated, tortuous retinal veins in all four quadrants. The presence of RAPD, macular edema, and disc edema also suggests an acute phase of CRVO [88–90]. CWS in CRVO form a ring around the optic disc in the distribution of the radial peripapillary capillaries (Fig. 16.12f, g). The cilioretinal arteriolar insufficiency (CRAI) may be present in up to 4% of the CRVOs. The chronic phase of CRVO is characterized by optic disc collaterals, macular edema, anterior segment neovascularization, retinal or optic disc neovascularization, and neovascular glaucoma. There are two types of CRVO, nonischemic CRVO, and ischemic CRVO. Ischemic CRVO presents with visual acuity less than 20/200, RAPD, extensive retinal hemorrhages in the posterior pole, angiography showing capillary non-perfusion in an area of >10 disc diameters, and poor visual prognosis due to macular ischemia and neovascular glaucoma [90, 91].

BRVO The occlusion of a main BRVO may present asymptomatic or with painless diminution of vision and sectorial scotoma. The occlusion of a macular branch presents an important diminution of central vision with preserved peripheral vision [87]. In the acute phase, they will present with dot-blot hemorrhages, hard and soft exudates, retinal and macular edema, and with sectorial venous tortuosity and dilatation [92] (Fig. 16.12i). The visual prognosis is good, most of the patients present with a final vision of 20/40 or better, but it is important to understand that vision depends on the site and severity of the vascular occlusion as well as on the development of collaterals.

16.8 Retinal Detachment

Retinal detachment is defined as the separation of the neurosensory retina from the underlying retinal pigment epithelium [32, 93]. The retinal detachments are classified as rhegmatogenous, tractional, and exudative.

Rhegmatogenous retinal detachments (RRDs) are caused by fluid passing from the vitreous cavity through a retinal break into the potential interspace between the sensory retina and the RPE [32, 93, 94]. Some risk factors for RRD include myopia, family history, fellow eye retinal tear or RRD, recent posterior vitreous detachment (PVD), peripheral predisposing lesions, and vitreoretinal degenerations. Patients may present with photopsia, floaters, and with diminution of vision. On clinical examination, IOP may be reduced, the retina will be detached, presenting with convex borders and contours, and with a corrugated appearance. In cases of chronic RRD, fixed folds result from proliferative vitreoretinopathy (PVR). The location of a retinal break may be defined with the help of the Lincoff rules, which correlate the location and configuration of the subretinal fluid with the position of the retinal break [95, 96].The principles in surgical management include a detailed assessment to find all the retinal breaks, the creation of a chorioretinal adhesion, and closure of retinal breaks (scleral buckling, vitrectomy, or pneumatic retinopexy) [93–95].

Tractional retinal detachments (TRD) develop when vitreous membranes pull the neurosensory retina away from the RPE. Vitreous membranes may develop after open-globe injuries or proliferative retinopathies (diabetic retinopathy or PVR). Interestingly, TRD presents a concave configuration and can be focal or extensive, central or peripheral. In such a scenario, a TRD may resolve if the traction is released by PPV [93, 97]. In some cases, the traction may develop a retinal tear and produce a combined retinal detachment (tractional and rhegmatogenous), in which the retinal mobility will be limited compared to the RRD due to the proliferating tissue. In addition, corrugations, extensive subretinal fluid, subretinal hemorrhages, and subretinal bands indicate rhegmatogenous components. In cases of combined retinal detachment, PPV or combined PPV with a scleral buckle are the preferred procedures. Figure 16.13 shows a histopathological specimen of epiretinal membrane with silicon oil globules in a case of recurrent retinal detachment.

Exudative retinal detachment (ERD) occurs when the blood-retinal barrier (retinal blood vessels or the RPE) is disrupted, allowing fluid to

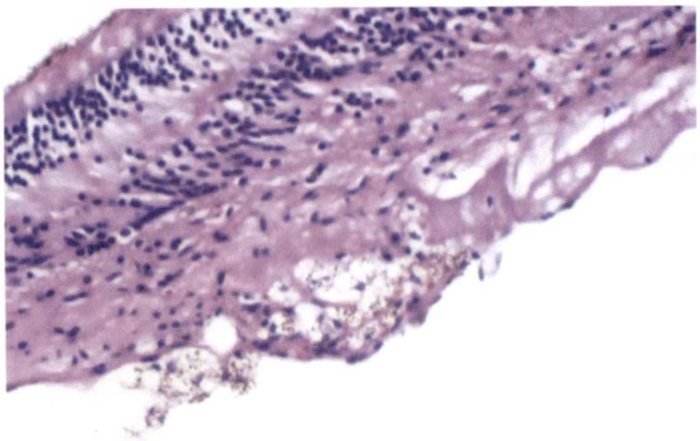

Fig. 16.13 Epiretinal membrane with silicon oil globules in a case of phthisis bulbi following end stage recurrent retinal detachment

pass into the subretinal space [98]. Inflammatory diseases and tumors are the leading causes of ERD. The ERD is characterized by shifting subretinal fluid and smoothness of the detached retinal surface. The treatment of ERD is nonsurgical.

16.9 Posterior Segment Manifestations of Ocular Trauma

Ocular trauma is a known cause of preventable monocular blindness and represents a great burden worldwide. Of particular interest is the posterior segment ocular trauma which may be present in open- or closed-globe injuries [99].

To unify the terms and compare clinical studies, Kuhn et al. developed a standardized classification for ocular injuries [100]. This classification was the base for the integration of the mechanical ocular injury classification which is useful to evaluate the functional status of the injured eye. This system is known as Birmingham Eye Trauma Terminology (BETT) [100]. The BETT classifies the ocular trauma as open in the presence of a full-thickness wound of the eyeball wall and as closed trauma when there is no full-thickness wound. Further, ocular traumas are classified according to the mechanism of injury. This system also assesses four different prognostic parameters for final vision including the type of injury, grade (initial visual acuity), the pupil (afferent pupillary defect), and zone.

For final visual acuity prognosis, the Ocular Trauma Score (OTS) is the scale of choice, which can be found elsewhere [101, 102].

Some of the injuries may manifest as subhyaloid hemorrhage. Valsalva retinopathy is characterized by subhyaloid hemorrhage over the macula (asterisk) or inferior hemorrhage along the inferotemporal arcade (Fig. 16.14a). It is important to understand that posterior segment trauma may be present in both, closed-globe (Fig. 16.14b–d) and open-globe injuries. The following list shows some of the pathologies most frequently found in ocular trauma.

The different types of closed-globe injuries are mentioned in Table 16.8. [101–111]

Open-globe injuries [100, 101, 112]

- Penetrating trauma: A penetrating wound is described as a full-thickness lesion of the eyewall caused by a sharp object where an entry site is observed, which can be single or multiple (Figs. 16.14e, f). A special characteristic is that these wounds are caused by sharp or pointed objects and present with clean and regular margins.
- Ocular rupture: It is caused by blunt objects or blunt trauma due to a sudden increase in the intraocular pressure. Ocular rupture will present with a significant disruption of the eyewall and the intraocular structures with a wound of irregular margins.
- Perforating trauma: This type of trauma presents with an entrance wound and an emerging wound. It is usually caused by a foreign body that penetrates and crosses the vitreous cavity emerging outside the eyeball through a different wound generally located in the posterior sclera.
- Intraocular foreign body: This type of wound has an entry site and an intraocular foreign body (IOFB). The IOFB can be anywhere in the eye including the anterior or posterior segment. It is important to rule out the presence of IOFB in all open-globe injuries (Fig. 16.14g, h).

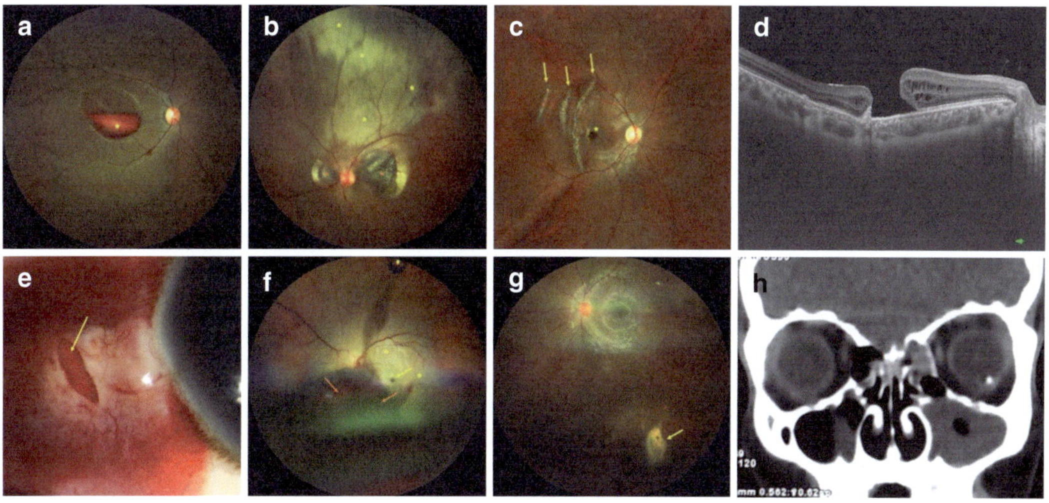

Fig. 16.14 Posterior segment manifestations in ocular trauma. (**a**) represents a case of Valsalva retinopathy; note the subhyaloid hemorrhage over the macula (asterisk) and the inferior hemorrhage along the inferotemporal arcade. Different cases of closed-globe injuries are shown in (**b**–**d**). (**b**) presents a case where subretinal hemorrhage (white asterisks) is observed at the macula and nasally to the optic disc, suggestive of choroidal ruptures. Observe the superior retinal whitening related to commotio retinae (yellow asterisks). (**c**) shows a case of multiple circumferential crescent-like lesions observed temporal to the fovea, indicating choroidal ruptures (yellow arrows); note the presence of a large traumatic macular hole (yellow asterisk) confirmed and detailed in the SS-OCT scan shown in (**d**). (**e**) and (**f**) present a case of penetrating trauma. In (**e**) a nasal conjunctival tear (yellow arrow) with hemorrhagic chemosis is present. Note the presence of vitreous hemorrhage (white arrow), posterior pole retinal whitening (yellow asterisk), and the presence of cherry red spot (yellow arrow) shown in (**f**). (**g** and **h**) show a case of intraocular foreign body (IOFB). In (**g**) an encapsulated IOFB is observed at the inferotemporal retina (yellow arrow) with localized vessel sclerosis and multiple hypopigmentary dot-like lesions. The CT scan revealed an intraocular hyperdense lesion compatible with a metallic IOFB shown in (**h**)

Table 16.8 Different types of closed-globe injuries

Valsalva retinopathy	Is a preretinal hemorrhage secondary to a sudden increase in the intrathoracic pressure as in Valsalva maneuvers which translates to an increase in the intraocular venous pressure which causes spontaneous rupture of retinal capillaries Features: Pre-macular hemorrhage under the internal limiting membrane Management: Spontaneous reabsorption and observation. ND: YAG laser hyaloidotomy and pars plana vitrectomy may be considered in cases of important hemorrhage extension
Battered-child syndrome	Suspect when there is an association with body trauma or when there is a discrepancy between the versions of how the accident happened Features: Bilateral retinal hemorrhages in the presence of cranioencephalic trauma Management: Notify authorities. Hemorrhages will spontaneously resolve in weeks. In cases of retinal detachment or retinal dialysis, vitreoretinal surgery is the preferred choice
Purtscher retinopathy	Bilateral and asymmetrical alterations in the retina product of retinal endothelial injury due to a sudden increase in the intraluminal pressure, embolus damage, and/or vitreoretinal interphase alterations due to trauma. Features: Macular and retinal edema, peripapillary cotton wool spots, preretinal and intraretinal hemorrhages, and optic disc edema Management: Observation with spontaneous resolution of hemorrhages and edema
Terson syndrome	Encompass any intraocular hemorrhage in the presence of intracranial hemorrhage and a sudden increase of the intracranial pressure Features: Subretinal, intraretinal, preretinal, subhyaloid, and/or vitreous hemorrhage. Papilledema may be present. A subhyaloid hemorrhage is the classic finding Management: Observation. In case of delayed reabsorption, PPV may be an option

(continued)

Table 16.8 (continued)

Chorioretinitis sclopetaria	Chorioretinal injury due to secondary shock in a direct or indirect impact on the eyeball Features: Retinal and choroidal rupture with bare sclera in an area that coincides with the external area of impact Management: Observation, of the scarring of the lesion borders, will prevent retinal detachment; laser photocoagulation is not required
Commotio retinae	Transitory whitening and opacification of the retina secondary to globe trauma. Retinal thickening and outer retinal layer disruption at OCT Features: Retinal whitening with irregular and ill-defined borders, of variable size that is apparent in the contralateral side of the impact Management: Observation. Avoid the usage of steroids
Choroidal rupture	Refers to the choroidal, Bruch's membrane, and RPE fracture secondary to trauma. It is considered a direct rupture when it occurs at the site of impact and its configuration is parallel to the ora serrata (anterior), and it is indirect when it occurs concentrically to the optic disc Features: Concentric curvilinear subretinal lesion with scleral show. In late phases, fibrotic tissue with RPE hyperplasia may be apparent Management: Observation. In case of neovascular membrane, anti-VEGF injection is the treatment of choice
Traumatic macular hole	Is a defect in the retina that involves all the retinal layers. The cause is the anteroposterior or tangential traction secondary to the trauma and the deformity of the eyeball during the impact, and also related to the retinal atrophy seen in these cases Features: Full-thickness defect in the macula with poor visual acuity Management: Observation for 3 to 6 months, a large proportion of cases spontaneously close. If the macular hole does not close spontaneously, then a PPV with gas tamponade is the treatment of choice

Financial Disclosures None for all authors.

Funding Hyderabad Eye Research Foundation.

References

1. Gupta MP, Herzlich AA, Sauer T, Chan CC. Retinal anatomy and pathology. Dev Ophthalmol. 2016;55:7–17. https://doi.org/10.1159/000431128. Epub 2015 Oct 26. PMID: 26502225
2. Sadda SVR, Hinton DR, Schachat AP, et al. Ryan's retina. 7th ed. Canada: Elsevier; 2022. https://doi.org/10.1016/C2010-1-69566-1.
3. Barishak YR. Embryology of the eye and its adnexae. Dev Ophthalmol. 1992;24:1–142. PMID: 1628748
4. Saint-Geniez M, D'Amore PA. Development and pathology of the hyaloid, choroidal and retinal vasculature. Int J Dev Biol. 2004;48(8–9):1045–58. https://doi.org/10.1387/ijdb.041895ms.
5. Sebag J. The vitreous. 1st ed. New York: Springer; 1989. https://doi.org/10.1007/978-1-4613-8908-8.
6. Goldberg MF. Persistent fetal vasculature (PFV): an integrated interpretation of signs and symptoms associated with persistent hyperplastic primary vitreous (PHPV). LIV Edward Jackson memorial lecture. Am J Ophthalmol. 1997;124(5):587–626.
7. Mary-Sinclair MN, Wang X, Swanson DJ, et al. Varied manifestations of persistent hyperplastic primary vitreous with graded somatic mosaic deletion of a single gene. Mol Vis. 2014;20:215–30. PMID: 24623965; PMCID: PMC3945809
8. Haddad R, Font RL, Reeser F. Persistent hyperplastic primary vitreous. A clinicopathologic study of 62 cases and review of the literature. Surv Ophthalmol. 1978;23(2):123–34.
9. Bakker R, Wagstaff EL, Kruijt CC, et al. The retinal pigmentation pathway in human albinism: not so black and white. Prog Retin Eye Res. 2022;91:101091. https://doi.org/10.1016/j.preteyeres.2022.101091. Epub 2022 Jun 18. PMID: 35729001
10. Kubasch AS, Meurer M. Okulokutaner und okulärer Albinismus [Oculocutaneous and ocular albinism]. Hautarzt. 2017;68(11):867–75. https://doi.org/10.1007/s00105-017-4061-x. German. PMID: 29018889
11. Marmoy OR, Blackwell C, Cornelius S, Thompson DA, Henderson RH. Diffuse bear-track retina: profound, bilateral, grouped congenital pigmentation of the retinal pigment epithelium in an infant. J AAPOS. 2020;24(6):384–6. https://doi.org/10.1016/j.jaapos.2020.08.003. Epub 2020 Oct 22. PMID: 33289665
12. Lingam G. Pattern of blood vessels in eyes with coloboma. Indian J Ophthalmol. 2013;61(12):743–8. https://doi.org/10.4103/0301-4738.122910. PMID: 24413826; PMCID: PMC3917394

13. Mohamed A, Chaurasia S, Ramappa M, Jalali S. Corneal thickness in uveal coloboma with microcornea. Eye (Lond). 2018;32(3):586–9. https://doi.org/10.1038/eye.2017.258. Epub 2017 Dec 1. PMID: 29192683; PMCID: PMC5848287
14. Lieb W, Rochels R, Gronemeyer U. Microphthalmos with colobomatous orbital cyst: clinical, histological, immunohistological, and electronmicroscopic findings. Br J Ophthalmol. 1990;74(1):59–62.
15. Lingam G, Sen AC, Lingam V, Bhende M, Padhi TR, Xinyi S. Ocular coloboma-a comprehensive review for the clinician. Eye (Lond). 2021;35(8):2086–109. https://doi.org/10.1038/s41433-021-01501-5. Epub 2021 Mar 21. PMID: 33746210; PMCID: PMC8302742
16. Fei P, Zhang Q, Li J, et al. Clinical characteristics and treatment of 22 eyes of morning glory syndrome associated with persistent hyperplastic primary vitreous. Br J Ophthalmol. 2013;97:1262–7.
17. Edwards AO. Clinical features of the congenital vitreoretinopathies. Eye. 2008;22(10):1233–42.
18. Shaimova VA, Shaimov T, Shaimov R, Galin A. Peripheral retinal degenerations. 2nd ed. Cham: Springer; 2017.
19. Byer NE. Lattice degeneration of the retina. Surv Ophthalmol. 1979;23(4):213–48.
20. Byer NE. Long-term natural history of lattice degeneration of the retina. Ophthalmology. 1989;96(9):1396–402.
21. Burton TC. The influence of refractive error and lattice degeneration on the incidence of retinal detachment. Trans Am Ophthalmol Soc. 1989;87:143.
22. Mizuno H, Fukumoto M, Sato T, et al. Involvement of the retinal pigment epithelium in the development of retinal lattice degeneration. Int J Mol Sci. 2020;21(19):7347. https://doi.org/10.3390/ijms21197347. PMID: 33027920; PMCID: PMC7583762
23. Wilkinson CP. Interventions for asymptomatic retinal breaks and lattice degeneration for preventing retinal detachment. Cochrane Database Syst Rev. 2014;2014(9):CD003170. https://doi.org/10.1002/14651858.CD003170.pub4. PMID: 25191970; PMCID: PMC4423540
24. Ulfik-Dembska K, Teper S, Dembski M, Nowińska A, Wylęgała E. Peripheral retinal degenerations and idiopathic epiretinal membrane: analysis with ultra-wide-field scanning laser ophthalmoscopy. J Clin Med. 2021;10(17):3876. https://doi.org/10.3390/jcm10173876. PMID: 34501323; PMCID: PMC8432095
25. O'Malley P, Allen RA, Traatsma BRS, O'Malley CC. Paving-stone degeneration of the retina. Arch Ophthalmol. 1965;73(2):169–82.
26. Jones WL. Atlas of the peripheral ocular fundus. Butterworth-Heinemann Medical; 1998.
27. Shukla M, Ahuja OP. A possible relationship between lattice and snail track degenerations of the retina. Am J Ophthalmol. 1981;92(4):482–5.
28. Kumar V, Kumar P, Roy S, Padhy SK. Pars plana cysts. Ophthalmic Surgery, Lasers Imaging Retin. 2018;49(10):e169–70.
29. Ghazi NG, Knape RM. Optical coherence tomography of peripheral retinal lesions in enucleated human eye specimens with histologic correlation II. Curr Eye Res. 2006;31(12):1047–9.
30. De Jong PTVM. Age-related macular degeneration. N Engl J Med. 2006;355(14):1474–85.
31. Haddad S, Chen CA, Santangelo SL, Seddon JM. The genetics of age-related macular degeneration: a review of progress to date. Surv Ophthalmol. 2006;51(4):316–63.
32. Yanoff M, Duker JS. Ophthalmology. 5th ed. Elsevier Health Sciences; 2019.
33. Sarks SH, Arnold JJ, Killingsworth MC, Sarks JP. Early drusen formation in the normal and aging eye and their relation to age related maculopathy: a clinicopathological study. Br J Ophthalmol. 1999;83(3):358–68.
34. Zhang X, Sivaprasad S. Drusen and pachydrusen: the definition, pathogenesis, and clinical significance. Eye. 2021;35:121–33. https://doi.org/10.1038/s41433-020-01265-4.
35. Ibbett P, Goverdhan SV, Pipi E, et al. A lasered mouse model of retinal degeneration displays progressive outer retinal pathology providing insights into early geographic atrophy. Sci Rep. 2019;9:7475. https://doi.org/10.1038/s41598-019-43906-z.
36. Curcio CA. Soft drusen in age-related macular degeneration: biology and targeting via the oil spill strategies. Invest Ophthalmol Vis Sci. 2018;59(4):AMD160.
37. Johnson PT, Lewis GP, Talaga KC, et al. Drusen-associated degeneration in the retina. Invest Ophthalmol Vis Sci. 2003;44(10):4481–8.
38. Naumann GOH, Naumann LR. Intraocular inflammations. In: Pathology of the eye. New York: Springer-Verlag; 1986. p. 99–184.
39. Miller JR, Hanumunthadu D. Inflammatory eye disease: an overview of clinical presentation and management. Clin Med (Lond). 2022;22(2):100–3. https://doi.org/10.7861/clinmed.2022-0046. PMID: 35304367; PMCID: PMC8966833
40. Li JJ, Yi S, Wei L. Ocular microbiota and intraocular inflammation. Front Immunol. 2020;23(11):609765. https://doi.org/10.3389/fimmu.2020.609765. PMID: 33424865; PMCID: PMC7786018
41. Jabs DA, Nussenblatt RB, Rosenbaum JT. Standardization of uveitis nomenclature for reporting clinical data. Results of the first international workshop. Am J Ophthalmol. 2005;140(3):509–16. https://doi.org/10.1016/j.ajo.2005.03.057.
42. Nayak S, Das T, Parameswarappa D, et al. Sight-threatening intraocular infection in patients with COVID-19 in India. Indian J Ophthalmol. 2021;69(12):3664.

43. Dave VP, Das T. Definition, signs, and symptoms of endophthalmitis. In: Endophthalmitis. Singapore: Springer; 2018. p. 3–8.
44. Das T, Dave VP, Dogra A, Joseph J, Sharma S. EMS working group. Endophthalmitis management study. Report #1. Protocol. Indian J Ophthalmol. 2021;69(7):1936–41. https://doi.org/10.4103/ijo.IJO_199_21. PMID: 34146061; PMCID: PMC8374761
45. Vitrectomy E. Results of the endophthalmitis vitrectomy study. Arch Ophthalmol. 1995;113:1479–96.
46. Clark WL, Kaiser PK, Flynn HW Jr, Belfort A, Miller D, Meisler DM. Treatment strategies and visual acuity outcomes in chronic postoperative Propionibacterium acnes endophthalmitis. Ophthalmology. 1999;106(9):1665–70.
47. Pastor-Idoate S, Bonshek R, Irion L, et al. Ultrastructural and histopathologic findings after pars plana vitrectomy with a new hypersonic vitrector system. Qualitative preliminary assessment. PLOS one. 2017;12(4):e0173883.
48. Murthy SI, Takkar B, Bhate M, Mishra DK, Sheba E, Sharma S. Herpes simplex virus anterior uveitis in a child presenting as a hypopyon in a white eye. Ocul Immunol Inflamm. 2022;30(7–8):1992–4.
49. Sung CH, Chuang JZ. The cell biology of vision. J Cell Biol. 2010;190:953–63.
50. Nash BM, Wright DC, Grigg JR, Bennetts B, Jamieson RV. Retinal dystrophies, genomic applications in diagnosis and prospects for therapy. Transl Pediatr. 2015;4(2):139–63. https://doi.org/10.3978/j.issn.2224-4336.2015.04.03. PMID: 26835369; PMCID: PMC4729094
51. Hamosh A, Scott AF, Amberger J, Valle D, McKusick VA. Online mendelian inheritance in man (OMIM) https://www.omim.org/
52. Daiger SP, Sullivan LS, Bowne SJ. RetNet Retinal Information Network https://web.sph.uth.edu/RetNet/
53. Campbell JP, Zhang M, Hwang TS, et al. Detailed vascular anatomy of the human retina by projection-resolved optical coherence tomography angiography. Sci Rep. 2017;10(7):42201. https://doi.org/10.1038/srep42201. PMID: 28186181; PMCID: PMC5301488
54. Osborne NN, Casson RJ, Wood JP, Chidlow G, Graham M, Melena J. Retinal ischemia: mechanisms of damage and potential therapeutic strategies. Prog Retin Eye Res. 2004;23(1):91–147. https://doi.org/10.1016/j.preteyeres.2003.12.001. PMID: 14766318
55. Dattilo M, Newman NJ, Biousse V. Acute retinal arterial ischemia. Ann Eye Sci. 2018;3:28. https://doi.org/10.21037/aes.2018.05.04. Epub 2018 Jun 6. PMID: 30198015; PMCID: PMC6124502
56. Wong TY, Mitchell P. Hypertensive retinopathy. N Engl J Med. 2004;351(22):2310–7. https://doi.org/10.1056/NEJMra032865. PMID: 15564546
57. AlTalbishi A, Khateb S, Amer R. Elschnig's spots in the acute and remission stages in preeclampsia: spectral-domain optical coherence tomographic features. Eur J Ophthalmol. 2015;25(5):e84–7. https://doi.org/10.5301/ejo.5000586. PMID: 25743779
58. Antonetti DA, Klein R, Gardner TW. Mechanisms of disease diabetic retinopathy. N Engl J Med. 2012;366(13):1227–39.
59. Early Treatment Diabetic Retinopathy Study Research Group. Photocoagulation for diabetic macular edema. Early treatment diabetic retinopathy study report number 1. Arch Ophthalmol. 1985;103:1796–806.
60. Relhan N, Flynn HW. The early treatment diabetic retinopathy study historical review and relevance to today's management of diabetic macular edema. Curr Opin Ophthalmol. 2017;28(3):205–12.
61. Sulochana KN, Biswas J, Ramakrishnan S. Eales' disease: increased oxidation and peroxidation products of membrane constituents chiefly lipids and decreased antioxidant enzymes and reduced glutathione in vitreous. Curr Eye Res. 1999;19(3):254–9.
62. Fung AT, Galvin J, Tran T. Epiretinal membrane: a review. Clin Experiment Ophthalmol. 2021;49(3):289–308. https://doi.org/10.1111/ceo.13914. Epub 2021 Mar 24. PMID: 33656784
63. Gandorfer A, Rohleder M, Grosselfinger S, Haritoglou C, Ulbig M, Kampik A. Epiretinal pathology of diffuse diabetic macular edema associated with vitreomacular traction. Am J Ophthalmol. 2005;139(4):638–52.
64. Nicoletti VG, Nicoletti R, Ferrara N, Meli G, Reibaldi M, Reibaldi A. Diabetic patients and retinal proliferation: an evaluation of the role of vascular endothelial growth factor (VEGF). Exp Clin Endocrinol Diabetes. 2003;111(04):209–14.
65. Ishida S, Shinoda K, Kawashima S, Oguchi Y, Okada Y, Ikeda E. Coexpression of VEGF receptors VEGF-R2 and neuropilin-1 in proliferative diabetic retinopathy. Invest Ophthalmol Vis Sci. 2000;41(7):1649–56.
66. Coucha M, Elshaer SL, Eldahshan WS, Mysona BA, El-Remessy AB. Molecular mechanisms of diabetic retinopathy: potential therapeutic targets. Middle East Afr J Ophthalmol. 2015;22(2):135–44. https://doi.org/10.4103/0974-9233.154386. PMID: 25949069; PMCID: PMC4411608
67. Hollborn M, Francke M, Iandiev I, Bühner E, Foja C, Kohen L, et al. Early activation of inflammation- and immune response-related genes after experimental detachment of the porcine retina. Invest Ophthalmol Vis Sci. 2008;49(3):1262–73. pmid:1832
68. Tamiya S, Kaplan HJ. Role of epithelial-mesenchymal transition in proliferative vitreoretinopathy. Exp Eye Res. 2016;142:26–31. https://doi.org/10.1016/j.exer.2015.02.008. PMID: 26675400
69. Das A, McGuire PG, Eriqat C, et al. Human diabetic neovascular membranes contain high levels of urokinase and metalloproteinase enzymes. Invest Ophthalmol Vis Sci. 1999;40(3):809–13. PMID: 10067990

70. Das A, McGuire PG. Retinal and choroidal angiogenesis: pathophysiology and strategies for inhibition. Prog Retin Eye Res. 2003;22(6):721–48.
71. Sadaka A, Giuliari GP. Proliferative vitreoretinopathy: current and emerging treatments. Clin Ophthalmol Auckl NZ. 2012;6:1325–33. https://doi.org/10.2147/OPTH.S27896.
72. Idrees S, Sridhar J, Kuriyan AE. Proliferative vitreoretinopathy: a review. Int Ophthalmol Clin. 2019;59(1):221–40. https://doi.org/10.1097/IIO.0000000000000258. PMID: 30585928; PMCID: PMC6310037
73. Wiedemann P, Hilgers RD, Bauer P, Heimann K. Adjunctive daunorubicin in the treatment of proliferative vitreoretinopathy: results of a multicenter clinical trial. Daunomycin study group. Am J Ophthalmol. 1998;126(4):550–9.
74. Wickham L, Bunce C, Wong D, McGurn D, Charteris DG. Randomized controlled trial of combined 5-fluorouracil and low-molecular-weight heparin in the management of unselected rhegmatogenous retinal detachments undergoing primary vitrectomy. Ophthalmology. 2007;114(4):698–704. https://doi.org/10.1016/j.ophtha.2006.08.042.
75. Chang YC, Hu DN, Wu WC. Effect of oral 13-cis-retinoic acid treatment on postoperative clinical outcome of eyes with proliferative vitreoretinopathy. Am J Ophthalmol. 2008;146(3):440–6. https://doi.org/10.1016/j.ajo.2008.05.002. Epub 2008 Jul 2. PMID: 18599016
76. Dong L, Han H, Huang X, et al. Idelalisib inhibits experimental proliferative vitroretinopathy. Lab Investig. 2022;102:1296–303. https://doi.org/10.1038/s41374-022-00822-7.
77. Xin T, Han H, Wu W, Huang X, Cui J, Matsubara JA, et al. Idelalisib inhibits vitreous-induced Akt activation and proliferation of retinal pigment epithelial cells from epiretinal membranes. Exp Eye Res. 2020;190:107884.
78. Scott IU, Campochiaro PA, Newman NJ, Biousse V. Retinal vascular occlusions. Lancet. 2020;396(10266):1927–40. https://doi.org/10.1016/S0140-6736(20)31559-2. PMID: 33308475; PMCID: PMC9546635
79. Biousse V, Nahab F, Newman NJ. Management of acute retinal ischemia. Follow the guidelines! Ophthalmology. 2018;125:1597–607.
80. Amarenco P. Transient ischemic attack. N Engl J Med. 2020;382:1933–41.
81. Hayreh SS. Acute retinal arterial occlusive disorders. Prog Retin Eye Res. 2011;30:359–94.
82. Varma DD, Cugati S, Lee AW, Chen CS. A review of central retinal artery occlusion: clinical presentation and management. Eye (Lond). 2013;27(6):688–97. https://doi.org/10.1038/eye.2013.25. Epub 2013 Mar 8. PMID: 23470793; PMCID: PMC3682348
83. Mac Grory B, Schrag M, Biousse V, et al. Management of central retinal artery occlusion: a scientific statement from the American heart association. Stroke. 2021;52:e282–94.
84. Mac Grory B, Nackenoff A, Poli S, et al. Intravenous fibrinolysis for central retinal artery occlusion: a cohort study and updated patient-level meta-analysis. Stroke. 2020;51:2018–25. https://doi.org/10.1161/STROKEAHA.119.028743.
85. Schrag M, Youn T, Schindler J, Kirshner H, Greer D. Intravenous fibrinolytic therapy in central retinal artery occlusion: a patient-level meta-analysis. JAMA Neurol. 2015;72(10):1148–54. https://doi.org/10.1001/jamaneurol.2015.1578.
86. Mason JO 3rd, Shah AA, Vail RS, Nixon PA, Ready EL, Kimble JA. Branch retinal artery occlusion: visual prognosis. Am J Ophthalmol. 2008;146(3):455–7. https://doi.org/10.1016/j.ajo.2008.05.009. Epub 2008 Jul 2. PMID: 18599018
87. Rehak J, Rehak M. Branch retinal vein occlusion: pathogenesis, visual prognosis, and treatment modalities. Curr Eye Res. 2008;33(2):111–31. https://doi.org/10.1080/02713680701851902. PMID: 18293182; PMCID: PMC2430176
88. Hayreh SS, Klugman MR, Beri M, Kimura AE, Podhajsky P. Differentiation of ischemic from non-ischemic central retinal vein occlusion during the early acute phase. Graefes Arch Clin Exp Ophthalmol. 1990;228(3):201–17. https://doi.org/10.1007/BF00920022.
89. Nicholson L, Talks SJ, Amoaku W, et al. Retinal vein occlusion (RVO) guideline: executive summary. Eye. 2022;36:909–12. https://doi.org/10.1038/s41433-022-02007-4.
90. Nicholson L, Vazquez-Alfageme C, Patrao NV, Triantafyllopolou I, Bainbridge JW, Hykin PG, et al. Retinal nonperfusion in the posterior pole is associated with increased risk of neovascularization in central retinal vein occlusion. Am J Ophthalmol. 2017;182:118–25.
91. Tsui I, Kaines A, Havunjian MA, Hubschman S, Heilweil G, Prasad PS, et al. Ischemic index and neovascularization in central retinal vein occlusion. Retina. 2011;31:105–10.
92. Lee YH, Kim YC. Clinical characteristics of branch retinal vein occlusion with increased retinal haemorrhage during treatment for macular oedema. Sci Rep. 2020;10:10272. https://doi.org/10.1038/s41598-020-67395-7.
93. Steel D. Retinal detachment. BMJ Clin Evid. 2014;3(2014):710. PMID: 24807890; PMCID: PMC3940167
94. Polkinghorne PJ, Craig JP. Northern New Zealand Rhegmatogenous retinal detachment study: epidemiology and risk factors. Clin Experiment Ophthalmol. 2004;32:159–63.
95. Sultan ZN, Agorogiannis EI, Iannetta D, Steel D, Sandinha T. Rhegmatogenous retinal detachment: a review of current practice in diagnosis and management. BMJ Open Ophthalmol. 2020;5(1):e000474. https://doi.org/10.1136/bmjophth-2020-000474. Erratum in: BMJ Open Ophthalmol 2021 Mar 14;6(1):e000474corr1. PMID: 33083551; PMCID: PMC7549457

96. Yoshida I, Shiba T, Hori Y, Maeno T. Relationships between retinal break locations and the shapes of the detachments. Clin Ophthalmol. 2018;31(12):2213–22. https://doi.org/10.2147/OPTH.S177594. Erratum in: Clin Ophthalmol 2019 Oct 10;13:1997. PMID: 30464382; PMCID: PMC6217139
97. Iyer SSR, Regan KA, Burnham JM, Chen CJ. Surgical management of diabetic tractional retinal detachments. Surv Ophthalmol. 2019;64(6):780–809. https://doi.org/10.1016/j.survophthal.2019.04.008. Epub 2019 May 9. PMID: 31077688
98. Amer R, Nalcı H, Yalçındağ N. Exudative retinal detachment. Surv Ophthalmol. 2017;62(6):723–69. https://doi.org/10.1016/j.survophthal.2017.05.001. Epub 2017 May 13. PMID: 28506603
99. Kuhn F. Ocular trauma: from epidemiology to war-related injuries. Graefes Arch Clin Exp Ophthalmol. 2011;249(12):1753–4. https://doi.org/10.1007/s00417-011-1834-1842. Epub 2011 Oct 14. PMID: 21997539
100. Kuhn F, Morris R, Witherspoon CD. Birmingham eye trauma terminology (BETT): terminology and classification of mechanical eye injuries. Ophthalmol Clin N Am. 2002;15(2):139–43. https://doi.org/10.1016/s0896-1549(02)00004-4. PMID: 12229228
101. Kuhn F, Maisiak R, Mann L, Mester V, Morris R, Witherspoon CD. The ocular trauma score (OTS). Ophthalmol Clin N Am. 2002;15(2):163–5. https://doi.org/10.1016/s0896-1549(02)00007-x. PMID: 12229231
102. Kuhn F, Morris R, Witherspoon CD, Heimann K, Jeffers JB, Treister G. A standardized classification of ocular trauma. Ophthalmology. 1996;103(2):240–3. https://doi.org/10.1016/s0161-6420(96)30710-0. PMID: 8594508
103. Rohowetz LJ, Patel V, Sridhar J, Yannuzzi NA. Valsalva retinopathy: clinical features and treatment outcomes. Retina. 2023;43(8):1317–20. https://doi.org/10.1097/IAE.0000000000003772. PMID: 36893442
104. Eisenbrey AB. Retinal hemorrhage in the battered child. Childs Brain. 1979;5(1):40–4. https://doi.org/10.1159/000119800. PMID: 109252
105. Hansen JB, Killough EF, Moffatt ME, Knapp JF. Retinal hemorrhages: abusive head trauma or not? Pediatr Emerg Care. 2018;34(9):665–70. https://doi.org/10.1097/PEC.0000000000001605. PMID: 30180101
106. Joshi C, Shuckett P, Stockl F. A picture worth remembering: posttraumatic Purtscher's retinopathy in a child. J Child Neurol. 2008;23(3):353–5. https://doi.org/10.1177/0883073807308700. Epub 2007 Dec 13. PMID: 18079317
107. Aboulhosn R, Raju B, Jumah F, et al. Terson's syndrome, the current concepts and management strategies: a review of literature. Clin Neurol Neurosurg. 2021;210:107008. https://doi.org/10.1016/j.clineuro.2021.107008. Epub 2021 Oct 27. PMID: 34775364
108. Kamboj A, Hwang CJ, Kulenkamp JE, et al. Chorioretinitis sclopetaria and orbital emphysema caused by a high-velocity liquid missile. Retin Cases Brief Rep. 2023;17(3):305–8. https://doi.org/10.1097/ICB.0000000000001161. PMID: 34001762
109. Wangsathaporn K, Tsui I. Commotio retinae resulting from rubber band injury in two girls. Ophthalmic Surg Lasers Imaging Retina. 2019;50(5):309–13. https://doi.org/10.3928/23258160-20190503-08. PMID: 31100162
110. Lupidi M, Muzi A, Castellucci G, et al. The choroidal rupture: current concepts and insights. Surv Ophthalmol. 2021;66(5):761–70. https://doi.org/10.1016/j.survophthal.2021.01.014. Epub 2021 Feb 2.PMID: 33545177
111. Miller JB, Yonekawa Y, Eliott D, Vavvas DG. A review of traumatic macular hole: diagnosis and treatment. Int Ophthalmol Clin. 2013;53(4):59. https://doi.org/10.1097/IIO.0b013e3182a26efe. PMID: 24088933
112. Scanzera AC, Leiderman YI, Cortina MS, Shorter ES. Open globe injuries from projectile impact: initial presentation and outcomes. Indian J Ophthalmol. 2022;70(3):860–4. https://doi.org/10.4103/ijo.IJO_797_21. PMID: 35225531; PMCID: PMC9114545

Orbital Lesions and Their Pathology

17

Dilip K. Mishra, Tarjani Vivek Dave,
and Neha Ghose

Contents

D. K. Mishra (✉)
Ophthalmic Pathology Laboratory, Kallam Anji
Reddy Campus, L V Prasad Eye Institute,
Hyderabad, Telangana, India
e-mail: dilipkumarmishra@lvpei.org

T. V. Dave · N. Ghose
Ophthalmic Plastic Surgery Service, Kallam Anji
Reddy Campus, L V Prasad Eye Institute,
Hyderabad, Telangana, India
e-mail: tarjani@lvpei.org

G. K. Vemuganti et al. (eds.), *Ocular Pathology*, https://doi.org/10.1007/978-981-96-8614-8_17

17.1 Introduction

The orbit is a complex structure that is enclosed within a pyramidal bony socket formed by four walls composed of seven bones. The main function of this bony orbit is to protect the eyeball and the soft tissue from mechanical injury. It houses the eyeball, extraocular muscles, fat, nerves, blood vessels, lacrimal gland and the orbital connective tissue.

The pathological processes in the orbit mirror those in the rest of the body. Approximately, 70% of all orbital tumors originate from the orbital tissue and 30% invade from the adjacent structures or metastasize to the orbit from a distant primary foci. Nonspecific inflammatory orbital diseases, orbital cysts and orbital lymphoid hyperplasia mimic true neoplasms and therefore fall under the broad category of "orbital tumors". Since the orbit is a very compact organ, the lesions, or tumors of the orbit present as a space occupying lesions (SOL). They can lead to an increase in the volume of orbit which results in proptosis of the eyeball and may at times disturb the visual and extraocular muscle function.

On histopathology the diagnosis of orbital tumors is difficult and requires immune stain, with an excellent clinic-radiologic correlation. The common orbital tumors include rhabdomyosarcoma, cavernous vascular malformation (cavernous hemangioma), lymphoid tumors and capillary hemangiomas.

17.2 Classification of Orbital Lesions

Classification of orbital tumors is based on demographics, site of origin, anatomic location within the orbit, histopathologic features, clinical course and imaging findings [1, 2]. Histologically orbital tumors can be classified into three broad categories that are benign, benign but locally aggressive, and malignant. Essentially, neoplasms of the orbit are primary when they originate from the orbital tissue and secondary when there is local invasion from adjacent structure or metastasis from distant organ.

Classification of Orbital Lesions

Tumors of the orbit

1. *Cystic lesions and teratoma*
   1.1. Dermoid cyst
   1.2. Epithelial cyst
   1.3. Teratoma
   1.4. Hematic cyst
   1.5. Paracytic cyst
   1.6. Lacrimal gland cyst
   1.7. Mucocele

   - 1.8. Microphthalmos with cyst
2. *Inflammatory tumors*
   - 2.1. Nonspecific inflammatory orbital disease (NSOID)
   - 2.2. Sarcoid nodule
   - 2.3. Ig4 Related orbital disease
   - 2.4. Fungal granuloma
   - 2.5. Myositis
3. *Hematolymphoid tumors*
   - 3.1. Reactive lymphoid hyperplasia
   - 3.2. Lymphoma
   - 3.3. Extramarginal zone lymphoma
   - 3.4. Follicular lymphoma
   - 3.5. Diffuse B-cell lymphoma (DLBL)
   - 3.6. Burkitt's lymphoma
   - 3.7. Acute lymphoblastic lymphoma/leukemia
4. *Myeloid sarcoma*
   - 4.1. Extra medullary myeloid sarcoma
5. *Lacrimal gland/Fossa tumor*
   - 5.1. Dacryoadenitis
   - 5.2. Ectopic lacrimal gland
   - 5.3. Epithelial tumors
   - 5.4. Dacryops
6. *Soft Tissue and Bone Tumors*
   - 6.1. *Soft Tissue tumors*
     - 6.1.1. *Fibroblastic tumor*
       - 6.1.2.1. Nodular fasciitis
       - 6.1.2.2. Solitary fibrous tumor (SFT)
       - 6.1.2.3. Inflammatory myofibroblastic tumor
     - 6.1.2. *Lipomatous tumor*
       - 6.1.2.1. Benign lipomatous tumor
       - 6.1.2.2. Malignanant lipomatous tumor or liposarcoma
     - 6.1.3. *Muscle tumor*
       - 6.1.3.1. *Skeltal muscle tumor*
       - 6.1.3.2. Rhabdomyosarcoma
       - 6.1.3.3. *Smooth muscle tumor*
       - 6.1.3.4. Leiomyoma
       - 6.1.3.5. Leiomyosarcoma
     - 6.1.4. *Vasculogenic tumor*
       - 6.1.4.1. Capillary hemangioma
       - 6.1.4.2. Cavernous malformation
       - 6.1.4.3. Arterio-venous (AV) malformation
       - 6.1.4.4. Orbital varix
       - 6.1.4.5. Lymphangioma
       - 6.1.4.6. Angiosarcoam
     - 6.1.5. *Peripheral nerve sheath tumor*
       - 6.1.5.1. Neurofibroma
       - 6.1.5.2. Schwannoma
       - 6.1.5.3. Malignant peripheral nerve sheath tumor (MPNST)
   - 6.2. *Tumors of orbital bone*
     - 6.2.1. *Tumors originating from bone (Osteogenic tumor)*
       - 6.2.1.1. Osteoma
       - 6.2.1.2. Osteosarcoma
       - 6.2.1.3. Ewing sarcoma
     - 6.2.2. *Tumors of chondrogenic origin*
       - 6.2.2.1. Primary mesenchymal chondrosarcoma
     - 6.2.3. *Fibro-osseus tumors*
       - 6.2.3.1. Fibrous histocytoma
       - 6.2.3.2. Fibrous dysplasia
       - 6.2.3.3. Fibrosarcoma
7. *Histiocytic Tumors*
   - 7.1. Rosai–Dorfman disease
   - 7.2. Langerhans cell histiocytosis (Eosinophilic granuloma)
   - 7.3. Juvenile xanthogranuloma
8. *Miscellaneous tumors*
   - 8.1. Alveolar soft part sarcoma
   - 8.2. Meningioma
   - 8.3. Metastatic tumors
   - 8.4. Synovial sarcoma
   - 8.5. Endodermal sinus tumor
   - 8.6. Melanocytic tumor

17.3 Cystic Lesions and Teratoma

17.3.1 Dermoid Cyst

Orbital dermoid cysts, the commonest orbital lesions in children, are congenital lesions representing closed sacs lined by an ectodermal epithelium. They are typically divided into deep (within the orbit) and superficial categories (adjacent to the orbital rim also called as angular dermoid). Dermoid

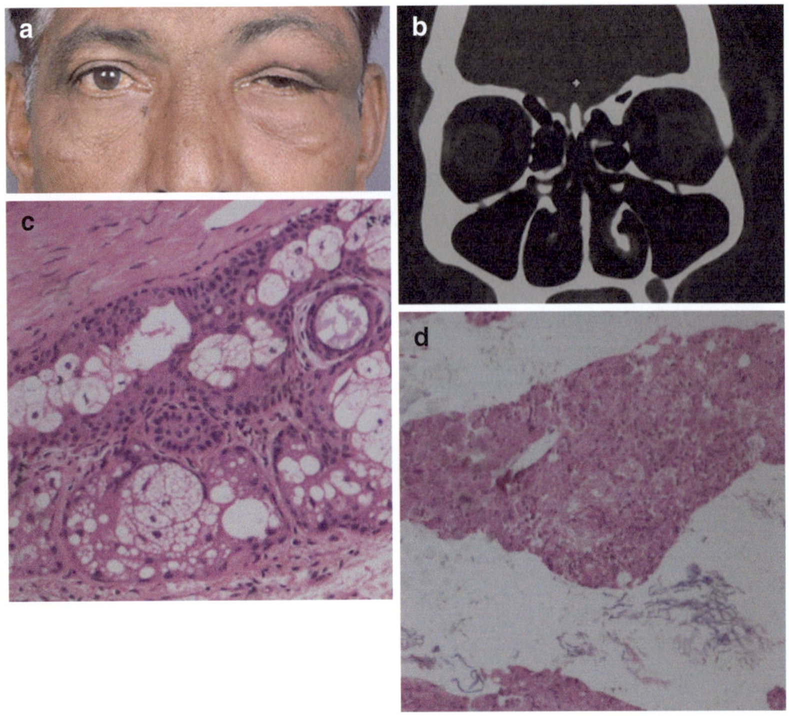

Fig. 17.1 Dermoid cyst. Clinical photograph of a 60-year-old gentleman with a small, nodular swelling over the left eyebrow since birth (**a**). Computed tomography (CT) scan of the orbit in the coronal view is suggestive of a hypodense cyst with an isodense lining along the temporal fossa (**d**). Histopathology showed a cyst filled with keratin flakes, and the surrounding cyst wall contains granuloma formation (**c**) and adnexal structure (**d**)

cysts are developmental choristomas comprising 3–9% of all orbital masses with an average incidence of 4–7% [3]. In the head and neck it has been postulated to arise from ectodermal rests "pinched off" at suture lines [4] (Fig. 17.1).

Superficial angular dermoid is usually diagnosed relatively early. As they grow slowly, less than 25% of them are identified at birth, and they usually manifest in the first decade of life. Clinical features include a painless subcutaneous mass at the fronto-zygomatic or the fronto-nasal suture line [5]. Over 80% of angular dermoids are at the fronto-zygomatic suture [6]. Deeper lesions are often identified as incidental masses, or they may occupy much of the orbit and manifest with proptosis in older children or adults.

Microscopically dermoid cysts contain a thick lining of epithelium and scant vascularity, and they may develop dystrophic calcification. The lining is composed of stratified squamous epithelium identical to that of the epidermis. By definition, the wall of a dermoid cyst contains additional ectodermal features, such as hair follicles or sebaceous glands, which are typically arranged in pilosebaceous units. The composition of dermoid cysts is complex, but all are derivatives of ectoderm. Thus, a dermoid inclusion cyst is monodermal which is derived from a single germ layer and is distinguished from a teratoma, which contains additional tissues of mesodermal or endodermal origin. The cystic cavity in dermoid cyst is filled with sebum, hair, and/or keratinous debris. A ruptured cyst may produce granulomatous inflammation.

17.3.2 Teratoma

In Greek word "teratoma" means monstrous growth. Teratomas are tumors composed of tissues derived from all three germ layers [7]. Orbital location is rare and comprises 0.8% of all orbital neoplasms [8]. The left orbit is more likely involved with a male: female ratio of 1:2 [9]. Orbital teratomas have been divided into four groups: (a) complete orbital fetus-in-fetus—orbitopagus parasiticus, (b) a portion of a second fetus in the orbit, (c) true orbital teratoma with all three germ layers, and (d) a tumor with only two germ cell lines [10]. Most orbital teratomas are sharply circumscribed, benign and well-differentiated histologically. On radiological examination most of the teratomas are benign and present with multiloculated, cystic masses with an admixture of tissues including calcification, fat, and ossification. Clinically, the tumor presents in healthy newborns with rapid growth, extreme unilateral proptosis, and marked stretching of the eyelids over a tense, fluctuating mass, with an increase in the palpebral fissure and transillumination of all or part of the orbital mass. The eye is usually normally formed but is displaced superiorly and proptosed. In rare cases, the eye is not formed, or only a rudimentary eye can be found. Kivelä and Tarkkanen classified orbital teratomas as: primary intraocular teratoma, primary orbital teratoma, combined orbital and extraorbital teratoma, and secondary orbital teratoma [11] (Fig. 17.2).

Microscopically, congenital orbital teratoma is comprised of tissues from all three embryonic germ cell layers and is categorized as mature or immature teratoma depending on the presence or absence of undifferentiated embryonic tissue. The predominant germ cell observed in orbital teratomas is surface ectoderm. The cyst is filled with keratin and adnexal structures, such as hair follicles and sweat glands. Neuroectodermal tissues such as primitive neural tubes, choroidal plexus, ganglia, and glial elements can be present. The mesoderm is the second most common germ cell layer, represented by muscle, bone, cartilage, and fat. The endoderm is the least common component of teratomas and may produce respiratory or gastrointestinal tissue cysts [12]. The immature or malignant teratoma contains variable amounts of mature elements from all three germ layers, admixed with immature elements that are commonly of neuroectodermal origin. Immature neuroepithelium can be spindled or sarcomatoid or with rosette, pseudorosette, and primitive tubule formation. Cells appear primitive, with scant cytoplasm, hyperchromatic nuclei and frequent mitoses, which helps differentiate the immature elements from mature brain tissue. Serum alpha-fetoprotein can be used in diagnosis of teratoma but its role is controversial as elevated levels of alpha-fetoprotein are common in neonates. However, a

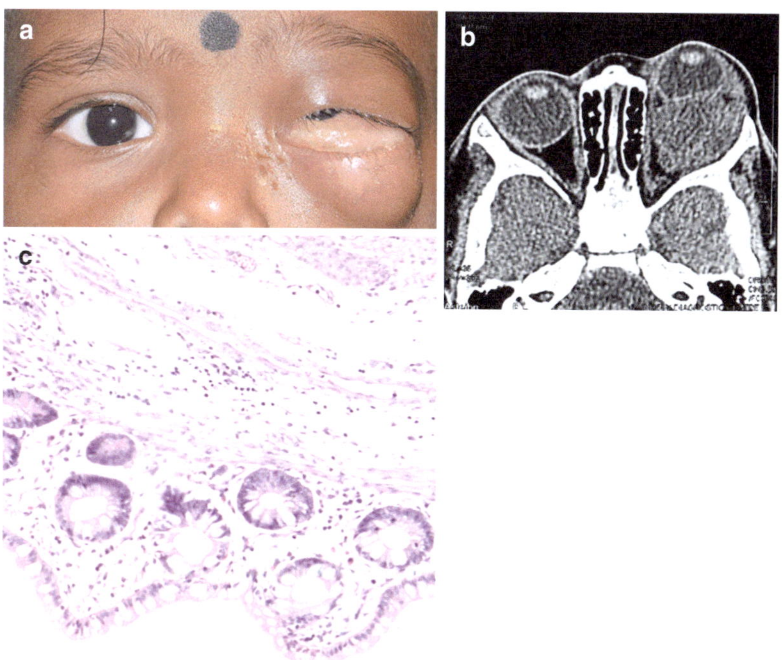

Fig. 17.2 Teratoma. Clinical photograph of a 2-year-old child with a large mass in the inferior orbit with proptosis and superior globe dystopia. CT orbit in the axial view showing a relatively well-defined isodense lesion in the left orbit indenting the globe posteriorly (**a**, **b**). Microscopy showed an intestinal gland of endodermal origin (**c**)

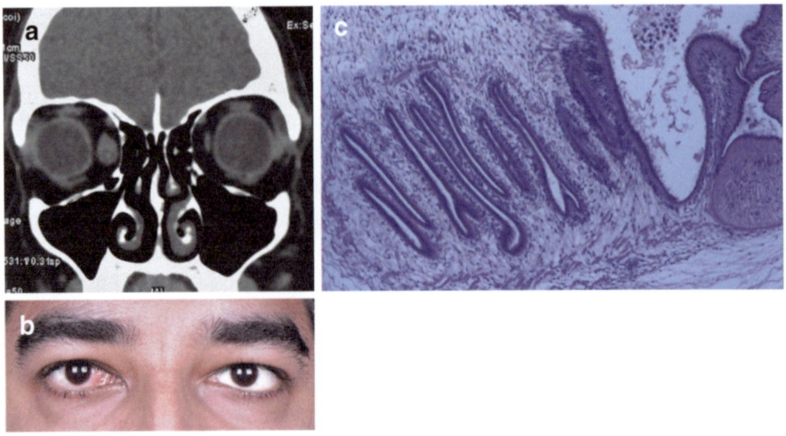

Fig. 17.3 Cysticercosis. Clinical photograph and CT scans of a 42-year-old gentleman with painful limitation of right eye movement with a circumscribed lesion in the medial rectus muscle which is isodense with a central hyperdensity (a and b). Microscopy showed larva of cysticercus forming a invaginated cyst wall and scolex (c)

persistent high level of serum alpha-fetoprotein in a treated case of malignant teratoma is indicative of recurrence of tumor or metastatic tumor.

17.3.3 Parasitic Cyst (Cysticercosis)

In 1829, Soemmering reported the first case of a live anterior chamber cysticercosis [13]. Cysticercus cellulosae, is a parasitic infestation caused by larval form of Taenia solium. Orbital and adnexal cysticercosis is reported in children and young adults with equal incidence in both genders [14]. Clinically, cysticercosis presents with periocular swelling, proptosis, ptosis, pain, diplopia, restriction of ocular motility due to extraocular muscle involvement, strabismus, decreased vision, lid edema, and orbital cellulitis. The superior rectus muscle is the most common muscle to be involved. Microscopic examination of cysticercosis shows a cystic cavity that contains the larval form of *Taenia solium*. The scolex is present at the cephalic region whereas a duct-like invagination seen at the caudal region which is lined by an eosinophilic membrane. The invaginated area is named as the scolex, and it contains a rostellum, suckers, and multiple hooklets. Host reaction is generally absent if the larva is viable. In a nonviable cyst, the cyst wall is thickened, and the scolex may degenerate into coarse mineralized granules. At this stage the host tissue responds to form granulomas composed of foreign body giant cells, epithelioid histocytes, and chronic inflammatory cells.

The serological tests used for the specific diagnosis are indirect hemagglutination, indirect immunofluorescence, and immune electrophoresis such as enzyme-linked immunosorbent assay (ELISA). Microscopic detection of adult worm in the stool may help in establishing the diagnosis (Fig. 17.3).

17.4 Inflammatory Tumors

17.4.1 Idiopathic Orbital Inflammatory Disease (IOID)

The moniker nonspecific orbital inflammatory disease (NSOID) is an idiopathic orbital inflammatory disease (IOID) also known as orbital pseudotumor. It is a benign, nonneoplastic, nonspecific, and noninfectious inflammatory disease of the orbit that may extend to peri-orbital tissues [15]. The incidence of IOID is 6–16% of orbital tumors [16]. It is more prevalent in third to sixth decade of life and more common in middle-aged women. Lacrimal gland is the most common epicenter for the inflammation [15]. IOID clinically present as periorbital edema, blepharoptosis, and a palpable mass. Radiographic imaging of the orbit shows evidence of a diffuse, poorly defined

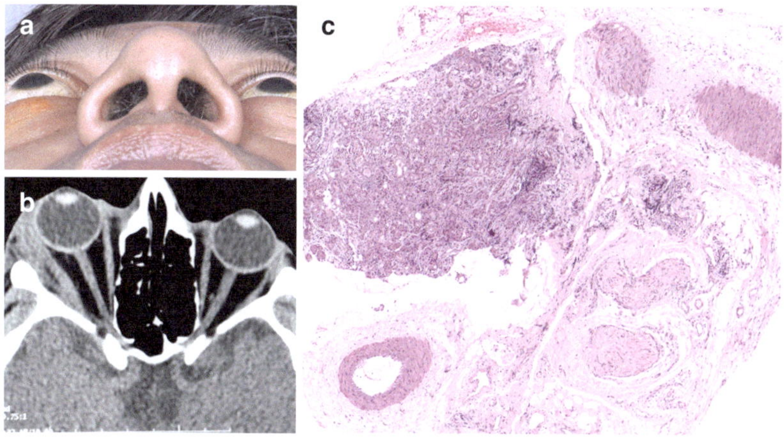

Fig. 17.4 NSOID. Clinical photograph and CT scans of a 48-year-old gentleman had painful protrusion of right eye with enlarged inferior rectus, lateral rectus and lacrimal gland (**a**, **b**). Microscopy showed chronic inflammatory cells with atrophic lacrimal gland (**c**)

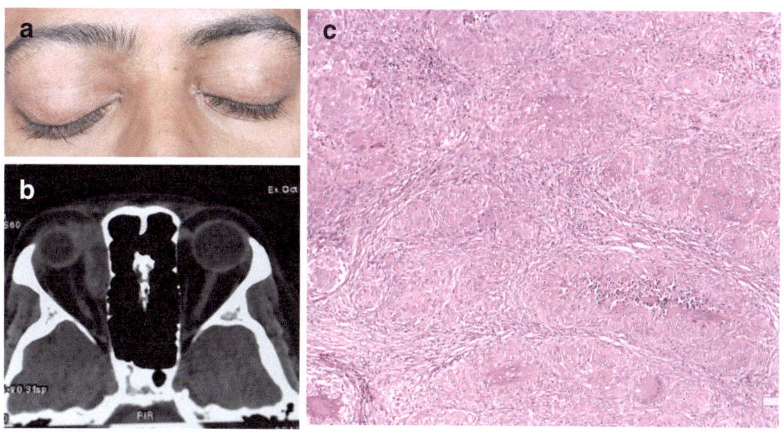

Fig. 17.5 Sarcoidosis. Clinical photograph and CT scans showed inferior dystopia and superomedial firm mass in right eye. Lesion was isodense (**a** and **b**). Microscopy showed granulomatous inflammation forming nodule-like area separated by fibrous septa (**c**)

SOL, myositis, dacryoadenitis, or perineuritis [16] (Fig. 17.4).

Histopathology of incision biopsy of the involved tissue along with ruling out specific orbital diseases is the cornerstone for forming a diagnosis of IOID. Therefore, it is likely a diagnosis of exclusion.

Microscopic examination of tissue shows polymorphic inflammatory response consisting of lymphocytes, plasma cells, macrophages, polymorphonuclear leucocytes, and eosinophils. Some of the lesions are associated with dense hyalinization and fibrovascular tissue and labelled as "sclerosing IOID".

The presence of necrosis, vasculitis, and granuloma formation almost excludes the NSOID. The close differential for IOID is IgG4-related disease for which tissue infiltration of plasma cells positive for IgG4 must be performed with immunohistochemistry stain, and serum levels of IgG4 must be examined in suspected cases.

17.4.2 Sarcoid Nodule (Sarcoidosis)

Sarcoidosis is a systemic disease of unknown etiology and is characterized by the presence of granulomas on histopathology in the affected organs. Ocular involvement is seen in about 25% of patients with sarcoidosis [17]. The most common ocular manifestation of sarcoidosis is uveitis, but any part of the eye, orbit, or lacrimal system can be involved with this disease [18] (Fig. 17.5).

Women are more likely to be affected by biopsy-proven sarcoidosis [19], and median age range varies from 45 to 55 years. Clinical manifestation of sarcoidosis are ptosis, proptosis, pain, loss of vision, palpable mass, diplopia, and eyelid swelling. In addition to these clinical findings globe displacement and tearing of eyes are other symptoms of this disease.

Microscopic examination of sarcoid nodule shows a granulomatous inflammation characterized by multiple discrete predominantly epithelioid granulomas. Classically these granulomas are of the "naked" type with few chronic inflammatory cells and rim of fibrosis and absence of necrosis. Schaumann (conchoidal) bodies, concentrically lamellated calcified nodules, are seen within the cytoplasm of multinucleated giant cells, or Asteroid bodies or star-shaped cytoplasmic inclusions may be found in some cases of sarcoidosis, but these findings are nonspecific for sarcoidosis. Chest X- ray for assessing the pulmonary involvement and elevated level of serum Angiotensin-Converting Enzyme (ACE) can be helpful in diagnosis of systemic sarcoidosis.

17.4.2.1 Fungal Granuloma (Orbital Mycosis)

Fungi are ubiquitous eukaryotic organisms found in dead, decaying vegetative matter, soil, and air. Orbital mycosis or fungal infections are lethal but rare infectious disease of orbit, and usually these infections spread to the orbit secondarily following inhalation and infection of sinuses. Orbital mycosis spread from sinuses through angioinvasion or infection from adjacent structures. Clinically they present as mass lesion which may cause delay and misdiagnosis, and patient may be treated with corticosteroid assuming the lesions are on the lines of idiopathic orbital inflammation. This may lead to a flare-up of infection and sometimes may cause death due to rapid spread of infection. *Mucorales* and *Aspergillus fumigatus* are the most common fungi to infect the orbit [20]. While fungal infections are common in the setting of a systemic immunocompromised state such as COVID-19 infection (recent pandemic), diabetes, chemotherapy for malignancy, and immunosuppressive treatment for the organ transplant [21], orbital fungal granulomas are common in immunocompetent individuals as well. Clinically orbital mycosis presents with orbital pain, periorbital edema, diplopia, ophthalmoplegia, chemosis, and decreased vision (Fig. 17.6).

Microscopically orbital mycosis shows granuloma formation which may or may not be associated with necrosis, depending on the virulence of fungus and host immunity. In immunocompromised host this infection may cause necrosis, acute fulminant disease associated with suppu-

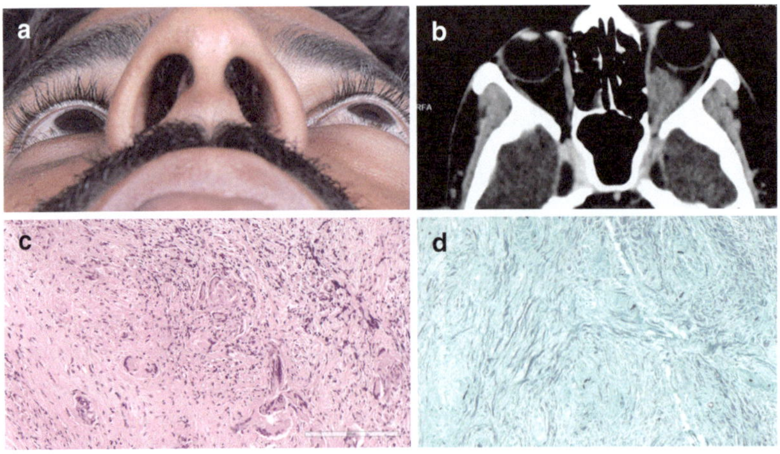

Fig. 17.6 Orbital mycosis. Clinical photograph showed left axial proptosis (**a**) and CT scan finding was well-defined hyperdense mass involving the inferior rectus muscle extending from apex to insertion (**b**) Microscopy showed granuloma formation contained multinucleated giant cells, chronic inflammatory cells and epithelioid histiocytes (**c**), and GMS confirmed the fungal filaments (**d**)

ration and necrosis of affected tissue. Angioinvasion is a prominent and diagnostic feature of mucormycosis. Special stains for fungus such as Periodic acid Schiff (PAS) and Grocott methenamine silver (GMS) stain clearly demonstrate the fungal hyphae and filaments (Fig. 17.6).

17.4.3 Hematolymphoid Tumors

Tumors of lymphoid origins or lymphoproliferative disorders of orbit or "Ocular adnexal lymphoproliferative disease" (OALD) is an umbrella term that varies from benign to malignant lesions. The lymphoproliferative lesions are the commonest primary orbital tumor among which orbital lymphoma is the most common, and it constitutes about 67–90% of all lymphoproliferative lesions. [22]

17.4.4 Reactive Lymphoid Hyperplasia/Lymphoid Hyperplasia (RLH or LH)

Orbit and adnexal structures are devoid of lymph nodes. However eyelid, conjunctiva, and lacrimal gland normally contain lymphoid tissue and lymphatic vessels from which lymphoid tissue and OALD originate. Saltzstein in 1963 first described a well-defined and differentiated lesion of lymphocytic tumors in lung which was composed of benign lymphocytes with well-formed germinal centers, and he used the term "pseudolymphoma" for these type of lesions [23] (Fig. 17.7).

The clinical presentation of low-grade lymphoma and orbital LH is similar, and it is difficult to differentiate solely on clinical presentation. These lesions generally present as a slowly progressive mass in the anterior orbit associated with minimal functional impairment since the mass tends to mold around the globe without producing an indentation on the globe. The presenting symptoms are usually tissue growth, ptosis, proptosis, and limitation in ocular motility. Few cases of orbital LH may present with inflammatory signs such as pain and redness. On clinical examination lacrimal gland lesions feel firm and rubbery, and their surface may be nodular or smooth on palpation.

Histologically, LH is characterized by dense lymphoid cell infiltrates with complete effacement of soft tissue histomorphology, and often these lymphoid cells are organized into secondary follicles of varying sizes [24]. These follicles contain well-organized zonal architecture with prominent germinal centers, and the follicles may show a starry sky appearance due to the presence of tingible body macrophages. On immune stains the lymphoid follicles contain mixture of small B- and T-cells. The Ki-67 staining reveals high mitotic activity usually restricted to germinal

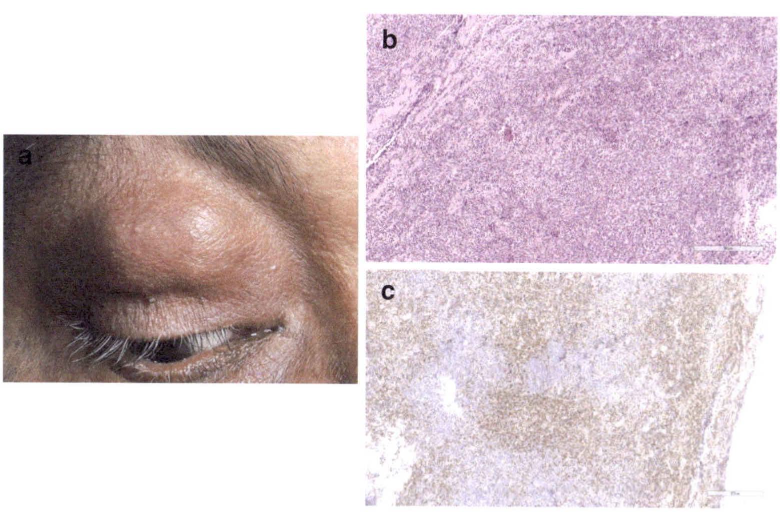

Fig. 17.7 Reactive lymphoid hyperplasia. Clinical photograph of a 52-year-old gentleman with a firm, circumscribed lesion in the upper eyelid (**a**). Histopathology showed monomorphic small round cell population (**b**), and immune stain for BCL-2 was not expressed in follicles (**c**)

centers that are usually eccentrically located near the follicle edge. The interfollicular area contains admixture of plasma cells, histiocytes, and lymphoid cells of predominantly T-cell origin (Fig. 17.7).

17.4.5 Lymphomas

Primary orbital lymphomas are very rare neoplasms of the orbit, and they constitute 1% of all non-Hodgkin's lymphoma (NHL) [25] and represent 8–10% of extranodal NHL. Over 95% are of B-cell origin [26]. Approximately 84% of orbital lymphomas are of low-grade variety, and only 16% are of high-grade on histology [27]. About 57% of orbital lymphomas are predominantly of mucosa-associated lymphoid tissue (MALT) or extranodal marginal zone lymphoma, and 19% are follicular type followed by diffuse large B-cell (DLBCL) and mantle-cell lymphomas [28].

17.4.6 Common Orbital Lymphomas

1. Extranodal marginal zone lymphoma or MALT type
2. Follicular lymphoma
3. Diffuse B-cell lymphoma

17.4.7 Extranodal Marginal Zone Lymphoma (ENMZL)

The most common subtype of primary ocular adnexal lymphomas (OALs) is extranodular marginal zone lymphoma (ENMZL) of mucosa-associated lymphoid tissue (MALT) type which constitute 35–80% of cases of all NHL.

EMZNL is commonly seen in the fifth to seventh decades of life with female predominance and in male/female ratio of 1:1.5/2. About 40% of EMZNL arise from the orbit, followed by conjunctiva in 35–40% cases, lacrimal gland in 10–15% cases, and eyelid in 10% of cases. In 10–15% of cases EMZNL is bilateral in presentation [29–31].

Orbital lymphoid proliferations clinically present as a palpable, firm to rubbery mass causing slowly, progressive proptosis which may be associated with periorbital edema, decreased visual acuity, motility disturbances, and diplopia (Fig. 17.8).

Conjunctival lymphoma typically presents as a mobile-pink or salmon-pink colored lesion in the fornices. This could be incidentally picked up, or the patient may present with redness and irritation. Lacrimal gland lymphomas can produce an inferior dystopia.

On histologic examination, extranodal marginal zone B-cell lymphoma of MALT type or MALTOMA or MALT lymphoma is characterized by monotonous population of lymphoid cells with poorly defined follicles. The characteristic histopathological feature of MALT lymphoma is lymphoepithelial lesions (LEL), defined by the infiltration and distortion of epithelial structures by aggregates of neoplastic lymphoid cells.

On immune stain the lymphoid cells in LEL and poorly defined follicles of MALT type are CD20 (corresponding to B-cell marker) positive and CD3-negative (corresponding to T-cell marker). Apoptotic marker BCL-2 overexpressed in lymphoid cells and LEL. Extramarginal marginal zone lymphomas are low-grade lymphomas having low Ki-67 index.

17.4.8 Follicular Lymphoma (FL)

Follicular lymphoma accounts for 5–10% of all ocular adnexal lymphoma [32, 33] and most ocular adnexal FLs occur in middle-aged and elderly patients with a female predominance in the female–male ratio of 1.6 [34].

In primary FL, the conjunctiva is the most common site of involvement (29% cases), followed by orbit (26% of cases) and the lacrimal gland (26%) [35]. FLs generally present with painless proptosis, diplopia, and a palpable mass. Clinical presentation is like the other ocular adnexal lymphomas.

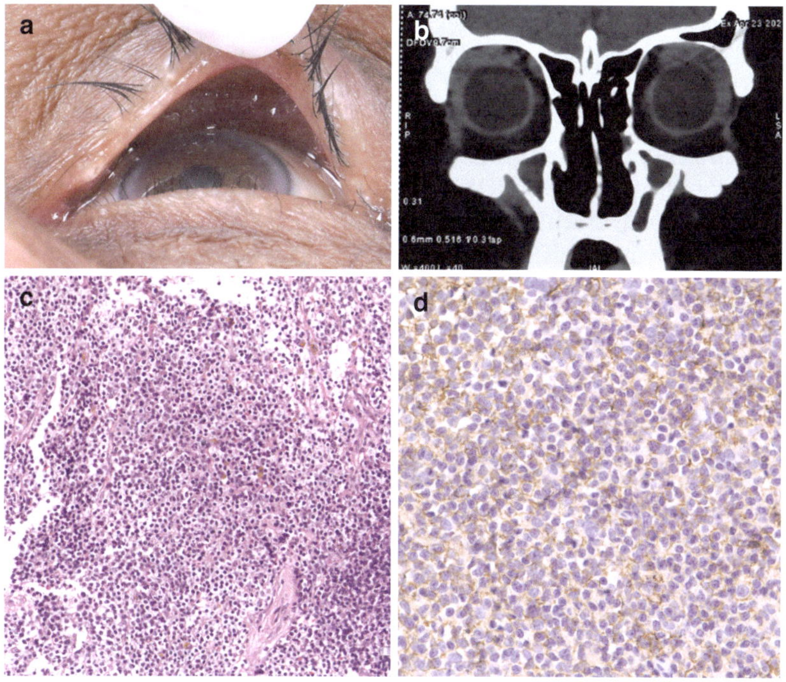

Fig. 17.8 Extramarginal zone lymphoma. Clinical photograph of a 65-year-old lady with a firm lesion noted in the superior sulcus with corresponding CT scan of both orbits showing molding of irregular isodense lesions around the globes in the superotemporal orbits (**a**, **b**). Microscopy showed small round cell infiltrates with complete effacement of soft tissue (**c**), these small round cells demonstrated diffuse membranous expression of CD20 (**d**)

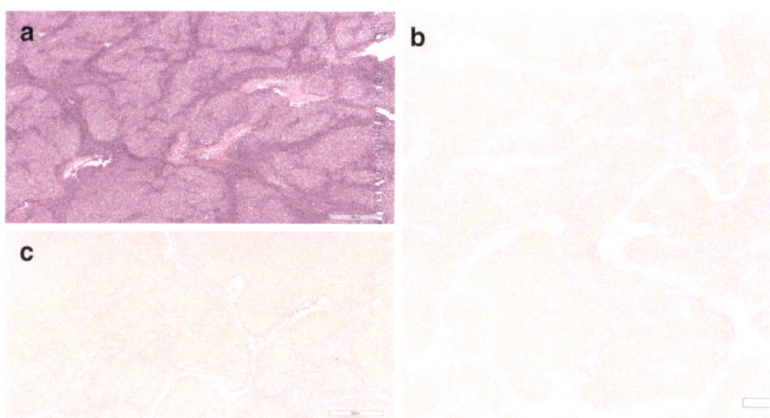

Fig. 17.9 Follicular lymphoma. Microscopic examination showed lymphoid cell population forming follicles (**a**), these neoplastic follicles expressed CD10 (**b**) and BCL-2 (**c**)

The histopathology finding in FL is complete effacement of soft tissue with infiltration of lymphoid cells predominantly composed of centrocytes and centroblasts. Nonpolarized lymphoid follicles of similar sizes with absent tingible body macrophages and absent mantle zone are mostly found in the cases of FL. Immune stain shows CD20 and BCL-2 expression in the neoplastic follicles with germinal center marker CD10 (Fig. 17.9).

Grading of follicular lymphoma is based on the number of centroblasts per high power field (Table 17.1). Depending on the number of centroblasts follicular lymphoma is classified into grade 1 to grade 3 (A&B).

(World Health Organization grading of follicular lymphoma)

Only histopathological findings are considered

Diffuse large B-cell lymphoma, not otherwise specified (DLBCL, NOS)

Diffuse large B-cell lymphomas (DLBCL) are aggressive lymphomas, and primary orbital and periorbital DLBCLs are an uncommon form of NHL. In all OALs, diffuse large B-cell lymphoma comprises 5–15% of cases and occurs most commonly in the orbit [36, 37].

Table 17.1 Grading of follicular lymphoma is based on the number of centroblasts per high power field

Grading	Number of centroblasts per high power field
1	0–5 centroblasts/high power field
2	6–15 centroblasts/high power field
3A	>15 centroblasts/high power field Centrocytes present
3B	>15 centroblasts/high power field Lack centrocytes

The usual clinical presentation of DLBCL is like any other OALs. The most frequent clinical presentation of DLBCL includes palpebral or orbital mass and exophthalmos.

The histopathology of DLBCL shows soft tissue infiltrate with diffuse sheets of large cells with irregular nuclear membranes and prominent nuclei. Numerous mitotic figures and intervening apoptotic cells are found between the large cells. These large cells are B-cells, and the 2008 WHO classification defines DLBCL as a diffuse growth of neoplastic large B lymphoid cells with nuclear size equal to or exceeding that of normal macrophage nuclei [38].

17.4.9 Immunohistochemistry

Cells in DLBCL are positive for CD20, PAX-5, CD19, and CD22. Variable BCL-2 and BCL-6 expression with a high Ki-67 index can be found (Fig. 17.10)

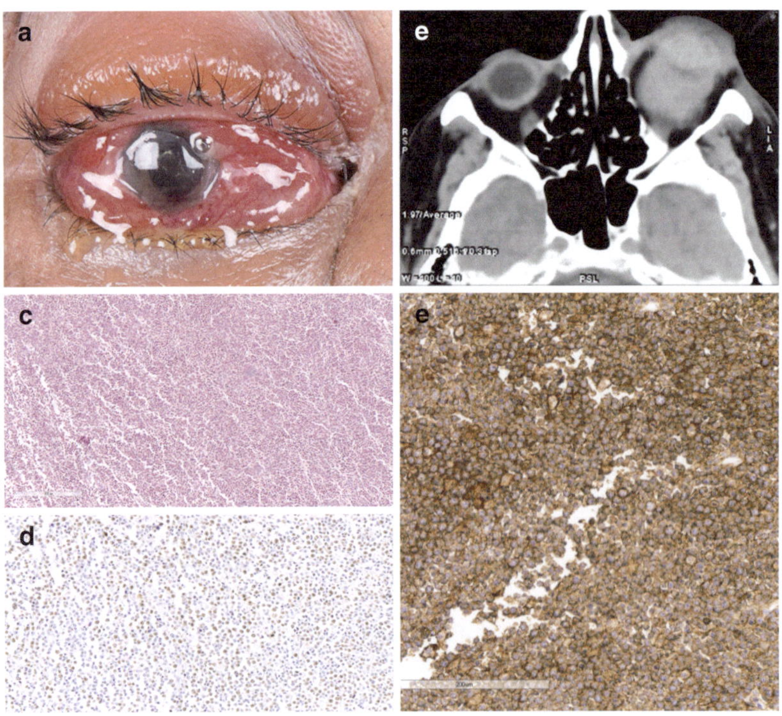

Fig. 17.10 Diffuse large B-cell lymphoma. High magnification photograph of the left eye and CT scan of a 60-year-old gentleman with left eye intraocular and orbital diffuse large B-cell lymphoma (**a**, **b**). Histopathology showed sheets of intermediate round cells having conspicuous nucleoli, irregular nuclear membrane infiltrating the soft tissue (**c**), and these round cells showed high Ki-67 index (**d**) and diffuse expression of CD20 (**e**)

17.4.10 Subclassification of DLBCLs

Morphologic variants of DLBCLs

- Centroblastic
- Immunoblastic
- T-cell/histiocyte rich
- Anaplastic

Based on gene expressions DLBCLs are:

- Germinal center B-cell like (GCB)
- Activated B-cell like (ABC)

17.4.11 Extramedullary Myeloid Sarcoma

Myeloid sarcoma (MS) is an extramedullary abnormal proliferation of primitive immature precursors of the granulocytic series of white blood cells which form solid tumor [39] (Fig. 17.11).

Myeloid sarcoma is a rare presentation of acute myeloid leukemia (AML) reported in 2.5–9.1% patients and is characterized by the presence of one or more tumors in extramedullary sites such as orbit, bone, lymph nodes, gastrointestinal tract, subcutaneous tissues, and central nervous system [40]. MS of orbit or other soft tissue can be diagnosed before the diagnosis of acute myeloid leukemia or hematologic malignancies.

The most frequent clinical manifestation of orbital MS is the unilateral exophthalmos, and other possible signs include painful lacrimal gland swelling, ptosis, tearing, and the presence of a conjunctival mass.

The histopathological examination of the orbital biopsy, malignant round cell tumor arranged in singly scattered, loose sheets, islands, or file pattern with thin fibrous septa. The individual tumor cells are round, ranging from intermediate to large in size, and contain scant cytoplasm, vesicular chromatin, and conspicuous nucleoli (blast cells). These round cells express myeloperoxidase, LCA (Leukocyte Common Antigen (need to expand), and CD68, which indicate their myeloid origin, and are negative for CD20 and CD3. A list of differentials for myeloid sarcoma and a panel of immune stains are essential to clinch the diagnosis.

17.4.12 Rosai–Dorfman Disease (RDD)

Rosai–Dorfman disease (RDD) is a rare, idiopathic, nonneoplastic, non-Langerhans cell type of histioproliferative disorder of unknown etiol-

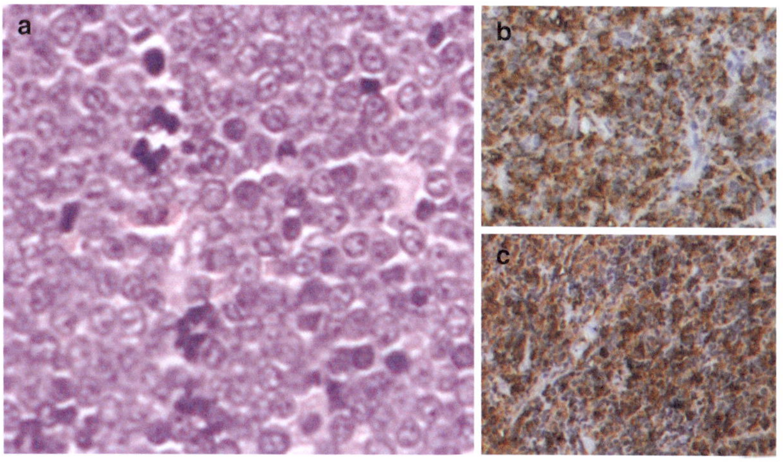

Fig. 17.11 Myeloid sarcoma. Histopathology showed sheets of round cells with prominent nucleoli (blast cells) (**a**) and these cells were positive for myeloperoxidase (MPO) (**b**) and CD68 (**c**)

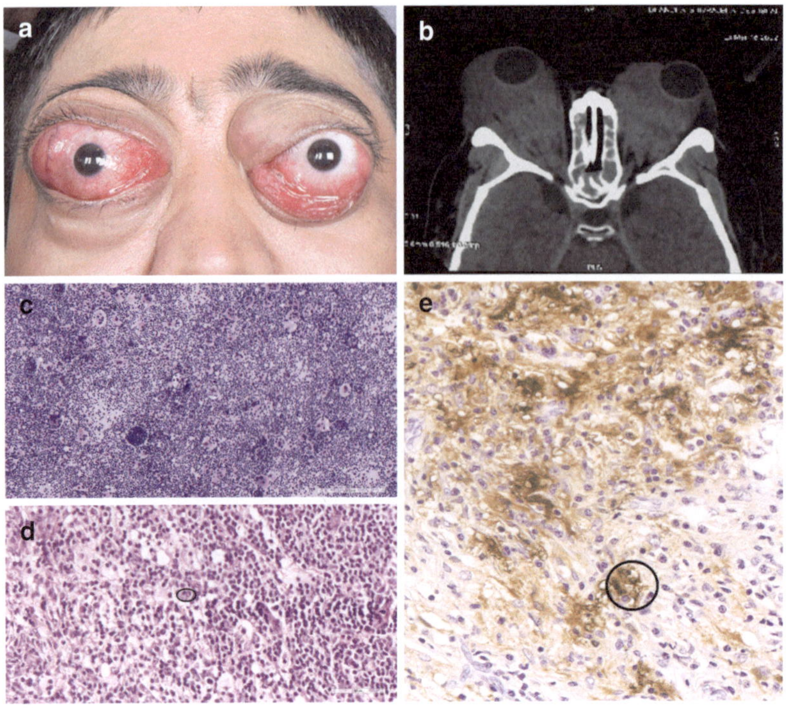

Fig. 17.12 Rosai–Dorfman disease. Clinical photograph and CT scan of a 28-year-old gentleman with Rosai–Dorfman disease involving both orbits leading to massive proptosis of both eyes (**a**, **b**). Fine needle aspiration and biopsy of the tissue showed lymphoid cells with lymphophagocytosis or emperipolesis (**c**, **d**). S-100 immune stain clearly demonstrated emperipolesis (**e**)

ogy. Extranodal RDD occurs rarely, and the common sites are eyes, ocular adnexa, and orbit [41]. Ocular RDD is a benign and self-limited disease, but clinically may simulate malignancy [42]. In 1969 Rosai and Dorfman described it as a separate entity for sinus histiocytosis with massive lymphadenopathy. The RDD is a rare pseudolymphomatous disorder characterized by persistent massive lymphadenopathy with increased histiocytes inside the lymph node sinuses [43] (Fig. 17.12).

The ophthalmic manifestations of RDD include presentation with orbital, eyelid, or epibulbar masses; lacrimal sac and/or duct obstruction; and rarely uveitis, scleritis, and compressive optic neuropathy [44].

Microscopically, the hallmark of RDD is emperipolesis which is characterized by the presence of intact cells mainly plasma cells or lymphocytes inside the histiocytes. Emperipolesis is different from phagocytosis. In the latter, histiocytes are engulfed by the cells and lysed by lysosomal enzymes. The soft tissue shows fibrosis and inflammatory cells (plasma cells and lymphocytes) admixed with histiocytes and emperipolesis. On immune stain RDD histiocytes are positive for CD68 and S-100. S-100 clearly demonstrates emperipolesis, whereas histiocytes are negative for CD1a which differentiates it from Langerhans' cell histiocytosis [45] (Fig. 17.12).

17.4.13 Vascular Lesions

Among all the space-occupying lesions of the orbit, vascular tumors and malformations account for 6.2–12.0% [46–50]. Based on the nature and for the convenience of management, vascular lesions were classified depending on the flow as static or dynamic, and according to distensibility and pulsatility (venous anomalies and arteriovenous anomalies). The diagnosis and management of vascular lesions sometimes lack clarity and may lead to mismanagement. To avoid these dif-

Table 17.2 The simple classification of orbital/ocular vascular lesions adopted from ISSVA (2014)

Vascular malformations		
Major blood vessel malformations	Simple malformations	Combined malformations
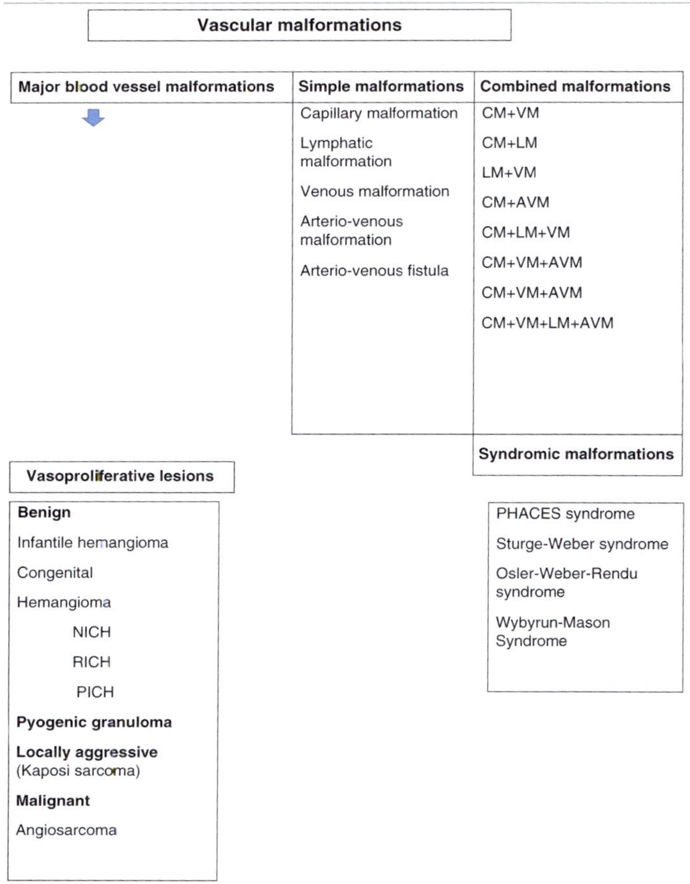	Capillary malformation Lymphatic malformation Venous malformation Arterio-venous malformation Arterio-venous fistula	CM + VM CM + LM LM + VM CM + AVM CM + LM + VM CM + VM + AVM CM + VM + AVM CM + VM + LM + AVM

(continued)

Table 17.2 (continued)

Vaso proliferative lesions		Syndromic malformations
Benign Infantile hemangioma Congenital Hemangioma NICH RICH PICH Pyogenic granuloma Locally aggressive (Kaposi sarcoma) Malignant Angiosarcoma		PHACES syndrome Sturge-Weber syndrome Osler-Weber-Rendu syndrome Wyburn-Mason Syndrome

Abbreviations: *CM* Capillary malformation, *VM* Venous malformation, *LM* Lymphatic Malformation, *AVM* Arterio-venous malformation, *NICH* Non-involuting congenital hemangioma, *PICH* Partially involuting congenital hemangioma, *RICH* Rapidly involuting congenital hemangioma ficulties, the International Society for the Study of Vascular Anomalies (ISSVA) in 2014 [51] reclassified all vascular lesions based on the clinical, radiological, and histological findings and natural history of the disease. Vascular lesions were broadly categorized into vasoproliferative tumors and vascular malformations. The simple classification of orbital/ocular vascular lesions adopted from ISSVA (2014) in Table 17.2.

17.4.14 Capillary Hemangioma

Capillary hemangioma is the most common orbital vascular tumor in infants, with an overall incidence of 5.6%. The occurrence of capillary hemangioma is more common in females (F:M, 3:2). The location of these vascular lesions is commonly extraconal, and they may extend intracranially through the optic canal or orbital fissures [52]. Clinically capillary hemangiomas may cause globe displacement, amblyopia, and or proptosis. The lesion appears blue when located subcutaneously and red when situated in superficial planes. The lesioned tissue displays proliferation of small capillary-sized blood vessels lined by benign endothelial cells. These blood vessels are separated by thin fibrous septa. We need to add the term strawberry nevus (Fig. 17.13).

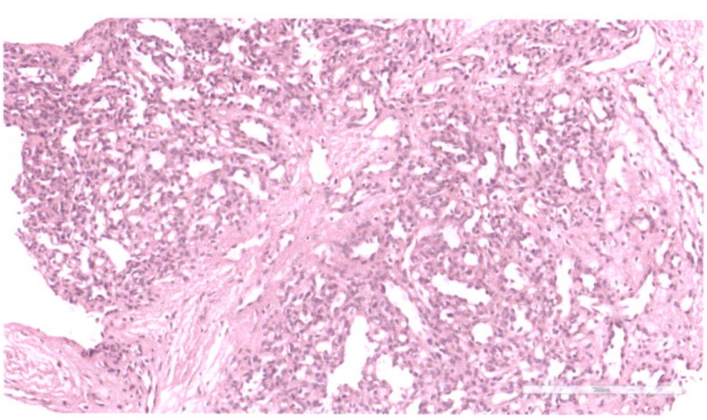

Fig. 17.13 Capillary hemangioma. Microscopic examination showed small-caliber blood vessels lined by endothelial cells, and these blood vessels are separated by thin fibrous septa (**c**)

17.4.15 Cavernous Hemangioma (Cavernous Vascular Malformation)

Cavernous hemangiomas are cavernous malformations and are the most common vascular lesions in adults. There is disagreement about the origin of cavernous hemangiomas; some authors suggest these lesions are of venous origin, and some contend they are low-flow arteriovenous malformation [53]. Cavernous hemangiomas are more common in women in the age range of 18–72 years [54]. Most of the cavernous malformations abruptly present with proptosis in females during puberty or pregnancy indicative of a possible role of hormone- or cytokine-mediated angiogenesis in the growth of these lesions [55]. These lesions are slowly progressive and clinically present as painless proptosis [53], and less common symptoms are lid swelling, palpable mass, diplopia, and visual disturbances [52]. The word cavernous is derived from "Cavern," which means a large hollow or cavity; hence cavernous hemangioma histologically has large blood-filled spaces which are lined by benign endothelial cells and separated by thin fibrous septa (Fig. 17.14).

17.4.16 Lymphangioma

Lymphangiomas are no-flow or low-flow vascular malformations. There are now termed as Veno-lymphatic malformations (VLM). The term VLM is used for these malformations that arise from pluripotent venous anlage which can differentiate into venous and lymphatic structures [56]. The incidence of these malformation is equal in male and female [57] and commonly present in infancy or childhood. These lesions clinically present as slow progressive proptosis, globe displacement, restrictions in eye mobility, and hemorrhage. Hemorrhage can occur with minor trauma or

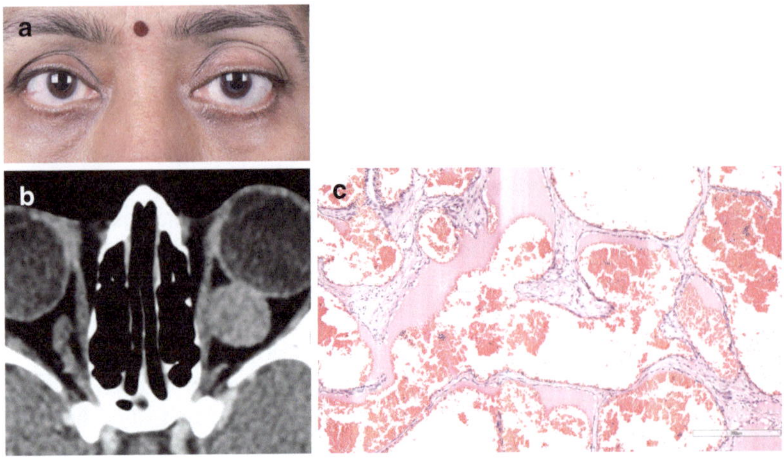

Fig. 17.14 Cavernous hemangioma. Cavernous vascular malformation). Clinical photograph and CT scan of a 50-year-old lady with proptosis of the left eye and a well-defined lesion posterior to the globe signifying a cavernous venous malformation (**a**, **b**). Microscopic examination showed large cystically dilated blood vessels lined by flattened endothelial cells and filled with blood (**c**)

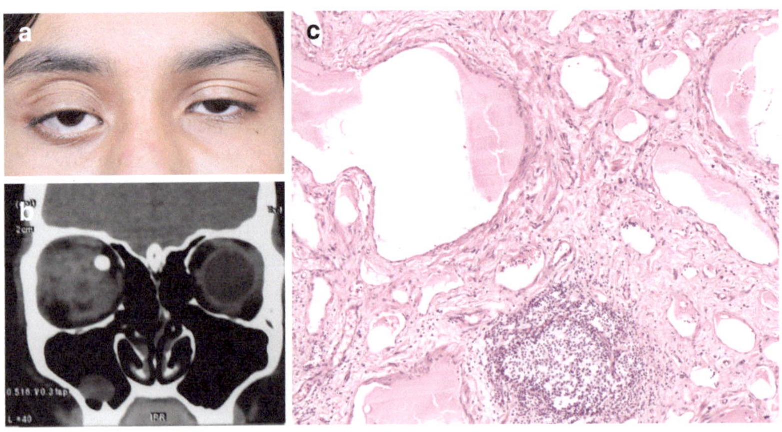

Fig. 17.15 Lymphangioma. Clinical photograph of a 25-year-old lady with inferior dystopia and proptosis of the right eye. CT scan shows a heterogenous multiloculated lesion with cystic spaces in the intra- and extraconal spaces (**a**, **b**). Histopathology showed irregular dilated vascular channels separated by fibrous septa and consisting of lymphoid cell aggregates focally. These vascular channels were filled with eosinophilic fluid (**c**)

infections. They present on histopathology as thin, delicate, irregularly spaced vascular channels of variable sizes ranging from capillary to cavernous caliber, and filled with colourless lymph. The luminal wall of vascular channels is lined by endothelial cells. The intervening septa of vascular channels contain lymphocytes and lymphoid follicles with neovascular tufts (Fig. 17.15).

17.4.17 Solitary Fibrous Tumor

Solitary fibrous tumors (SFTs) are rare mesenchymal spindle-cell neoplasms which commonly arise from the pleura and can also originate from liver, lungs, peritoneum, pericardium, kidney, and uncommonly from the head and neck origin [58]. Orbital SFT clinically causes slowly progressive painless proptosis. The common age of

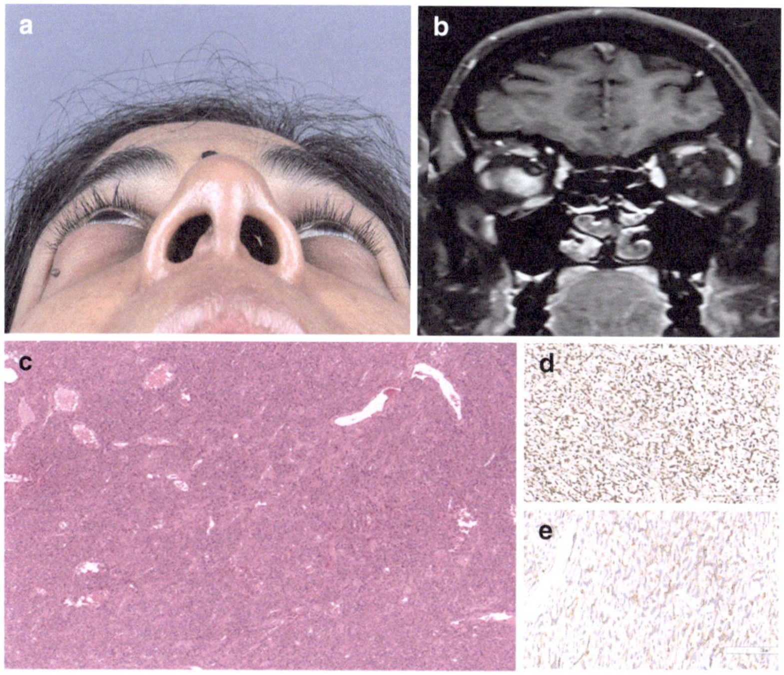

Fig. 17.16 Solitary fibrous tumor (SFT). Clinical image shows proptosis of right eye (**a**), and T1- and T2-weighted MRI shows hypo- and hyperdense heterogenous lesion involving anterior and mid-orbit with molding around posterior part of globe (**b**). Microscopic examination showed spindle cells arranged in a patternless pattern with entrapped staghorn-shaped blood vessels (**c**), and immune stain for STAT-6 (**d**) with CD34 (**e**) confirms the diagnosis of SFT

presentation is the fourth decade of life and age range of 9–76 years [59] (Fig. 17.16).

Microscopic examination of SFT generally shows a well-circumscribed, encapsulated cellular mass composed of spindle cells arranged in whorl or patternless pattern. These spindle cells contain moderate amount of cytoplasm with an indistinct cell border and mildly pleomorphic nuclei with inconspicuous to prominent nucleoli. In between the tumor cells entrapped blood vessels of varying caliber and staghorn pattern of blood vessels can also be found.

Immune stain for CD99, CD34 and BCL-2 are strongly expressed in spindle cells of SFT (Fig. 17.16).

17.4.18 Lacrimal Gland Tumor

In all space-occupying lesion (SOL) of orbit, lacrimal gland mass contributes 10% [60] and out of this 50% are epithelial origin and 50% are non-epithelial origin. The most common epithelial benign lesion of the lacrimal gland is the benign mixed tumor (pleomorphic adenoma), which generally presents as a painless mass, whereas malignant lesion of epithelial origin presents with painful swelling of the upper eyelid.

17.4.19 Benign Mixed Tumor (Pleomorphic Adenoma, PA)

Pleomorphic adenoma is the most common lacrimal gland tumor and constitutes 3–5% of all orbital tumors and 50% of all epithelial tumors of the lacrimal gland [61, 62]. Clinically PA presents as slowly painless progressive proptosis with inferonasal displacement of the eyeball. The most common age of presentation is fourth and fifth decades of life [60, 61].

Grossly PA appear as encapsulated grayish white nodular mass. The cut surface appears homogenous grayish white with myxoid substance.

Microscopically, PA contains a mixture of epithelial, myoepithelial, and stomal cells. Tumor cells are arranged in glandular, trabecular, and tubular patterns with areas of solid sheets and cystic patterns. The inner layer of tumor cells is lined by epithelial cells of cuboidal to basaloid

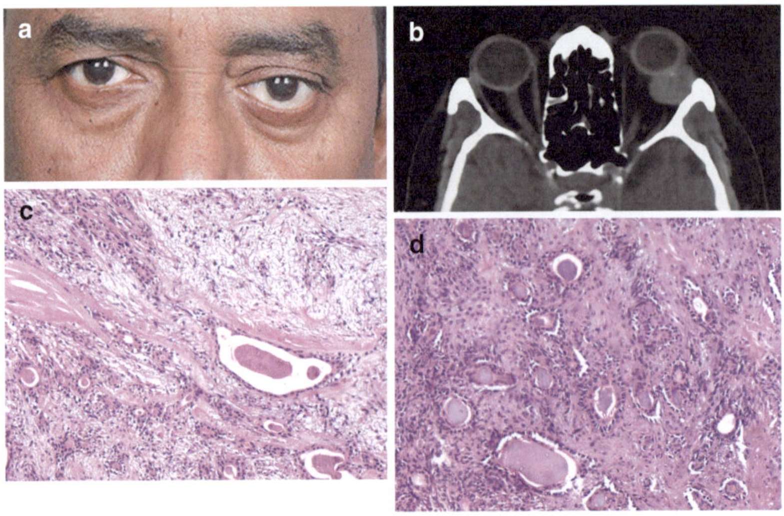

Fig. 17.17 Pleomorphic adenoma. Clinical photograph of a 48-year-old gentleman with inferior dystopia and proptosis of the left eye. CT scan shows a well-defined isodense lesion in the left lacrimal gland area without surrounding bone erosion or fossa formation (**a**, **b**). Microscopic examination showed epithelial and myoepithelial cells forming gland and tubules in which few glands were filled with eosinophilic fluid. Background was chondromyxoid substance (**c**, **d**)

cell type, and outer layer is lined by myoepithelial cells of plasmacytoid, spindle cells to stellate cells type. Stromal or mesenchymal components are myxoid to chondromyxoid to osseous substance. The tumor area may show adipose, sebaceous, osseous, or squamous (with keratinization and pearl) metaplasia (Fig. 17.17).

17.4.20 Adenoid Cystic Carcinoma (ACC)

The most common malignant tumor of lacrimal gland is adenoid cystic carcinoma, and it constitutes 1.6% of all orbital tumors [63, 64]. These tumors have no gender-predilection, and common age of clinical presentation is 40 years of age, with an age range of 6.5 to 80 years. Clinically ACC presents as rapid-onset temporal mass associated with globe displacement, diplopia, visual change, ptosis, and lacrimation. ACC has a tendency to invade nerves or perineural invasion, so these patients may present with pain. Microscopically ACC presents in three patterns, and these patterns are cribriform, tubular, and solid. Variable combination of these patterns can be seen in individual patients. Perineural involvement and lymphovascular emboli are characteristics of ACC (Fig. 17.18).

17.4.21 Cribriform Pattern

This is also called Swiss cheese or sieve-like pattern of tumor, and this pattern is the most common in ACC and almost found in all cases of adenoid cystic carcinoma, even in small focal areas. The tumor island shows basaloid or myoepithelial cells and form glandular area with lumen which are filled with eosinophilic PAS positive, diastase resistant, or alcian blue-positive basophilic myxoid substance. The basaloid cells are predominant type of neoplastic cells and contain angulated nuclei and scanty cytoplasm with indistinct cell borders.

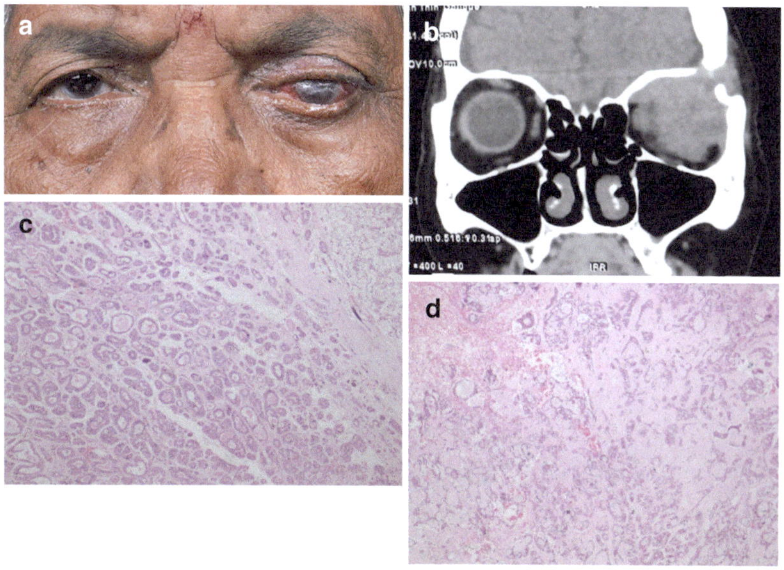

Fig. 17.18 Adenoid cystic carcinoma. Clinical photograph of a 67-year-old lady with left eye proptosis and inferior dystopia leading to exposure keratopathy. CT scan shows an ill-defined large isodense lesion in the left lacrimal gland area with surrounding bone erosion with extension into the temporal fossa (**a**, **b**). Microscopically tumor showed cribriform, acinar and solid pattern of neoplastic cells (**c**, **d**)

17.4.22 Tubular Pattern

The tumor forms elongated tubules and is lined by a single layer of ductal cells which are surrounded by single or multiple layers of basaloid cells. These tubules are strangulated as they are embedded in abundant hyaline material.

17.4.23 Solid Pattern

The tumor cells are basaloid type and closely packed to form aggregates. The stroma may not be seen. There is an absence of peripheral palisading of nuclei, and tumor cells show nuclear pleomorphism and mitotic activity.

17.4.24 Meningioma

Meningioma arises from the arachnoid layer of meninges and constitutes approximately 4% of all intraorbital tumors. Cells lining the intraorbital and intracanalicular portion of optic nerve give rise the primary lesions, and secondary lesions originate from the intracranial extension of meningioma to the orbit [65] (Fig. 17.19).

Intraorbital meningiomas are most common in young adult females [66]. Childhood meningiomas are more aggressive and tend to have poor prognosis in comparison to their adult counterparts. According to the WHO, the majority of meningiomas are benign and are categorized as grade 1 with the most common variant being meningothelial meningioma [65]. Meningioma usually presents with painless progressive proptosis and visual loss.

Microscopically, the tumor cells are cellular and arranged in a whorl pattern and contain syncytial cells having indistinct cell borders, eosinophilic cytoplasm, and uniform nuclei with pseudoinclusions. A few psammomatous calcification between the tumor cells can be found.

17.4.25 Other Tumors of Orbit

17.4.25.1 Rhabdomyosarcoma (RMS)

Rhabdomyosarcoma contributes 4% of all SOL of orbit in children, and the mean age of presentation or diagnosis is 6–8 years [66]. Previously

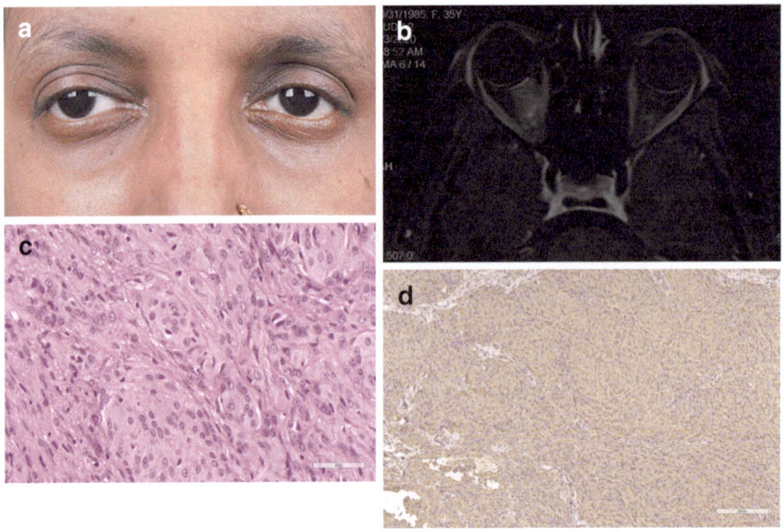

Fig. 17.19 Meningioma. Clinical photograph of a 35-year-old lady with right eye axial proptosis with mild resistance to retropulsion. T1-weighted MRI shows a well-defined intraconal lesion encasing right optic nerve (**a**, **b**). Histopathology showed whorl pattern of meningothelial cells having round to oval nuclei with eosinophilic cytoplasm and few of the cells also showed intranuclear inclusion (**c**). Tumor cells were positive for vimentin (**d**)

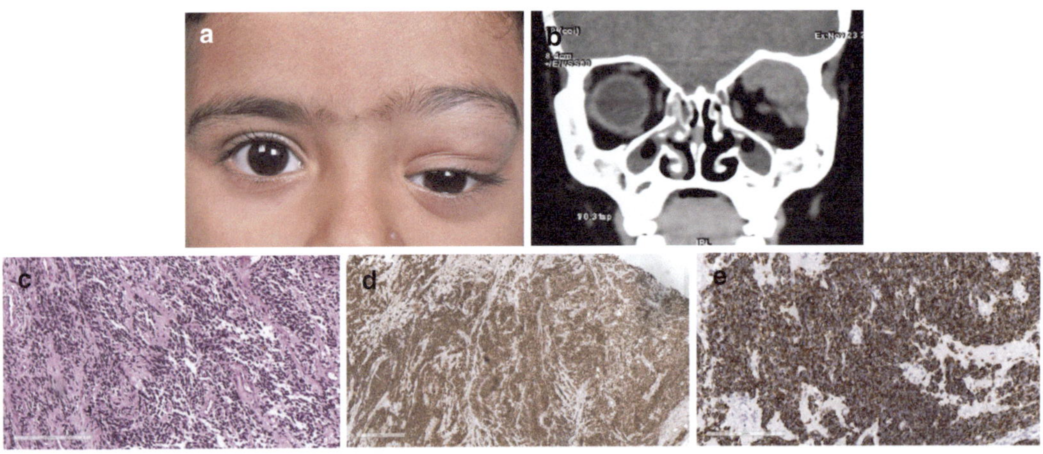

Fig. 17.20 Rhabdomyosarcoma. Clinical photograph showed proptosis of left eye and CT scan showed a dense mass lesion superolateral of orbit (**a**, **b**). Microscopic examination showed a tumor forming alveoli and nest and had oval to spindle cells with hyperchromatic nuclei (**c**). These tumor cells were positive for desmin and MyoD1 (**d**, **e**)

it was thought that RMS originated from extraocular muscles, but now it is believed that it originates from pluripotent mesenchymal cells which can differentiate into skeletal muscle (Fig. 17.20).

Orbital RMS clinically presents with rapidly progressive proptosis over weeks and or globe displacement predominantly downward and outward [67, 68].

17.4.25.2 Histopathological Features

On histopathologically embryonal, alveolar, and pleomorphic variants of RMS can be observed. In 1958, Horn and Enterline proposed that rhabdomyosarcomas could be subdivided into embryonal, alveolar, botryoid, and pleomorphic types [69]. Embryonal and alveolar RMS are common in children and adolescents, whereas pleomorphic RMS is common in adults.

17.4.25.3 Embryonal RMS (ERMS)

Embryonal RMS is a primitive myoblastic neoplasm mostly found in hollow visceral organs, the genitourinary tract, and the head and neck region. The histologic features of ERMS include round blue cells to spindle cells of mesenchymal origin arranged in loose sheets or fascicles with alternating hypocellular and hypercellular areas in myxoid background. These mesenchymal cells are in various stages of myogenesis, including primitive stellate cells, differentiating rhabdomyoblasts with elongated and eosinophilic, so-called tadpole or spider cells, and terminally differentiated cells with cross-striations or myotube formation [70]. On immunohistochemistry ERMS show positivity for desmin, patchy to moderate intensity for myogenin, and MyoD1. These tumor cells express high proliferation index (Ki-67) and are negative for *FOXO1* (*FKHR*) rearrangements demonstrated by Fluorescence in situ hybridization (FISH) method.

17.4.25.4 Alveolar RMS (ARMS)

On histomorphology of ARMS, tumor cells are blue round cells forming nests that are separated by fibrous septa and have a vague resemblance with fetus alveoli. Classic variant of ARMS have an alveolar arrangement of round cells, whereas the solid variant of ARMS may mimic ERMS. The cells in the solid variant are large and form nests and an alveolar pattern. Coagulative necrosis may be present. Myogenin is strongly expressed in ARMS, and 50% of cases also express cytokeratin and neuroendocrine markers chromogranin and synaptophysin [71]. ARMS exhibits typical cytogenetic characteristics, including t(2;13)(q35;q14) or t(1;13)(p36;q14), which result in *PAX3-FOXO1* or *PAX7-FOXO1* fusion genes. Detection of the fusion gene by RT-PCR or of the FOXO1 translocation by FISH is commonly used for molecular diagnosis [72].

17.4.25.5 Pleomorphic RMS

Pleomorphic RMS is a high-grade sarcoma composed of undifferentiated round and spindle cells that display skeletal-muscle differentiation without embryonal or alveolar components [73]. These tumors are aggressive in nature and have high propensity for visceral and bone metastasis.

17.4.26 Metastatic Tumors

Out of all orbital tumors metastatic orbital neoplasm constitute approximately 1–13% cases [74, 75].The most common mode of orbital metastasis is hematogenous route from the primary site and the most common primary sites from which tumor spread to orbit are breast, lung, and prostate [76]. Carcinomas from different primary sites are commonly metastasizes to the orbit whereas sarcoma or melanoma have rare tendency to metastasize to the orbit [77]. The mean age of presentation of orbital Metastasis is 60 years, and clinically these patients commonly present with diplopia, proptosis, pain, decreased vision, ptosis, and palpable mass [74]. As the orbit is a compact small structure, metastatic deposit rapidly causes symptoms and signs due to mass effect or invasion.

Anterior orbit is commonly invaded and reported to be involved in 66% of cases of orbital metastasis [75], whereas posterior orbit metastatic deposits less common than the anterior orbit [74].

For the confirmation of orbital metastasis radiological evaluation and biopsy with immune stain is essential. In most instances the metastatic tumor in orbit histopathologically resembles with the primary tumor, but sometimes poor differentiation or high grading of tumor makes it difficult to diagnose on histomorphological basis, in such cases panel of immune stains like cytokeratin, CK-7, and CK-20 provide some clue of primary origin of tumor [78]. Metastatic workup algorithm for tumor is provided in the following diagram.

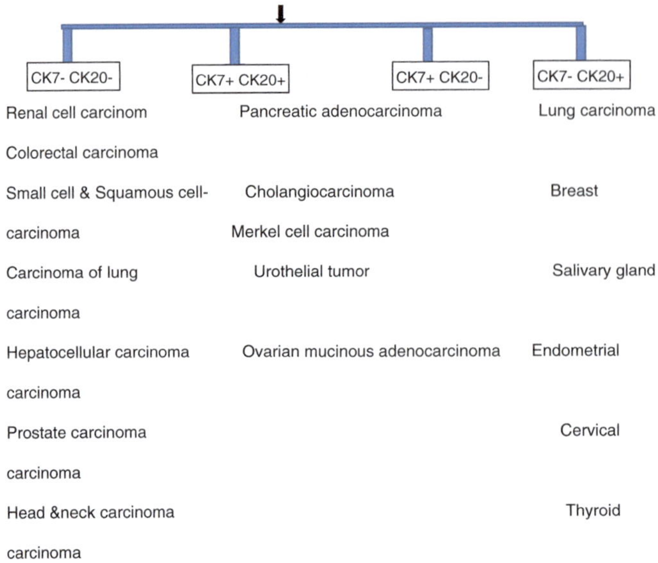

References

1. Yanoff M, Sassani JW. Ocular pathology. Elsevier Health Sciences; 2018 Dec 5.
2. Alkatan HM, Al Marek F, Elkhamary S. Demographics of pediatric orbital lesions: a tertiary eye center experience in Saudi Arabia. J Epidemiol Glob Health. 2019;9(1):3.
3. Grovc AS Jr. Orbital disorders: diagnosis and managemcnt. In: McCord Jr CD, editor. Oculoplastic. Surgery. Ncw York: Raven Press; 1981. p. 274–7.
4. Pfeiffcr RL, Nicholl RJ. Dcrmoid and cpidermoid tumours of the orbit. A rch Ophthal. 1948;40:639.
5. Pear BL. Epidermoid and dermoid sequestration cysts. Am J Roentgenol Radium Therapy, Nucl Med. 1970;110:148–55.
6. New GB, Drich JB. Dermoid cysts of the head and neck. Surg Gynecol Obstet. 1937;65:48–55.
7. Tapper D, Lack EE. Teratomas in infancy and childhood. A 54-year experience at the Children's Hospital Medical Center. Ann Surg. 1983;198:398–410.
8. Günalp I, Gündüz K. Cystic lesions of the orbit. Int Ophthalmol. 1996;20:273–7.
9. Choi SH, Han YB, Lee TJ. A case of congenital orbital teratoma. Korean J Ophthalmol. 1987;1:139–44.
10. Damato PJ, Damato FJ. Neonatal orbital teratoma. Br J Ophthalmol. 1962;46:685–91.
11. Kivelä T, Tarkkanen A. Orbital germ cell tumors revisited: a clinicopathological approach to classification. Surv Ophthalmol. 1994;38(6):541–54.
12. González C, Restrepo C, Salazar G, Monsalve P. Congenital orbital teratoma: case report. Colomb Med (Cali). 2012;43:82–5.
13. Sommering ST. Uber einen Cysticercus cellulosae im Men- schlichen Auge. Oken's Iseis. 1830;8:717–8.
14. Pushker N, Bajaj MS, Betharia SM. Orbital and adnexal cysticercosis. Clin Experiment Ophthalmol. 2002;30(5):322–33.
15. Eshraghi B, Sonbolestan SA, Abtahi MA, Mirmohammadsadeghi A. Clinical characteristics, histopathology, and treatment outcomes in adult and pediatric patients with nonspecific orbital inflammation. J Curr Ophthalmol. 2019;31(3):327–34.
16. Spindle J, Tang SX, Davies B, Wladis EJ, Piozzi E, Pellegrini M, Lally SE, Shields C, Shinder R. Pediatric idiopathic orbital inflammation: clinical features of 30 cases. Ophthalmic Plast Reconstr Surg. 2016;32(4):270–4.
17. Newman KL, Newman LS. Occupational causes of sarcoidosis. Curr Opin Allergy Clin Immunol. 2012;12(2):145.
18. Bradley D, Baughman RP, Raymond L, Kaufman AH. Ocular manifestations of sarcoidosis. Semin Respir Crit Care Med. 2002;6:543–8.
19. Rothova A, Alberts C, Glasius E, Kijlstra A, Buitenhuis HJ, Breebaart AC. Risk factors for ocular sarcoidosis. Doc Ophthalmol. 1989;72(3–4):287–96.
20. Bitar D, Van Cauteren D, Lanternier F, Dannaoui E, Che D, Dromer F, Desenclos JC, Lortholary O. Increasing incidence of zygomycosis (mucormycosis), France, 1997–2006. Emerg Infect Dis. 2009;15(9):1395.
21. Almyroudis NG, Sutton DA, Linden P, Rinaldi MG, Fung J, Kusne S. Zygomycosis in solid organ transplant recipients in a tertiary transplant center and review of the literature. Am J Transplant. 2006;6(10):2365–74.

22. Knowles DM, Jakobiec FA, McNally L, Burke JS. Lymphoid hyperplasia and malignant lymphoma occurring in the ocular adnexa (orbit, conjunctiva, and eyelids): a prospective multiparametric analysis of 108 cases during 1977 to 1987. Hum Pathol. 1990;21:959–73.
23. Saltzstein SL. Pulmonary malignant lymphomas and pseudolymphomas: classification, therapy, and prognosis. Cancer. 1963;16:928e55.
24. Fitzpatrick PJ, Macko S. Lymphoreticular tumors of the orbit. Int J Radiat Oncol Biol Phys. 1984;10(3):333–40.
25. Freeman C, Berg JW, Cutler SJ. Occurrence and prognosis of extra-nodal lymphomas. Cancer. 1972;29:252–60.
26. Bessel EM, Henk JM, Wright JE, et al. Orbital and conjunctival lymphoma: treatment and prognosis. Radiat Oncol. 1988;13:237–44.
27. Fung CY, Tarbell NJ, Lucarelli MJ, et al. Ocular adnexal lymphoma: clinical behaviour of distinct World Health Organization classification of subtypes. Int J Radiat Oncol Biol Phys. 2003;57:1382–91.
28. White WL, Ferry JA, Harris NL, Grove AS. Jr ocular adnexal lymphoma: a clinicopathologic study with identification of lymphomas of mucosa-associated lymphoid tissue type. Ophthalmology. 1995;102:1994–2006.
29. Moslehi R, Devesa SS, Schairer C, Fraumeni JF. Jr rapidly increasing incidence of ocular non-Hodgkin lymphoma. J Natl Cancer Inst. 2006;98:936–9.
30. Woo JM, Tang CK, Rho MS, Lee JH, Kwon HC, Ahn HB. The clinical characteristics and treatment results of ocular adnexal lymphoma. Korean J Ophthalmol. 2006;20:7–12.
31. Yoon JS, Ma KT, Kim SJ, Kook K, Lee SY. Prognosis for patients in a Korean population with ocular adnexal lymphoproliferative lesions. Ophthalmic Plast Reconstr Surg. 2007;23:94–9.
32. Eckardt AM, Lemound J, Rana M, Gellrich NC. Orbital lymphoma: diagnostic approach and treatment outcome. World J Surg Onc. 2013;11:73.
33. Coupland SE, Hellmich M, Auw-Haedrich C, Lee WR, Stein H. Prognostic value of cell- cycle markers in ocular adnexal lymphoma: an assessment of 230 cases. Graefes Arch Clin Exp Ophthalmol. 2004;242:130–45.
34. Rasmussen PK, Coupland SE, Finger PT, Graue GF, Grossniklaus HE, Honavar SG, McKelvie P, Mulay K, Prause JU, Ralfkiaer E, Sjö LD. Ocular adnexal follicular lymphoma: a multicenter international study. JAMA Ophthalmol. 2014;132(7):851–8.
35. Coupland SE, Hellmich M, Auw-Haedrich C, Lee WR, Stein H. Prognostic value of cell-cycle markers in ocular adnexal lymphoma: an assessment of 230 cases. Graefes Arch Clin Exp Ophthalmol. 2004;242(2):130–45.
36. Oh DE, Kim YD. Lymphoproliferative diseases of the ocular adnexa in Korea. Arch Ophthalmol. 2007;125(12):1668–73.
37. Rey-Porca C, Pérez-Encinas M, González F. Orbital lymphomas, presentation of nine cases. Arch Soc Esp Oftalmol. 2008;83(2):95–103.
38. Campo E, Swerdlow SH, Harris NL, Pileri S, Stein H, Jaffe ES. WHO classification of lymphoid neoplasms and beyond: evolving concepts and practical applications. Blood. 2008;117(19):5019–32.
39. Guermazi A, Feger C, Rousselot P. Granulocytic sarcoma (chloroma): imaging findings in adults and children. AJR. 2002;178(February):319–25.
40. Pileri SA, Ascani S, Cox MC. Myeloid sarcoma: clinico-pathologic, phenotypic and cytogenetic analysis of 92 adult patients. Leukemia. 2007;21:340–50.
41. Foucar E, Rosai J, Dorfman RF. The ophthalmologic manifestations of sinus histiocytosis with massive lymphadenopathy. Am J Ophthalmol. 1979;87:354.
42. Fernandes BF, Brazuna A, Moura LR, et al. Extranodal Rosai-Dorfman disease presenting as an epibulbar tumor. Cornea. 2008;27:378–81.
43. Rosai J, Dorfman RF. Sinus histiocytosis with massive lymphadenopathy. A newly recognized benign clinicopathological entity. Arch Pathol. 1969;87:63–70.
44. Foucar E, Rosai J, Dorfman R. Sinus histiocytosis with massive lymphadenopathy (Rosai-Dorfman disease): review of the entity. Semin Diagn Pathol. 1990;7:19–73.
45. McClellan SF, Ainbinder DJ. Orbital Rosai-Dorfman disease: a literature review. Orbit. 2013;32:341–6.
46. Shields JA, Bakewell B, Augsburger JJ, Flanagan JC. Classification and incidence of space-occupying lesions of the orbit. Arch Ophthalmol. 1984;102:1606–11.
47. Henderson JW, Campbell RJ, Farrow GM, Garrity JA. Orbital Tumors. New York: Raven Press; 1994. p. 43–52.
48. Günalp I, Gündüz K. Biopsy-proven orbital lesions in Turkey. A survey of 1092 cases over 30 years. Orbit. 1994;13:67–79.
49. Seregard S, Sahlin S. Panorama of orbital space-occupying lesions. The 24-year experience of a referral center. Acta Ophthalmol Scand. 1999;77:91–8.
50. Sen DK. Aetiological pattern of orbital tumors in India and their clinical presentations. A 20-year retrospective study. Orbit. 1990;9:299–302.
51. Wassef M, Blei F, Adams D, Alomari A, Baselga E, Berenstein A, et al. Vascular anomalies classification: recommendations from the international society for the study of vascular anomalies. Pediatrics. 2015;136:e203–14.
52. Bilaniuk LT. Orbital vascular lesions: role of imaging. Radiol Clin North Am. 1999;37:169–83.
53. Rootman J. Vascular malformations of the orbit:hemodynamic concepts. Orbit. 2003;22:103–20.
54. Ansari SA, Mafee MF. Orbital cavernous hemangioma: role of imaging. Neuroimaging Clin N Am. 2005;15:137–58.
55. Zauberman H, Feinsod M. Orbital hemangiomagrowth during pregnancy. Acta Ophthalmol (Copenh). 1970;48:929–33.

56. Katz SE, Rootman J, Vangveeravong S, et al. Combined venous lymphatic malformations of theorbit (so-called lymphangiomas): association withnoncontiguous intracranial vascular anomalies. Ophthalmology. 1998;105:176–84.
57. Harris GJ, Sakol PJ, Bonavolonta G, ConciliisC D. An analysis of thirty cases of orbital lymphangioma: pathophysiologic considerations and management recommendations. Ophthalmology. 1990;97:1583–92.
58. Brunnemann RB, Ro JY, Ordonez NG, Mooney J, El-Naggar AK, Ayala AG. Extrapleural solitary fibrous tumor: a clinicopathologic study of 24 cases. Mod Pathol. 1999;12:1034–42.
59. Krishnakumar S, Subramaniam N, Mohan ER, Mahesh L, Biswas J, Rao NA. Solitary fibrous tumor of the orbit: a clinicopathologic study of six cases with review of the literature. Surv Ophthalmol. 2003;48:544–54.
60. Shields CL, Shields JA, Eagle RC, et al. Clinicopathologic review of 142 cases of lacrimal gland lesions. Ophthalmology. 1989;96:431–5.
61. Duck Kim Y. Lacrimal gland tumors. In: Karcioglu ZA, editor. Orbital tumors, diagnosis and treatment. New York: Springer; 2005. p. 204–20.
62. Font RL, Smith SL, Bryan RG. Malignant epithelial tumors of the lacrimal gland. A clinicopathologic study of 21 cases. Arch Ophthalmol. 1998;116:613–6.
63. Font RL, Gamel JW. Epithelial tumors of the lacrimal gland: an analysis of 265 cases. In: Jacobiec FA, editor. Ocular and adnexal tumors. Birmingham: Aesculapius Publishing; 1978. p. 787–805.
64. Shields JA, Shields CL, Scartozzi R. Survey of 1264 patients with orbitaltumors and simulating lesions: the 2002 Montgomery lecture, part 1. Ophthalmology. 2004;111(5):997–1008.
65. Yanoff M, Fine BS. Ocular pathology. 5th edition,Chapter 14. St. Lious: Mosby; 2002. p. 501.
66. Rao AA, Naheedy JH, Chen JY, Robbins SL, Ramkumar HL. A clinical update and radiologic review of pediatric orbital and ocular tumors. J Oncol. 2013;2013:975908.
67. Shields JA, Shields CL. Rhabdomyosarcoma: review for the ophthalmologist. Surv Ophthalmol. 2003;48:39–57.
68. Conneely MF, Mafee MF. Orbital rhabdomyosarcoma and simulating lesions. Neuroimaging Clin N Am. 2005;15:121–36.
69. Horn RC Jr, Enterline HT. Rhabdomyosarcoma: a clinicopathological study and classification of 39 cases. Cancer. 1958;11:181–99.
70. WHO Classification of Tumours Editorial Board. WHO classification of tumours of soft tissue and bone. 5th ed. Lyon: IARC; 2020.
71. Cloutier BT, Costa FD, Tazelaar HD, Folpe AL. Aberrant expression of neuroendocrine markers in angiosarcoma: a potential diagnostic pitfall. Hum Pathol. 2014;45(8):1618–24.
72. Slater O, Shipley J. Clinical relevance of molecular genetics to paediatric sarcomas. J Clin Pathol. 2007;60:1187–94.
73. Fletcher C, Bridge JA, Hogendoorn PC, Mertens F. WHO classification of tumours of soft tissue and bone: WHO classification of Tumours, vol. 5. World Health Organization; 2013.
74. Ahmad SM, Esmaeli B. Metastatic tumors of the orbit and ocular adnexa. Curr Opin Ophthalmol. 2007;18:405–13.
75. Magliozzi P, Strianese D, Bonavolontà P, Ferrara M, Ruggiero P, Carandente R, et al. Orbital metastases in Italy. Int J Ophthalmol. 2015;8:1018–23.
76. Shields JA, Shields CL, Scartozzi R. Survey of 1264 patients with orbital tumors and simulating lesions: the 2002 Montgomery lecture, part 1. Ophthalmology. 2004;111:997–1008.
77. Shields JA, Shields CL, Brotman HK, Carvalho C, Perez N, Eagle RC Jr. Cancer metastatic to the orbit: the 2000 Robert M. Curts Lecture Ophthalmic Plast Reconstr Surg. 2001;17:346.
78. Varadhachary GR, Abbruzzese JL, Lenzi R. Diagnostic strategies for unknown primary cancer. Cancer. 2004;100(9):1776–85.

Optic Nerve and Its Disorders

18

Akshay Badakere, Swathi Vallabh,
Geeta K. Vemuganti, and Dilip K. Mishra

Contents

A. Badakere (✉)
Department of Pediatric Ophthalmology, Sankara Nethralaya, Chennai, India

S. Vallabh
Department of Glaucoma, Sankara Nethralaya, Chennai, India

G. K. Vemuganti
University of Hyderabad, Hyderabad, India
e-mail: gkvemuganti@gmail.com

D. K. Mishra
Ophthalmic Pathology Laboratory, LV Prasad Eye Institute, Hyderabad, India

G. K. Vemuganti et al. (eds.), *Ocular Pathology*, https://doi.org/10.1007/978-981-96-8614-8_18

18.1 Introduction

The optic nerve is subject to various pathologies secondary to inflammation, ischemia, trauma, and tumors. Some disorders may be congenital in origin. Not only are these disorders a threat to vision but they can also impact the life of the patient and may be an indicator of underlying systemic disease.

While majority of optic nerve disorders are detected by a good clinical examination, certain disorders like optic neuritis, traumatic optic neuropathy and congenital anomalies need imaging modalities to pick up associations; be it demyelination suggestive of multiple sclerosis, trauma to the skull, or certain central nervous system and endocrine disorders.

This chapter aims to provide a review of these disorders and their corresponding pathological changes.

Optic nerve and its disorders can be classified as

1. Congenital, developmental, inherited, and degenerative
   (a) Optic nerve hypoplasia
   (b) Excavations of optic disc
      - Optic disc coloboma
      - Morning glory disc (syndrome)
      - Peripapillary staphyloma
   (c) Leber's hereditary optic neuropathy
   (d) Optic nerve head drusen
2. Inflammatory
   (a) Typical demyelinating optic neuritis
   (b) Neuromyelitis optica spectrum disorders

    (c) Myelin oligodendrocyte glycoprotein antibody (MOG IgG) associated optic neuritis
    (d) Inflammatory optic neuritis
    (e) Infectious optic neuritis
3. Ischemic
    (a) Arteritic ischemic optic neuropathy
    (b) Nonarteritic ischemic optic neuropathy
4. Traumatic
5. Tumors
    A. Intrinsic tumors
        (a) Optic nerve glioma (benign and malignant),
        (b) Ganglioglioma
        (c) Medulloepithelioma
        (d) Hemangioblastoma
    B. The optic nerve sheath tumors
        (a) Optic nerve sheath meningioma
        (b) Schwannoma
        (c) Hemangiopericytoma

18.2 Congenital Anomalies

Congenital malformations of the optic nerve, especially those involving the optic nerve head and surrounding tissues, include a broad spectrum of malformations frequently associated with congenital blindness or significant visual impairment.

The principal congenital abnormalities of the optic disc that can significantly impair visual function are optic nerve hypoplasia and excavations of the optic disc.

Excavations of optic disc include

(a) Optic disc coloboma
(b) Morning glory disc
(c) Peripapillary staphyloma

18.2.1 Optic Nerve Hypoplasia

18.2.1.1 Definition

This is a congenital, nonprogressive, developmental anomaly characterized by a small optic disc, peripapillary double-ring sign, retinal nerve fiber layer thinning, and vascular tortuosity

18.2.1.2 Etiology

Largely a sporadic condition with no known cause. Histopathologically, the lack of degenerated neurons in ONH is indicative of axonal loss due to apoptosis during development. Known risk factors include [1, 2]:

- Young maternal age
- First pregnancies
- Maternal smoking
- Preterm birth
- Fetal alcohol syndrome
- Type 1 diabetes in mothers

18.2.1.3 Clinical Features

The typical features seen are a peripapillary ring around the optic nerve, tortuous retinal vessels.

DM- DD ratio- this is the ratio of the distance between the center of the disc to the center of the macula (DM) to diameter of optic disc (DD). A ratio more than 3 is suggestive of this condition, whereas a ratio more than 4 is possibly diagnostic [3, 4]. A relative afferent pupillary defect (RAPD) can be elicited when it is bilateral and asymmetric. Magnetic resonance imaging (MRI) may reveal decrease in size of optic nerve and chiasmal hypoplasia

18.2.1.4 Associations [5]

Ocular: microphthalmos, coloboma, aniridia, nystagmus, strabismus

Neurologic: Anencephaly, cerebral atrophy, basal encephaloceles, hypoplasia of the cerebellar vermis, cystic dilatation of the fourth ventricle, and posterior fossa cysts

Endocrinologic: dysfunctions of HPA axis causing deficiencies of thyroid, pituitary, growth and antidiuretic hormones

In children abnormal sexual development is noted, and the levels of luteinizing hormone, follicle-stimulating hormone, and testosterone should be tested.

Septo- Optic Dysplasia (SOD) which includes optic nerve hypoplasia, pituitary abnormalities, midline abnormalities of the brain are also to be looked for.

18.2.1.5 Treatment

A complete eye exam should be performed, and glasses should be prescribed, if there is a refractive error referred to appropriate specialties and undergo neuroimaging. In children occlusion therapy can also help. In view of the varied possible systemic associations, a patient with optic nerve hypoplasia must be referred to appropriate specialties [1, 5].

18.2.1.6 Clinicopathological Correlation

An 8-year-old girl was referred for amblyopia management. On examination her visual acuities were 20/100 for distance and N8 for near in the right eye and 20/20 N6 in the left eye. Dilated retinoscopy confirmed the absence of a refractive error. Pupil examination showed a grade 1 RAPD in the right eye. Fundus exam was essentially normal in the left eye and in the right eye there was a hypoplastic disc with vascular tortuosity (Figs. 18.1 and 18.2). She was referred to a pediatric endocrinologist for endocrine evaluation and advised to MRI of brain. Endocrine evaluation revealed decreased growth hormone levels and MRI revealed an absent septum pellucidum.

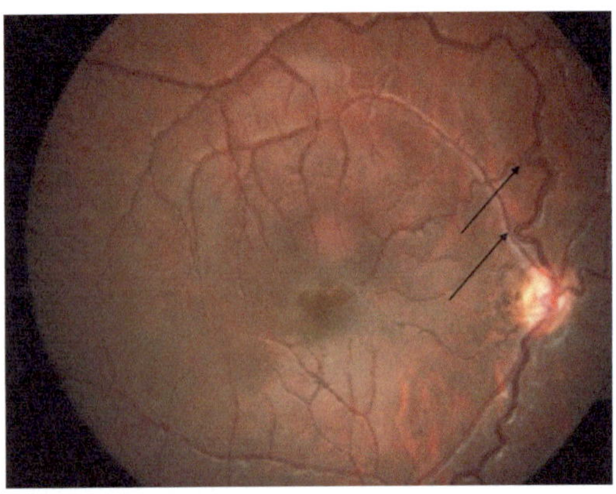

Fig. 18.1 Hypoplastic optic disc showing small-sized optic disc and vascular tortuosity (black arrows)

18.2.2 Excavations of Optic Disc [1]

These include

- Morning glory disc anomaly (MGDA)
- Optic disc coloboma
- Peripapillary staphyloma

MGDA [1, 5] is characterized by

- Conical excavation of optic disc and posterior pole
- Presence of the characteristic glial tissue on the optic disc (giving the appearance of the morning glory flower)
- Presence of annular pigmentation around the optic disc

18.2.2.1 Etiology

It is hypothesized that a failure in closure of the fetal fissure, dysgenesis of the optic stalk and its failure to close, and a primary mesenchymal abnormality may cause this anomaly [1].

18.2.2.2 Clinical Features

Usually unilateral, with a typical appearance of an excavated optic disc filled with glial tissue. Visual acuity may vary from no perception of light to 6/6 in rare cases.

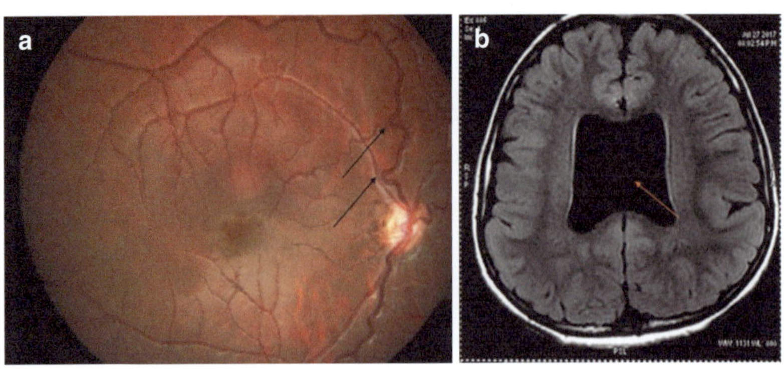

Fig. 18.2 (**a**) Hypoplastic optic disc—note a small optic disc with tortuous vessels. (**b**) MRI Brain axial section showing an absent septum pellucidum (yellow arrow)

18.2.2.3 Associations [1]

It is generally an isolated condition but may be associated with transsphenoidal encephaloceles and hypopituitarism, and these patients have characteristic facies with wide forehead, flattened nasal bridge, and hypertelorism.

Ocular complications like rhegmatogenous retinal detachment at disc margin or within the cup and subretinal neovascularization can be seen. Treatment includes a complete and thorough eye exam, correction of any refractive error, and occlusion therapy if needed. Appropriate referrals to specialty services to rule out any underlying systemic associations are also important.

18.2.2.4 Peripapillary Staphyloma

This is characterized by an excavation around the optic disc.

The precise etiology is unknown. It may arise because of a disturbance in scleral development at around 20 weeks of gestation [1]. It is suggested that the development of intraocular pressure causes herniation of scleral tissue leading to an excavation [1].

Clinical Features

The characteristic appearance is that of an optic disc placed in an excavation. The disc may be normal or may exhibit some temporal pallor. Vision may vary from 6/6 to very poor vision. Children may be myopic or emmetropic.

Associations [1]

In most cases, unilateral and isolated. Rarely may be associated with

- frontonasal dysplasia
- basal encephalocele
- facial capillary hemangioma or linear nevus sebaceous syndrome

As in other congenital anomalous discs, a complete eye exam should be performed with correction of underlying refractive error and patching if needed.

18.2.2.5 Optic Disc Coloboma

This is characterized by a bowl-shaped excavation of the optic disc and is generally decentered and present inferiorly.

Etiology

This is thought to result from abnormal fusion of the proximal ends of the optic cup. It is thought that insults to the developing fetus at the sixth week of gestation also play a role. It has two modes of inheritance sporadic and autosomal dominant. PAX 2 gene mutations are also thought to be involved since some of these are a part of the renal-coloboma syndrome [1].

Clinical Features

Visual acuity can be variable. Typical appearance of optic disc with coloboma being decentered and located inferiorly. May be associated with refractive errors.

Associations [1, 6]

- Internal carotid artery dysgenesis
- Transsphenoidal encephalocele
- Hypopituitarism
- CHARGE syndrome (C: colobomas, H: heart defects, A: Choanal Atresia, R: growth retardation, G: genitourinary abnormalities, E: ear abnormalities)
- Walker–Warburg syndrome
- Goltz focal dermal hypoplasia
- Aicardi syndrome, Goldenhar syndrome, and linear sebaceous naevus syndrome.

Treatment involves correction of underlying refractive error and patch therapy for amblyopia in children. Specialist referrals where indicated are important.

Clinicopathological correlation: An 8-year-old boy was brought by his parents after an incidental finding at a school screening. The school screening had revealed that the child could not read the vision chart with the right eye. On examination while his vision was 20/20 in the left eye, in the right eye, he could count fingers up to 2 meters. He had a grade 2 RAPD in the right eye and cycloplegic refraction revealed −2 diopter sphere refractive error in the right eye and plano in the left eye. Fundus exam revealed a normal disc and retina in the left eye, in the right eye there was a colobomatous disc (Fig. 18.3). He was prescribed glasses and advised left eye occlusion therapy with eye patches for 3 hours daily.

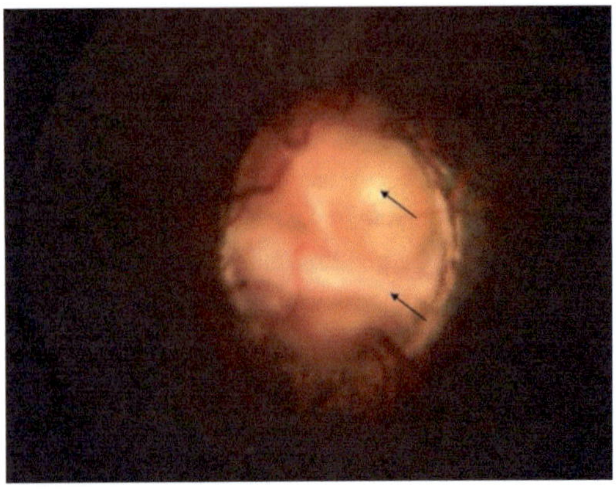

Fig. 18.3 Optic disc coloboma showing a colobomatous area temporally and inferiorly (arrows)

18.3 Optic Neuritis

Under this spectrum are included [7]

(a) Typical demyelinating optic neuritis
(b) Neuromyelitis optica spectrum disorders
(c) Myelin oligodendrocyte glycoprotein antibody (MOG IgG) associated optic neuritis
(d) Inflammatory optic neuritis
(e) Infectious optic neuritis

Clinicopathologic correlation: while typical demyelinating optic neuritis is often associated with multiple sclerosis (MS), atypical optic neuritis can be associated with autoimmune, inflammatory, or infectious etiology.

It is important to differentiate between the two, and the points enumerated in Table 18.1 can help.

Table 18.1 Clinical features of optic neuritis

Features	Typical optic neuritis	Atypical optic neuritis
Laterality	Unilateral	Unilateral or bilateral
Gender	Female	Male
Pain	Painful	Painless
Age	3rd decade	<18 years, >50 years
Optic disc	Normal, papillitis	Papillitis
Prognosis	Spontaneous improvement	Worsening of vision over 2 weeks

18.3.1 Typical Optic Neuritis

Typical optic neuritis is characterized by acute onset, unilateral, painful (rarely painless) vision loss due to demyelination. Patients classically present with vision loss, painful eye movements, loss of color vision, and decreased contrast sensitivity.

The vision begins to spontaneously improve within 2 weeks even without treatment. An optic disc evaluation shows papillitis or a normal-appearing disc. Pupil examination reveals a relative afferent pupillary defect on the affected side. Diagnosis is based on these clinical features. An MRI brain and orbit with contrast should be done to look for post-contrast enhancement of the optic nerve and for demyelinating lesions suggestive of MS. [7]

Typical optic neuritis improves spontaneously, and hence observation without initiating intravenous methyl prednisolone can be a chosen line of management. IV steroids as shown by Optic Neuritis Treatment Trial (ONTT) aid in faster visual recovery over 1 month, but at 6 months there is not much difference as compared to observation [7].

Treatment with oral steroids alone is not advised since it has been shown to increase recurrence [7].

18.3.1.1 Clinicopathological Correlation

A 22-year-old male presented to us with a sudden and painful loss of vision in the right eye. His visual acuity was 20/40, N6 in the right eye and 20/20, N6 in the left eye. Pupil evaluation revealed a grade 2 RAPD in the right eye. Fundus examination of the left eye was essentially normal while in the right eye it revealed a hyperemic disc with surrounding RNFL edema (Fig. 18.4). We requested an MRI of the brain and orbits with contrast. The MRI scans of the orbit revealed the presence of post-contrast enhancement of the right optic nerve (Fig. 18.4b). The MRI scan of the Brain did not reveal any lesions suggestive of multiple sclerosis. He was treated with intravenous methyl prednisolone 500 mg twice a day for

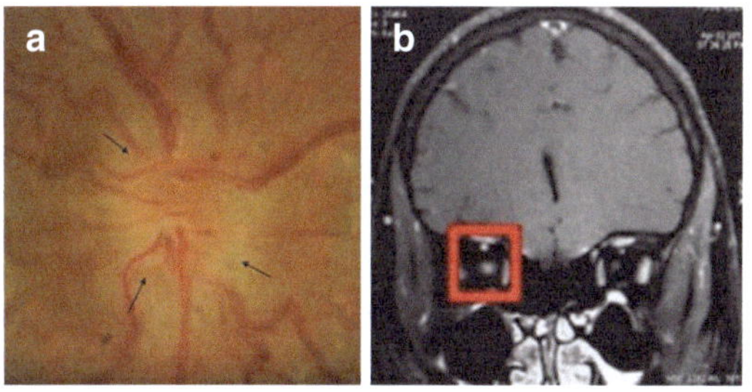

Fig. 18.4 (**a**) Papillitis in a case of optic neuritis showing a hyperemic disc with surrounding RNFL edema (arrows denote RNFL edema); (**b**) MRI orbit coronal section showing post-contrast enhancement of the right optic nerve (shown within the red square)

3 days followed by oral steroids 1 mg per kg body weight for 11 days as per the ONTT protocol. On completion of treatment, he had regained 20/20 vision in the right eye.

18.3.2 Neuromyelitis Optica Spectrum Disorders (NMOSD) [7]

Neuromyelitis Optica (NMO) also known as Devic disease is an inflammatory and demyelinating disorder of the central nervous system affecting the optic nerve and spinal cord. It is characterized by antibodies directed against the aquaporin-4 water channel present in astrocytes or against myelin oligodendrocyte glycoprotein (MOG).

Some of the typical presentations of NMO include

- Severe and bilateral optic neuritis
- Longitudinally extensive transverse myelitis
- Area postrema syndrome

18.3.2.1 Clinical Features

Typically presents with rapid and profound vision loss in an older age group and has a female prediliction. Vision loss tends to be rapid and profound. MRI of the brain and orbit shows a longer segment of optic nerve involvement, posterior portion of optic nerve, and/or chiasmal involvement. An MRI spine shows transverse myelitis with intramedullary spinal cord involvement spanning more than three segments. MRI may also show lesions in the cerebral cortex, diencephalon, and brainstem.

NEMOS (Neuromyelitis Optica Study group) recommends intravenous (IV) methyl prednisolone 1 gram per day for 5 days as in the acute phase. Worsening despite IV steroids may be an indication for plasma exchange (PLEX) [8].

Following treatment of acute phase, long-term immunosuppression with rituximab, mycophenolate mofetil, or azathioprine is indicated to prevent or decrease recurrence rates.

18.3.3 Myelin Oligodendrocyte Glycoprotein Antibody (MOG IgG)-Associated Optic Neuritis

Although a distinct clinical entity from NMO, it shares features like severe and profound vision loss. Compared to NMO and MS, MOG-associated optic neuritis tends to be more steroid dependent. When compared to NMO, it also has a better prognosis.

On MR Imaging, MOG optic neuritis can also have extensive optic nerve involvement, although chiasmal involvement is less common. Perineural involvement is more common in MOG optic neuritis.

18.3.3.1 CRION [7]

Chronic Relapsing Inflammatory Optic Neuropathy is a steroid-dependent optic neuropathy.

These patients have favorable outcomes following long-term steroid therapy.

18.3.4 Infectious Optic Neuritis [7]

A host of bacterial, viral, parasitic, and fungal infections can lead to optic neuritis. Mycobacterium tuberculosis, Leptospira, West Nile virus, HIV—to name a few—can all cause optic neuritis. The presence of fever, signs of atypical optic neuritis as mentioned in Table 18.1, or a history of travel should raise the suspicion of infectious optic neuritis.

18.3.5 Granulomatous Noninfectious Causes: Less Commonly Cause Neuritis

Sarcoidosis, eosinophilic granuloma, granulomatosis polyangiitis, non-specific orbital inflammatory disease.

18.4 Ischemic Optic Neuropathy (ION)

This is an optic neuropathy that results from ischemic damage due to vascular insufficiency [9].

Ischemic neuropathies can be classified as anterior ION (90% of cases are anterior ION) and posterior ION depending upon the site of optic nerve damage. These are further subclassified as arteritic and nonarteritic. Arteritic is usually as a result of giant cell arteritis (GCA), and nonarteritic is as a result of ischemic damage or hypoperfusion [9, 10].

18.4.1 Arteritic ION

18.4.1.1 Arteritic Anterior ION (AAION)

The main cause is GCA which is a systemic vasculitis affecting medium- and small-sized arteries. The posterior ciliary artery is affected in AAION, and this can result in profound vision loss.

The other vasculitides affecting the optic nerve are Polyarteritis Nodosa, Systemic Lupus Erythematosus, and Herpes Zoster [10].

18.4.1.2 Arteritic Posterior ION

Like its anterior variant, GCA is the most common cause. The main arteries affected are the orbital arteries. APION is rare when compared to AAION [10].

18.4.2 Nonarteritic ION

18.4.2.1 Nonarteritic Anterior ION (NAAION)

It is caused by one of the two following proposed mechanisms: [9, 10]

1. Nonperfusion or hypoperfusion of the optic nerve head

   Predisposing factors for these are systemic conditions like Diabetes mellitus, hyperlipidemia, atherosclerosis, arteriosclerosis, nocturnal hypotension, migraine, and sleep apnea. Anatomical factors like a small and cupless optic disc or a "crowded disc" are also risk factors. Some of the other associated risk factors are optic nerve drusen, markedly raised intraocular pressure and the location of the watershed zone of the optic nerve and the posterior ciliary arteries.
2. Embolic occlusion

   Embolism of the vessels supplying the optic nerve, although rare, may cause profound visual loss [10].

18.4.2.2 Surgical Posterior ION- [9, 10]

This is seen following prolonged surgical procedures, especially spinal and orthopedic surgeries, neck surgeries, and surgeries for penetrating trauma of the thorax and abdomen.

Although the exact cause is not known, it could be hypotension caused by any one or a combination of

- Blood loss
- Trauma
- Prolonged general anesthesia

Also implicated as possible causes are hemodilution caused by intravenous fluids and prolonged prone positioning leading to orbital compression.

Clinical Features

AAION

Certain specific signs and symptoms include sudden, severe vision loss, headache, jaw claudication. These may be associated with tenderness over the scalp and over the temporal artery [10].

Pupil evaluation reveals a relative afferent pupillary defect (RAPD). An optic nerve examination reveals a classic chalky white disc edema with peripapillary hemorrhages in few cases.

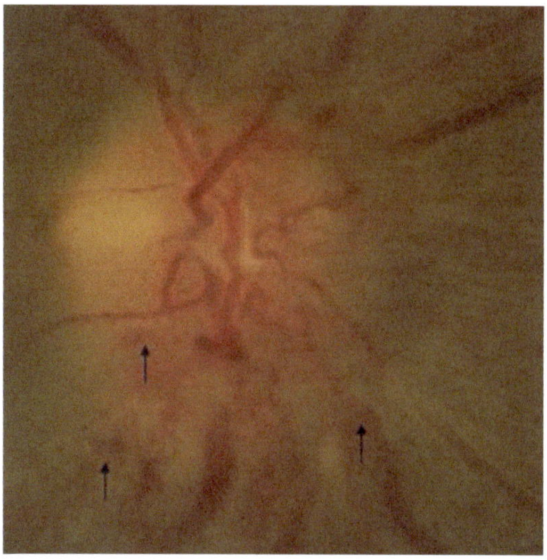

Fig. 18.5 Case of NAAION shows sectoral edema with hyperemia and peripapillary hemorrhages (peripapillary hemorrhages denoted by arrows)

NAAION

Here the visual acuity may vary from 20/20 to very poor vision. These patients have a RAPD on examination. Optic disc exam reveals sectoral disc edema with hyperemia, attenuated blood vessels, and in some cases peripapillary hemorrhages. Examination of the fellow eye may reveal the presence of a small, crowded disc which also known as a disc at risk.

Visual field evaluation reveals an inferior altitudinal defect in most cases (Fig. 18.5).

Figure 5 case of NAAION shows sectoral edema with hyperemia (long arrow) and peripapillary hemorrhages (arrow heads)

AAION is an ophthalmic emergency, and the goal of treatment is to prevent vision loss in the fellow eye which can happen in a matter of hours to few days. An immediate evaluation of ESR and CRP must be done which is elevated in GCA. AAION due to GCA is responsive to corticosteroids, and hence intravenous steroids can limit damage in the afflicted eye and prevent vision loss in the fellow eye [9, 10].

NAAION at present does not have any proven treatment. Many therapeutic modalities have been tried such as steroids, intravitreal anti-VEGF agents like bevacizumab, neuroprotection, etc., but at present there is no proven gold standard for treatment. These patients should be investigated for underlying systemic diseases, and these should be managed.

18.5 Traumatic Optic Neuropathy

Traumatic optic neuropathy (TON) is a disorder which threatens vision and is caused by ocular and/ or head trauma [11, 12].

Based on the modes of injury, it is classified as Direct and Indirect TON [11, 12]

18.5.1 Direct TON

This is caused by anatomical disruption of optic nerve either due to laceration or severe contusion or concussion injury. Vision loss tends to be severe, and prognosis is generally poor.

18.5.2 Indirect TON [12]

Here although the exact mechanism of optic nerve injury is debatable, it tends to be a combination of

- Shear injury to axons
- Contusion necrosis from ischemic damage
- Compression from edema
- Apoptosis of injured and intact neurons
- Diffuse axonal injury

Vision loss tends to be less severe, although prognosis remains guarded.

18.5.3 Clinical Features

Patients present with a sudden vision loss. On clinical examination, if the injury is unilateral or bilateral but asymmetric, there is a relative afferent pupillary defect. A dilated exam of the optic disc may reveal a normal-looking disc initially or optic atrophy. Visual acuity can vary and can even result in no perception of light.

It is important to examine for coexistent ocular, facial, and head injuries and assess the level of consciousness of the patient.

Visual field assessment can be done if possible and can show variable visual field afflictions.

Neuroimaging should ideally be done to look for optic canal injuries and to look for fracture fragments impinging on the optic nerve. This also helps guide further surgical intervention. CT scan orbit is the imaging modality of choice for the above.

Although treatment regimens vary, they consist of a combination of [11, 12] steroid therapy, surgical decompression of the optic nerve canal, where indicated, or combination of the two.

18.6 Tumors of the Optic Nerve (Schematic Diagram of Nerve with Tumor Outside and Tumor Within Would Be Useful)

Optic nerve tumors can be classified as intrinsic tumors and tumors of the optic nerve sheath.

The intrinsic or primary tumors of optic nerve include optic nerve glioma (benign and malignant), ganglioglioma, medulloepithelioma, and hemangioblastoma.

The optic nerve sheath tumors include optic nerve sheath meningioma, schwannoma, and hemangiopericytoma [13].

18.6.1 Optic Nerve Glioma

These comprise about 1% of all intracranial tumors. They are largely sporadic but are seen to be familial especially when associated with Neurofibromatosis type 1. These tumors have a female predilection and are generally seen in childhood. In studies by Chutorian and associates and Rush and associates, it has been seen that the median age at presentation was about 11 years, and most patients were symptomatic in childhood [14, 15].

18.6.1.1 Clinical Features

A typical case presents with proptosis and decreased visual acuity. On clinical examination there is a relative afferent pupillary defect on the side involved along with optic atrophy. In long-standing cases there maybe signs of compression like central retinal vein obstruction, presence of optico ciliary shunts and neovascularization of the iris.

There may be associated features of NF1 and must be looked for.

Diagnosis is made by a combination of clinical findings and neuroimaging. Computed Tomography (CT) or Magnetic Resonance Imaging (MRI) can be used. A fusiform enlargement of the optic nerve can be seen in patients with NF1, while a kinked and buckled appearance is seen in those without NF1. MRI can also be used to look for involvement of the chiasm [13].

Histologically three patterns can be seen [16]:

Transitional area—here the tumor merges with the normal optic nerve tissue. There is an increase in size and number of glial cells with enlarged nerve bundles and a reticulated appearance Coarsely reticulated and myxomatous area—these result from necrosis resulting in cystoid spaces. Astrocytic areas—these show features similar to juvenile astrocytomas of the cerebellum and show spindle formation (Fig. 18.6a), presence of Rosenthal fibers. The tumor cells are immunoreactive to Glial Fibrillary Acidic Protein (GFAP) antibody (Fig. 18.6b). These are benign lesions and are self-limited and may regress over time. Long-term studies have shown that over time most patients maintain good visual function. The role of surgery, chemotherapy, and radiotherapy is limited.

NF1 patients with unilateral optic nerve gliomas may be followed up with neuroimaging at regular intervals. Proptosis causing cosmetic deformities, deteriorating visual function, and extension of tumor may be indications for surgical excision.

18.6.1.2 Malignant Optic Nerve Glioma [13]

Malignant gliomas can involve the anterior visual pathway causing visual loss, neurological signs and can be fatal and are generally seen in adults between the second and eighth decades.

The clinical features include those due to optic nerve compression like vision loss, RAPD and

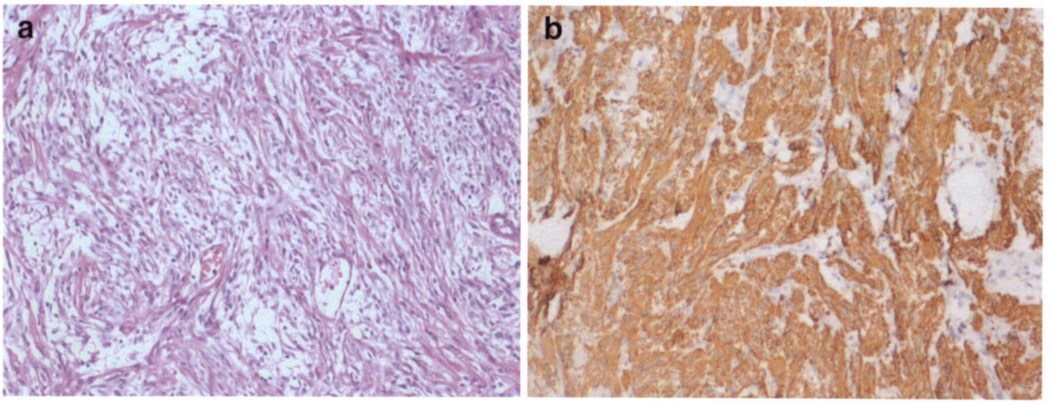

Fig. 18.6 Astrocytoma (W.H.O grade-I).Tumor is composed of spindle cells with long cytoplasmic process in fibrillary background (**a**) and these spindle cells strongly expressed glial fibrillary acidic protein, (GFAP)(**b**)

optic atrophy, and those due to neurological manifestations like hemiplegia and hypothalamic dysfunction.

Malignant optic nerve gliomas may involve the proximal or the distal optic nerve, and although the clinical features are similar, in the latter, the optic disc may initially look normal.

The MRI/CT findings can be nonspecific with diffuse thickening of the optic nerve.

The tumor tends to be vascular with areas of necrosis and almost always involves the entire portion of the optic nerve. Histopathologically there is cellular pleomorphism and hyperchromaticity of nuclei, with areas of necrosis and hemorrhage.

These tumors carry a poor prognosis with death occurring in most cases.

18.6.1.3 Ganglioglioma

These are ganglion cell tumors which arise from the optic nerve substance.

These have similar presentations to optic nerve gliomas, and a distinction can only be made on excision biopsy. Histopathologically this tumor is made up of large ganglion cells and glial stroma. Immunohistochemistry shows the presence of synaptophysin and neurofilament protein [13].

18.6.1.4 Medulloepitheliomas [13]

Although most commonly seen to arise from the brain and spinal cord, they can also be seen arising from the optic nerve.

Clinical Features

These depend upon the location of the tumor with anterior involvement causing symptoms and signs similar to an optic nerve glioma and posterior tumors causing vision loss with an initially normal appearing optic nerve.

MRI and CT features resemble an optic nerve glioma with fusiform enlargement being seen.

Histopathologically, it shows the presence of multilaminar columnar cells in tubes and cords with strands of cells interspersed giving a "net" like appearance.

Anaplastic areas and mitoses may be seen in varying degrees. A medulloepithelioma may be simple when made up of medullary epithelium and structures from the optic vesicle or may be teratoid with cartilage and striated muscle. The teratoid version may be benign or malignant. The treatment consists of complete excision, although recurrences and metastases are known to occur.

18.6.1.5 Hemangioblastoma [13, 17]

These arise within the optic nerve substance and may be seen in those patients who are diagnosed with Von Hippel–Lindau disease, although it may be seen in isolation.

The clinical features and imaging findings are similar to those seen in optic nerve gliomas.

Histopathologically, the tumor is made up of endothelial cells and interstitial cells.

These tumors are benign, and treatment involves complete removal if possible.

18.6.2 Optic Nerve Sheath Tumors

18.6.2.1 Optic Nerve Sheath Meningioma

Optic nerve sheath can be classified as primary or secondary depending upon their site of origin. While the primary tumors arise from the intraorbital or intracanalicular portions, secondary tumors arise from the sphenoid ridge or the tuberculum sellae or the olfactory groove and then involve the adjacent optic canal to involve the optic nerve.

Clinical Features

This tumor has a predilection for middle-aged women. Patients may complain of blurred vision or, sometimes, of transient visual obscurations. Dutton and associates have reported that vision at presentation can be 20/40 or better in up to 45% of cases [17]. The other clinical features are similar to any compressive optic neuropathy with RAPD, color vision loss, and a possible pale optic disc. A careful fundus evaluation may reveal optico ciliary shunt vessels. The triad of vision loss, optic atrophy, and optico ciliary shunt vessels strongly suggests the presence of an optic nerve sheath meningioma.

There also may be proptosis and limited extraocular motility.

Once these clinical findings are noted, neuroimaging in the form of CT scans or MRI of the brain and orbit helps in confirming diagnosis. The classical findings on neuroimaging include calcification around the optic nerve with tubular or bulbous enlargement.

Histopathology reveals meningoendothelial cells arising from the arachnoid mater. Gross examination reveals a tumor with well-defined borders compressing adjacent tissue. Histologically they can have syncytial, fibroblastic, transitional, psammomatous, secretory, or microcystic patterns [18]. Histopathology of meningothelial meningioma mostly shows whorl like pattern of meningothelial cells (Fig. 18.7). Fractionated radiotherapy is the treatment of choice in most cases. Those cases with significant intracranial spread may need to be considered for craniotomy and removal of tumor to prevent it from involving the contralateral optic nerve.

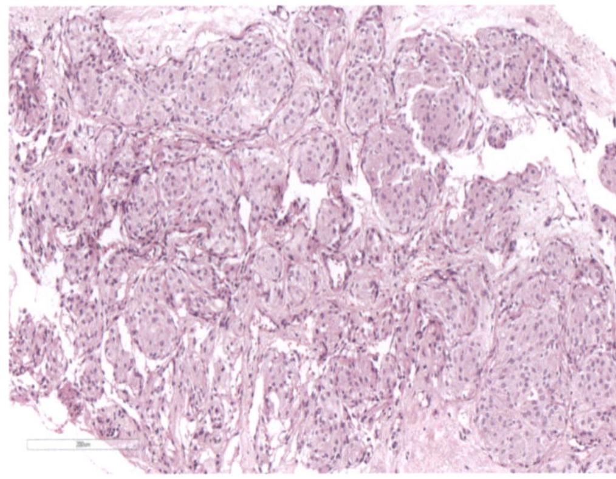

Fig. 18.7 Meningioma (W.H.O grade-I).Typical whorl pattern of meningothelial cells in meningothelial meningioma

18.6.2.2 Schwannoma [13]

These are benign tumors which arise from the Schwann cells, and although commonly arise from the vestibular nerve, they can arise from the optic nerve as well. It is thought that in the optic nerve they arise from the sympathetic nerves that adhere to the optic nerve sheath. The clinical and radiological features are like those of an optic nerve glioma, and histopathology is required to confirm diagnosis. Histologically the classic biphasic pattern with spindle cells forming palisades and Verocay bodies is seen (Antoni A areas). These are intermixed with paucicellular areas with hyalization and cystoid degeneration. Rarely cellular variants are seen earlier referred to as ancient schwannoma. The tumor cells are immunoreactive to S-100. Treatment involves surgery or stereotactic radiotherapy.

18.6.2.3 Hemangiopericytoma [13]

These are made up of pericytes of blood vessels and can arise from any tissue that has capillaries. These tumors have no gender predilection.

Clinical features are seen around the fifth decade and resemble any compressive optic neuropathy. Histopathological examination shows spindle-shaped cells and varying differentiation. The treatment of choice is complete surgical excision.

18.7 Conclusion

Optic nerve pathologies may be congenital or may be acquired as a result of ischemia, inflammation, trauma, or tumors. Many of these conditions may be associated with underlying systemic conditions. While some of these conditions can be diagnosed based on clinical examination, some like tumors may need neuroimaging and histopathological examination.

References

1. Dutton GN. Congenital disorders of the optic nerve: excavations and hypoplasia. Eye. 2004;18(11):1038–48.
2. Tornqvist K, Ericsson A, Källén B. Optic nerve hypoplasia: risk factors and epidemiology. Acta Ophthalmol Scand. 2002;80(3):300–4.
3. Zeki SM, Dudgeon J, Dutton G. Reappraisal of the ratio of disc to macula/disc diameter in optic nerve hypoplasia. Br J Ophthalmol. 1991;75(9):538–41.
4. Barr DB, Weir CR, Purdie AT. An appraisal of the disc–macula distance to disc diameter ratio in the assessment of optic disc size. Ophthalmic Physiol Opt. 1999;19(5):365–75.
5. Amador-Patarroyo MJ, Pérez-Rueda MA, Tellez CH. Congenital anomalies of the optic nerve. Saudi J Ophthalmol. 2015;29(1):32–8.
6. Brodsky MC. Congenital optic disc anomalies. In: Pediatric neuro-ophthalmology. New York: Springer; 2010. p. 59–96.
7. Abel A, McClelland C, Lee MS. Critical review: typical and atypical optic neuritis. Surv Ophthalmol. 2019;64(6):770–9.
8. Trebst C, Jarius S, Berthele A, Paul F, Schippling S, Wildemann B, Borisow N, Kleiter I, Aktas O, Kümpfel T. Update on the diagnosis and treatment of neuromyelitis optica: recommendations of the Neuromyelitis Optica Study Group (NEMOS). J Neurol. 2014;261(1):1–6.
9. Biousse V, Newman NJ. Ischemic optic neuropathies. N Engl J Med. 2015;372(25):2428–36.
10. Hayreh SS. Management of ischemic optic neuropathies. Indian J Ophthalmol. 2011;59(2):123.
11. Karimi S, Arabi A, Ansari I, Shahraki T, Safi S. A systematic literature review on traumatic optic neuropathy. J Ophthalmol. 2021;2021
12. Yu-Wai-Man P. Taiwan Journal of Ophthalmology. Taiwan J Ophthalmol. 2015;5:3e8.
13. Miller NR. Primary tumours of the optic nerve and its sheath. Eye. 2004;18(11):1026–37.
14. Chutorian AM, Schwartz JF, Evans RA, Carter S. Optic gliomas in children. Neurology. 1964;14(2):83.
15. Rush JA, Younge BR, Campbell RJ, MacCarty CS. Optic glioma: long-term follow-up of 85 histopathologically verified cases. Ophthalmology. 1982;89(11):1213–9.
16. Yanoff M, Sassani JW. Ocular pathology. Philadelphia: Elsevier Health Sciences; 2018.
17. Dutton JJ. Optic nerve gliomas and meningiomas. Neurol Clin. 1991;9(1):163–77.
18. Frosch MP, Anthony DC, De Girolami U. The central nervous system. In: Kumar V, et al., editors. Robbins and Cotran pathologic basis of disease. Philadelphia: Elsevier Inc; 2010. p. 1279–344.

Pathology of Intraocular Tumors

19

Saumya Jakati, Vijitha S. Vempuluru,
and Swathi Kaliki

Contents

S. Jakati (✉)
Ophthalmic Pathology Laboratory, Kallam Anji Reddy campus, L V Prasad Eye Institute, Hyderabad, Telangana, India
e-mail: saumyajakati@lvpei.org; saumya.jakati@gmail.com

V. S. Vempuluru · S. Kaliki
Ophthalmic Plastics, Ocular Oncology, Dacryology, and Aesthetics Services, Kallam Anji Reddy Campus, L V Prasad Eye Institute, Hyderabad, Telangana, India

Operation Eyesight Universal, Kallam Anji Reddy campus, L V Prasad Eye Institute, Hyderabad, Telangana, India
e-mail: vijitha.vempuluru@lvpei.org; swathikaliki@lvpei.org

G. K. Vemuganti et al. (eds.), *Ocular Pathology*, https://doi.org/10.1007/978-981-96-8614-8_19

19.1 Introduction

Eyeball has uniquely designed intraocular structures which aid in facilitating neurosensory function. Aqueous and vitreous humor help in maintaining the ideal contour of the globe. The various intraocular structures of eye include iris, ciliary body, choroid, retina, retinal pigment epithelium, and optic disc. Iris, ciliary body, and choroid are pigmented tissues, and these structures together constitute the "uvea." The specialized structures derived from the neuroectoderm include the retina, retinal pigment epithelium, ciliary body epithelium, and iris pigment epithelium. Retina is a neurosensory organ which is derived embryologically from neural crest cells and has specialized light-sensing receptors, rods, and cones. Optic disc is the area wherein the axons of retinal nerves form the optic nerve. These intraocular structures have unique histomorphology and pathologies. Advanced imaging tools help in understanding and better visualization of the intraocular tumors. Tools in aid are ultrasound biomicroscopy (UBM), ultrasound sonography (A-scan and B-scan), optical coherence tomography, fluorescein angiography, and indocyanine green angiography.

19.2 Classification

Intraocular tumors have a distinct histomorphology. Broadly, the intraocular tumors are classified into benign or malignant categories and based on the tumor location. Lesions confined to the intraocular space have better prognosis than those which have extraocular direct extension or spread; for example, orbital retinoblastomas, that is, retinoblastomas with extraocular extension tend to have a poorer prognosis than intraocular tumors [1]. An overview of benign and malignant intraocular lesions is provided in Table 19.1.

Table 19.1 Overview of benign and malignant intraocular lesions

Site	Benign	Malignant
Iris	Melanocytic nevus Ocular melanocytosis Lisch nodule Pigment epithelial cyst Implantation cyst	Iris melanoma Histiocytic tumors
Ciliary body	Uveal melanocytoma Ciliary body adenoma Adenomatous hyperplasia Reactive epithelial hyperplasia Leiomyoma Schwannoma Glioneuroma Ganglioneuroma Medulloepithelioma – (a) Teratoid (b) Nonteratoid	Adenocarcinoma
Choroid	Naevi Uveal melanocytic hyperplasia Neurofibroma Schwannoma Hemangioma Ganglioneuroma Osteoma	Melanoma Primary choroidal lymphoma Secondary lymphomatous infiltration Leukemic infiltration Secondary tumors
Retina	Retinocytoma Astrocytic hamartoma Nodular and massive gliosis Hemangioblastoma Cavernous hemangioma	Retinoblastoma Vitreoretinal lymphoma Leukemic infiltration Secondary tumors
Retinal pigment epithelium	Adenoma Reactive hyperplasia Simple and combined hamartomas Congenital hypertrophy	Adenocarcinoma
Optic disc	Astrocytic hamartoma Melanocytoma	Secondary tumors

19.3 Tumors and Tumor Like Lesions of Uveal Tissue

19.3.1 Iris

19.3.1.1 Benign Tumors

Melanocytic Nevus

Melanocytic nevus is a benign proliferation of melanocytes and is common in Caucasians. Clinically, they appear as flat to elevated lesions with effacement of the iris stromal architecture. Most commonly seen in the inferior aspect of the iris, these lesions can be well circumscribed to ill defined and vary in size, shape, and degree of pigmentation. They can occasionally be associated with secondary changes such as irregular pupil, secondary cysts, or cataract [2]. Melanocytoma or magnocellular nevus is an uncommon variant of iris nevus with distinct clinical and pathological features such as deep pigmentation, tendency for spontaneous necrosis, and glaucoma [3]. Etiopathogenesis of melanocytic nevus is multifactorial. On histopathology, nevi cells are benign and are spindle with elongated nucleus with intranuclear grooves or intranuclear inclusions. Long-standing cases show documented increase in size of the lesions [3]. They are indolent lesions and require periodic evaluations to detect malignant transformation into a melanoma. The most frequent mutations encountered are *GNA11* or *GNAQ* similar to melanomas [4].

Ocular Melanocytosis

Ocular melanocytosis or melanosis oculi or Nevus of Ota is a congenital pigmentary abnormality associated with increased melanocytes cells in uveal tract and other ocular structures such as sclera, conjunctiva, and optic nerve. Ocular melanocytosis with associated skin pigmentation is termed oculodermal melanocytosis. Orbital tissues, meninges, palate, and tympanic membrane can also be involved [5].

The condition manifests most commonly as unilateral to rarely bilateral flat, slate gray to brown patches of pigmentation on the sclera. Iris appears hyperchromic and has a velvety appearance. Hyperpigmentation of the uveal tissue can be partial, sectoral, or total [6]. Histopathology of iris and ciliary body shows heavily pigmented melanocytes. About 1 in 400 patients with oculodermal melanocytosis run the risk of development of uveal melanoma, occasionally in childhood and can have an aggressive clinical course. Similar to melanocytic nevus *GNA11* or *GNAQ* are found in these lesions [4].

Lisch Nodule

Lisch nodules are melanocytic hamartomas of the iris, most commonly associated with neurofibromatosis type-1 (NF-1) also known as von Recklinghausen disease. These tumors are also known as Sakurai–Lisch nodule and serve as one of the essential diagnostic parameters for NF-1. Etiology includes genetic predisposition to *NF-1* gene mutation and UV radiation [7]. These lesions are often associated with ocular lesions associated with NF-1 such as neurofibromas, gliomas, and choroidal nevi. Denovo mutations in NF are 42%. Neurofibromatosis has autosomal dominant pattern of inheritance with 100% penetrance and wide variable presentation. The inactivation of protein neurofibromin which is a RAS GTPase-activating protein causes increased signaling of *RAS* oncogenes [8].

The prevalence of Lisch nodules in NF-1 increases with age and is seen in >90% of patients at 30 years of age [9]. They are usually multiple, bilateral, and distributed all over the iris and appear as 1–2 mm dome-shaped nodules on the surface of iris. Color of Lisch nodules varies with ethnicity and ranges from yellow to brown [9]. Histopathologically, they are melanocytic hamartomas with elements of neural crest origin and show no atypia [9].

Iris Pigment Epithelial (IPE) Cyst

Primary cysts of the iris are sporadic can arise from the iris pigment epithelium or the iris stroma. The former arise from the posterior pigment epithelium of the iris and can be classified into central or pupillary, midzonal or retro-iridic, peripheral or iridociliary, dislodged, freely floating types based on their location [10].

Central IPE cysts can be unilateral and solitary or bilateral and multifocal. They appear as brown well-defined lesions along the pupillary margin. When they collapse spontaneously, they form irregular lesions termed "iris flocculi" [10]. Congenital iris flocculi have been associated aortic dissection as a result of mutation in smooth muscles common to iris and aorta.

Midzonal IPE cysts appear as round to fusiform brown lesions posterior to the pupillary margin and are better visualized after pupillary dilatation. They rarely cause visual impairment which can be managed by aspiration to collapse the cyst.

Peripheral IPE cysts are the most common type of IPE cysts but are detected less often due to their location. They can be unilateral or bilateral and manifest as anterior bowing of iris stroma or visualized on gonioscopy but are best visualized on ultrasound biomicroscopy [10].

Microscopically, these cysts are lined by pigment epithelium with intracystic clear fluid. Occasionally keratin flakes may be noted. Iris stromal cyst, melanocytoma, melanoma, and ciliary body medulloepithelioma are common differentials.

Implantation Cyst

Epithelial implantation cysts of iris most commonly occur secondary to trauma or penetrating injury. Secondary implantation cysts are usually symptomatic resulting in pain, redness, or photophobia. Based on the clinical appearance, they are classified as serous cysts with thin translucent membranes that are occasionally septate with clear to hazy cyst fluid; pearl cysts comprising keratin debris lined by an opaque wall embedded within the iris; and epithelial downgrowth which shows epithelial sheets, cysts, and pearls. Large-sized cysts can obliterate the angle [11]. Histopathologically, these cysts are lined by stratified nonkeratinized squamous epithelium with or without goblet cells.

19.3.1.2 Malignant Lesions

Iris Melanoma

Iris melanoma is a malignant tumor that arises from the melanocytes of the iris stroma, which are derivatives of the neural crest. More common in Caucasians, these tumors often arise in the inferior quadrants of the iris and can be of circumscribed, diffuse, tapioca or trabecular meshwork types in morphology. While a circumscribed melanoma appears as a well-defined lesion with variable pigmentation, diffuse melanomas manifest as hyperchromic heterochromia. Ring melanoma is a variant of diffuse melanoma which is largely confined to trabecular meshwork with minimal iris involvement (Fig. 19.1). Tapioca melanoma refers to a variant of iris melanoma which comprises multiple amelanotic lesions on the surface of the iris. Iris melanoma can be associated with corectopia, ectropion uveae, secondary glaucoma, seeding or extension to the anterior chamber angle, hyphema, and extraocular extension [12].

Histologic description and genetics of all melanomas are given under choroidal melanoma.

Histiocytic Tumors

Histiocytic tumors include juvenile xanthogranuloma, Rosai–Dorfman disease, Langerhans cell histiocytosis, and Erdheim–Chester disease.

19.3.2 Ciliary Body

19.3.2.1 Leiomyoma

Leiomyoma of ciliary body is a benign tumor of neural crest origin. Literature supports a female preponderance, usually in the reproductive age group. Uveal leiomyomas are unilateral and unifocal with ciliary body being the most common site of involvement. Ciliary body leiomyomas are most often located in the temporal quadrant and are typically slow-growing. Patients can present with blurred vision as a result of subluxation of lens and/or secondary retinal detachment. When asymptomatic, tumors may be incidentally detected on routine clinical examination. Clinical signs include focal angle closure, iridodialysis, focal tumor infiltration of the angle structures, lens subluxation, and tumor-related cataract. On transillumination, leiomyomas have been classically described to transmit light, but this can be variable subject to overlying pigmentation. Ultrasound biomicroscopy aids in identification

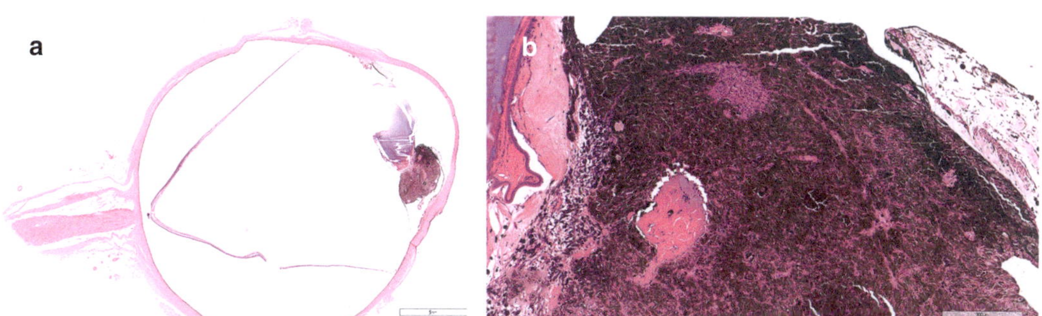

Fig. 19.1 Photomicrograph showing (**a**) the scanner view of the Iris melanoma (H&E; scanner view); (**b**) melanoma arising from the posterior pigment epithelium and touching the lens capsule and causing wrinkling of the capsule (H&E;×300)

of the tumor location, and tumors demonstrate variable internal reflectivity. On magnetic resonance imaging, the tumor appears isointense to hyperintense on T1-weighted images with marked signal enhancement with gadolinium and hypointense on T2-weighted images [12]. Owing to overlapping imaging features with uveal melanoma, a biopsy may be warranted for confirmation of the diagnosis [13]. On gross morphology, the lesion is a well-circumscribed, gray-white, fleshy growth arising from ciliary body which rarely grows beyond one centimeter. Microscopically, lesional cells are spindle cells with abundant cytoplasm and oval, fine-granular nucleus with mild pleomorphism. Cells show diffuse and strong expression with SMA, MSA, h-caldesmon, desmin, and calponin. Intraocular pigmented uveal leiomyomas are known to occur and can be confused with uveal melanomas. IHC with SMA would be diagnostic of the former [13].

19.3.2.2 Adenoma

Ciliary body adenoma is a benign lesion that can arise from the pigmented or nonpigmented epithelium. Adenoma of the pigment epithelium of the ciliary body is rare and is often misdiagnosed as a ciliary body melanoma. Tumors are often unilateral and unifocal, dome-shaped, gray to black in color, with abruptly elevated margins and can be associated with secondary cataract and vitreous hemorrhage [14]. Acquired tumors of the nonpigmented ciliary epithelium are rare and are seen in adults. Though benign they can exhibit growth leading to a mass effect, cataract, subluxation of lens and secondary glaucoma [15]. These tumors are often misdiagnosed as a ciliary body melanoma wherein histopathological examination aids in establishing a diagnosis.

Similar to adenocarcinomas, these benign counterparts exhibit similar variants of solid, papillary, and pleomorphic morphology. S100 is diffuse and intensely expressed by lesional cells. Expression of pancytokeratin is variable [16]. Changes in chromosome 6, loss of opticin and *BRAF* mutations are a few of the listed genetic implications [17].

Case illustration: (Figs. 19.2)A 28-year-old male presented with whitish appearance in the black portion of the left eye. On examination, ciliary body lesion was seen in the inferior portion of the ciliary body. Mass is dome-shaped, gray to black in color with abrupt elevated margins. Gross morphology revealed a fleshy gray white to tan colored mass. Lesional cells were polygonal with abundant cytoplasm on histology and showed positivity for S100.

19.3.2.3 Medulloepithelioma: (a) Teratoid and (b) Non-teratoid

Medulloepithelioma is primary intraocular embryonal tumor arising from the nonpigmented ciliary epithelium [18]. These are also known as diktyomas or teratoneuromas. Primitive medullary epithelial anlage of optic cup is considered to be the cell of origin.

Most often diagnosed within the first decade of life, no gender or racial predilection has been identified [19]. Small tumors can be asymptomatic, and secondary effects such as cataract or glaucoma may be evident before the tumor can be visualized. Most common symptoms include poor vision, leukocoria, glaucoma, painful red eye, or a visible mass within the eye [19]. However, these cases are often misdiagnosed or missed which delay the management [20]. On examination, the lesion appears pink, gray white to yellow mass in the region of the ciliary body often with intratumoral cysts. Associated features include iris/angle neovascularization, corectopia, ectropion uveae, neovascular glaucoma, focal cataract, lens subluxation, lens coloboma, cyclitic membrane, or retrolental membranes. About 5% of patients with medulloepithelioma have a history of pleuropulmonary blastoma, a part of familial cancer syndrome, Pleuropulmonary Blastoma Family Tumor and Dysplasia Syndrome [19].

Medulloepitheliomas can be classified as shown in Fig. 19.3:

On gross morphology, these are solid cystic masses with intralesional cysts which are the major pointers to diagnosis. Extraocular spread

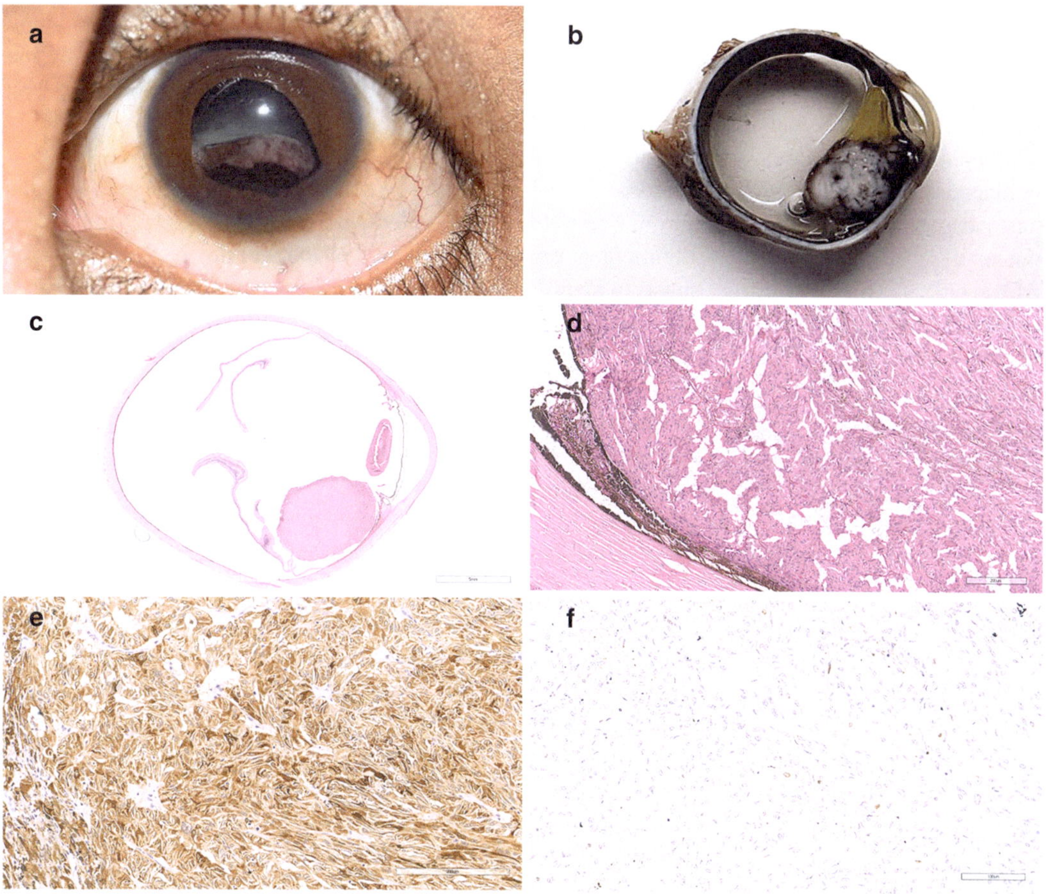

Fig. 19.2 Photomicrographs show (**a**) External photograph showing pigmented lesion in the inferior portion of the ciliary body region; (**b**) Gross picture showing the ciliary body lesion which is fleshy, gray white, and focally pigmented; (**c**) scanner view of the well-circumscribed lesion (H&E; scanner view); (**d**) Lesion arising from ciliary body and is composed large, polygonal cells with abundant cytoplasm(H&E;×40); (**e**) Lesional cells showing strong of expression S100 (diaminobenzidine chromogen; ×200); and (f) no expression of pancytokeratin (diaminobenzidine chromogen; ×200)

Fig. 19.3 Classification of medulloepitheliomas

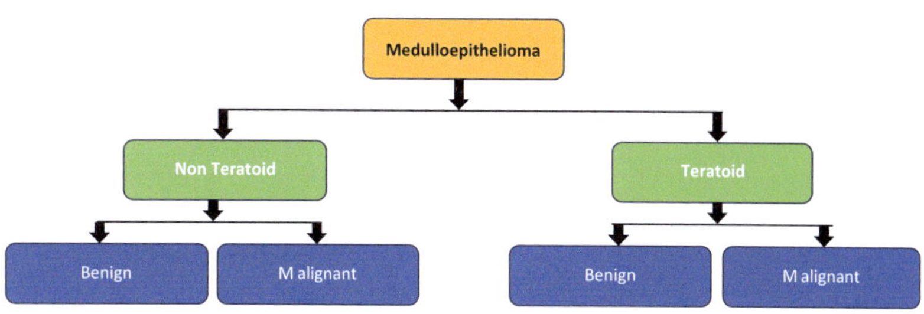

can occur through the shunts introduced to treat neovascular glaucoma. On histopathology, lesion is composed of cells arranged in cords, trabeculae, rosettes, and parallel ribbons of primitive neuroepithelial cells in the form of fish net (diktyomatous) pattern. Background shows acellular, pale basophilic, myxoid, hyaluronidase-rich mucopolysaccharides which is highlighted on Alcian blue. There can be diffuse sheets of neuroepithelial cells with Homer–Wright and Flexner–Wintersteiner rosettes. Features of malignancy include invasion of adjacent ocular tissues, extraocular extension, sarcomatous change, marked pleomorphism, atypia, and increased mitosis [21]. The present WHO classifies them into grade 1, benign; grade 2, lesion with pleomorphism, increased mitotic activity, and local invasion; grade 3, lesions associated with malignant transformation and metastatic potential. Lesions with presence of heterologous elements such as cartilage (most common), muscle, myoblasts, and glial tissue are categorized as teratoid. Malignancy can occur in the non-teratoid medulloepitheliomas also. On IHC, these lesional cells are positive for pan CK and CK18. They are negative for CK7, CK20, EMA, NSE, or Vimentin. Focal positivity is known for GFAP, S100, and HMB45. The differential diagnosis includes retinoblastoma and persistent fetal vasculature. Metastasis is known to occur in the brain in rare cases [22]. Medulloepitheliomas are known to have germline mutation of DICER-1 gene located on long arm of Chromosome 14,q32.13 and are known to develop pleuropulmonary blastomas, Sertoli-Leydig cell tumors, multinodular goiter, cystic nephroma, embryonal rhabdomyosarcoma, nasal epithelial hamartomas, pituitary blastomas, pineoblastomas, and other tumors [23–25]. Hence, these patients must undergo testing and active surveillance [26].

Case illustration: (Figs. 19.4) A 2-year-old female presented with whitish lesion in the left eye since past six months. On examination, amelanotic lesion was seen in the angle with vitreous membranes. Biopsy of the mass was attempted elsewhere. On magnetic resonance imaging, retrolenticular mass was seen. Histopathology revealed benign teratoid medulloepithelioma with lesion showing histology of skin, intestine, and adnexal structures.

Case illustration: (Figs. 19.5) A 17-year-old male presented with redness of the eye and whitish appearance in the anterior portion of the left eye for the past 8 months. On examination, white membrane like structures were noted in the ciliary body region. On gross morphology, a translucent lesion was seen arising from the superior aspect of ciliary body region. Histopathology of the enucleation specimen revealed a malignant nonteratoid medulloepithelioma.

Case illustration: (Figs. 19.6)A 2-year-old boy presented with a fleshy mass occupying the entire black portion of right eye. On examination, amelanotic mass was noted in the anterior chamber. B-scan showed a noncalcific intraocular mass. Histopathology of the enucleated eye showed a malignant teratoid medulloepithelioma.

19.3.2.4 Adenocarcinoma

Adenocarcinoma of ciliary body is a malignant epithelial tumor arising from pigmented or non-pigmented epithelium of ciliary body. These are exceptionally rare tumors, often associated with chronic ocular inflammation or phthisical eyes. Clinically, they can be amelanotic or pigmented lesions within the ciliary body. They can extend anteriorly to involve the iris and can present with secondary glaucoma. Establishing a clinical diagnosis can be challenging, and the presence of extraocular spread has a poor prognosis [27].

On gross morphology, these are seen as irregular dark colored masses, solid, and homogeneous. As the lesional growth is toward the lens, it might cause lens subluxation or cataractous changes. Microscopically, the lesional cells are arranged in acinar pattern, cords, and tubules. The lesional cells are large, cuboidal to polygonal with a large nucleus, and prominent nucleoli [28]. Extracellular material deposit is seen in the background which is hyaluronidase-sensitive mucopolysaccharide and highlighted on

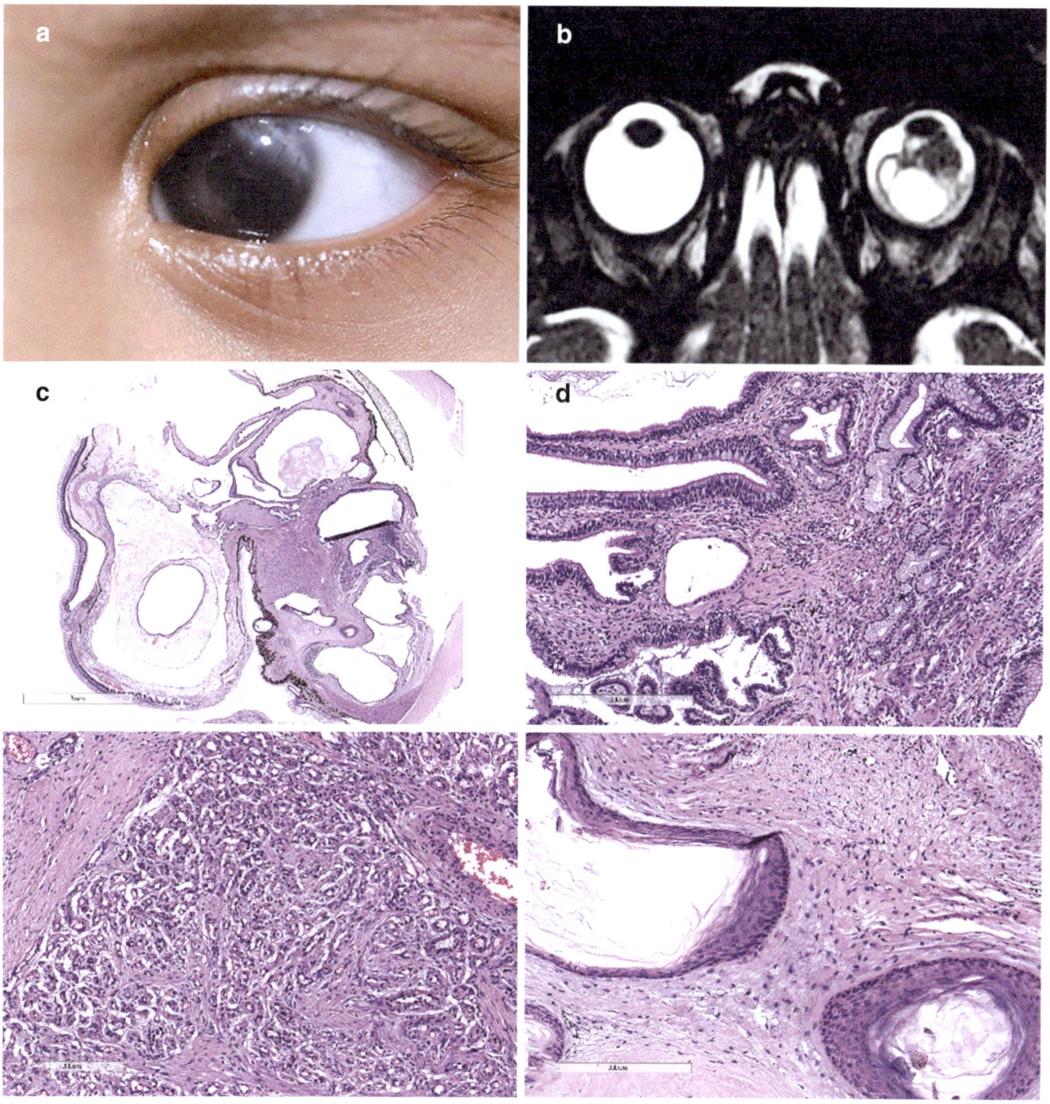

Fig. 19.4 Photomicrographs show (**a**) External photograph of the left eye showing corneal sutures present from 11 to 3 o clock hours, status post-incisional biopsy; amelanotic pink lesion from 12:30 to 1:30 in the angle of anterior chamber; elevated ciliary lesion with overlying pigment from 10:30 to 3:00 with whitish membrane inferotemporally; (**b**) Magnetic resonance imaging of the orbits revealed retrolental intraocular mass; (**c**) Lesion showing arising from the ciliary body and occupying the posterior chamber (H&E; scanner view); (**d**) Intralesional intestinal tissue (H&E;×40); (**e**) Acinar or glandular structures (H&E;×40); (**f**) Keratin cysts (H&E;×40)

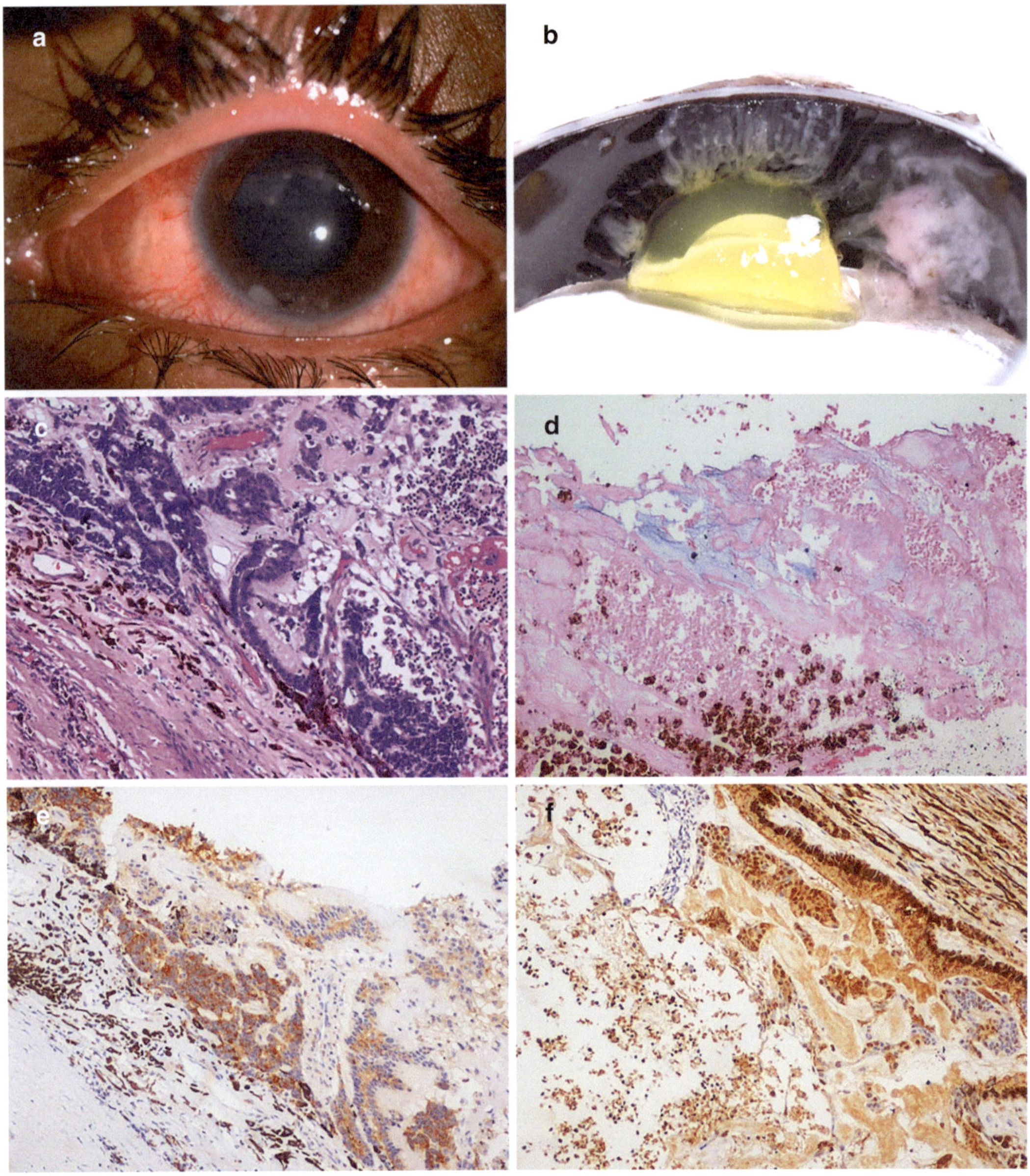

Fig. 19.5 Photomicrographs show (**a**) External photograph of left eye showing conjunctival congestion and tumor infiltration in the anterior chamber inferiorly; (**b**) Gross image of the enucleated eyeball showing pink, fluffy, translucent lesion in the ciliary body region; (**c**) Photomicrograph showing the lesion arising from ciliary body and is arranged in papillae, acini, and cords in the background of basophilic myxoid stroma (H&E; ×100); (**d**) Extracellular myxoid stroma highlighted on Alcian blue (Alcian blue; ×100); (**e**) Strong cytoplasmic expression of cytokeratin (Diaminobenzidine chromogen; ×100); and (**f**) Synaptophysin (Diaminobenzidine chromogen; ×100)

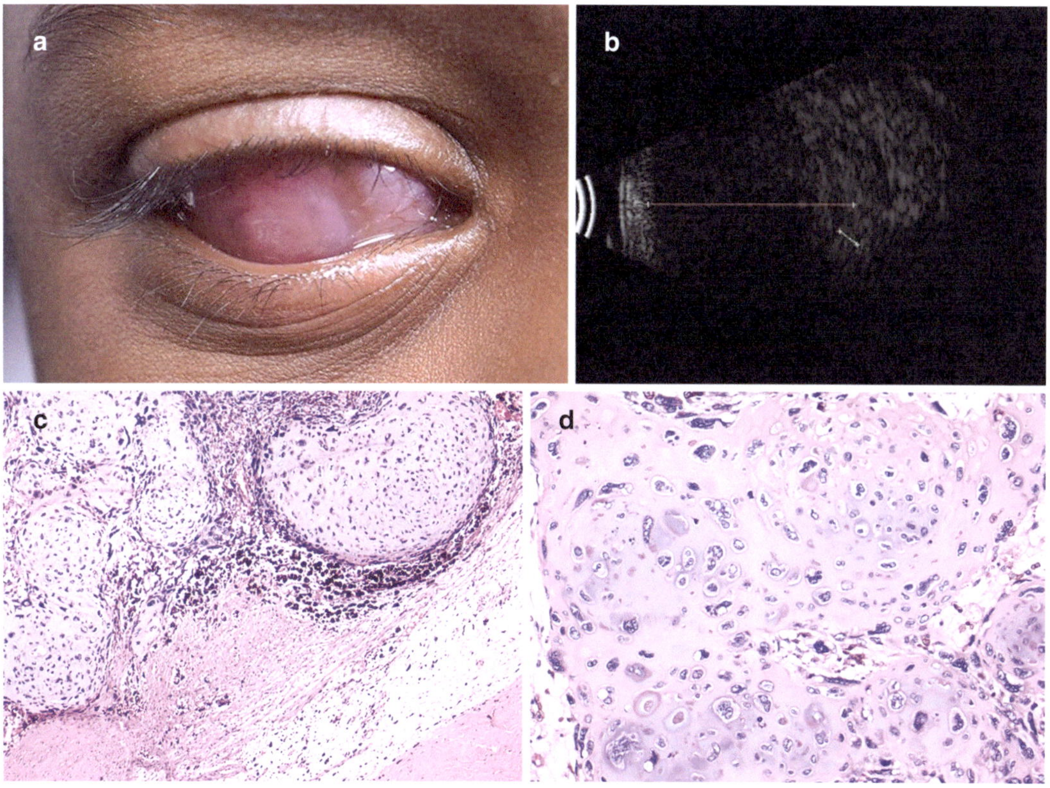

Fig. 19.6 Photomicrographs show (**a**) External photograph showing amelanotic mass filling the entire anterior chamber; (**b**) B-scan ultrasonography showing intraocular mass without calcification; (**c**) Photomicrograph showing pleomorphic lesion arising from the adjacent ciliary body arranged in lobules (H&E; ×40); (**d**) Lesional cells are markedly pleomorphic and bizarre with hyperchromatic to vesicular nuclei with prominent nucleoli in chondroid background (H&E; ×100)

periodic acid Schiff's stain. Solid, pleomorphic, and papillary are the variants included. The pigmented adenocarcinomas can be differentiated from ciliary body melanomas, as pancytokeratin is expressed by the former lesion, whereas HMB45, S100, and Melan A are not. However, pleomorphic adenocarcinomas can be negative for pancytokeratin [29]. Genetic profile includes 6p gain, 6q loss, and *BRAF* mutations in a few cases [30].

19.3.3 Choroid

19.3.3.1 Benign Tumors

Hemangioma

A benign hamartomatous vascular proliferation of the choroid, choroidal hemangioma can occur as a circumscribed lesion or as a diffuse tumor, commonly unilateral, commonly seen in patients with Sturge–Weber syndrome [31].

Circumscribed choroidal hemangioma is unilateral, usually involving the posterior uvea and may involve up to half of the choroid, posterior to equator [32]. On examination, the lesion appears orange-red with well-defined borders. Rarely, they can be multifocal [33]. Associated features include subretinal fluid, cystoid retinal degeneration, retinal pigment epithelial hyperplasia or fibrous metaplasia, retinoschisis, and occasionally neovascular glaucoma following total retinal detachment [31]. The differential diagnosis includes amelanotic melanoma (amelanotic), metastasis, choroidal granuloma, and choroidal osteoma [34]. Fluorescein angiography is characteristic with hyperfluorescence in pre-arterial phase and late diffuse staining. Indocyanin angiography shows early filling of the lesion with a "wash-out" hypercyanescence in late phase. On ultrasound, the tumor appears a well-defined choroidal mass with high internal reflectivity [34] (Fig. 19.7).

Diffuse choroidal hemangiomas are usually associated with ipsilateral nevus flammeus, as a part of Sturge–Weber syndrome. Usually diagnosed in childhood, they can be associated with secondary retinal detachment or anisometropic amblyopia. Bright red reflex is noted known as a "tomato catsup fundus". The involved eye shows diffuse thickening of the choroid. Associated features include cystoid degeneration, retinal detachment, and secondary glaucoma [31, 35, 36].

Histopathologically, choroidal hemangiomas are seen as proliferation of thin walled blood vessels lined by endothelial cells and are often confused with melanomas clinically and on imaging [37].

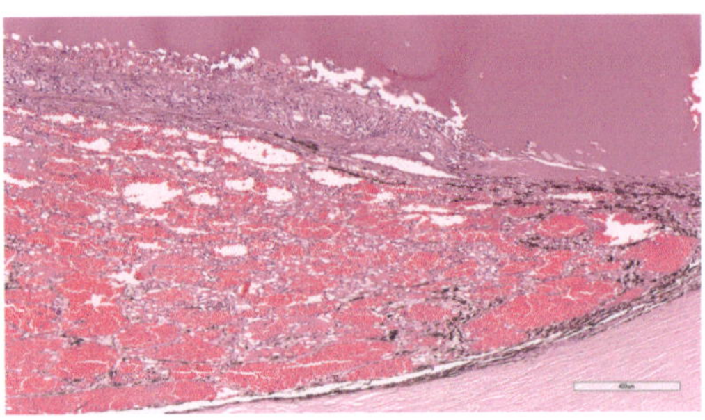

Fig. 19.7 Photomicrograph showing lesion in the choroid showing proliferating vessels arranged back to back and are lined by thin-walled capillary channels (H&E; ×40)

Schwannoma

Schwannoma is a benign peripheral nerve sheath tumor arising from Schwann cells, commonly seen in middle-aged women [38]. Clinically schwannomas appear as yellow to white lesions with subretinal fluid and may also be associated with exudation and retinal feeder vessels [38, 39]. These lesions can extend into the ciliary body. Patients primarily present with vision loss or a painful eye with intraocular mass. Differential diagnosis includes amelanotic melanoma and choroidal hemangioma [38]. Indocyanine angiography differentiates a schwannoma from a hemangioma by the absence of late washout phenomenon [38]. Microscopically, these tumors have compact and hypercellular Antoni A areas with occasional Verocay bodies along with hypocellular Antoni B areas which comprise mononuclear cells. Ancient schwannomas show nuclear atypia which are degenerative changes [38–40].

Neurofibroma and Ganglioneuroma

Neurofibroma is a nerve sheath tumor which can occur in the background of NF-1 and is detected in childhood. It involves the choroidal nerves and ciliary nerves. Choroidal involvement is one of the major criteria for diagnosis of NF-1. Choroidal nodules are seen in >80% of patients with neurofibromatosis and comprise proliferating Schwann cells around axons. Choroidal nodules are best visualized on near-infrared reflectance imaging wherein they appear as bright patches [41]. Histopathology shows proliferation of Schwann cells with fibroblasts and melanocytes [42].

Ganglioneuromas of the choroid are extremely rare, and reports suggest incidental diagnosis in enucleated/eviscerated ocular specimens in patients with neurofibromatosis 1. Histopathology shows spindle cells along with clusters of ganglion cells that have abundant cytoplasm, large vesicular nuclei, and prominent nucleoli [43] (Fig. 19.8).

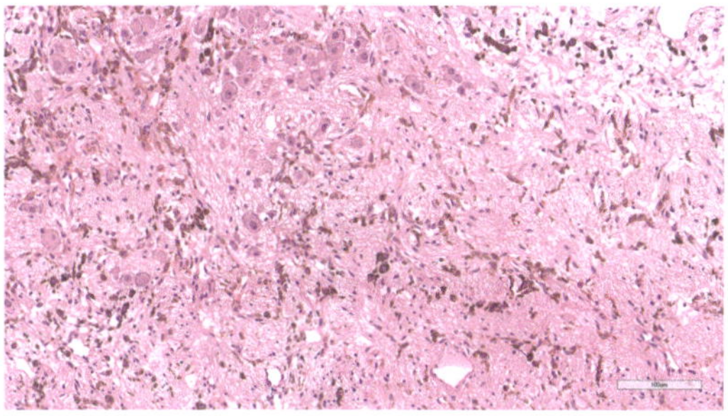

Fig. 19.8 Photomicrograph showing lesion within the choroid composed of choroidal melanocytes admixed with large Ganglion cells in fibrillary background (H&E;×100)

Osteoma

Osteomas are benign ossifying tumors of unknown etiology. They are more often unilateral than bilateral and seen in young women. Symptoms when present include blurred vision and visual field defects. Choroidal osteomas are seen in the juxta-papillary and macular areas of choroid. They appear as deep, orange-red, well-defined lesions with scalloped edges. Older lesions tend to appear more yellow from depigmentation of retinal pigment epithelium. Choroidal neovascularization is a known secondary complication to choroidal osteomas [44]. Ultrasonography, optical coherence tomography and computed tomography can demonstrate the calcification within the lesion. Microscopically, these lesions are similar to osteomas elsewhere in the body composed of irregular bony trabeculae lined by osteoblastic rimming with intervening spaces showing loose connective tissue. This should be distinguished from osseous metaplasia seen in phthisical eyes as the osseous metaplastic change occurs on the inner surface of retinal pigment epithelium [34].

19.3.3.2 Malignant Tumors

Ciliochoroidal Melanoma

These are the primary malignant melanocytic tumors arising from the choroid and ciliary body. Uveal melanoma is the most common primary intraocular tumor in adults and 90% involved the choroid. Mean age-adjusted is about 5 per million per year. Risk factors include light eye color, fair skin, lack of ability to tan, and cutaneous or uveal nevi. Melanomas can arise de novo or from preexisting nevi and systemic associations include congenital ocular or oculodermal melanocytosis, dysplastic nevus or BAP1 tumor predisposition syndrome [45]. *GNA11* or *GNAQ* driver mutations are detected in almost all the melanomas. However, *BRAF* mutation is rare. Metastatic uveal melanomas show loss of chromosome 3 in association with polysomy 8q and *BAP1* mutations [4]. Other mutations seen in uveal melanomas include *SF3B1* and *EIF1AX* [46]. Based on gene expression profiling, uveal melanomas are categorized into two classes. Class 1 is subcategorized into 1A (low risk of metastasis) and 1B (intermediate risk of metastasis). Class 2 tumors show high risk of metastasis [47].

Most common symptoms encountered with ciliochoroidal melanoma are blurred vision, flashes of light or photopsia, floaters, visual field loss, visible mass lesion, and metamorphopsia. While patients can also be asymptomatic, large tumors induce pain, redness, and raised intraocular pressure. Clinically, choroidal melanoma appears as a dome-shaped tumor with variable pigmentation. Associated features include retinal detachment, vitreous hemorrhage, and sometimes extrascleral tumor extension. Ancillary investigations such as optical coherence tomography (dome-shaped choroidal tumor with shaggy photoreceptors and subretinal fluid), ultrasonography (acoustic hollowing, choroidal excavation, and orbital shadowing), and fundus fluorescein or indocyanine angiography (double circulation) aid in diagnosing a small choroidal melanoma [45].

On gross morphology, melanomas are seen as a dome-shaped or a mushroom-shaped elevated mass extending into vitreous cavity arising from the choroid or ciliary body. Mushroom is classically seen as the lesion breaks through the Bruch's membrane of RPE. The overlying retina appears detached, degenerated, and fragmented with focal subretinal exudates (Fig. 19.9).

Microscopically, choroidal melanomas can be categorized per Callendar classification into spindle, epithelioid and mixed of which epithelioid type is considered to be highly aggressive and invasive. Presently, modified version of this

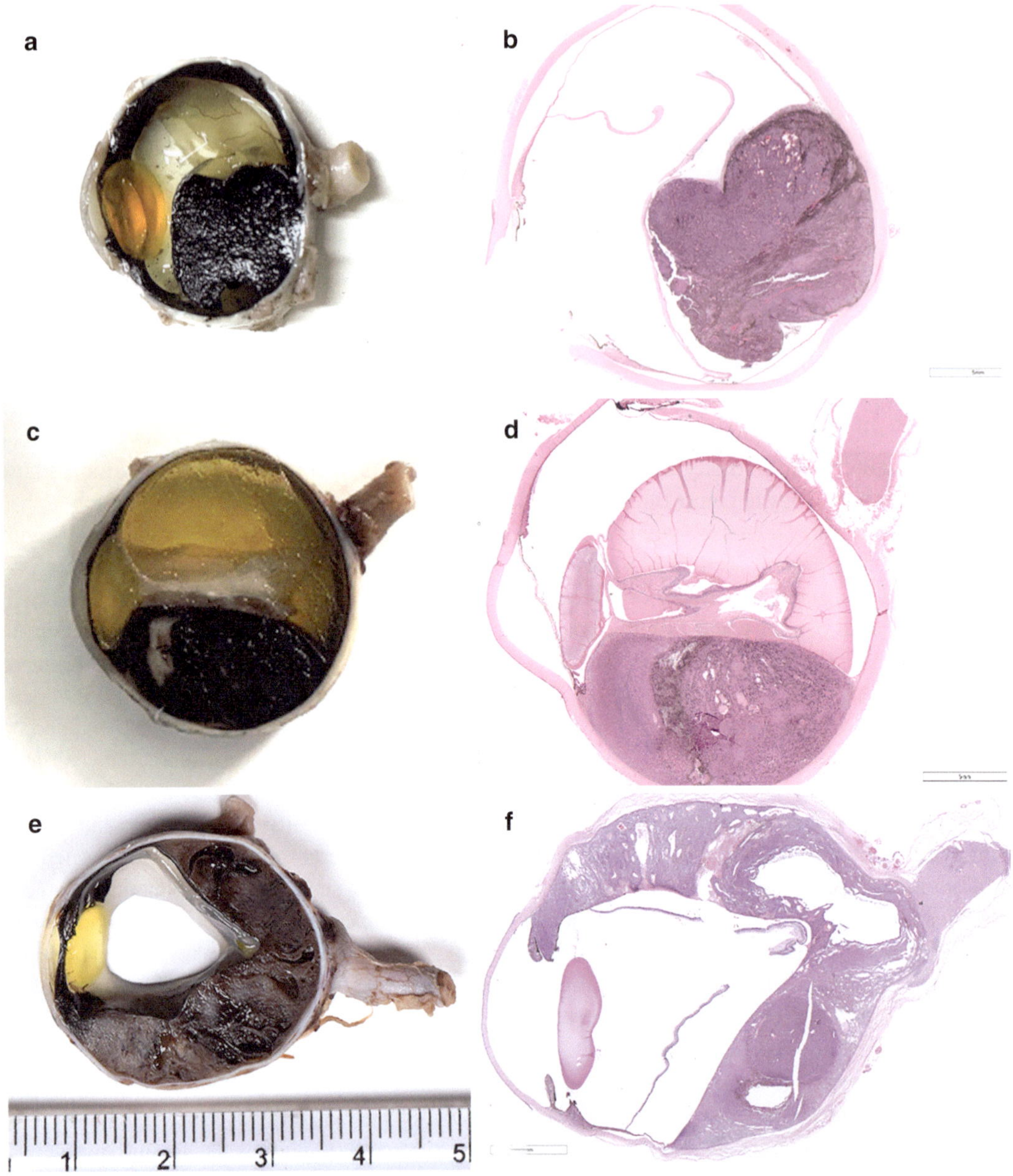

Fig. 19.9 Corresponding gross and microscopic images of choroidal melanomas (**a**) mushroom or collar button-shaped melanoma; (**b**) Dome-shaped lesion; (**c**) Diffuse involvement

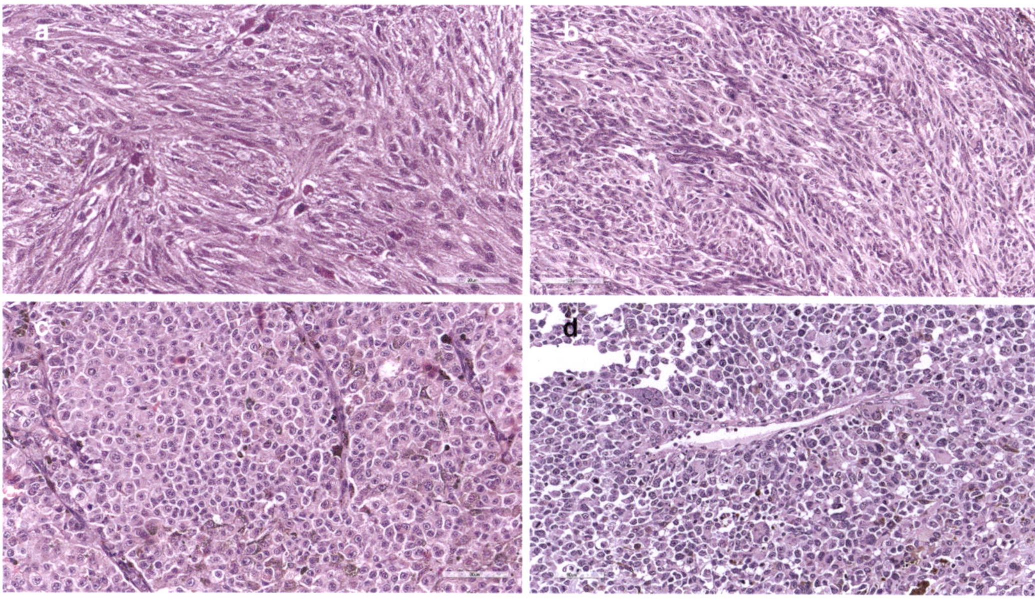

Fig. 19.10 Photomicrograph showing the melanoma cell type through modified Callender classification: (**a**) Spindle A cells (naevoid- like which are slender elongated), (**b**) Spindle B cells, (**c**) Epithelioid cells, and (**d**) Epithelioid cells with severe anaplasia

classification is used wherein the lesions are classified into spindle A, spindle B, epithelioid and Mixed [48] (Fig. 19.10). Spindle A cells are cohesive elongated, spindle, with central intranuclear grooves. Spindle B cells are cohesive, plump spindle with cigar-shaped nuclei. Epithelioid cells are discohesive and are enlarged polygonal with abundant eosinophilic cytoplasm [48]. The melanin pigment production is variable ranging from amelanotic to densely pigmented lesions. Spindle cell melanomas should contain >90% of spindle cells. Epithelioid cell melanomas have the worst prognosis whereas pure spindle cell tumor have the best prognosis [48]. Rarely, uveal melanomas undergo spontaneous necrosis due to insufficient blood supply and are termed as "Ghost cell melanoma" [49] (Fig. 19.11). Necrotic cells cause release of cytokines and tumor necrosis factor-1. Pigment dispersion is also noted within the ciliochoroidal capillaries and induces pigmentary glaucoma. All the sections must be meticulously assed for extrascleral and optic nerve extension (Fig. 19.12). Hemorrhagic choroid melanomas are also reported which show large areas of intraocular hemorrhage. "Balloon cells" in melanoma are induced after radiotherapy and show foamy cytoplasm. Other variants of melanoma include diffuse melanomas, ring melanoma, amelanotic melanoma, and clear cell melanoma. Choroidal melanomas invariably express HMB45, S100, Melan A, tyrosinase, SOX10, and Ki-67. Vascular pattern in melanomas is well-documented. Vasculogenic mimicry or the vascular patterns in melanomas which can be parallel, straight, parallel with crosslinking, arcs, arcs with branching, closed vascular loops are predictors of metastasis. Over the last decade, molecular workup for genetic mutations as well as molecular prognostic factors that can classify them as Class 1 and Class 2 tumors have now become a routine feature specially in western world where it is more common [47] Like retinoblastoma, choroidal melanomas are observed to show vitreous seeding [50]. Differential diagnosis includes melanocytoma, bilateral diffuse uveal melanocytoma, and metastasis [50–52].

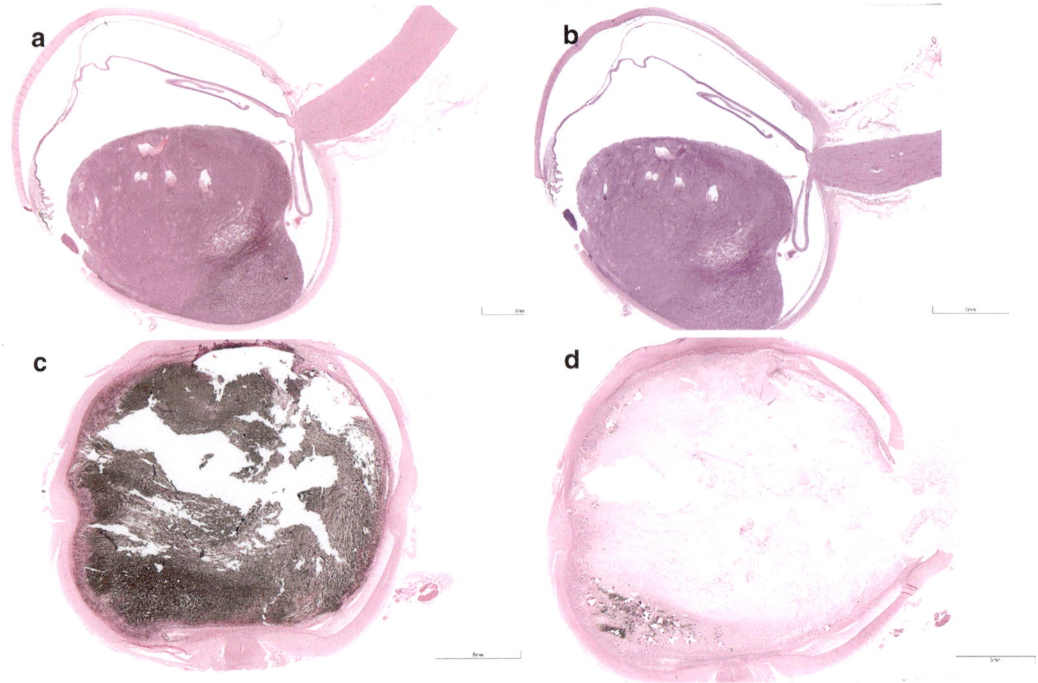

Fig. 19.11 Photomicrograph showing **a&b**) H&E stained spindle cell ciliochoroidal melanoma and the corresponding bleached section on scanner view in comparison to **c&d**) Ghost cell melanoma showing dense pigmentation of posterior chamber and the corresponding bleach section showing no viable lesion

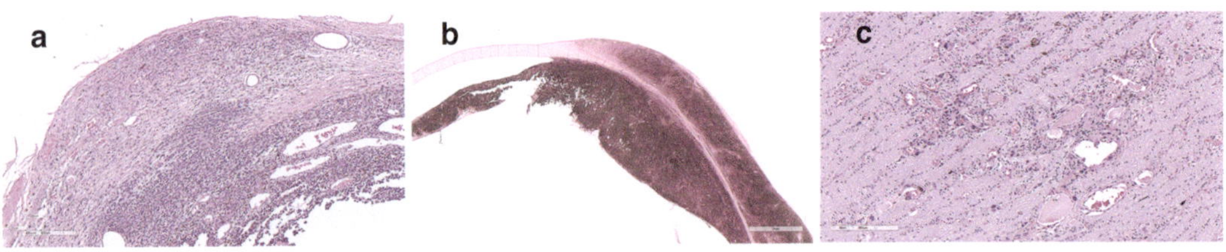

Fig. 19.12 Photomicrograph showing Epithelioid melanoma involving various intraocular structures (**a**) Sclera (H&E; ×40); (**b**) Choroidal melanoma involving adjacent ciliary body, iris and sclera (H&E;×40); (**c**) Retrolaminar involvement of optic nerve (H&E; ×100)

19.4 Salient Features

Always examine the globe after enucleation for pigmentation over sclera and enlarged emissary veins.

All pigmented lesions should be complemented by bleached sections for better visualization of lesional cellular morphology after removal of intracytoplasmic pigment. This would also help distinguish lesional cells from pigment-laden macrophages.

19.5 Leukemic Infiltration

Leukemic infiltration of choroid occurs secondary to the systemic leukemic involvement with a slight male predominance [53]. Choroid might act as sanctuary site similar to testis in these cases [53]. Clinically, this presents as vision loss from serous retinal detachment in the macular region [54]. These lesions are seen in the posterior choroid and can be seen in cases of subleukemic or aleukemic leukemia; hence examination of eyes is an essential part of the systemic workup in patients with leukemia [53].

19.6 Tumors and Tumor-Like Lesions of Retina

19.6.1 Benign

19.6.1.1 Retinocytoma

Retinocytoma is a presumed benign variant of retinoblastoma and has also been termed spontaneous regressed/ arrested retinoblastoma. About 2–10% of patients with retinoblastoma harbor retinocytoma which is usually diagnosed within the second decade of life. Retinocytoma appears as a gray white translucent lesion with calcification and associated features include retinal pigment epithelial alterations and chorioretinal atrophy. They are mostly unilateral and may be occasionally bilateral [55].

Lesions comprise only photoreceptor-differentiated cells forming fleurettes (flower like) with thick neurofibrillary processes without any lumen and bland nuclei [56].

Salient Features

- Alcian blue stains the background and the matrix of the retinocytoma cells

19.6.1.2 Retinal Capillary Hemangioma

Case illustration: (Fig. 19.13)

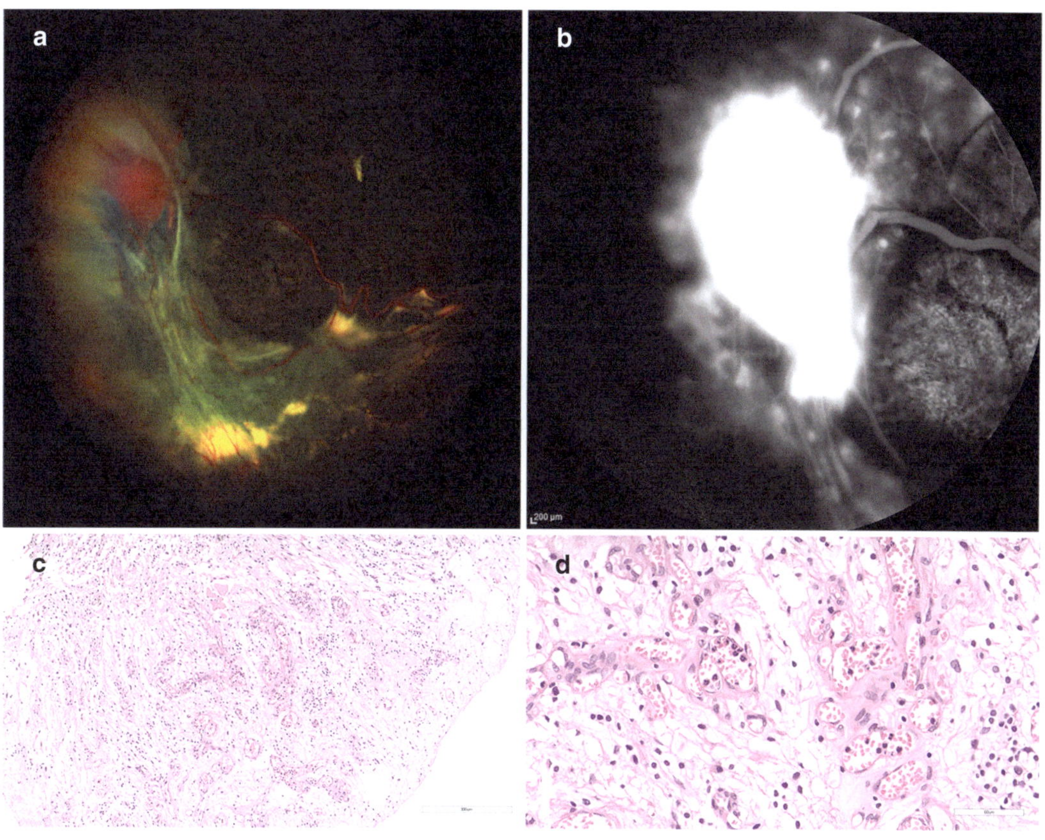

Fig. 19.13 Photomicrographs show (**a**) Color fundus photograph of the right eye showing reddish-lesion in the temporal periphery with a dilated feeder artery and a draining vein; (**b**) Fluorescent angiography late phase of the lesion showing leakage and staining; (**c**) Photomicrograph showing proliferating capillary-sized vessels in retina (H&E;×100); (**d**) Higher magnification of capillary-sized vessels lined by thin-walled blood vessels with intraluminal RBCs (H&E;×200). Fundus photograph (Panel A) and fluorescent angiography (Panel B). Courtesy: Dr Vishal Raval, Anant Bajaj Retina Institute, Kallam Anji Reddy campus, L V Prasad Eye Hospital

19.6.2 Malignant

19.6.2.1 Retinoblastoma

Retinoblastoma (RB) is the most common intraocular pediatric malignancy with a prevalence of one in 16,000 to 18,000 live births. Etiopathogenesis is attributed to somatic or germline mutations in chromosome 13. RB is a small blue round cell tumor originating from the primitive neuroectoderm. Affected individuals are also prone to other secondary cancers such as osteosarcoma, soft tissue sarcomas and melanomas [57].

The median age of presentation ranges from 12 to 24 months and is bilateral in 30–40% of the cases. Clinical features include white eye reflex or leukocoria which is the most common presenting symptom followed by strabismus, decreased vision, red eye, or proptosis in advanced cases [57, 58] (Fig. 19.14). The diagnosis of RB is largely clinical by visualization of the tumors on indirect ophthalmoscopy. Intraocular tumors present as well-defined yellow-white tumors which grow into the vitreous or the subretinal space. Associated features include tumor seeding, retinal detachment, neovascular glaucoma, buphthalmos, and extraocular extension or proptosis in advanced cases [57].

On gross morphology, RB appears friable whitish mass extending into the vitreous cavity. Large, globe-filling tumors can show extension into the adjacent choroid, sclera, ciliary body, iris, anterior chamber and trabecular meshwork (Fig. 19.15).

Microscopically the lesion can be endophytic, exophytic (arising from the outer retinal layers) or mixed (Fig. 19.16). Endophytic tumors arise from inner retinal layers and grow into the vitreous cavity. Tumor differentiation denotes the level of photoreceptor differentiation of cancer-

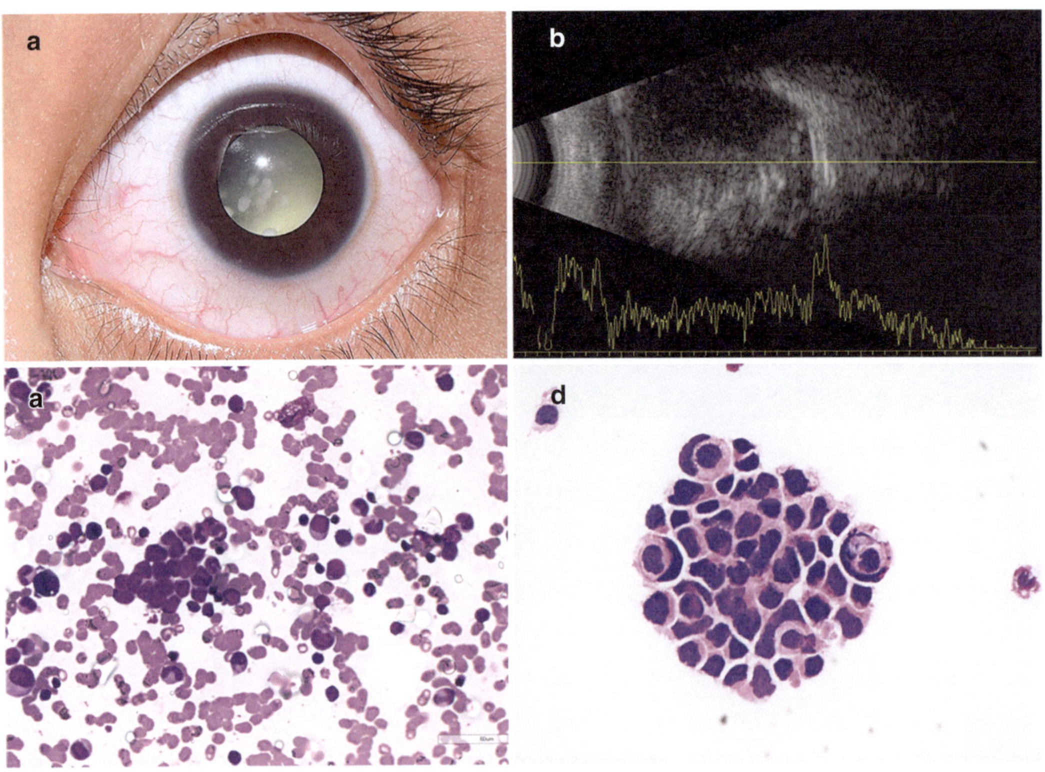

Fig. 19.14 Photomicrographs show (**a**) External photograph of the left eye showing leukocoria due to large endophytic tumor with vitreous seeds. (**b**) Ultrasonography of the left eye showing a large intraocular mass with an area of calcification causing high amplitude spikes and sound attenuation. C&D) Retinoblastoma infiltrates in bone marrow aspirate (Giemsa; ×100) and CSF (Giemsa; ×400)

ous cell (Fig. 19.17). Necrosis and calcification are very common in these lesions. Rarely, the inflammatory markers released from necrotic component can induce pseudocellulitis and are associated with high-risk features [58–62]. Azzopardi phenomenon is a mechanism in which the DNA from the necrosed tumor cells is deposited in the walls of the blood vessels. All the high-risk features must be keenly observed such as choroidal involvement (> or <3 mm, optic nerve involvement (beyond lamina cribrosa; resected margin and meninges), scleral invasion, extrascleral involvement iris and ciliary body involvement, anterior chamber and trabecular meshwork involvement [59] (Fig. 19.18). The most crucial microscopic parameters include tumor at the transected end of optic nerve, involvement of the meningeal spaces of optic nerve, full-thickness scleral involvement, and extrascleral extension. Sometimes, tiny isolated clusters of tumor cells detach themselves from the main tumor body giving rise to vitreous seeds which are usually refractory to treatment. These vitreous seeds have been recently classified based on histopathology as dust, sphere, and cloud. Similarly, the aqueous seeds have also been classified as dust, sphere, and cloud [63–65]. Additional findings such as cataractous changes and secondary glaucomatous changes can also be seen. Post-chemotherapy enucleation shows variable areas of viable tumor cells, tumoral calcinosis, and large areas of

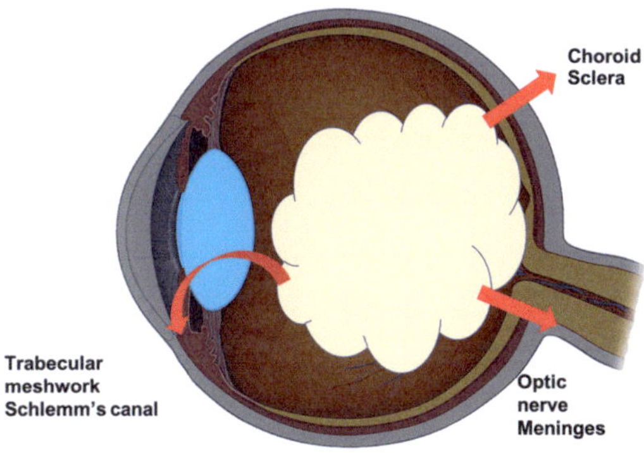

Fig. 19.15 Routes of spread of retinoblastoma (1) through optic nerve and meninges, (2) through choroid and sclera, and (3) through aqueous drainage

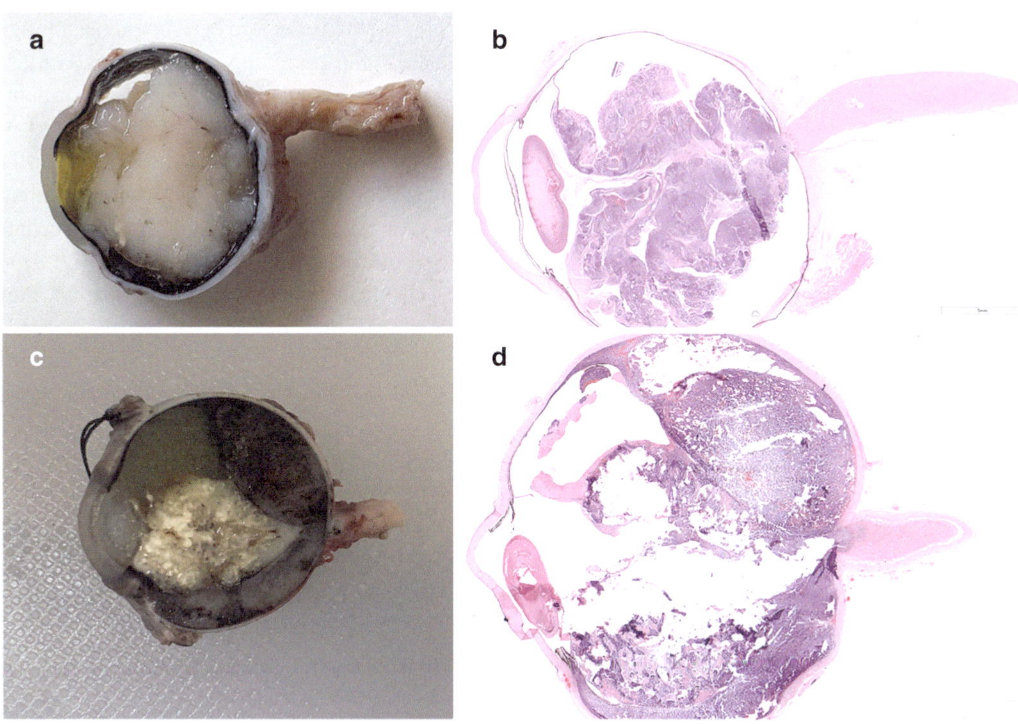

Fig. 19.16 Gross images and the corresponding photomicrographs of the P–O sections (central calottes) (H&E; scanner view) (**a**) Exophytic growth and (**b**) Endophytic and exophytic growth

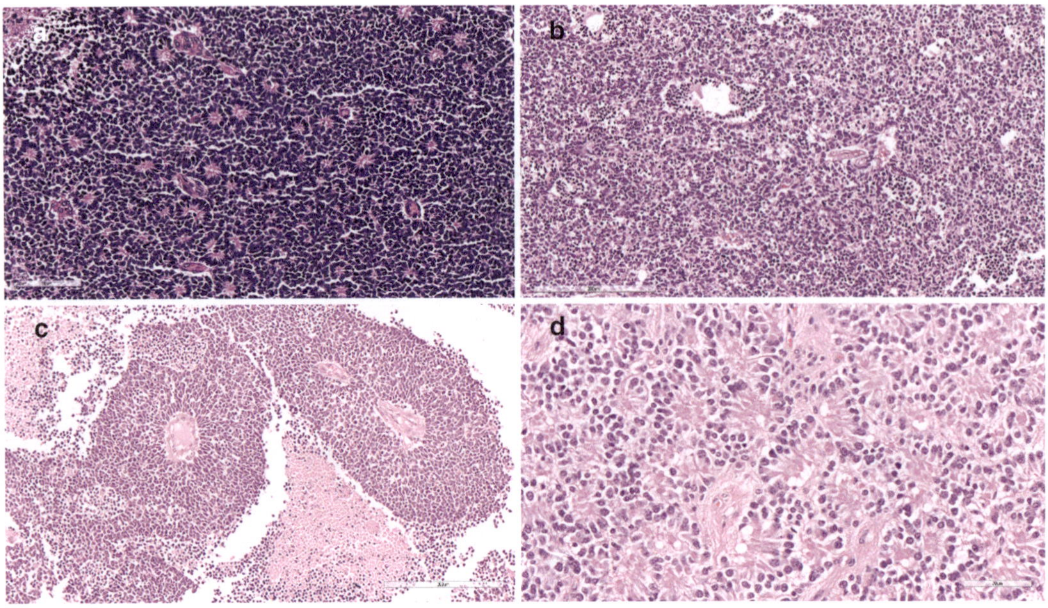

Fig. 19.17 Microscopic images of showing differentiation of retinoblastoma Panel (**a**) well differentiated with Flexner Wintersteiner rosettes (H&E; ×200) Panel (**b**) Poorly differentiated (H&E; ×200) Panel (**c**) Peritheliomatous pattern (H&E; ×200) and Panel (**d**) Retinocytoma like areas (H&E; ×400)

necrosis [66] (Fig. 19.19). Secondary sarcomas such as osteosarcomas are delayed or late complications of retinoblastoma.

In addition to the TNM staging, 8th edition of the AJCC has added hereditable trait as the new category in classification with subcategories of HX, HO, and H1 based on the status of *RB1* gene mutation. *MYCN* amplification (*MYCN*^{A}) is also noted in a few of the unilateral retinoblastomas [67].

Salient Features

- On gross morphology, enlargement of emissary vein or enlarged optic nerve head should be documented and examined for involvement on histopathology
- Periodic acid Schiff's stain helps in the identification of Bruch's membrane breach to rule in or rule out focal choroidal invasion in RB
- IHC with synaptophysin can be performed to identify the suspicious crushed cells at the transected end of optic nerve

19.6.2.2 Primary Intraocular Lymphoma

Intraocular lymphomas are heterogeneous malignant lesions and often clinically present as masquerade and uveitis not responding to treatment, being the most common [68]. Coupland et al. have classified intraocular lymphomas primarily based on their anatomic location, whether they are uveal or retinal. Uveal lymphomas are further classified into choroid, ciliary body, and iris, whereas retinal lymphomas are classified into vitreal, retinal, and vitreoretinal [69]. Choroidal lymphomas are further classified into primary and secondary. Most often the intraocular lymphomas are B-cell lymphomas. The retinal lymphomas tend to be high grade and aggressive (DLBCL) whereas the choroidal lymphomas are low grade and have a very indolent course (EMZL) [69]. Lymphomas are rare in ciliary body. Iris lymphomas are mixed cell lymphomas [69].

19.6.2.3 Primary Vitreoretinal Lymphoma

Primary vitreoretinal lymphomas (PVRLs) are an extremely rare disease usually seen in adults with

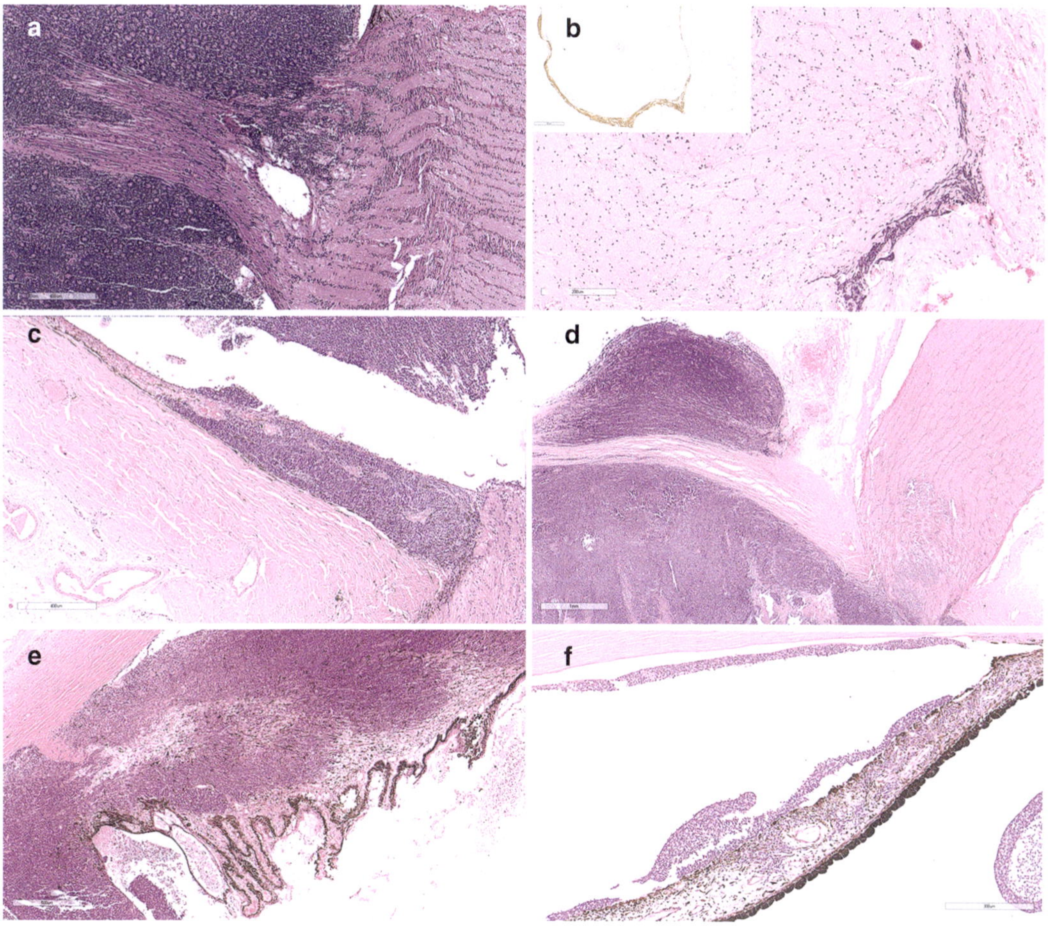

Fig. 19.18 Photomicrographs showing various high risk features (**a**) pre-laminar invasion of optic nerve (H&E;×40); (**b**) Involvement of the transected end of optic nerve (H&E; ×400) with synaptophysin expression in lesional cells (inset synaptophysin; ×400); (**c**) Choroidal involvement (H&E; ×40); (**d**) Extrascleral extension (H&E; ×40); (**e**) Infiltration of ciliary body and iris (H&E;×40); (**f**) Anterior chamber seeds with iris involvement (H&E; ×40)

a slight female predominance. Predisposing factors for PVRL would be an immunocompromised state such as HIV or EBV infection.

PVRL is usually bilateral. Long-standing decreased vision with floaters is often the presenting symptom. The presence of headache, altered sensorium and seizures suggests concomitant occurrence of primary CNS lymphomas (PCNSL) must be ruled out, as PVRL is considered as the subset or extension of the PCNSL. Clinical examination shows sheets and clusters of cells in vitreous and proliferating lymphoma cells in the retina and in the subretinal space which appear as creamy lesions. Islands of pigment gives a "leopard spot" appearance. The deposits also tend to accumulate perivascular in location and are often seen as perivascular sheathing [69]. Associated features include retinal pigment epithelial atrophy, perivascular sheathing, subretinal fibrosis, and less commonly contiguous spread to optic nerve, choroid, and sclera. Owing to the presence of deposits of lymphoma cells within the retina and subretinal space, the ideal biopsy of choice is a chorioretinal biopsy. Differential diagnosis includes acute retinal necrosis, intraocular infections such as herpes simplex, cytomegalovirus, and varicella [70].

Undiluted vitreous biopsy sample submitted for cytological analysis serves as the diagnostic and prognostic sample. Cytology smears of PVRL show large atypical lymphoid cells with background necrosis. Cytology is usually com-

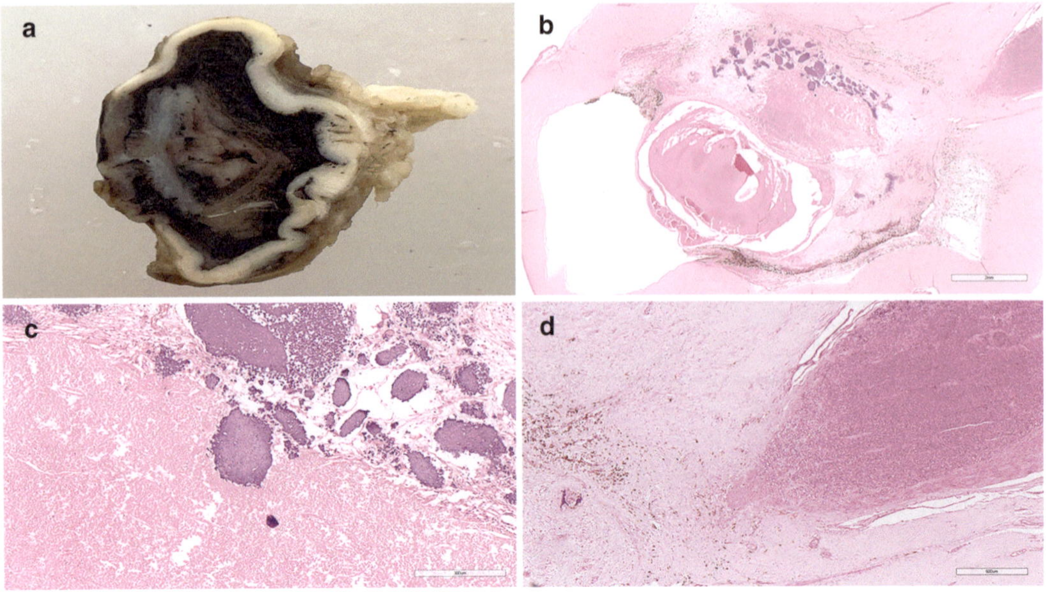

Fig. 19.19 Post-chemotherapy (secondary) enucleation of retinoblastoma: (**a**) Gross image showing shrunken, irregular, disorganized globe; (**b**) Scanner view of the globe with disorganized vitreous cavity, calcified lesion, deep anterior chamber and cataractous lens (H&E; scanner view); (**c**) Lesion with tumoral calcinosis and necrosis (H&E; ×200); (**d**) Optic involvement (H&E; ×40)

plemented by immunohistochemistry by using CD markers or by molecular diagnostic techniques including flow cytometry or PCR analysis. PVRL is almost always diffuse large B-cell lymphomas. Histopathology of a chorioretinal biopsy shows classic perivascular pattern of atypical lymphoid proliferation [71]. PCR for MYD88 mutation is noted in about 70% PVRL. Bone marrow biopsy and positron emission tomography–computed tomography are performed as part of the staging protocol to rule out systemic involvement. Leukemic infiltrates and secondary tumors (metastasis) are extremely rare [72].

Salient Features

- The atypical lymphoid cells are deposited around the vessels, clinically seen as perivascular sheathing.

19.6.2.4 Primary Choroidal Lymphoma:

Primary choroidal lymphomas are rare, low-grade, and indolent lymphomas. Classically seen after 60 years of age, they are usually unilateral and present with slowly progressive vision loss [72]. Clinically, they are visible as cream colored choroidal infiltrates resembling multifocal choroidopathy and can extend into the adjacent ciliary body and iris, emissary canals, and subconjunctival space. Serous retinal detachment is seen. Extension into the optic nerve gives a classic ultrasound appearance termed as whale tail sign [73].

Microscopically, there is monotonous clonal proliferation of small round cells similar to low-grade lymphomas. Ancillary techniques are required for a definitive diagnosis. These lesions should be distinguished from all the reactive proliferations of lymphomononuclear cells [73].

19.6.2.5 Secondary Choroidal Lymphomas

These lymphomas occur secondary to systemic lymphomas and are confined to choroid. Rarely there can be retinal and anterior segment involvement [69]. Most common secondary lymphomas are diffuse large B-cell lymphomas, plasma cell dyscrasias (multiple myeloma and plasmacytomas), lymphoplasmacytic lymphomas, marginal zone B-cell lymphomas, and chronic lymphocytic leukemia. Orbital Burkitt's lymphoma with intraocular extension has also been reported [74–76].

19.6.2.6 Primary Iris and Ciliary Body Lymphomas

Both iris and ciliary body are rare locations [77, 78]. Ciliary body lymphomas tend to low-grade EMZL, whereas iris lymphomas are high-grade [69, 77, 78].

19.6.2.7 Secondary Lymphomatous Infiltration

Lymphomatous infiltration is secondary to the underlying systemic lymphomas. The neoplastic cells are limited to choroid by Bruch's membrane and appear as diffusely expansile lesions. These lesions extend into ciliary body and iris causing involvement of anterior chamber and subsequently secondary glaucoma. Most cases undergo enucleation which on gross examination show diffuse infiltration of choroid with invasion of intraocular and extraocular structures. The subgrouping of lymphomas is done as per the WHO classification of tumors of hematopoietic and lymphoid tissues based on the ancillary techniques [79].

19.6.2.8 Leukemic Infiltration

These lesions may occur in conjunction with choroidal lymphomas and show focal to diffuse involvement by monomorphic atypical lymphoid cells. Diffuse large B-cell lymphomas is the most common occurring lymphoid neoplasm in the eye.

19.7 Tumors and Tumor-Like Lesions of Retinal Pigment Epithelium

19.7.1 Benign

19.7.1.1 Simple and Combined Hamartomas

Hamartomas of RPE and retina are extremely rare. They are categorized into simple hamartomas when limited to RPE, whereas the combined ones are seen in both retina and RPE (CHR-RPE). These lesions are noted in the adolescent age group and are often unilateral and sporadic. CHR-RPE is associated with NF-1, NF-2, and Gorlin syndrome. They usually occur in the peripapillary location and have progressive vision loss. They appear as flat to raised or elevated, well-circumscribed, pigmented lesions with vascularization. CHR-RPE are more vascular than simple hamartomas. Microscopically both the lesions show disorganized RPE or retinal cells with gliosis and vascularity. Differential diagnosis includes melanocytoma and uveal melanomas [80].

19.7.1.2 Congenital Hypertrophy

Congenital hypertrophy of RPE (CHRPE) is benign hypertrophy of the epithelium with macro-melanosomes and is usually seen in adults with female predominance. Lesions are asymptomatic, seen in the peripheral fundus, and are benign. Solitary CHRPE are seen as well-delineated, flat to raised black lesions with typical depigmented lacunae surrounded by a "halo" [81]. Microscopically these are markedly hypertrophied RPE cells with large round melanosomes (normally the melanosomes are ellipsoidal in RPE) (Fig. 19.20). Differential diagnosis includes nevus, melanoma, and congenital grouped pigmentation. Multifocal CHRPE manifests as groups of slate gray lesions which are smaller than solitary CHRPE and lack the classic lacunae or halo.

19.7.1.3 Adenoma

Adenoma is the benign tumor of the retinal pigment epithelium and is generally diagnosed in the sixth decade of life. There is no sex or race predilection. Lesions are usually solitary and unilateral small, dark brown to black tumors which are slow-growing. Associated features include intraretinal or subretinal exudation, presence of a feeding artery and draining vein, and retinal invasion. Adenoma of the RPE is known to arise from solitary CHRPE [80].

Microscopically, the lesion is arranged in cords and tubules separated by thin fibrous septae

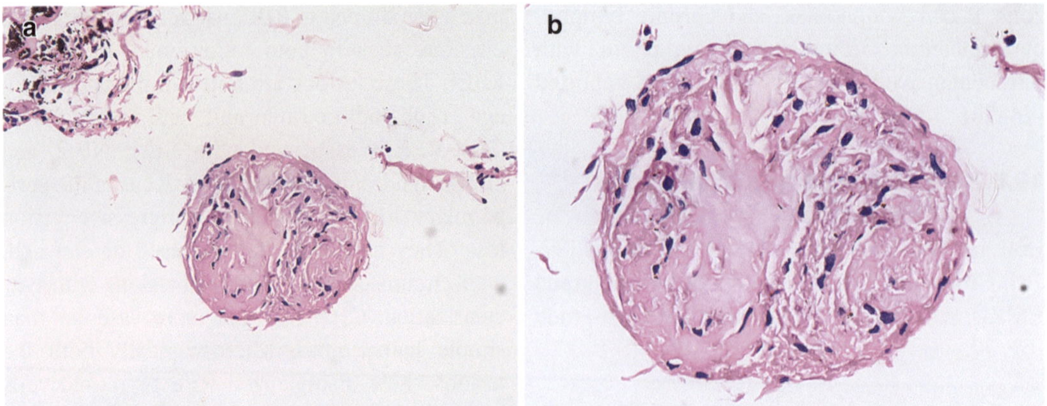

Fig. 19.20 Photomicrograph shows (**a**) well-circumscribed lesion arising from the adjacent retinal pigment epithelium (H&E; ×40); (**b**) Lesion on higher magnification shows proliferation of the fibrous metaplasia (or gliosis) (H&E; ×400)

which are PAS positive. Lesional cells are large, polygonal with moderate to abundant granular cytoplasm. Nuclei are oval to round and uniform. These cells can invade into the overlying retina.

19.7.2 Malignant

19.7.2.1 Adenocarcinoma

Adenocarcinoma is a malignant epithelial tumor of RPE. These tumors are and have been described in chorioretinal scars, phthisical eyes, and CHRPE lesions. Clinical features include vision loss, presence of pigmented or pale subretinal tumor with subretinal exudation, and retinal detachment; and can be mistaken for choroidal melanoma. Occasionally a dilated retinal feeder vessel may be seen which is not seen with choroidal melanoma. Microscopically, atypical epithelial cells are arranged in a solid pattern. The cells can be linearly arranged over choroid and may form tubules, lobules, or pseudoacinar pattern. Marked pleomorphism, nuclear atypia, and increased mitotic activity are noted. Invasion into underlying choroid is the differentiating feature of adenocarcinoma from adenoma [82].

Acknowledgments The authors would like to acknowledge the technical team at Ophthalmic Pathology Laboratory. A special thanks to Mr. B. Sreedhar Rao, Mr. G. Chenchu Naidu, Mr M. Thirupati Rao, and Ms. K. Anusha.

References

1. Rootman J, Ellsworth RM, Hofbauer J, Kitchen D. Orbital extension of retinoblastoma: a clinicopathological study. Can J Ophthalmol. 1978;13(2):72–80. PMID: 647466
2. Shields JA, Shields CL. Melanocytic tumors of iris stroma. In: Intraocular tumors: an Atlas and textbook. 3rd ed. Wolters Kluwer. p. 54–6.
3. Demirci H, Mashayekhi A, Shields CL, Eagle RC Jr, Shields JA. Iris melanocytoma: clinical features and natural course in 47 cases. Am J Ophthalmol. 2005;139(3):468–75. https://doi.org/10.1016/j.ajo.2004.10.008. PMID: 15767055.
4. Decatur CL, Ong E, Garg N, Anbunathan H, Bowcock AM, Field MG, Harbour JW. Driver mutations in uveal melanoma: associations with gene expression profile and patient outcomes. JAMA Ophthalmol. 2016;134(7):728–33. https://doi.org/10.1001/jamaophthalmol.2016.0903. PMID: 27123562; PMCID: PMC4966162.
5. Shields CL, Kaliki S, Livesey M, et al. Association of ocular and oculodermal melanocytosis with the rate of uveal melanoma metastasis: analysis of 7872 consecutive eyes. JAMA Ophthalmol. 2013;131(8):993–1003. https://doi.org/10.1001/jamaophthalmol.2013.129.
6. Shields JA, Shields CL. Congenital ocular melanocytosis. In: Intraocular tumors: an Atlas and textbook. 3rd ed. Wolters Kluwer. p. 25–6.
7. Zehavi C, Romano A, Goodman RM. Iris (Lisch) nodules in neurofibromatosis. Clin Genet. 1986;29(1):51–5.
8. Ratner N, Miller SJ. A RASopathy gene commonly mutated in cancer: the neurofibromatosis type 1 tumour suppressor. Nat Rev Cancer. 2015;15(5):290–301. https://doi.org/10.1038/nrc3911. Epub 2015 Apr 16. PMID: 25877329; PMCID: PMC4822336
9. Senthilkumar VA, Tripathy K. Lisch Nodules. [Updated 2022 Feb 21]. In: StatPearls [Internet].

Treasure Island (FL): StatPearls Publishing; 2022 Jan-. Available from: https://www.ncbi.nlm.nih.gov/books/NBK557560/.
10. Shields JA, Shields CL. Cysts of the iris pigment epithelium. What is new and interesting? The 2016 Jose Rizal International Medal Lecture. Asia Pacific J Ophthalmol. 2017;6(1):64–9.
11. Venkateswaran N, Ching SST, Fischer W, Lee F, Yeaney G, Hindman HB. The diagnostic and therapeutic challenges of posttraumatic iris implantation cysts: illustrative case presentations and a review of the literature. Case Rep Ophthalmol Med. 2015:Article ID 375947, 11 pages, 2015. https://doi.org/10.1155/2015/375947.
12. Shields CL, Kaliki S, Shah SU, et al. Iris melanoma: features and prognosis in 317 children and adults. J AAPOS. 2012;16(1):10–6.
13. Tomar AS, Finger PT, Iacob CE. Intraocular leiomyoma: current concepts. Surv Ophthalmol. 2020;65(4):421–37.
14. Shields JA, Shields C, Gunduz K, Eagle RC. Adenoma of the ciliary body pigment epithelium: the 1998 Albert Ruedemann, Sr, Memorial Lecture, Part 1. Arch Ophthalmol. 1999;117(5):592–7.
15. Shields JA, Augsburger JJ, Wallar PH, Shah HG. Adenoma of the nonpigmented epithelium of the ciliary body. Ophthalmology. 1983;90(12):1528–30.
16. Lieb WE, Shields JA, Eagle RC Jr, Kwa D, Shields CL. Cystic adenoma of the pigmented ciliary epithelium. Clinical, pathologic, and immunohistopathologic findings. Ophthalmology. 1990;97(11):1489–93.
17. Mori T, Sukeda A, Sekine S, Shibata S, Ryo E, Okano H, Suzuki S, Hiraoka N. SOX10 expression as well as BRAF and GNAQ/11 mutations distinguish pigmented ciliary epithelium neoplasms from uveal melanomas. Invest Ophthalmol Vis Sci. 2017;58(12):5445–51. https://doi.org/10.1167/iovs.17-22362. PMID: 29059311.
18. Kaliki S, Shields CL, Eagle RC Jr, Vemuganti GK, Almeida A, Manjandavida FP, Mulay K, Honavar SG, Shields JA. Ciliary body medulloepithelioma: analysis of 41 cases. Ophthalmology. 2013;120(12):2552–9.
19. Tadepalli SH, Shields CL, Shields JA, Honavar SG. Intraocular medulloepithelioma- a review of clinical features, DICER 1 mutation, and management. Indian J Ophthalmol. 2019;67(6):755–62.
20. Alkatan H, Al-Amry M, Al-Hussain H, Al-Dhibi H, Al-Mesfer S. Medulloepithelioma of the ciliary body: the delay in diagnosis and frequent initial mismanagement. Can J Ophthalmol. 2011;46(5):431–8.
21. Shields JA, Eagle RC Jr, Ferguson K, Shields CL. Tumors of the nonpigmented epithelium of the ciliary body: the Lorenz E. Zimmerman Tribute Lecture. Retina. 2015;35(5):957–65.
22. Ho YF, Tsai YJ, Wu SY. Malignant ciliary body medulloepithelioma with brain and parotid metastasis. J Pediatr Ophthalmol Strabismus. 2017;54:e18–22.
23. Hořínová V, Drábová K, Nosková H, Bajčiová V, Šoukalová J, Černá L, Hůrková V, Slabý O, Štěrba J. DICER1 syndrome. Klin Onkol. 2019;32(Supplementum2):123–7.
24. Kramer GD, Arepalli S, Shields CL, Shields JA. Ciliary body medulloepithelioma association with pleuropulmonary blastoma in a familial tumor predisposition syndrome. J Pediatr Ophthalmol Strabismus. 2014;51(Online):e48–50.
25. Laird PW, Grossniklaus HE, Hubbard GB. Ciliary body medulloepithelioma associated with pleuropulmonary blastoma. Br J Ophthalmol. 2013;97(8):1079, 1086-7.
26. Schultz KAP, Williams GM, Kamihara J, Stewart DR, Harris AK, Bauer AJ, Turner J, Shah R, Schneider K, Schneider KW, Carr AG, Harney LA, Baldinger S, Frazier AL, Orbach D, Schneider DT, Malkin D, Dehner LP, Messinger YH, Hill DA. *DICER1* and associated conditions: identification of at-risk individuals and recommended surveillance strategies. Clin Cancer Res. 2018;24(10):2251–61.
27. Kopsidas K, Mudhar H, Sisley K, et al. Adenocarcinoma with bilateral lung metastases: histological, molecular, genetic and clinical aspects. Ocular Oncol Pathol. 2019;5:79–84.
28. Dryja TP, Zakov ZN, Albert DM. Adenocarcinoma arising from the epithelium of the iris and ciliary body. Int Ophthalmol Clin. 1980;20(2):177–90.
29. Grossniklaus HE, Zimmerman LE, Kachmer ML. Pleomorphic adenocarcinoma of the ciliary body. Immunohistochemical and electron microscopic features. Ophthalmology. 1990;97(6):763–8.
30. Nicolò M, Nicolò G, Zingirian M. Pleomorphic adenocarcinoma of the ciliary epithelium: a clinicopathological, immunohistochemical, ultrastructural, DNA-ploidy and comparative genomic hybridization analysis of an unusual case. Eur J Ophthalmol. 2002;12(4):319–23. https://doi.org/10.1177/112067210201200412. PMID: 12220004.
31. Witschel H, Font RL. Hemangioma of the choroid. A clinicopathological study of 71 cases and a review of literature. Surv Ophthalmol. 1976;20:415–31.
32. Mashayekhi A, Shields CL. Circumscribed choroidal hemangioma. Curr Opin Ophthalmol. 2003;14(3):142–9. https://doi.org/10.1097/00055735-200306000-00006. PMID: 12777933.
33. Vempuluru VS, Kaliki S. Multifocal circumscribed choroidal hemangioma. BMJ Case Rep. 2020;13(2):e233222.
34. Alameddinee RM, Mansour AM, Kahtani E. Review of choroidal osteomas. Middle East Afr J Ophthalmol. 2014;21:244–50.
35. Sullivan TJ, Clarke MP, Morin JD. The ocular manifestations of the Sturge Weber syndrome. J Pediatr Ophthalmol Strabismus. 1992;29:349–56.
36. Susac JO, Smith JL, Scelfo RJ. The "tomato-catsup" fundus in Sturge-Weber syndrome. Arch Ophthalmol. 1974;92:69–70.
37. Shields JA, Stephens RF, Eagle RC Jr, Shields CL, De Potter P. Progressive enlargement of a circumscribed choroidal hemangioma. A clinicopathologic correla-

tion. Arch Ophthalmol. 1992;110(9):1276–8. https://doi.org/10.1001/archopht.1992.01080210094033. PMID: 1520116.
38. Jajapuram SD, Mishra DK, Kaliki S. Choroidal schwannoma presenting with neovascular glaucoma: a report of two cases. Oman J Ophthalmol. 2019;12(2):125–8.
39. Damato B, Damato EM, Konstantinidis L, Heimann H, Coupland SE. Choroidal schwannoma: a case series of five patients. Br J Ophthalmol. 2014;98(8):1096–100.
40. Yu Y, Cheng Y, Wang K, Sun K, Shen D, Liang J. Intraocular schwannoma: a case series of 3 patients. Oncol Lett. 2019;17(1):1274–8.
41. Viola F, Villani E, Natacci F, et al. Choroidal abnormalties detected by near-infrared reflectance imaging as a new diagnostic criterion for neurofibromatosis 1. Ophthalmology. 2012;119:369–75.
42. Shields JA, Sanborn GE, Kurz GH, Augsburger JJ. Benign peripheral nerve tumor of the choroid: a clinicopathologic correlation and review of the literature. Ophthalmology. 1981;88(12):1322–9.
43. Shome D, Vemuganti GK, Honavar SG. Choroidal ganglioneuroma in a patient with neurofibromatosis type 1: a case report. Eye (Lond). 2006;20(12):1450–1.
44. Aylward GW, Chang TS, Pautler SE, Gass JD. A long-term follow-up of choroidal osteoma. Arch Ophthalmol. 1998;116(10):1337–41. https://doi.org/10.1001/archopht.116.10.1337. PMID: 9790633.
45. Kaliki S, Shields CL. Uveal melanoma: relatively rare but deadly cancer. Eye (Lond). 2017;31(2):241–57.
46. Afshar AR, Damato BE, Stewart JM, Zablotska LB, Roy R, Olshen AB, Joseph NM, Bastian BC. Next-generation sequencing of uveal melanoma for detection of genetic alterations predicting metastasis. Transl Vis Sci Technol. 2019;8(2):18. https://doi.org/10.1167/tvst.8.2.18. PMID: 31024753; PMCID: PMC6472431.
47. Onken MD, Worley LA, Ehlers JP, Harbour JW. Gene expression profiling in uveal melanoma reveals two molecular classes and predicts metastatic death. Cancer Res. 2004;64(20):7205–9.
48. McLean IW, Foster WD, Zimmerman LE, Gamel JW. Modifications of callender's classification of uveal melanoma at the Armed Forces Institute of Pathology. Am J Ophthalmol. 2018;195:lvi–lx.
49. Thareja S, Rashid A, Grossniklaus HE. Spontaneous necrosis of choroidal melanoma. Ocul Oncol Pathol. 2014;1(1):63–9. https://doi.org/10.1159/000366559. Epub 2014 Sep 10. PMID: 27175363; PMCID: PMC4864576.
50. Raval V, Bowen RC, Soto H, Biscotti C, Yeaney G, Sears J, Singh A. Vitreous seeding of choroidal melanoma. Retina. 2021;41(4):890–4. https://doi.org/10.1097/IAE.0000000000002989. PMID: 33009220.
51. Chattopadhyay C, Kim DW, Gombos DS, Oba J, Qin Y, Williams MD, Esmaeli B, Grimm EA, Wargo JA, Woodman SE, Patel SP. Uveal melanoma: from diagnosis to treatment and the science in between. Cancer. 2016;122(15):2299–312.
52. Oellers P, Wolkow N, Jakobiec FA, Kim IK. Hemorrhagic choroidal melanoma. Am J Ophthalmol Case Rep. 2018;(10):105–7.
53. Reddy SC, Jackson N, Menon BS. Ocular involvement in leukemia–a study of 288 cases. Ophthalmologica. 2003;217(6):441–5. https://doi.org/10.1159/000073077. PMID: 14573980.
54. Adam MK, Pitcher JD, Shields CL, Maguire JI. Enhanced depth imaging optical coherence tomography of precursor cell leukemic choroidopathy before and after chemotherapy. Middle East Afr J Ophthalmol. 2015;22(2):249–52.
55. Singh AD, Santos MCM, Shields CL, Shields JA, Eagle RC. Observations on 17 patients with retinocytoma. Arch Ophthalmol. 2000;118(2):199–205.
56. Margo C, Hidayat A, Kopelman J, Zimmerman LE. Retinocytoma: a benign variant of retinoblastoma. Arch Ophthalmol. 1983:96315–20.
57. Gupta AK, Meena JP. A narrative review of retinoblastoma and recent advances in its management. Pediatr Med. 2020;3:20.
58. Singh L, Kashyap S. Update on pathology of retinoblastoma. Int J Ophthalmol. 2018;11(12):2011–6.
59. Vemuganti G, Honavar S, John R. Clinicopathological profile of retinoblastoma patients in Asian Indians. Invest Ophthalmol Vis Sci. 2000;41(S):790.
60. Nalcı H, Gündüz K, Erden E. Necrotic intraocular retinoblastoma associated with orbital cellulitis. Surv Ophthalmol. 2018;63(1):114–8.
61. Martino F, Gelmi MC, Galluzzi P, De Francesco S, Miracco C, Hadjistilianou D. Orbital pseudocellulitis: a retinoblastoma-associated masquerade syndrome. Ocul Oncol Pathol. 2020;6(6):430–7.
62. Kaliki S, Jakati S, Vempuluru VS, Mallu A, Mishra DK. Retinoblastoma associated with orbital pseudocellulitis and high-risk retinoblastoma: a study of 32 eyes. Int Ophthalmol. 2021;42:19.
63. Kaliki S, Srinivasan V, Gupta A, Mishra DK, Naik MN. Clinical features predictive of high-risk retinoblastoma in 403 Asian Indian patients: a case-control study. Ophthalmology. 2015;122(6):1165–72. https://doi.org/10.1016/j.ophtha.2015.01.018. Epub 2015 Apr 1. PMID: 25841975.
64. Amram AL, Rico G, Kim JW, Chintagumpala M, Herzog CE, Gombos DS, Chévez-Barrios P. Vitreous seeds in retinoblastoma: clinicopathologic classification and correlation. Ophthalmology. 2017;124(10):1540–7. https://doi.org/10.1016/j.ophtha.2017.04.015. Epub 2017 May 17. PMID: 28528011.
65. Jakati S, Kaliki S. Aqueous seeding in retinoblastoma: classification and clinicopathologic correlation. Ophthalmol Retina. 2022;6(5):421–8. https://doi.org/10.1016/j.oret.2021.12.013. Epub 2021 Dec 24. PMID: 34958963.
66. Biewald EM, Bornfeld N, Metz KA, Schlüter S, Kiefer T, Radbruch A, Göricke S, Sirin S, Ketteler P, Bechrakis NE. Histopathology of retinoblastoma eyes enucleated after intra-arterial chemotherapy. Br J Ophthalmol. 2020;104(8):1171–5.

67. Rushlow DE, Mol BM, Kennett JY, Yee S, Pajovic S, Thériault BL, Prigoda-Lee NL, Spencer C, Dimaras H, Corson TW, Pang R, Massey C, Godbout R, Jiang Z, Zacksenhaus E, Paton K, Moll AC, Houdayer C, Raizis A, Halliday W, Lam WL, Boutros PC, Lohmann D, Dorsman JC, Gallie BL. Characterisation of retinoblastomas without RB1 mutations: genomic, gene expression, and clinical studies. Lancet Oncol. 2013;14(4):327–34. https://doi.org/10.1016/S1470-2045(13)70045-7. Epub 2013 Mar 13. PMID: 23498719.
68. Coupland SE, Perez-Canto A, Hummel M, Stein H, Heimann H. Assessment of HOPE fixation in vitrectomy specimens in patients with chronic bilateral uveitis (masquerade syndrome). Graefes Arch Clin Exp Ophthalmol. 2005;243(9):847–52. https://doi.org/10.1007/s00417-005-1166-1. Epub 2005 May 21. PMID: 15909161.
69. Coupland SE, Damato B. Understanding intraocular lymphomas. Clin Experiment Ophthalmol. 2008;36(6):564–78. https://doi.org/10.1111/j.1442--9071.2008.01843.x. PMID: 18954321.
70. Mulay K, Narula R, Honavar SG. Primary vitreoretinal lymphoma. Indian J Ophthalmol. 2015;63(3):180–6.
71. Sobolewska B, Chee SP, Zaguia F, Goldstein DA, Smith JR, Fend F, Mochizuki M, Zierhut M. Vitreoretinal Lymphoma. Cancers (Basel). 2021;13(16):3921.
72. Mashayekhi A, Dalvin LA, Lim LS, Ancona-Lezama D, Mazloumi M, Chang M, Shields CL, Shields JA. Association of vitreoretinal lymphoma with systemic lymphoma. Retina. 2021;41(2):259–65.
73. Kam AW, Galvin J, Cherepanoff S, Miller AA, Fung AT. Primary choroidal lymphoma diagnosed with 27-guage pars plana vitrectomy choroidal biopsy. Case Rep Ophthalmol. 2019;10(2):213–20.
74. Feman SS, Niwayama G, Hepler RS, Foos RY. "Burkitt tumor" with intraocular involvement. Surv Ophthalmol. 1969;14(2):106–11. PMID: 5350356.
75. Payne T, Karp LA, Zimmerman LE. Intraocular involvement in Burkitt's lymphoma. Arch Ophthalmol. 1971;85(3):295–8. https://doi.org/10.1001/archopht.1971.00990050297009. PMID: 5100804.
76. Wysenbeek YS, Nissenkorn I, Cohen S, Ben-Sira I, Stark B, Zaizov R. Intraocular involvement of Burkitt's lymphoma in a Bedouin child. Pediatr Hematol Oncol. 1987;4(4):309–14. https://doi.org/10.3109/08880018709141283. PMID: 3152936.
77. Raju VK, Green WR. Reticulum cell sarcoma of the uvea. Ann Ophthalmol. 1982;14(6):555–60. PMID: 7051936
78. Velez G, de Smet MD, Whitcup SM, Robinson M, Nussenblatt RB, Chan CC. Iris involvement in primary intraocular lymphoma: report of two cases and review of the literature. Surv Ophthalmol. 2000;44:518–26.
79. Grossniklaus HE, Eberhart CG, Kivela TT, editors. WHO classification of tumors of the eye. 4th ed. Internal Agency for Research on Cancer: Lyon; 2018.
80. Shields JA, Shields CL. Tumors and related lesions of the pigmented epithelium. Asia Pac J Ophthalmol (Phila). 2017;6(2):215–23.
81. Shields CL, Mashayekhi A, Ho T, Cater J, Shields JA. Solitary congenital hypertrophy of the retinal pigment epithelium: clinical features and frequency of enlargement in 330 patients. Ophthalmology. 2003;110(10):1968–76.
82. Mori H, Takahashi K. A case of adenocarcinoma of the retinal pigment epithelium: an immunohistochemical and electron microscopic study. Ocul Oncol Pathol. 2017;4(1):38–43.

Eye and Systemic Disorders

20

Akshay Badakere

Contents

A. Badakere (✉)
Pediatric Ophthalmology Department, Sankara Nethralaya, Chennai, India

G. K. Vemuganti et al. (eds.), *Ocular Pathology*, https://doi.org/10.1007/978-981-96-8614-8_20

20.1 Introduction

The eye can often be the first organ involved in a systemic disease or may harbor signs indicative of an underlying systemic disorder and identifying this will help in early and timely diagnoses. These signs may involve either or both of the anterior and posterior segment of the eye [1].

The eye can also get involved as a part of the spectrum of drug-induced disorders and early recognition of these is vital [2].

Broadly it is useful to classify systemic disorders involving the eye as (Table 20.1)

1. Congenital/Developmental
2. Acquired

Table 20.1 enlists systemic disorders involving eye.

20.2 Congenital

20.2.1 Phacomatoses

Phacomatoses refer to a group of heterogeneous neurocutaneous disorders affecting tissues that develop from the neuroectoderm. These syndromes typically affect the central and peripheral nervous system, skin, and other organ systems. Diagnosis is based on identification of clinical features, imaging (Magnetic Resonance Imaging, Computed Tomography, Ultrasonography, etc.), and family screening to establish a genetic pattern [3, 4].

Phacomatoses include:

Neurofibromatosis types 1 and 2
Tuberous sclerosis
Sturge–Weber syndrome
Von Hippel–Lindau syndrome

Table 20.1 Classification of systemic disorders involving the eye

Type of disorder	Categories of diseases	Name of disease
Congenital	1. Phacomatoses 2. Ectopia lentis 3. Inherited metabolic disorders 4. Retinal dystrophies	Neurofibromatosis types 1 and 2 Marfan syndrome, Ehlers–Danlos syndrome Mucopolysaccharidoses, Galactosemia Retinitis Pigmentosa
Acquired	Vascular Autoimmune and Connective tissue disease Endocrine disorders Infectious Drug induced	Systemic hypertension Systemic lupus Erythematosus, Rheumatoid arthritis Diabetes Mellitus, Thyroid eye disease Viral and bacterial infections

Miscellaneous (uncommon): Ataxia Telangiectasia, Incontinentia Pigmenti, Neurocutaneous Melanosis, and Hypomelanosis of Ito.

20.2.1.1 Neurofibromatosis Type 1 (NF1)

NF1 is the most common phacomatoses with an incidence of 1 in 2700–3300 live births. It results from mutations in NF1 gene on chromosome 17q11.2. It is inherited in an autosomal dominant pattern with complete penetrance and variable expressivity.NF1 encodes neurofibromin, a tumor suppressor gene. This is a negative regulator of the RAS protein [4].

The most common clinical feature of NF1 are the café-au-lait spots and are the earliest manifestations. Optic nerve gliomas are the most common central nervous system tumors. Neurofibromas involving the scalp, neck, spine, and orbits can also be seen. These can be discrete or in the form of plexiform neurofibromas which are diffuse. Bony deformities in the form of dysplasia of the greater wing of sphenoid can also be present.

The clinical criteria for diagnosis of NF1 have been defined by the National Institute of health. Table 20.2 lists these criteria. At least two or more criteria must be fulfilled for diagnosis [3, 4].

Table 20.2 Diagnostic criteria for Neurofibromatosis type 1

Clinical criteria	Details
Café-au-lait spots	Six or more Pre-pubertal >5 mm in diameter Post-pubertal >15 mm in greatest diameter
Neurofibromas	Two or more dermal Or 1 Plexiform
Skin fold freckling	Axillary or inguinal
Optic pathway gliomas	
Lisch nodules	Two or more
Bony lesions	Sphenoid wing dysplasia Pseudoarthrosis
Family history	First-degree relative with NF1 or any of the above criteria

Clinical Features- [4]

(a) Cutaneous
(b) Ophthalmic
(c) Oncologic
(d) Cardiovascular
(e) Musculoskeletal

(a) *Cutaneous Features*
1. Café-au-lait spots: These are pigmented macules that can occur anywhere on the body, although they are rare on the scalp, palms, and soles. Attention should be paid to the number of macules since up to 26% of the general population can have 1–5 spots. In those children with more than six spots up to 95% can develop by the age of 8 years [4].
2. Intertriginous freckling: Axillary and inguinal freckling is seen in up to 77% of individuals and helps in diagnosis of NF1 in individuals with multiple Café-au-lait spots [4].
3. Dermal neurofibromas: these are peripheral nerve tumors which are benign and are the hallmark of NF1 [4].

(b) *Ophthalmic Features:*
1. Lisch nodules: These are pigmented hamartomas of the iris. These are dome-shaped lesions about 1–2 mm in diameter and can vary in color from clear to brown in appearance [3, 4].
2. Choroidal nodules: These are separate lesions seen in the choroid and need near infrared reflectance imaging to visualize these. Kumar V and associates have highlighted the role of Swept-source OCT and OCT Angiography to demonstrate choroidal nodules in a case of NF1 [5].

(c) *Oncologic*- [4]:

Table 20.3 briefly enlists the oncologic features seen in NF1

(d) *Cardiovascular/Disorders of CNS* [4]
1. Coarctation of aorta
2. Pulmonary stenosis
3. Moyamoya disease
4. Aneurysms

(e) Musculoskeletal: two commonly seen features are sphenoid wing dysplasia and pseudoarthrosis of the long bones. The other

Table 20.3 The oncologic features seen in Neurofibromatosis 1

Oncologic features
Benign peripheral nerve sheath tumors
Typically seen in NF1
Can be localized or diffuse
"bag of worms" on palpation
Method of choice to detect them is MRI
Malignant Peripheral Nerve Sheath Tumors
These are sarcomas developing from the nerve sheath
Can develop within an existing plexiform neurofibroma
Seen generally in the second or third decade
Risk factors are prior radiotherapy, family history, whole or microdeletions of NF1
Optic Pathway Gliomas
Most common CNS tumor in NF1
Seen in up to 20% of NF1 patients
Seen as fusiform dilatation of the optic nerves
May involve the chiasm, optic tracts, and optic radiations

features include osteopenia, scoliosis, and macrocephaly [4].

20.2.1.2 Neurofibromatosis Type 2 (NF2)

NF2 is an autosomal dominant disorder. The gene involved is the NF2 gene on chromosome 22q12. The prevalence is lower than NF1 (1 in 25,000–40,000) [3, 4].

The diagnostic criteria are as follows: [3]

NF2 diagnosis requires any one of the following two criteria

1. Bilateral vestibular schwannomas (characteristic of NF2)
2. Family history of NF1 with
   (a) Unilateral vestibular schwannoma
   (b) Any two among—Meningioma, Glioma, Neurofibroma, schwannoma, or juvenile posterior subcapsular cataracts

20.2.1.3 Tuberous Sclerosis (TS) [3]

Autosomal dominant multisystem disorder, with a prevalence of 1 in 6,000–10,000. Typical triad consists of

1. Facial angiofibroma
2. Seizure
3. Mental retardation

A classical feature of TS is hamartomas in multiple organ systems.

Intracranial manifestations

1. Cortical tubers—most common intracranial lesion

Commonly involve the frontal gyri

Seen in up to 95% cases

2. Subependymal nodules

These are hamartomas classically seen in the region of the lateral ventricles

3. Other lesions
   (a) Subependymal giant cell astrocytomas
   (b) Radial migration lines

These are white matter lesions extending from subependymal nodules to the cortical tubers

Other lesions

(a) Pulmonary lymhangioleiomyomatosis—thin cystic lesions in the lung parenchyma
(b) Renal angiomyolipoma
(c) Renal cell carcinoma (rarely)

20.2.1.4 Sturge–Weber syndrome- [3]

This entity is characterized by vascular involvement of the face, leptomeninges and eye. It affects both sexes equally with an incidence of 1 in 40,000–50,000 and its classical lesion is the port-wine stain which is an angioma on the face seen typically along the distribution of the ophthalmic division of the trigeminal nerve.

There may be angiomas in the pia mater which may obstruct venous flow leading to ischemia.

20.2.1.5 Von Hippel–Lindau Syndrome [3]

This is an autosomal dominant disease, due to deletion of the VHL gene on the short arm of chromosome 3 with incidence is 1 in 36,000. It is characterized by hemangioblastomas of the brain and spinal cord. The cerebellum is the most common site for a hemangioblastoma. Patients are prone to develop multiple tumors of the visceral organs. The most common findings are cysts involving the pancreas (up to 90%) and renal cysts and can also develop renal cell carcinoma, pheochromocytoma, and neuroendocrine tumors of the pancreas.

20.2.2 Ectopia Lentis

This is a condition in which the lens is displaced from its normal position. The displacement could be a subluxation, where the lens is partially displaced and some part of the lens remains in the pupillary area or it may be dislocated, where the lens is no longer attached to the zonules and is displaced completely [6]. Figure 20.1 is an example of a dislocated lens (yellow arrow) into the anterior chamber.

The conditions where ectopia lentis are seen are the following [6]

1. With systemic association
   (a) Marfan syndrome
   (b) Ehlers–Danlos syndrome
   (c) Weill–Marchesani Syndrome
   (d) Homocystinuria
   (e) Hyperlysinemia
   (f) Sulfite oxidase deficiency
2. Isolated/without systemic associations
   (a) Simple ectopia lentis
   (b) Ectopia lentis et pupillae:

Table 20.4 describes the various disorders associated with ectopia lentis [6–8].

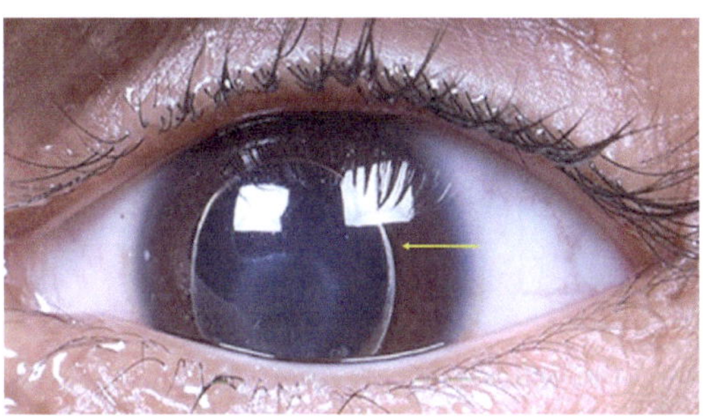

Fig. 20.1 A lens (yellow arrow) dislocated into the anterior chamber

20.2.3 Inherited Metabolic Disorders (IMD)

The eye is the fourth most common organ involved in genetic disorders. Inherited metabolic disorders are a heterogeneous group of disorders affecting pathways of metabolism with an underlying genetic defect [10].

IMD can affect the following structures of the eye [10, 11]

Cornea
Lens
Retina
Optic nerve

Details of ocular affliction in IMDs can be referred to in the chapter on this topic.

20.3 Acquired

20.3.1 Thyroid Eye Disease (TED)

Thyroid eye disease affects up to 50% patients with Graves' disease, and a small subgroup can have severe disease. It is not associated with thyroid function and may be seen in hypo/eu or hyperthyroidism [2].

TED is up to six-fold more common in women but is generally more severe in men. It is more severe in smokers than nonsmokers.

The exact pathogenesis, although not well known, is hypothesized to be an autoimmune response linked to cross-reactivity against antigens in the thyroid and orbit. During the acute phase orbital fibroblasts differentiate into myofibroblasts and adipocytes and lay down hyaluronan. Hence during this active phase, there is increased extracellular matrix production as well as release of cytokines and pro-inflammatory substances.

Hence, while the acute phase is characterized by a congested and inflamed eye, the chronic phase is characterized by a quiet eye with fibrotic changes.

The most common clinical features include [2] (Figs. 20.2, 20.3, 20.4, and 20.5)
(a) lid retraction
(b) proptosis

Table 20.4 Various disorders associated with ectopia lentis

Condition	Ocular findings	Systemic findings	Inheritance	Gene involved
Marfan syndrome	Ectopia lentis Axial myopia Increased axial length Iridodonesis Phacodonesis Poorly dilating pupils Retinal detachment	Tall stature Pectus excavatum Scoliosis Hypermobile joints Arachnodactyly Aortic root dilatation Aneurysm of aorta (risk of dissection) Mitral valve prolapse	AD	FBN1 gene (15q21)
Ehlers–Danlos syndrome classic type	*Common ocular features* Ectopia lentis Axial and/or lenticular myopia Keratoconus Fragile sclera Angioid streaks Retinal tears	Cardinal features Skin hyperextensibility Widened atrophic Scarring Smooth and velvety skin Joint hypermobility	AD	COL5A1/ COL5A2
Hypermobility		Generalized joint hypermobility skin involvement soft skin	AD	TNX-B, COL5A1
Vascular		Excessive bruising Thin, translucent skin Arterial/intestinal/uterine fragility or rupture Characteristic facial appearance	AD	COL3A1
Vascular like		Skin extensibility Arterial rupture Osteopenia Easy bruising Atrophic scarring	AD	COL1A1
Cardiac valvular		Severe cardiac valvular disease Skin hyperextensibility Joint hypermobility	AR	COL1A2
Kyphoscoliotic		Muscular hypotonia Generalized joint laxity Kyphoscoliosis at birth	AR	LH-1
EDS/OI overlap syndrome		Joint hypermobility Mild skin involvement Increased bone fragility	AD	COL1A1/ COL1A2
Arthrochalasis type		Severe generalized joint hypermobility recurrent subluxations Congenital bilateral hip dislocation Skin hyperextensibility Widened, atrophic scars	AD	COL1A1/ COL1A2
Dermatosparaxis type		Fragile skin Sagging, redundant skin Excessive bruising *Characteristic facies* Eyelid edema down slanting palpebral fissures epicanthic folds blue sclerae gingival hyperplasia, micrognathia short hands and feet Umbilical hernia Delayed closure of fontanelles	AR	ADAMTS2
Weill–Marchesani syndrome	Ectopia lentis Microspherophakia Glaucoma Lenticular myopia	Brachydactyly Stiff joints Patent ductus arteriosus Pulmonary valve stenosis Thoracic artery aneurysm	AD AR	FBN1 gene ADAMTS10, ADAMTS17, LTBP2

(continued)

Table 20.4 (continued)

Condition	Ocular findings	Systemic findings	Inheritance	Gene involved
Homocystinuria	Ectopia lentis Iridodonesis Phacodonesis Axial/ lenticular myopia Glaucoma Retinal detachment	Marfanoid habitus Developmental delay Seizures Risk of thrombosis (especially during surgery)	AR	Chr 21q22.3 (deficiency of cyatathione b synthase)
Simple ectopia lentis (Isolated EL)	Ectopia lentis Refractive errors Enlarged iris processes Abnormal iridocorneal angle Lens coloboma Amblyopia Glaucoma Retinal detachment	None	AD AR	FBN1 (15q21.1) ADAMTSL4(1q21.2)
Ectopia lentis et pupillae [9]	Ectopia lentis Slit like pupils Poorly dilating pupils Iridodonesis and transillumination Microspherophakia Persistent pupillary membranes Raised IOP Cataract Retinal detachment	None	AR	

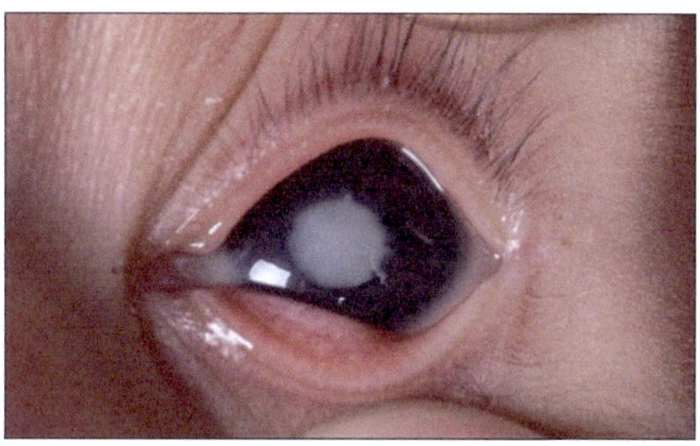

Fig. 20.2 Total lenticular opacity in an infant with galactosemia

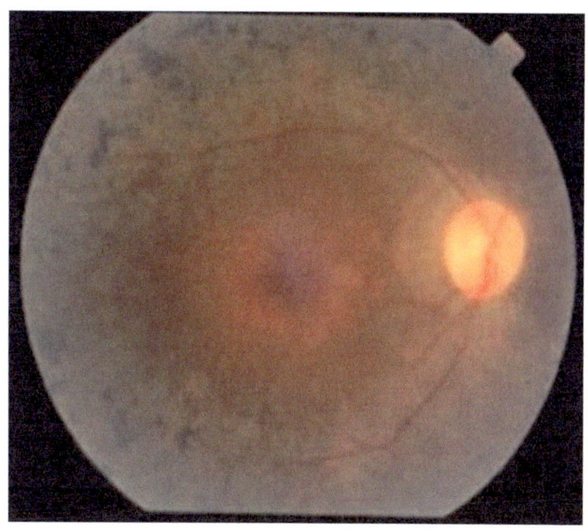

Fig. 20.3 Fundus photo of a patient with Retinitis Pigmentosa

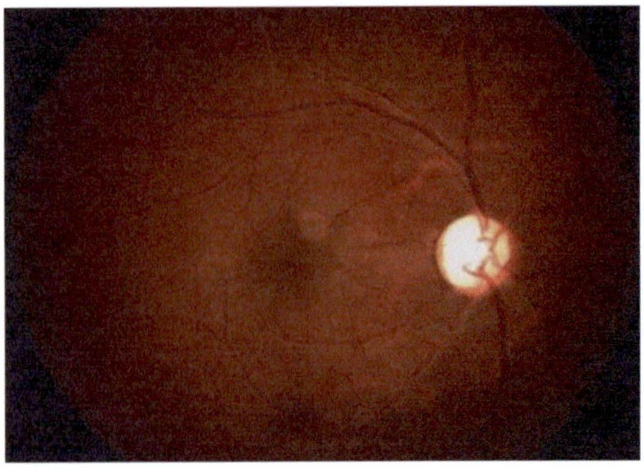

Fig. 20.4 Pale Optic disc in a patient with Leber's Hereditary Optic Neuropathy

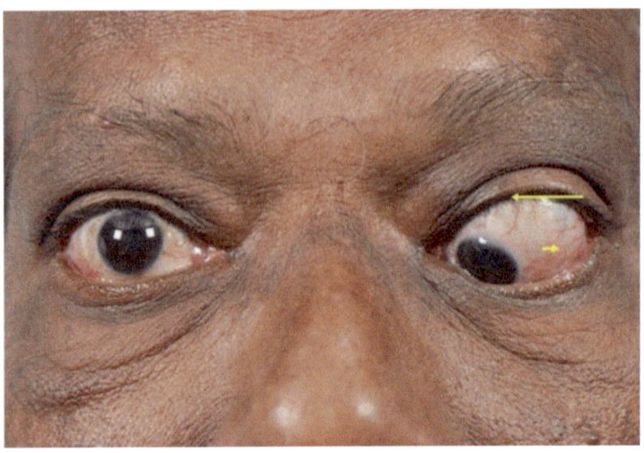

Fig. 20.5 Patient with TED with lid retraction (long arrow) and conjunctival congestion (small arrow) with a downward and inward displacement of the left eye

(c) restricted ocular movements leading to diplopia

There can be a threat to vision due to

(a) Compressive optic neuropathy (swollen extraocular muscles compressing the optic nerve at the apex)
(b) Exposure keratopathy due to lid retraction

The European Group on Graves' Ophthalmopathy (EUGOGO) classifies TED as [2]

- Mild disease
- Moderate to severe
- Severe disease

Mild disease

This is characterized by the following clinical features

(a) Mild soft tissue involvement.
(b) Mild lid retraction <2 mm.
(c) Proptosis <3 mm.
(d) no diplopia, optic nerve, or corneal involvement

Moderate to severe disease

(a) Moderate to severe soft tissue involvement.
(b) Lid retraction >2 mm.
(c) Proptosis >3 mm.
(d) Diplopia

Severe disease

(a) Optic neuropathy
(b) Exposure keratopathy leading to corneal melt

Management

According to EUGOGO therapy depends upon the stage of the disease

- *Mild disease*
  Mainly supportive therapy in the form of lubricants, head-end elevation, and ice compresses. Selenium 200 μg/day can be added to treatment, since this being an antioxidant is needed for conversion of T4 to T3
- *Moderate Disease:*
  Immunosuppressive therapy with systemic steroids and/or orbital radiation
- *Severe Disease*
  Is an emergency and systemic steroids followed by orbital decompression if needed
  Cosmetic surgery to the orbit, eyelids and muscles can be considered once the disease is in the quiescent phase.

20.3.2 Systemic Vasculitis Affecting the Eye

'Vasculitis' refers to a wide range of disorders characterized by [12]

(a) Inflammation of blood vessels with/without necrosis
(b) Ischemia of the affected organ

(c) Presence of circulating autoantibodies
(d) Each vasculitis has predilection for vessels of a particular size

Systemic vasculitis depending on vessel size is given in Table 20.5 [13].

Ocular features of systemic inflammatory disease may be due to the disease process itself or the drugs used.

Table 20.6 describes the ocular features secondary to the disease process [13].

Table 20.5 Classification of systemic vasculitis

Vessels	Disease
Large arteries	Giant cell arteritis Takayasu's arteritis Aortitis in Rheumatoid arthritis
Medium arteries	Polyarteritis Nodosa Kawasaki disease
Small- and medium-sized vessels	Granulomatosis with Polyangiitis Eosinophilic granulomatosis with Polyangiitis (Churg–Strauss syndrome) Microscopic polyangiitis Systemic lupus erythematosus Sjogren's syndrome
Small vessels	Henoch–Schoenlein purpura Cryoglobulinemia Cutaneous leukocytoclastic angiitis

Table 20.6 Ocular features secondary to systemic disease

Ocular feature	Systemic disease
Scleritis	Rheumatoid arthritis Granulomatosis with polyangiitis Relapsing polychondritis
Keratitis	Rheumatoid arthritis Granulomatosis with polyangiitis
Uveitis	Sarcoidosis Bechet's syndrome Vogt–Koyanagi–Harada disease
Retinal vasculitis	Systemic lupus erythematosus Polyarteritis Nodosa Microscopic polyangiitis Granulomatosis with polyangiitis
Orbital inflammation	Polyarteritis Nodosa Granulomatosis with polyangiitis
Optic neuropathy	Giant cell arteritis Churg–Strauss syndrome

20.3.3 Drugs and the Eye

There are several drugs used in systemic conditions that can affect the eye and vice versa [2]. Table 20.7 represents an example to highlight these effects.

20.3.4 Disorders Affecting the Skin and the Eye

There exists a wide variety of multisystem diseases which can affect both the eyes and skin. These diseases may be in the form of connective tissue disorders and vasculitides as mentioned in Table 20.5 or in the form of mucocutaneous disorders like reactive arthritis, sarcoidosis, necrobiotic xanthogranuloma, and amyloidosis. Another important systemic disease which involves the skin and the eye is Albinism.

Table 20.8 gives a list of diseases apart from connective tissue diseases and vasculitides, which can have ocular manifestations

20.3.4.1 Reactive Arthritis (Reiter's syndrome)

Reactive arthritis (also known as Reiter's syndrome) has multiple systemic features and is characterized by seronegative arthritis, eye, and

Table 20.7 Ocular adverse effects of systemic drugs

Drug	Effects
Ethambutol	Toxic optic neuropathy
Chloroquine	Maculopathy
Amiodarone	Vortex keratopathy
Acetazolamide	Paresthesia, renal stones
Corticosteroids	Cataract, glaucoma
Vitamin A, retinoids	Idiopathic intracranial hypertension

Table 20.8 Cutaneous disorders with ocular manifestations

Cutaneous disorders with ocular manifestations
Reactive arthritis
Sarcoidosis
Necrobiotic xanthogranuloma
Albinism

cutaneous manifestations. It is classically described as a triad of conjunctivitis, urethritis, and arthritis. A number of organisms have been implicated, and these include *Chlamydia trachmatis*, *Shigella flexneri*, *Salmonella*, etc [14, 15].

The etiopathology, although not entirely clear, is thought to be due to an immune response to the infection and is suggested by the presence of bacteria in synovium of affected individuals. Up to 80% of affected individuals are positive for HLA-B27

20.3.4.2 Clinical Features [14]

Symptoms begin as early as a week or several months after primary infection. The clinical features can be generalized and systemic like fever, weight loss, and malaise. There can also be urethritis, cervicitis, and inflammation of the prostate. Connective tissue affliction in the form of arthritis and enthesitis are seen. The mucocutaneous manifestations are circinate balanitis, keratoderma blennorrhagicum, and oral stomatitis. Children may have diarrhea episodes preceding systemic manifestations.

Ocular manifestations include conjunctivitis, anterior uveitis (these are two most common), posterior uveitis, cystoid macular edema, and cataract formation. Anterior uveitis may cause synechiae formation leading to raised intraocular pressure.

Diagnosis: This is based on the spectrum of clinical findings. For microbiological workup urine analysis in the form of cultures, PCR and ELISA may be needed. Stool culture in children can help identify the organism involved. HLA B 27 testing, although not mandatory, can be done.

Treatment [14]: The initial line of therapy for arthritis includes rest, analgesics, and nonsteroidal anti-inflammatory drugs (NSAIDs) and intra-articular steroids. Certain severe and recalcitrant cases may need methotrexate. The role of antibiotics and immunosuppressives like TNF inhibitors is debatable.

20.3.4.3 Sarcoidosis

Sarcoidosis is a chronic inflammatory multisystem disorder of unknown etiology characterized by noncaseating granulomas [16, 17].

The basic pathology of this disorder is these granulomas which destroy normal tissue leading to scarring and fibrosis of the affected organ system. Although the exact etio-pathogenesis is not known, it is thought that an altered immune response to various pathogens ranging from dust to bacteriae (*P ropionibacterium acne, Mycobacteria* sp., etc.), viruses lead to the disease [18].

The most common organ system involved is the pulmonary (up to 95%) followed by skin, lymph nodes, and eye.

20.3.4.4 Clinical Presentation

As in any multisystem disorder patients tend to have generalized symptoms and signs like fatigue, fever, weight loss, and night sweats. Patients may also have cough which is nonproductive. Some may present with a fulminant form called Lofgren's syndrome characterized by high fever, arthralgia, lymphadenopathy, and erythema nodosum. They may have uveitis as well [19]. Uveo-parotid fever or Heerfordt syndrome refers to the constellation of fever, parotid gland inflammation, uveitis, and facial nerve palsy [20].

Cutaneous manifestations commonly seen are subcutaneous nodules, lupus pernio, macules, and papules. Erythema nodosum is a subcutaneous nodule seen over the shin and is a nonspecific sarcoid sign.

Uveitis: The most common ocular involvement is in the form of uveitis (anterior> posterior> intermediate> pan-uveitis). There may be conjunctival nodules, mutton fat keratic precipitates and iris nodules, vitritis, and perivasculitis. "Candle wax drippings" is a term used to describe the perivenous exudation in the posterior segment. There may be "snowball opacities" in the vitreous in patients with intermediate uveitis.

There may be adnexal involvement in the form of lacrimal gland infiltration, and over time this can lead to dry eye. Sarcoid may involve the optic nerve in the form of an infiltrative or compressive optic neuropathy.

Other ocular features include neovascularization, cataracts, and cystoid macular edema.

20.3.4.5 Diagnosis

The clinical signs and the organ systems involved aid in diagnosis. Blood investigations include a complete blood count, serum Calcium, and serum Angiotensin Converting Enzyme levels. CT chest or chest radiography and pulmonary function tests need to be done as well.

Vitamin D levels need to be tested since sarcoid granulomas can convert Vitamin D 25 to the active form dihydroxy Vitamin D 1,25. ECG and echocardiography should be done to rule out cardiac involvement. Skin biopsies from nodules aid in diagnosis and is easier and less invasive than biopsies from lung.

20.3.4.6 Treatment

This depends upon severity of disease and the number of organ systems involved. In some patients, the condition may resolve spontaneously and they may be asymptomatic [14].

Steroids play an important role in treatment. They may be given systemically in multisystem involvement, and for ocular sarcoid they can be given as topical medications if limited to anterior uveitis. Optic nerve or posterior segment affliction warrants systemic steroid therapy. Immunomodulation with antimalarial agents, monoclonal antibodies, methotrexate, TNF inhibitors, and thalidomide can be used in the presence of refractory disease.

20.3.5 Necrobiotic Xanthogranuloma

This is a chronic multisystem granulomatous disease which is progressive and characterized by xanthomatous plaques and is associated with paraproteinemia and lymphoproliferative disease [14, 21]. Although the exact etiopathology is unknown, it is hypothesized that an abnormal immune response to the paraprotein causes a granuloma with necrobiosis. An alternate hypothesis suggests that the paraprotein behaves like a lipoprotein activating monocytes resulting in xanthomas and granulomatous response [22].

The clinical features result from systemic/visceral, ocular, and cutaneous manifestations. The systemic manifestations can be in the form of giant cell myocardial disease, IgG gammopathy, multiple myeloma and can involve the spleen, liver, kidneys and ovaries [14].

Cutaneous involvement is seen in the form of macules and papules. These can coalesce to form nodules and plaques. Oral mucosal lesions and periorbital lesions can also be present.

Ocular features can be seen in close to 80% of patients with necrobiotic xanthogranuloma. Eyelid nodules and plaques can cause cicatricial changes. The anterior segment manifestations include conjunctivitis, episcleritis, keratitis, and scleritis. Lesions in the orbit can cause proptosis.

Initial workup must include a complete blood count, erythrocyte sedimentation rate, C-reactive protein along with serum lipid levels, a metabolic panel, and serum electrophoresis. Biopsy of skin and bone marrow may be needed in certain cases. Echocardiography and imaging to look for orbital lesions are important considerations [14].

Histopathology examination reveals granulomatous inflammation in the dermis extending up to subcutaneous fat with areas of necrobiosis and giant cells. Infiltration with plasma cells and lymphocytes is also seen. Characteristically cholesterol clefts are seen in the necrobiotic areas.

20.3.5.1 Treatment [14]

Intralesional steroids for cutaneous lesions and ablative lasers have been used. Surgical excision of cutaneous nodules can also be done. Chemotherapy may be needed to control systemic disease.

20.3.5.2 Amyloidosis

The term amyloidosis encompasses localized and systemic disorders characterized by extracellular deposition of fibrillar proteins in tissues and end organs. Amyloid deposits may consist of fibrils, serum amyloid P, or a protein-derived amyloid fiber in the form of β-pleated sheets.

The disease can be classified as primary and secondary systemic amyloidosis, hemodialysis-associated, heredofamilial, and primary cutaneous and secondary cutaneous types [23–25].

20.3.5.3 Clinical Presentation [14]

Primary systemic amyloidosis is seen in plasma cell disorders like Waldenstrom macroglobulinemia and multiple myeloma. The clinical features depend upon the organ involved. Patients may present with heart failure, generalized edema due to hypoalbuminemia, and proteinuria. They also have weight loss and fatigue in the initial period. Other features include autonomic neuropathy, malabsorption syndromes, and hepatomegaly. Rarely they can develop carpal tunnel syndrome and arthropathies.

Mucocutaneous manifestations are due to infiltration of skin and mucosa and include waxy papules, nodules, plaques, and macroglossia commonly. The rare features include alopecia, bullae formation, nail dystrophy, and cutis laxa.

20.3.5.4 Ocular Features

Although rare, amyloidosis may occur in the form of eyelid and periorbital nodules. Purpura around eyelids causing the typical raccoon eyes are also seen. Amyloid may rarely infiltrate the lacrimal gland.

Diagnosis is largely based on clinical features aided by biopsy. Biopsy of the mucocutaneous lesions, or abdominal fat pad biopsies, can be tested for amyloid. Amyloid is PAS positive, and on routine-staining procedures reveals an eosinophilic pink amorphous material. The other stains that can be used include Congo red, Crystal violet, and thioflavin T [14, 26]. Serum and urine electrophoresis is an important test and can detect abnormal proteins in up to 90% of patients. If electrophoresis fails to pick up abnormal proteins, a bone marrow biopsy can be done to look for monoclonal plasma cells. Scintigraphy with labeled serum amyloid P helps to know the extent of disease and prognosis.

20.3.5.5 Treatment

Treatment in most cases involves multiple specialties. Immunosuppressive agents like cyclophosphamide, melphalan, and steroids have a role in managing systemic disease. Coexisting features like cardiac failure, renal, and hematologic issues need to be addressed.

20.3.6 Albinism

Albinism encompasses a heterogeneous group of congenital hypomelanotic disorders and is divided into three general categories: ocular albinism, oculocutaneous albinism, and albinoidism [27, 28].

20.3.6.1 Etiopathology

Melanin accounts for pigmentation of the skin, hair, and eyes and is produced by subcellular organelles called melanosomes within melanocytes. The melanocytes are derived from the neural crest and the optic cup. Melanocytes originating in the neural crest migrate to the skin, eyes, and hair follicles. The melanocytes of the RPE are derived from neuroectoderm as cells originating from the outer layer of the optic vesicle. If the cells from the neural crest are affected, oculocutaneous albinism (OCA) results; if melanosomes from neural-ectoderm are affected, ocular albinism (OA) results.

Thus, to simplify it

- Regional hypopigmentation involving neuroectoderm ➔ Ocular Albinism (OA)
- Neural crest cell ➔ Albinoidism
- Both ➔ Oculocutaneous albinism (OCA)

The enzyme critical to melanin production is tyrosinase; although there are also a number of post-tyrosinase factors and enzymes that regulate the quantity and quality of melanin produced, the rate-limiting step in human melanogenesis is the conversion of tyrosine to dopa and dopaquinone by tyrosinase. If tyrosinase is absent, the rate-limiting step is blocked, and no eumelanin or pheomelanin are produced. If tyrosinase is downregulated but not completely inactive, there will be a preferential shunting to the pheomelanin pathway, giving the patient a yellow, orange, or reddish pigmentation [27].

20.3.6.2 Clinical Features

Individuals with albinism can present with the following symptoms.

Hypopigmentation of skin, hair, and eye (Fig. 20.6a, b), nystagmus, photophobia, reduced

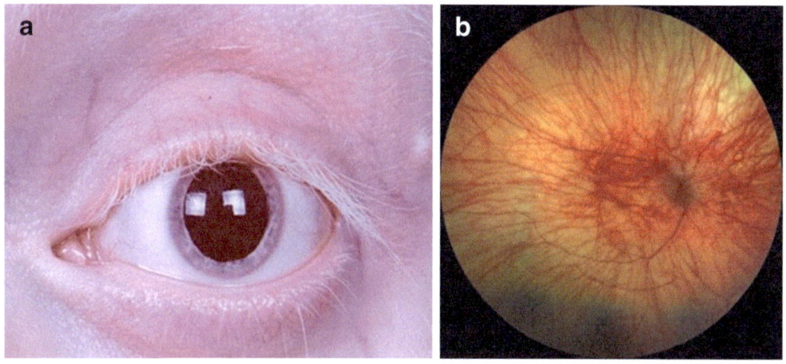

Fig. 20.6 a and b Light colored eyelashes, hypochromic iris, and typical albinotic fundus

vision, abnormal head posture, strabismus, rashes on skin, and occasionally repeated infections.

20.3.6.3 Treatment

Treatment involves a complete and thorough ocular exam which includes a cycloplegic refraction. To address photophobia tinted glasses are to be prescribed. Patients with albinism are at higher risk of squamous cell and basal cell cancers in sun-exposed areas and thus should be strongly encouraged to limit their sun exposure through avoiding outdoor activities and through using sun-protective products such as appropriate clothing, large-brim hats, sunglasses, and sunscreen agents. They should be advised to use appropriate sunblock during the period of prolonged sun exposure. Consultation with a dermatologist may be useful. Patients with albinism rarely can have associated bleeding diathesis or repeated infections due to syndromes like Hermansky–Pudlak or Chediak–Higashi, which must be ruled out.

Last but not least are two commonly seen systemic disorders with systemic implications. They are Diabetes Mellitus and Systemic Hypertension.

20.3.7 Diabetic Mellitus

Diabetes is a major cause of preventable blindness. Diabetics are 25 times more prone to develop blindness than nondiabetics [29]. Diabetes may be type 1 or type 2. The former is due to an autoimmune process causing destruction of the beta cells of the pancreas, and the latter is due to insulin resistance caused by lifestyle issues.

20.3.7.1 Pathophysiology

Ocular morbidity occurs as a result of diabetic retinopathy which represents end-organ microvascular damage of the retina. It is of two types: Nonproliferative diabetic retinopathy (NPDR) and Proliferative diabetic retinopathy (PDR).

Although the exact pathophysiology is unknown, it is thought to be an interplay between electrolyte imbalance, histologic changes at the basement membrane of capillaries, circulatory changes, and role of vaso-proliferative factors.

Electrolyte imbalance occurs due to increased levels of aldose reductase leading to death of retinal pericytes. This leads to microaneurysm formation. There is deposition of extracellular matrix, breakdown of blood retinal barrier, and thickening of capillary basement membrane contributing to edema at the macula. Leukocytosis at the retina leads to capillary dropout, occlusions, and endothelial damage. There is upregulation of vaso-proliferative factors like the vascular endothelial growth factor, caused by retinal ischemia which can lead to neovascularization characteristic of proliferative diabetic retinopathy [29].

20.3.7.2 Clinical Features

Nonproliferative diabetic retinopathy (NPDR) is characterized microaneurysms which are located in the inner nuclear layer of the retina, dot and blot hemorrhages, in the middle retinal layers, hard exudates, located between the inner plexiform and inner nuclear layer of the retina, soft exudates which are nerve fiber infarcts and are due capillary occlusion at the retinal nerve fiber layer, intraretinal microvascular abnormalities (IRMA), these are dilated capillaries which func-

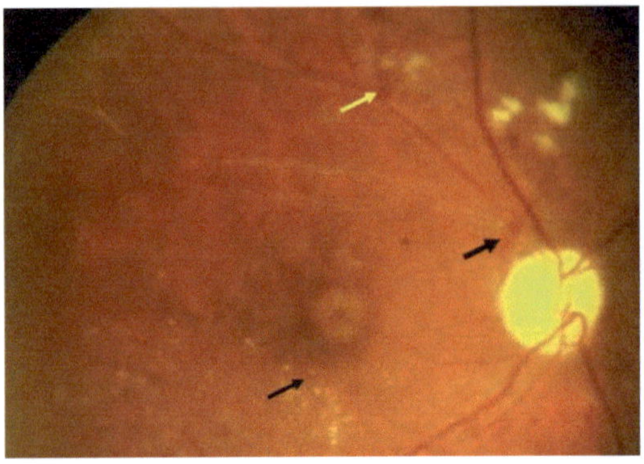

Fig. 20.7 Fundus photograph of a patient with NPDR showing hard exudates (small black arrow), dot hemorrhages (yellow arrow), and blot hemorrhages (broad black arrow)

tion as collateral, retinal edema characterized by accumulation of fluid between the outer plexiform layer and inner nuclear layer. Figure 20.7 is a fundus photograph of an eye with NPDR.

Based on the extent to which these signs are seen, NPDR is classified as [30]

(a) *Mild NPDR*: Presence of occasional microaneurysms
(b) *Moderate NPDR*: Increased number of microaneurysms with dot and blot hemorrhages, IRMA, venous beading, and soft exudates may be present
(c) *Severe NPDR*: This can be remembered by the "4-2-1 rule"

4 quadrants of hemorrhages and microaneurysms or 2 or more quadrants of venous beading or IRMA in 1 or more quadrants

(d) *Very Severe NPDR*: 2 or more changes of severe NPDR

Proliferative Diabetic Retinopathy This is characterized by signs of neovascularization of the disc (NVD), along the major vascular arcades (NVE–neovascularization elsewhere). PDR can be classified as [30]

Early PDR: Presence of new vessels but not satisfying the HRC (high-risk criteria)

High-risk PDR: Includes any of the following:

(a) neovascularization of disc (NVD) involving >1/3rd to 1/4th disc diameter
(b) NVD < 1/3rd to 1/4th disc diameter with vitreous and/or preretinal hemorrhage
(c) NVE with vitreous and/or preretinal hemorrhage

High-risk PDR is an ophthalmic emergency and warrants immediate treatment to prevent vision loss.

Diabetic macular edema (DME) is often seen in patients with diabetic retinopathy and can be a cause for vision loss. DME is characterized by the presence of retinal thickening within 2 disc diameters of the center of the macula. DME may be called Clinically Significant Macular Edema (CSME) when there is [31]

1. Retinal thickening at or within 500 microns from the center of macula.
2. Hard exudates at or within 500 microns from the center of macula associated with adjacent retinal thickening.
3. Retinal thickening at least one disc area in size, at least a part of which is within one disc diameter of the center of macula.

Investigations needed include fasting and postprandial blood sugars, hemoglobin A1c, lipid profile, renal function tests and certain special ocular investigations like Ocular Coherence tomography (to aid in diagnosis and follow up of DME), and Fundus Fluorescein Angiography (FFA) (to look for areas of retinal nonperfusion, new vessels).

20.3.7.3 Treatment [29]

NPDR can be managed conservatively with strict control over glycemic levels, control of coexistent hypertension, dyslipidemia, and regular dilated fundus examinations by an ophthalmologist. Depending on the severity of NPDR, follow-up is advised.

DME is managed with focal lasers and/or intravitreal anti-VEGF injections along with the measures described for NPDR.

PDR, as mentioned above, is an ophthalmic emergency and needs immediate pan-retinal photocoagulation (PRP) to decrease VEGF levels and promote regression of new vessels. This may be done in combination with anti-VEGF agents intravitreally.

Depending on the severity and presence of vitreous hemorrhage, tractional retinal detachment surgery in the form of vitrectomy may also be needed.

20.3.8 Systemic Hypertension

Systemic hypertension can affect multiple organ systems, and these include cardiovascular, renal, brain and central nervous system, and ocular. Although retina is the chief site of affliction in the ocular system, it can affect the choroid and the optic nerve [32].

20.3.8.1 Pathophysiology

Hypertensive retinopathy goes through three phases based on the extent of control of blood pressure, and these are vasoconstrictive, sclerotic, and exudative [32].

In the vasoconstrictive phase, there is retinal arteriole narrowing and vasospasm. The sclerotic phase, as the name suggests, is characterized by vessel wall thickening, arteriovenous (AV) crossing changes, and silver and copper wiring of the vessels. In the exudative phase, there is damage to the blood retinal barrier causing exudation, hemorrhages, and retinal ischemia.

20.3.8.2 Clinical Features

The most common clinical signs include tortuosity and constriction of retinal arterioles, dot and blot and flame-shaped hemorrhages, and cotton wool spots (Fig. 20.8). There can also be localized edema and in cases where the blood pressure is very high there may be bilateral optic disc edema. In long-standing cases of systemic hypertension there may be some subtle signs on examining the retinal arteriole like AV crossing changes, copper and silver wiring, which occur due to thickening of the vessel walls causing an increased light reflex on ophthalmoscopy.

Fibrinoid necrosis of arterioles in the choroid with subsequent infarction of the choriocapillaris is a feature of malignant hypertension. This can lead to the formation of hyperpigmented patches called Elschnig pearls or linear streaks over the choroidal arteries, known as Siegrist streaks. There may also be pockets of serous retinal detachment in malignant hypertension.

Classification of Hypertensive Retinopathy [32, 33]

There are two main classifications

Keith–Wagner–Barker classification

Scheie classification

Keith–Wagner–Barker Classification

Group 1—slight constriction of retinal arterioles

Group 2—changes seen in Group 1 + focal narrowing of retinal arterioles+ AV nicking

Group 3—changes seen in Group 2 + flame shaped hemorrhages + hard exudates + cotton wool spots

Group 4—changes seen in group 3 + optic disc swelling

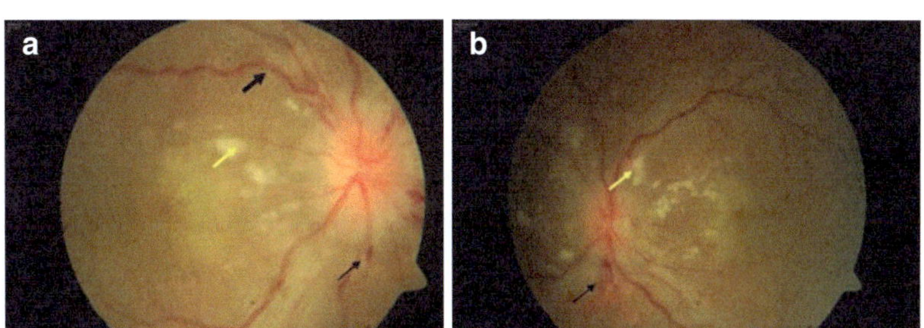

Fig. 20.8 Fundus photograph of a patient with hypertensive retinopathy showing cotton wool spots (yellow arrows), splinter hemorrhages (thin black arrows), and vascular tortuosity (broad black arrow).

Scheie Classification

This classifies hypertensive retinopathy and arteriosclerosis into the following stages:

For hypertensive retinopathy

Stage 0: No visible abnormalities

Stage 1: Diffuse arteriolar narrowing

Stage 2: Stage 1 + focal arteriolar constriction

Stage 3: Stage 2 + retinal hemorrhage

Stage 4: Stage 3 + hard exudates + retinal edema+ optic disc swelling

Arteriosclerosis

Stage 0: Normal

Stage 1: Broadening of arteriolar light reflex

Stage 2: Stage 1 + AV crossing changes

Stage 3: Copper wiring of arterioles

Stage 4: Silver wiring of arterioles

20.3.8.3 Treatment

As in any systemic condition, control of blood pressure, along with lifestyle modifications, is advised.

20.4 Conclusion

The eye can get involved in a plethora of systemic disorders. Patients may initially present with ocular manifestations as is seen in systemic vasculitis and endocrine disorders like hyper or hypothyroidism, or it may get involved later on in disease, sometimes as a result of therapy. Communication between various streams in medicine can ensure complete care for a patient.

References

1. Nowinska AK, Machalińska A, Módis L, Koprowski R, Rechichi M. Ocular manifestations of systemic diseases. Cham: Springer.
2. Lenake M, Du Toit N. The eye in systemic disease: CPD article. S Afr Fam Pract. 2014;56(1):8–14.
3. Swarup MS, Gupta S, Singh S, Prakash A, Mehndiratta A, Garg A. Phakomatoses: a pictorial review. Indian J Radiol Imaging. 2020;30(2):195.
4. Becker B, Strowd RE. Phakomatoses. Dermatol Clin. 2019;37(4):583–606.
5. Kumar V, Singh S. Multimodal imaging of choroidal nodules in neurofibromatosis type-1. Indian J Ophthalmol. 2018;66(4):586.
6. Sadiq MA, Vanderveen D. Genetics of ectopia lentis. In: Seminars in ophthalmology, Vol. 28, No. 5–6. Taylor & Francis; 2013. p. 313–20.
7. Callewaert B, Malfait F, Loeys B, De Paepe A. Ehlers-Danlos syndromes and Marfan syndrome. Best Pract Res Clin Rheumatol. 2008;22(1):165–89.
8. Perez-Roustit S, Nguyen DT, Xerri O, Robert MP, De Vergnes N, Mincheva Z, Benistan K, Bremond-Gignac D. Ocular manifestations in Ehlers-Danlos syndromes: clinical study of 21 patients. Journal francais d'ophtalmologie. 2019;42(7):722–9.
9. Byles DB, Nischal KK, Cheng H. Ectopia lentis et pupillae: a hypothesis revisited. Ophthalmology. 1998;105(7):1331–6.
10. Rajappa M, Goyal A, Kaur J. Inherited metabolic disorders involving the eye: a clinico-biochemical perspective. Eye. 2010;24(4):507–18.
11. Poll-The BT, de Buy Wenniger-Prick CM. The eye in metabolic diseases: clues to diagnosis. Eur J Paediatr Neurol. 2011;15(3):197–204.
12. Jain AP, Jaru-Ampornpan P, Douglas RS. Thyroid eye disease: redefining its management—a review. Clin Experiment Ophthalmol. 2021;49(2):203–11.
13. Menezo V, Lightman S. The eye in systemic vasculitis. Clin Med. 2004;4(3):250.
14. McCluskey P, Powell RJ. The eye in systemic inflammatory diseases. Lancet. 2004;364(9451):2125–33.
15. Wanat KA, Kim B, Rosenbach M. Multisystem diseases affecting the skin and eye. Clin Dermatol. 2016;34(2):214–41.
16. Fendler C, Laitko S, Sörensen H, Gripenberg-Lerche C, Groh A, Uksila J, Granfors K, Braun J, Sieper J. Frequency of triggering bacteria in patients with reactive arthritis and undifferentiated oligoarthritis and the relative importance of the tests used for diagnosis. Ann Rheum Dis. 2001;60(4):337–43.
17. Yamamoto M. The concept, definition and diagnostic criteria of sarcoidosis. Nihon rinsho. Jpn J Clin Med. 1994;52(6):1426–32.
18. American Thoracic Society. Statement on sarcoidosis. Joint Statement of the American Thoracic Society (ATS), the European Respiratory Society (ERS) and the World Association of Sarcoidosis and Other Granulomatous Disorders (WASOG) adopted by the ATS Board of Directors and by the ERS Executive Committee, February 1999. Am J Respir Crit Care Med. 1999;160(2):736–55.
19. Haimovic A, Sanchez M, Judson MA, Prystowsky S. Sarcoidosis: a comprehensive review and update for the dermatologist: part I. Cutaneous disease. J Am Acad Dermatol. 2012;66(5):699–e1.
20. Nunes H, Bouvry D, Soler P, Valeyre D. Orphanet J Rare Dis. Sarcoidosis. 2007;2(1):46.
21. Rao DA, Dellaripa PF. Extrapulmonary manifestations of sarcoidosis. Rheum Dis Clin. 2013;39(2):277–97.

22. Fernández-Herrera J, Pedraz J. Necrobiotic xanthogranuloma. In: Seminars in cutaneous medicine and surgery, Vol. 26, No. 2. W.B. Saunders; 2007. p. 108–13.
23. Bullock JD, Bartley GB, Campbell RJ, Yanes B, Connelly PJ, Funkhouser JW. Necrobiotic xanthogranuloma with paraproteinemia: case report and a pathogenetic theory. Ophthalmology. 1986;93(9):1233–6.
24. Falk RH, Comenzo RL, Skinner M. The systemic amyloidoses. N Engl J Med. 1997;337(13):898–909.
25. Fernandez-Flores A. Cutaneous amyloidosis: a concept review. Am J Dermatopathol. 2012;34(1):1–7.
26. Pinney JH, Hawkins PN. Amyloidosis. Ann Clin Biochem. 2012;49:229–41.
27. Schreml S, Szeimies RM, Vogt T, Landthaler M, Schroeder J, Babilas P. Cutaneous amyloidoses and systemic amyloidoses with cutaneous involvement. Eur J Dermatol. 2010;20(2):152–60.
28. Levin AV, Stroh E. Albinism for the busy clinician. J Am Assoc Pediatr Ophthalmol Strabismus. 2011;15(1):59–66.
29. Wright KW, Spiegel PH, editors. Pediatric ophthalmology and strabismus. Springer Science & Business Media; 2013.
30. Singh R, Ramasamy K, Abraham C, Gupta V, Gupta A. Diabetic retinopathy: an update. Indian J Ophthalmol. 2008;56(3):179.
31. Early Treatment Diabetic Retinopathy Study Research Group. Fundus photographic risk factors for progression of diabetic retinopathy: ETDRS report number 12. Ophthalmology. 1991;98(5):823–33.
32. Grading diabetic retinopathy from stereoscopic color fundus photographs—an extension of the modified Airlie House classification. ETDRS report number 10. Early treatment diabetic retinopathy study research group. Ophthalmology. 1991;98(5 Suppl):786–806.
33. Modi P, Arsiwalla T. Hypertensive retinopathy. (Updated 2019 Jan 23). StatPearls (Internet). Treasure Island (FL): StatPearls Publishing. 2018

MIX
Papier aus verantwortungsvollen Quellen
Paper from responsible sources
FSC® C105338

If you have any concerns about our products,
you can contact us on
ProductSafety@springernature.com

In case Publisher is established outside the EU,
the EU authorized representative is:
Springer Nature Customer Service Center GmbH
Europaplatz 3, 69115 Heidelberg, Germany

Printed by Libri Plureos GmbH
in Hamburg, Germany